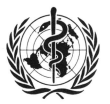

World Health Organization Classification of Tumours

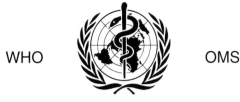

WHO   OMS

International Agency for Research on Cancer (IARC)

Pathology and Genetics of Tumours of the Urinary System and Male Genital Organs

Edited by

John N. Eble

Guido Sauter

Jonathan I. Epstein

Isabell A. Sesterhenn

IARCPress

Lyon, 2004

World Health Organization Classification of Tumours

Series Editors   Paul Kleihues, M.D.
                  Leslie H. Sobin, M.D.

Pathology and Genetics of Tumours of the Urinary System and Male Genital Organs

Editors   John N. Eble, M.D.
           Guido Sauter, M.D.
           Jonathan I. Epstein, M.D.
           Isabell A. Sesterhenn, M.D.

Coordinating Editors   Figen Soylemezoglu, M.D.
                        Wojciech Biernat, M.D.

Editorial Assistant   Stéphane Sivadier

Layout   Lauren A. Hunter
          Allison L. Blum
          Lindsay S. Goldman

Illustrations   Thomas Odin

Printed by   Team Rush
              69603 Villeurbanne, France

Publisher   IARCPress
             International Agency for
             Research on Cancer (IARC)
             69008 Lyon, France

This volume was produced in collaboration with the

International Academy of Pathology (IAP)

The WHO Classification of Tumours of the Urinary System and Male Genital Organs presented in this book reflects the views of a Working Group that convened for an Editorial and Consensus Conference in Lyon, France, December 14-18, 2002.

Members of the Working Group are indicated
in the List of Contributors on page 299.

The WHO Working Group on Tumours of the Urinary System and Male Genital Organs pays tribute to Dr F. Kash Mostofi (1911-2003), outstanding pathologist, who through his vision, teachings and personality influenced generations of physicians worldwide.

Published by IARC Press, International Agency for Research on Cancer,
150 cours Albert Thomas, F-69008 Lyon, France

Format for bibliographic citations:
Eble J.N., Sauter G., Epstein J.I., Sesterhenn I.A. (Eds.): World Health Organization
Classification of Tumours. Pathology and Genetics of Tumours of the Urinary System
and Male Genital Organs. IARC Press: Lyon 2004

IARC Library Cataloguing in Publication Data

Pathology and genetics of tumours of the urinary system and male genital organs /
    editors J.N. Eble... [et al.]

    (World Health Organization classification of tumours ; 6)

    1. Bladder neoplasms - genetics 2. Bladder neoplasms - pathology
    3. Genital neoplasms, male - genetics 4. Genital neoplasms, male - pathology
    5. Kidney neoplasms - genetics 6. Kidney neoplasms - pathology
    7. Prostatic neoplasms – genetics 8. Prostatic neoplasms - pathology
    I. Eble, John N. II. Series

    ISBN 92 832 2412 4   (NLM Classification: WJ 160)

Contents

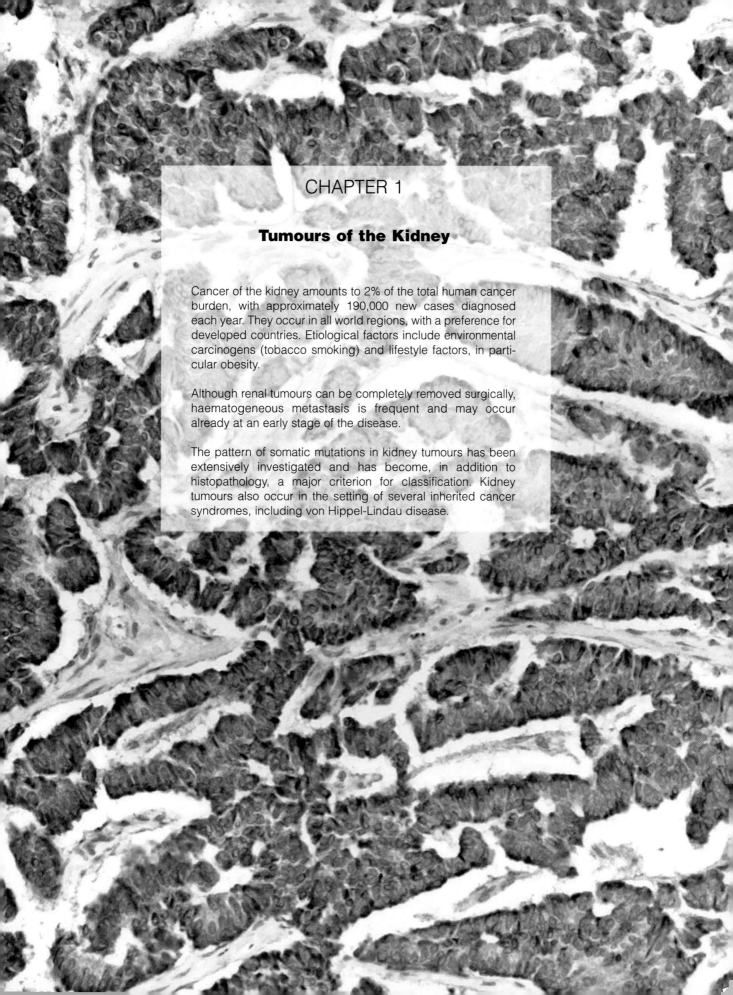

CHAPTER 1

Tumours of the Kidney

Cancer of the kidney amounts to 2% of the total human cancer burden, with approximately 190,000 new cases diagnosed each year. They occur in all world regions, with a preference for developed countries. Etiological factors include environmental carcinogens (tobacco smoking) and lifestyle factors, in particular obesity.

Although renal tumours can be completely removed surgically, haematogeneous metastasis is frequent and may occur already at an early stage of the disease.

The pattern of somatic mutations in kidney tumours has been extensively investigated and has become, in addition to histopathology, a major criterion for classification. Kidney tumours also occur in the setting of several inherited cancer syndromes, including von Hippel-Lindau disease.

WHO histological classification of tumours of the kidney

Renal cell tumours
Clear cell renal cell carcinoma   8310/3[1]
Multilocular clear cell renal cell carcinoma   8310/3
Papillary renal cell carcinoma   8260/3
Chromophobe renal cell carcinoma   8317/3
Carcinoma of the collecting ducts of Bellini   8319/3
Renal medullary carcinoma   8319/3
Xp11 translocation carcinomas
Carcinoma associated with neuroblastoma
Mucinous tubular and spindle cell carcinoma
Renal cell carcinoma, unclassified   8312/3
Papillary adenoma   8260/0
Oncocytoma   8290/0

Metanephric tumours
Metanephric adenoma   8325/0
Metanephric adenofibroma   9013/0
Metanephric stromal tumour   8935/1

Nephroblastic tumours
Nephrogenic rests
Nephroblastoma   8960/3
    Cystic partially differentiated nephroblastoma   8959/1

Mesenchymal tumours
Occurring Mainly in Children
    Clear cell sarcoma   9044/3
    Rhabdoid tumour   8963/3
    Congenital mesoblastic nephroma   8960/1
    Ossifying renal tumour of infants   8967/0

Occurring Mainly in Adults
    Leiomyosarcoma (including renal vein)   8890/3
    Angiosarcoma   9120/3
    Rhabdomyosarcoma   8900/3
    Malignant fibrous histiocytoma   8830/3

Haemangiopericytoma   9150/1
Osteosarcoma   9180/3
Angiomyolipoma   8860/0
    Epithelioid angiomyolipoma
Leiomyoma   8890/0
Haemangioma   9120/0
Lymphangioma   9170/0
Juxtaglomerular cell tumour   8361/0
Renomedullary interstitial cell tumour   8966/0
Schwannoma   9560/0
Solitary fibrous tumour   8815/0

Mixed mesenchymal and epithelial tumours
Cystic nephroma   8959/0
Mixed epithelial and stromal tumour
Synovial sarcoma   9040/3

Neuroendocrine tumours
Carcinoid   8240/3
Neuroendocrine carcinoma   8246/3
Primitive neuroectodermal tumour   9364/3
Neuroblastoma   9500/3
Phaeochromocytoma   8700/0

Haematopoietic and lymphoid tumours
Lymphoma
Leukaemia
Plasmacytoma   9731/3

Germ cell tumours
    Teratoma   9080/1
    Choriocarcinoma   9100/3

Metastatic tumours

---

[1] Morphology code of the International Classification of Diseases for Oncology (ICD-O) {808} and the Systematized Nomenclature of Medicine (http://snomed.org). Behaviour is coded /0 for benign tumours, /3 for malignant tumours, and /1 for borderline or uncertain behaviour.

TNM classification of renal cell carcinoma

TNM classification [1,2]

T – Primary Tumour

TX	Primary tumour cannot be assessed
T0	No evidence of primary tumour

T1	Tumour 7 cm or less in greatest dimension, limited to the kidney
T1a	Tumour 4 cm or less
T1b	Tumour more than 4 cm but not more than 7 cm
T2	Tumour more than 7 cm in greatest dimension, limited to the kidney
T3	Tumour extends into major veins or directly invades adrenal gland or perinephric tissues but not beyond Gerota fascia
T3a	Tumour directly invades adrenal gland or perinephric tissues[a] but not beyond Gerota fascia
T3b	Tumour grossly extends into renal vein(s)[b] or vena cava or its wall below diaphragm
T3c	Tumour grossly extends into vena cava or its wall above diaphragm
T4	Tumour directly invades beyond Gerota fascia

Notes: [a] Includes renal sinus (peripelvic) fat
[b] Includes segmental (muscle-containing) branches

N – Regional Lymph Nodes

NX	Regional lymph nodes cannot be assessed
N0	No regional lymph node metastasis
N1	Metastasis in a single regional lymph node
N2	Metastasis in more than one regional lymph node

M – Distant Metastasis

MX	Distant metastasis cannot be assessed
M0	No distant metastasis
M1	Distant metastasis

Stage grouping

Stage	T	N	M
Stage I	T1	N0	M0
Stage II	T2	N0	M0
Stage III	T3	N0	M0
	T1, T2, T3	N1	M0
Stage IV	T4	N0, N1	M0
	Any T	N2	M0
	Any T	Any N	M1

---

[1] {944,2662}.
[2] A help desk for specific questions about the TNM classification is available at http://www.uicc.org/tnm

Renal cell carcinoma

J.N. Eble
K. Togashi
P. Pisani

Definition

Renal cell carcinoma is a group of malignancies arising from the epithelium of the renal tubules.

Epidemiology of renal cell cancer

Renal cell cancer (RCC) represents on average over 90% of all malignancies of the kidney that occur in adults in both sexes. Overall it is the 12th most common site in men and 17th in women. In males living in industrialized areas including Japan, it is as common as non-Hodgkin lymphoma ranking 6th, while in less developed areas it ranks 16th, in the same order of magnitude as carcinoma of the nasopharynx. In women it ranks 12th and 17th in developed and developing countries respectively {749}. The incidence is low in the African and Asian continents but not in Latin America where around 1995 Uruguay recorded one of the highest rates in the world. The highest rates in both men and women were observed in the Czech Republic with 20 and 10 annual new cases per 100,000 population respectively, age standardized {2016}. The lowest rates recorded were less that 1 new case per 100,000 showing a 10-fold variation in the risk of the disease. The latest systematic analyses of time trends of the incidence of kidney cancer indicate a general increase in both sexes in all monitored regions, up until the mid-80s {481}. These trends were paralleled by mortality, which thereafter began to slow down or even fall in some high risk countries {2843}. After the low peak in children due to nephroblastoma, the incidence of renal cell cancer increases steadily after age 40 years as most epithelial tumours but the risk levels off or even declines from age 75 in both sexes. It is two to three times more common in men than in women in both high and low risk countries {2016}.

Etiology

Tobacco smoking is a major cause of kidney cancer and accounts for at least 39% of all cases in males {2015}. Exposure to carcinogenic arsenic compounds in industrial processes or through drinking water increases the risk of renal cancer by 30% {1150}. Several other environmental chemicals have been addressed as possible carcinogens for the kidney but definitive evidence has not been established. These include asbestos, cadmium, some organic solvents, pesticides and fungal toxins. Some steroidal estrogens and the nonsteroidal diethylstilboestrol induce tumours in hamster {1150,1154}, but to date an excess has not been reported in exposed humans. Estrogens could be involved in the mechanism that induces RCC in overweight and obese individuals. Several epidemiological studies both prospective and retrospective, conducted in many different populations have established that the risk of kidney cancer increases steadily with increasing body mass index (BMI), the most common measure of overweight {1156}. The incidence of RCC in obese people (BMI>29 kg/m^2) is double that of normal individuals and about 50% increased if overweight (BMI 25-30 kg/m^2) {221}. The same authors estimated that in Europe

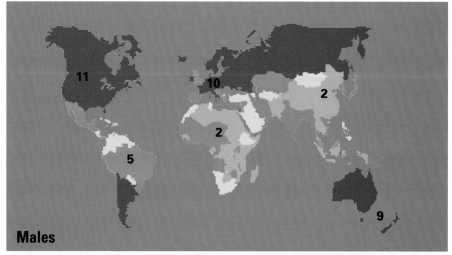

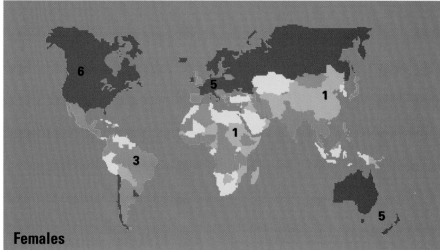

Fig. 1.01 Estimates of the age-standardized incidence rates of kidney cancer, adjusted to the world standard age distribution (ASR). From Globocan 2000 {749}.

one quarter of kidney cancers in both sexes are attributable to excess weight. The association has been reported as stronger in women than in men in some but not all studies.

The incidence of RCC is significantly increased in people with a history of blood hypertension that is independent of obesity and tobacco smoking {458,962,2912}. The association with the use of diuretics instead is referable to hypertension, while a small but consistent excess of RCC has been established with exposure to phenacetin-containing analgesics that also cause cancer of the renal pelvis {1150}.

Parity is a factor that has been investigated in several studies but results are discordant {1430}. A real association would be supported by estrogen-mediated carcinogenesis that is documented in animal models. Conversely, it could be a confounded effect of excess body weight that is often increased in women who had many children. Other exposures that have been addressed are a family history of kidney cancer {829}, birth weight {221}, low consumption of fruits and vegetables {2841} and the use of antihypertensive drugs other than diuretics. The significance of these associations remain however unclear.

Few studies have investigated the hypothesis that genetic characteristics may modulate the effect of exposure to chemical carcinogens. In one study the effect of tobacco smoking was stronger in subjects with slow acetylator genotypes as defined by polymorphisms in the N-acetyltransferase 2 gene that is involved in the metabolism of polycyclic aromatic hydrocarbons {2359}. Conversely, RCC was not associated with the glutatione S-transferase (GST)

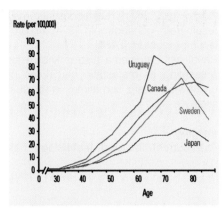

Fig. 1.02 Age-specific incidence rates of renal cell cancer in selected countries.

M1 null genotype that is also involved in the metabolism of several carcinogens, but was significantly decreased in either smokers and non-smokers having the GST T1 null genotype {2544}.

Clinical features

Signs and symptoms
Haematuria, pain, and flank mass are the classic triad of presenting symptoms, but nearly 40% of patients lack all of these and present with systemic symptoms, including weight loss, abdominal pain, anorexia, and fever {870}. Elevation of the erythrocyte sedimentation rate occurs in approximately 50% of cases {634}. Normocytic anaemia unrelated to haematuria occurs in about 33% {438,902}. Hepatosplenomegaly, coagulopathy, elevation of serum alkaline phosphatase, transaminase, and alpha-2-globulin concentrations may occur in the absence of liver metastases and may resolve when the renal tumour is resected {1441}. Systemic amyloidosis of the AA type occurs in about 3% of patients {2705}.

Renal cell carcinoma may induce paraneoplastic endocrine syndromes {1441,2525}, including humoral hypercalcemia of malignancy (pseudohyperparathyroidism), erythrocytosis, hypertension, and gynecomastia. Hypercalcemia without bone metastases occurs in approximately 10% of patients and in nearly 20% of patients with disseminated carcinoma {736}. In about 66% of patients, erythropoietin concentration is elevated {2526}, but less than 4% have erythrocytosis {902,2526}. Approximately 33% are hypertensive, often with elevated renin concentrations in the renal vein of the tumour-bearing

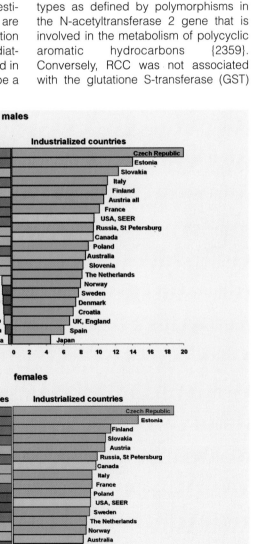

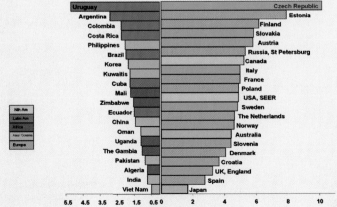

Fig. 1.03 Age-standardized incidence rates of renal cell cancer recorded by population-based cancer registries around 1995. From D.M. Parkin et al. {2016}.

kidney {902,2491}. Gynecomastia may result from gonadotropin {904} or prolactin production {2486}.

Renal cell carcinoma also is known for presenting as metastatic carcinoma of unknown primary, sometimes in unusual sites.

Imaging

The current imaging technology has altered the management of renal masses as it enables detection and characterization of very small masses. Radiological criteria established by Bosniak assist management of renal masses {283}. Ultrasonography is useful for detecting renal lesions and if it is not diagnostic of a simple cyst, CT before and after IV contrast is required. Plain CT may confirm a benign diagnosis by identifying fat in angiomyolipoma {284}. Lesions without enhancement require nothing further, but those with enhancement require follow-ups at 6 months, 1 year, and then yearly {258}. Increased use of nephron-sparing and laparoscopic surgery underscores the importance of preoperative imaging work-up. Routine staging work-up for renal cell carcinoma includes dynamic CT and chest radiography.

Familial renal cell carcinoma

M.J. Merino
D.M. Eccles
W.M. Linehan
F. Algaba
B. Zbar
G. Kovacs
P. Kleihues

A. Geurts van Kessel
M. Kiuru
V. Launonen
R. Herva
L.A. Aaltonen
H.P.H. Neumann
C.P. Pavlovich

The kidney is affected in a variety of inherited cancer syndromes. For most of them, the oncogene / tumour suppressor gene involved and the respective germline mutations have been identified, making it possible to confirm the clinical diagnosis syndrome, and to identify asymptomatic gene carriers by germline mutation testing {2510}. Each of the inherited syndromes predisposes to distinct types of renal carcinoma. Usually, affected patients develop bilateral, multiple renal tumours; regular screening of mutation carriers for renal and extrarenal manifestations is considered mandatory.

Von Hippel-Lindau disease (VHL)

Definition
The von Hippel-Lindau (VHL) disease is inherited through an autosomal dominant trait and characterized by the development of capillary haemangioblastomas of the central nervous system and retina, clear cell renal carcinoma, phaeochromocytoma, pancreatic and inner ear tumours. The syndrome is caused by germline mutations of the *VHL* tumour suppressor gene, located on chromosome 3p25–26. The VHL protein is involved in cell cycle regulation and angiogenesis.

Approximately 25% of haemangioblastomas are associated with VHL disease {1883}.

MIM No.
193300 {1679}.

Synonyms and historical annotation
Lindau {1506} described capillary haemangioblastoma, and also noted its association with retinal vascular tumours, previously described by von Hippel {2752}, and tumours of the visceral organs, including kidney.

Incidence
Von Hippel-Lindau disease is estimated

Table 1.01
Major inherited tumour syndromes involving the kidney. Modified, from C.P. Pavlovich et al. {2032}

Syndrome	Gene Protein	Chromosome	Kidney	Skin	Other tissues
von Hippel-Lindau	*VHL* pVHL	3p25	Multiple, bilateral clear-cell renal cell carcinoma (CCRCC), renal cysts	-	Retinal and CNS haemangioblastomas, phaeochromocytoma, pancreatic cysts and neuroendocrine tumours, endolymphatic sac tumours of the inner ear, epididymal and broad ligament cystadenomas
Hereditary papillary renal cancer	*c-MET* HGF-R	7q31	Multiple, bilateral papillary renal cell carcinomas (PRCC) Type 1	-	-
Hereditary leiomyomatosis and RCC	*FH* FH	1q42-43	Papillary renal cell carcinoma (PRCC), non-Type 1	Nodules (leiomyomas)	Uterine leiomyomas and leiomyosarcomas
Birt-Hogg-Dubé	*BHD* Folliculin	17p11.2	Multiple chromophobe RCC, conventional RCC, hybrid oncocytoma, papillary RCC, oncocytic tumours	Facial fibrofolliculomas	Lung cysts, spontaneous pneumothorax
Tuberous sclerosis	*TSC1* Hamartin *TSC2* Tuberin	9q34 16p13	Multiple, bilateral angiomyolipomas, lymphangioleiomyomatosis	Cutaneous angiofibroma ('adenoma sebaceum') *peau chagrin*, subungual fibromas	Cardiac rhabdomyomas, adenomatous polyps of the duodenum and the small intestine, lung and kidney cysts, cortical tubers and subependymal giant cell astrocytomas (SEGA)
Constitutional chromosome 3 translocation	Unknown		Multiple, bilateral clear-cell renal cell carcinomas (CCRCC)	-	-

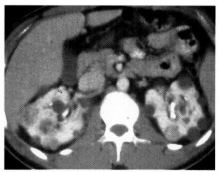

Fig. 1.04 Familial renal carcinoma. CT scan of a patient with von Hippel-Lindau disease with multiple, bilateral cystic renal lesions.

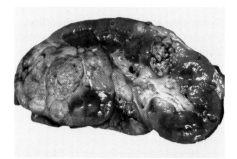

Fig. 1.05 Renal cell carcinoma in a patient with von Hippel-Lindau disease. The large tumour has the characteristic yellow appearance of clear cell renal cell carcinoma. Small cysts are present in the cortex, and a second tumour is seen in the lower pole.

to occur at rates of 1: 36 000 {1598} to 1: 45 500 population {1589}.

Diagnostic criteria

The clinical diagnosis of von Hippel-Lindau disease is based on the presence of capillary haemangioblastoma in the CNS or retina, *and* the presence of one of the typical VHL-associated extraneural tumours *or* a pertinent family history. In VHL disease, germline *VHL* mutations can virtually always be identified {2510}.

Kidney tumours associated with VHL

The typical renal manifestation of VHL are kidney cysts and clear-cell renal cell carcinomas (CCRCC). Multiple kidney tumours of other histological types rule out the diagnosis of VHL {2032}. Histological examination of macroscopically inconspicuous renal tissue from VHL patients may reveal several hundred independent tumours and cysts {2773}.

Clinical Features

Renal lesions in carriers of VHL germline mutations are either cysts or CCRCC. They are typically multifocal and bilateral. The mean age of manifestation is 37 years versus 61 years for sporadic CCRCC, with an onset age of 16 to 67 years {2032}. There is a 70% chance of developing CCRCC by the age of 70 years {1597}. The diagnostic tools of choice are CT and MR imaging. Metastatic RCC is the leading cause of death from VHL {2384}.

The median life expectancy of VHL patients was 49 years {1279,1883}. In order to detect VHL-associated tumours in time, analyses for germline mutations of the *VHL* gene have been recommended in every patient with retinal or CNS haemangioblastoma, particularly in those of younger age and with multiple lesions. Periodic screening of VHL patients by MRI should start after the age of ten years {328}.

Extrarenal manifestations

Retinal haemangioblastomas manifest earlier than kidney cancer (mean age, 25 years) and thus offer the possibility of an early diagnosis. CNS haemangioblastomas develop somewhat later (mean, 30 years); they are predominantly located in the cerebellum, further in brain stem and spinal chord. Both lesions are benign and rarely life threatening. Phaeochromocytomas may constitute a major clinical challenge, particularly in VHL families with predisposition to the development of these tumours. They are often associated with pancreatic cysts. Other extrarenal manifestations include neuroendocrine tumours, endolymphatic sac tumours of the inner ear, and epididymal and broad ligament cystadenomas.

Genetics

The *VHL* gene is located at chromosome 3p25–26. The *VHL* tumour suppressor gene has three exons and a coding sequence of 639 nucleotides {1445}.

Gene expression

The *VHL* gene is expressed in a variety of human tissues, in particular epithelial cells of the skin, the gastrointestinal, respiratory and urogenital tract and endocrine and exocrine organs {500,2277}. In the CNS, immunoreactivity for pVHL is prominent in neurons, including Purkinje cells of the cerebellum {1559,1864}.

Function of the VHL protein

Mutational inactivation of the *VHL* gene in affected family members is responsible

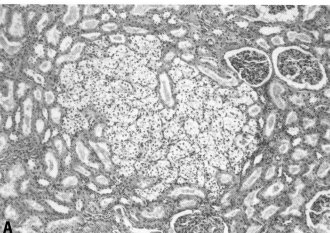
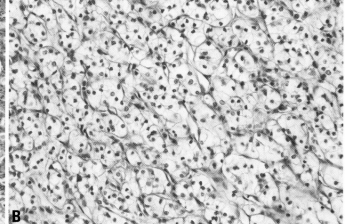

Fig. 1.06 VHL disease. **A** Small, initial clear cell RCC. **B** Higher magnification of a typical clear cell RCC.

Table 1.02
Genotype - phenotype correlations in VHL patients.

VHL-type	Phenotype	Predisposing mutation
Type 1	Without phaeochromocytoma	686 T -> C Leu -> Pro
Type 2A	With phaeochromocytoma and renal cell carcinoma	712 C -> T Arg -> Trp
Type 2B	With phaeochromocytoma but without renal cell carcinoma	505 T-> C Tyr -> His 658 G-> T Ala -> Ser

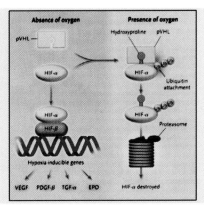

Fig. 1.07 Control of Hypoxia-inducible factor (HIF) by the gene product of the von Hippel-Lindau gene (pVHL). From D.J. George and W.G. Kaelin Jr. {855}. Copyright © 2003 Massachusetts Medical Society.

for their genetic susceptibility to renal cell carcinoma and capillary haemangioblastoma, but the mechanisms by which the suppressor gene product, the VHL protein (pVHL), causes neoplastic transformation, have remained enigmatic. Several signalling pathways appear to be involved {1942}, one of which points to a role of pVHL in protein degradation and angiogenesis. The alpha domain of pVHL forms a complex with elongin B, elongin C, Cul-2 {1533,2028,2488} and Rbx1 {1264} which has ubiquitin ligase activity {1188}, thereby targeting cellular proteins for ubiquitinization and proteasome-mediated degradation. The domain of the *VHL* gene involved in the binding to elongin is frequently mutated in VHL-associated neoplasms {2488}. The beta-domain of pVHL interacts with the alpha subunits of hypoxia-inducible factor 1 (HIF-1) which mediates cellular responses to hypoxia. Under normoxic conditions, the beta subunit of HIF is hydroxylated on to one of two proline residues. Binding of the hydroxylated subunit pVHL causes polyubiquitination and thereby targets HIF-alpha for proteasome degradation {855}. Under hypoxic conditions or in the absence of functional VHL, HIF-alpha accumulates and activates the transcription of hypoxia-inducible genes, including vascular endothelial growth factor (VEGF), platelet-derived growth factor (PDGF-beta), transforming growth factor (TGF-alpha) and erythropoietin (EPO). Constitutive overexpression of VEGF explains the extraordinary capillary component of VHL associated neoplasms {1650}. VEGF has been targeted as a novel therapeutic approach using neutralizing anti-VEGF antibody {1654}. Induction of EPO is responsible for the

occasional paraneoplastic erythrocytosis in patients with kidney cancer and CNS haemangioblastoma.
Additional functions of the VHL protein may contribute to malignant transformation and the evolution of the phenotype of VHL associated lesions. Recent studies in renal cell carcinoma cell lines suggest that pVHL is involved in the control of cell cycle exit, i.e. the transition from the G_2 into quiescent G_0 phase, possibly by preventing accumulation of the cyclin-dependent kinase inhibitor p27 {2027}. Another study showed that only wild-type but not tumour-derived pVHL binds to fibronectin. As a consequence, VHL-/- renal cell carcinoma cells showed a defective assembly of an extracellular fibronectin matrix {1943}. Through a down-regulation of the response of cells to hepatocyte growth factor / scatter factor and reduced levels of tissue inhibitor of metalloproteinase 2 (TIMP-2), pVHL deficient tumours cells exhibit a significantly higher capacity for invasion {1353}. Further, inactivated pVHL causes an overexpression of transmembrane carbonic anhydrases that are involved in extracellular pH regulation {1186} but the biological significance of this dysregulation remains to be assessed.

Gene mutations and VHL subtypes
Germline mutations of the VHL gene are spread all over the three exons. Missense mutations are most common, but nonsense mutations, microdeletions / insertions, splice site mutations and large deletions also occur {1882, 1958,2927}. The spectrum of clinical manifestations of VHL reflects the type of germline mutation. Phenotypes are based on the absence (type 1) or presence (type 2) of phaeochromocytoma.

VHL type 2 is usually associated with missense mutations and subdivided on the presence (type 2A) or absence (2B) of renal cell carcinoma {136,421, 893,1883}. In contrast to loss of function variants in VHL type 1, mutations predisposing to pheochromocytoma (VHL type 2) are mainly of the missense type predicted to give rise to conformationally changed pVHL {2804,2927}. In addition, VHL type 2C has been used for patients with only phaeochromocytoma {2201, 2804}; however several years later some of these cases developed other VHL manifestations.
According to its function as a tumour suppressor gene, VHL gene mutations are also common in sporadic haemangioblastomas and renal cell carcinomas {1268,1931}.

Hereditary papillary renal carcinoma (HPRC)

Definition
Hereditary papillary renal carcinoma (HPRC) is an inherited tumour syndrome characterized with an autosomal dominant trait, characterized by late onset, multiple, bilateral papillary renal cell tumours.

MIM No.   179755 {1679}.

Diagnostic criteria
The diagnosis of HPRC is based on the occurrence of multiple, bilateral kidney tumours. It has been estimated that approximately 50% of affected family

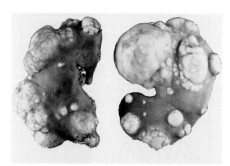

Fig. 1.08 Hereditary papillary renal cancer (HPRC) with multiple, bilateral papillary RCC.

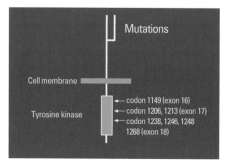

Fig. 1.09 Germline mutations of the *MET* oncogene in hereditary papillary renal cell carcinoma (HPRC).

members develop the disease by the age of 55 years {2327}. Extrarenal manifestations of HPRC have not been identified.

Papillary renal cell carcinoma
BHD patients develop myriad papillary tumours, ranging from microscopic lesions to clinically symptomatic carcinomas {1979}. The histological pattern has been termed papillary renal carcinoma type 1 and is characterized by papillary or tubulo-papillary architecture very similar to papillary renal cell carcinoma, type 1.

Genetics
Responsible for the disease are activating mutations of the *MET* oncogene which maps to chromosome 7q31. *MET* codes for a receptor tyrosine kinase {799,1212,1213,1570,2326,2327,2926, 2928}. Its ligand is hepatocyte growth factor (HGFR). Mutations in exons 16 to 19, ie the tyrosine kinase domain causes a ligand-independent constitutive activation.

Duplication of the mutant chromosome 7 leading to trisomy is present in a majority of HPRC tumours {768,845,1996,2032, 2937}.

Management
For patients with confirmed germline mutation, annual abdominal CT imaging is recommended.

Hereditary leiomyomatosis and renal cell cancer (HLRCC)

Definition
Hereditary leiomyomatosis and renal cell cancer (HLRCC, MIN no: 605839) is an autosomal dominant tumour syndrome caused by germline mutations in the FH gene. It is characterized by predisposition to benign leiomyomas of the skin and the uterus. Predisposition to renal cell carcinoma and uterine leiomyosarcoma is present in a subset of families.

MIM No.   605839 {1679}.

Diagnostic criteria
The definitive diagnosis of HLRCC relies on FH mutation detection. The presence of multiple leiomyomas of the skin and the uterus papillary type 2 renal cancer, and early-onset uterine leiomyosarcoma are suggestive {51,52,1330,1450,1469, 2632}.

Renal cell cancer
At present, 26 patients with renal carcinomas have been identified in 11 families out of 105 (10%) {52,1329,1450,1469, 2632}. The average age at onset is much earlier than in sporadic kidney cancer; median 36 years in the Finnish and 44 years in the North American patients, (range 18-90 years). The carcinomas are typically solitary and unilateral {1450, 2632}. The most patients have died of metastatic disease within five years after diagnosis. The peculiar histology of renal cancers in HLRCC originally led to identification of this syndrome {1450}. Typically, HLRCC renal carcinomas display papillary type 2 histology and large cells with abundant eosinophilic cytoplasm, large nuclei, and prominent inclusion-like eosinophilic nucleoli. The Fuhrman nuclear grade is from 3 to 4. Most tumours stain positive for vimentin and negative for cytokeratin 7. Recently, three patients were identified having either collective duct carcinoma or oncocytic tumour {52,2632}. Regular screening for kidney cancer is recommended, but optimal protocols have not yet been determined. Computer tomography and abdominal ultrasound have been proposed {1328,2632}. Moreover, as renal cell carcinoma is present only in a subset of families, there are no guidelines yet, whether the surveillance should be carried out in all FH mutation families.

Leiomyomas of the skin and uterus
Leiomyomas of the skin and uterus are the most common features of HLRCC, the penetrance being approximately 85% {1328,2632}. The onset of cutaneous leiomyomas ranges from 10-47 years, and uterine leiomyomas from 18-52 years (mean 30 years) {2632}. Clinically, cutaneous leiomyomas present

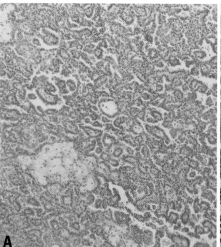
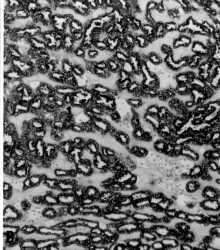

Fig. 1.10 Hereditary papillary renal cell carcinoma (HPRC) **A** Tumours have a papillary or tubulo-papillary architecture very similar to papillary renal cell carcinoma, type 1. Macrophages are frequently present in the papillary cores. **B** Hereditary papillary renal cell carcinoma frequently react strongly and diffusely with antibody to cytokeratin 7.

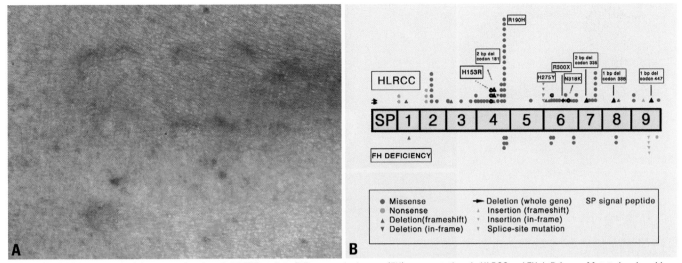

Fig. 1.11 A Multiple cutaneous leiomyomas in a female HLRCC patient. **B** Fumarate hydratase (FH) gene mutations in HLRCC and FH deficiency. Mutated codons identified in the families with RCC and/or uterine leiomyosarcoma are indicated.

as multiple firm, skin-coloured nodules ranging in size from 0.5-2 cm. Uterine leiomyomas in HLRCC are often numerous and large. Cutaneous leiomyomas are composed of interlacing bundles of smooth muscle cells with centrally located blunt-ended nucleus. Uterine leiomyomas are well-circumscribed lesions with firm and fibrous appearance. Histologically, they are composed of interlacing bundles of elongated, eosinophilic smooth muscle cells surrounded by well-vascularized connective tissue. Leiomyomas with atypia may also occur.

Leiomyosarcoma of the uterus

Predisposition to uterine leiomyosarcoma is detected in a subset of HLRCC families (3 out of 105 families) {1450,1469}. The cases have been diagnosed at 30-39 years. Uterine leiomyosarcomas invade the adjacent myometrium and are not well demarcated from normal tissue. The tumours are densely cellular and display spindle cells with blunt-ended nuclei, eosinophilic cytoplasm, and a variable degree of differentiation.

Genetics

Gene structure and function
FH is located in chromosome 1q42.3-q43, consists of 10 exons, and encodes a 511 amino acid peptide. The first exon encodes a mitochondrial signal peptide. {661,662,2623}, but processed FH (without the signal peptide) is present also in the cytosol. Mitochondrial FH acts in the tricarboxylic acid (Krebs) cycle catalyzing conversion of fumarate to malate. FH is also known to be involved in the urea cycle. However, the role of cytosolic FH is still somewhat unclear. Biallelic inacti-

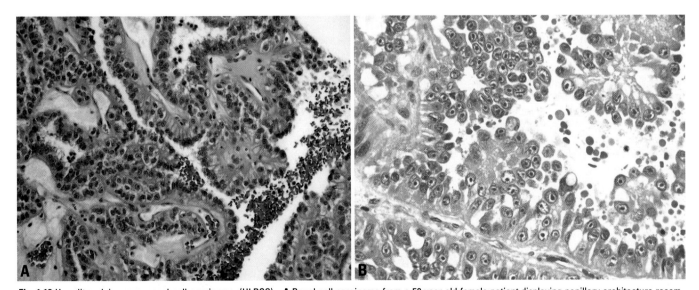

Fig. 1.12 Hereditary leiomyoma renal cell carcinoma (HLRCC). **A** Renal cell carcinoma from a 50 year old female patient displaying papillary architecture resembling papillary renal cell carcinoma, type 2 (H&E staining, magnification x10). **B** Thick papillae are covered by tall cells with abundant cytoplasm, large pseudostratified nuclei and prominent nucleoli.

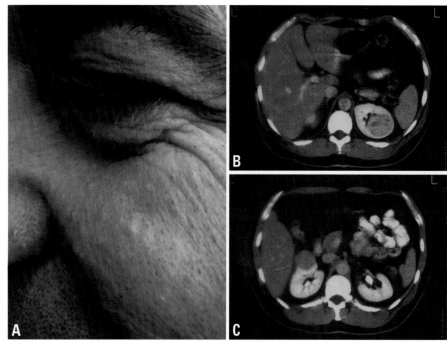

Fig. 1.13 A Early facial fibrofolliculomas in BHD syndrome. **B,C** CT scan images of abdomen in BHD patient showing multiple bilateral renal carcinomas which necessitated bilateral nephrectomy and subsequent renal transplant.

vation of FH has been detected in almost all HLRCC tumours {52,1329,1330,1450}.
FH mutations
Germline mutations in FH have been found in 85% (89/105) of the HLRCC families {52,1330,1469,2627,2632}. Altogether 50 different germline mutations have been identified. Two founder mutations have been detected in the Finnish population, a missense mutation H153R (in 3 out of 7 families) and a 2-bp deletion in codon 181 (in 3 out of 7 families). Most of the families with these mutations included renal cell cancer and/or uterine leiomyosarcoma {1330,1469,2627}. A splice site mutation IVS4+1G>A was detected in families of Iranian origin {465}. In addition, a missense mutation R190H was reported in 35% of the families from North America.
To date, the role of FH in sporadic tumorigenesis has been evaluated in three different studies {169,1330,1469}. Somatic FH mutations seem to be rare, but have been found in uterine leiomyomas and a high-grade sarcoma.

FH deficiency
This is a recessive disease caused by biallelic germline mutations in FH. The syndrome is characterized by neurological impairment, growth and developmental delay, fumaric aciduria and absent or reduced enzyme activity in all tissues. Heterozygous parents are neurologically asymptomatic heterozygous carries of the mutation with a reduced enzyme activity (approximately 50%). Tumour predisposition similar to HLRCC is likely {2627}. Thus far, 10 different FH mutations have been reported in 14 FH deficiency families (Fig 3.).

Genotype-phenotype correlations
No clear pattern has emerged to date. Three mutations (K187R, R190C, and R190H) have been reported in both HLRCC and FH deficiency. Renal cell cancer and uterine leiomyosarcoma occur only in a minority of families, but the same mutations (a 2-bp deletion in codon 181, R190H, and H275Y) have been identified in families with or without malignancies.
Because some families appear to have high risk of cancer at early age, and others little or no risk, modifying gene/s could play a key role in the development of renal cancer and uterine leiomyosarcoma in HLRCC {697,2627,2632}.

Birt-Hogg-Dubé syndrome (BHD)

The BHD syndrome conveys susceptibility to develop renal epithelial tumours resembling mainly chromophobe and clear cell renal carcinomas and renal oncocytomas as well as fibrofolliculomas and pulmonary cysts {246,1891,2033, 2631,2924}.

Definition
Birt-Hogg-Dubé (BHD) syndrome is a syndrome characterised by benign skin tumours, specifically fibrofolliculomas, trichodiscomas and acrochordons. Multiple renal tumours and spontaneous pneumothoraces are frequent in patients with BHD syndrome.

MIM No. 135150 {1679}.

Diagnostic criteria
Renal tumours
Renal pathology may vary in individuals with BHD syndrome. Tumours can be multiple and bilateral. Renal oncocytoma is well described and is usually thought of as a benign tumour. Other histopathologies have been described including papillary and chromophobe adenocarcinoma with a mixed population of clear and eosinophillic cells. The age at clinical manifestation is approximately 50 years and the mean number of tumours present is 5 per patient. Metastatic disease is rare and appears to only occur if the primary tumour has a diameter of >3 cm {2031}.

Skin tumours
Fibrofolliculomas (FF), trichodiscomas (TD) and acrochordons are the classical skin lesions in BHD syndrome. The FF and TD lesions look the same and present as smooth dome-shaped, skin coloured papules up to 5mm in diameter over the face, neck and upper body with onset typically in the third or fourth decade of life. Skin lesions are initially subtle but remain indefinitely and become more obvious with increasing age as illustrated by Toro et al 1999 {2631}. Acrochordons (skin tags) are not always present. Biopsy will usually demonstrate an epidermis with aberrant follicular structures, thin columns of epithelial cells and small immature sebocytes clustered within the epithelial cords. Alcian blue demonstrates the presence of abundant mucin within the stroma.

Other lesions
Spontaneous pneumothorax and the

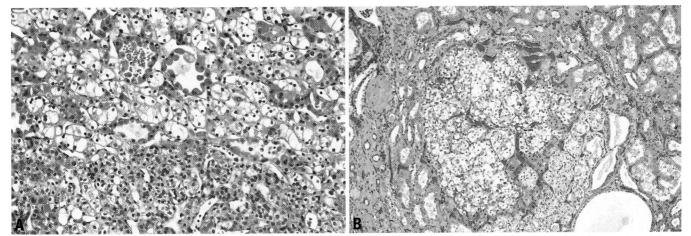

Fig. 1.14 Birt-Hogg-Dubé syndrome (BHD). **A** Hybrid oncocytic tumour composed of a mixture of clear cells and cells with abundant eosinophilic cytoplasm. **B** Small cluster of clear cells is surrounded by normal tubules. These lesions can be found scattered through the renal parenchyma.

presence of pulmonary cysts are recognised features of BHD syndrome. Multiple lipomas and mucosal papules have been described {2361}. A reported association with colonic neoplasia has not been confirmed in subsequent studies, there may be a slight increase in the incidence of other neoplasia although this remains unclear {1307}.

Genetics
BHD syndrome is a rare autosomal dominant condition with incomplete penetrance. The BHD gene maps to chromosome 17p11.2 {1306,2328}. It codes for a novel protein called folliculin whose function is unknown currently {1891}.

Affected family members typically show frameshift mutations, ie insertions, stop codons, deletions {1891}. A mutational hot spot present in more than 40% of families was identified in a tract of 8 cytosines {2032}.

LOH analyses and assessment of promoter methylation indicate that BHD is also involved in the development of a broad spectrum of sporadic renal cancers {1308}.

Management
Surveillance for all first-degree relatives of an affected individual is advocated. Skin examination to determine diagnosis from the third decade. For those with skin features or found to have the characteristic dermatological features, annual renal MRI scan would be the investigation of choice to detect any renal malignancy at as early a stage as possible and to facilitate minimal renal surgery where possible to conserve renal function. In tumour predisposition syndromes where a second somatic muta-

tion in the normally functioning wild type gene will leave no functioning protein in the cell, repeated examinations involving ionising radiation may carry a risk of inducing malignancy.

Constitutional chromosome 3 translocations

Definition
Inherited cancer syndrome caused by constitutional chromosome 3 locations with different break points, characterized by an increased risk of developing renal cell carcinomas (RCC).

MIM No. 144700 {1679}.

Diagnostic criteria
Occurrence of single or multiple, unilateral or bilateral RCC in a member of a family with a constitutional chromosome 3 translocation. The association of RCC with a chromosome 3 translocation alone is not diagnostic since this genetic alteration is also observed in sporadic cases.

Pathology
Tumours show histologically the typical features of clear cell RCC.

Table 1.03
Familial renal cell cancer associated with chromosome 3 constitutional translocation. From F. van Erp et al. {2695}.

Translocation	Number of RCC cases	Generations Involved	Mean age	Reference
t(3:8)(p14:q24)	10	4	44	Cohen et al. {476}
t(3:6)(p13:q25.1)	1	3	50	Kovacs et al {1371}
t(2:3)(q35:q21)	5	3	47	Koolen et al. {1355}
t(3:6)(q12:q15)	4	4	57.5	Geurts van Kessel et al. {862}
t(3:4)(p13:p16)	1	3	52	Geurts van Kessel et al. {862}
t(2:3)(q33:q21)	7	3	n.i.	Zajaczek et al. {2917}
t(1:3)(q32:q13.3)	4	4	66.7	Kanayama et al. {1265}

Genetics

The first family was described by Cohen et al. {476} with 10 RCC patients over 4 generations. All patients were carriers of a t(3;8)(p14;q24). In a second RCC family a t(3;6)(p13;q25) was found to segregate and, as yet, only one person in the first generation developed multiple bilateral RCCs {1371}. Additionally, a single sporadic case with a constitutional t(3;12)(q13;q24) was reported {1374}.

Seven families have now been reported; translocations are different but in all families the breakpoints map to the proximal p-and q-arms of chromosome 3.

Affected family members carry a balanced chromosomal translocation involving chromosome 3. The mode of inheritance is autosomal dominant. Translocations vary among different families and this may affect penetrance. Loss of the derivative chromosome 3 through genetic instability is considered the first step in tumour development, resulting in a single copy of VHL. The remaining VHL copy may then be mutated or otherwise inactivated. However, this mechanism involving VHL is hypothetical as affected family members do not develop extra-renal neoplasms or other VHL manifestations.

The identification of at least 7 families strongly supports the notion that constitutional chromosome 3 translocations may substantially increase the risk to develop renal cell carcinoma and this should be taken into account in the framework of genetic counselling.

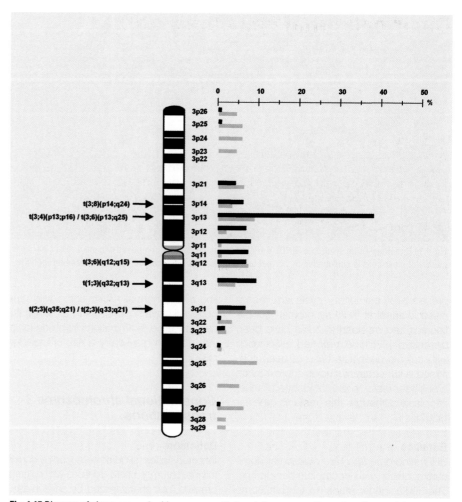

Fig. 1.15 Diagram of chromosome 3 with seven constitutional chromosome 3 translocations and the respective breakpoint positions (left). On the right side, breakpoint frequencies (%) of chromosome 3 translocations in 93 Dutch families are shown (grey bars), in addition to somatic chromosome 3 translocations in 157 sporadic RCCs (black bars). From F. van Erp et al. {2695}.

Clear cell renal cell carcinoma

D.J. Grignon
J.N. Eble
S.M. Bonsib
H. Moch

Definition
Clear cell renal cell carcinoma is a malignant neoplasm composed of cells with clear or eosinophilic cytoplasm within a delicate vascular network.

ICD-O code   8310/3

Synonym
The term "granular cell renal cell carcinoma" was used for many years for renal cell carcinomas with eosinophilic cytoplasm and high nuclear grade {1845}. Some renal neoplasms of this morphology are now included among the clear cell type, but similar appearing cells occur in other tumour types, and so the term "granular cell renal cell carcinoma" should no longer be used. {2514}. Historically, the terms Grawitz tumour and hypernephroma have also been used for clear cell renal cell carcinoma.

Macroscopy
Clear cell renal cell carcinomas (RCCs) are solitary and randomly distributed cortical tumours that occur with equal frequency in either kidney. Multicentricity and/or bilaterality occur in less than 5 percent of cases {1193}. Multicentricity and bilaterality and early age of onset are typical of hereditary cancer syndromes such as von Hippel-Lindau syndrome.
Clear cell RCCs are typically globular tumours which commonly protrude from the renal cortex as a rounded, bosselated mass. The interface of the tumour and the adjacent kidney is usually well demarcated, with a "pushing margin" and

pseudocapsule. Diffuse infiltration of the kidney is uncommon. The average size is 7 cm in diameter but detection of small lesions is increasing in countries where radiologic imaging techniques are widely applied. Size itself is not a determinant of malignancy though increasing size is associated with a higher frequency of metastases. All kidney tumours of the clear cell type are considered malignant tumours. The clear cell renal cell carcinoma is typically golden yellow due to the rich lipid content of its cells; cholesterol, neutral lipids, and phospholipids are abundant. Cysts, necrosis, haemorrhage, and calcification are commonly present. Calcification and ossification occur within necrotic zones and have been demonstrated radiologically in 10 to 15 percent of tumours {209,822}.

Tumour spread and staging
About 50% of clear cell RCCs are stage 1 and 2 and less than 5% stage 4. Invasion of perirenal and sinus fat and/or extension into the renal vein occurs in about 45% {1753}. Recognition of stage pT3a requires detection of tumour cells in direct contact with perinephric or renal sinus fat. Clear cell RCCs most commonly metastasize hematogenously via the vena cava primarily to the lung, although lymphatic metastases also occur. Retrograde metastasis along the paravertebral veins, the v. testicularis/v. ovarii, intrarenal veins, or along the ureter may also occur. Clear cell RCC is well known for its propensity to metastasize to unusual sites, and late metastasis, even af-

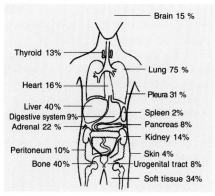

Fig. 1.17 Frequency of organ involvement by haematogenous metastasis in patients with metastatic renal cell carcinoma (n=636) at autopsy. H. Moch (unpublished).

ter ten years or more, is not uncommon. Prognosis of patients with clear cell RCC is most accurately predicted by stage. Within stages, grade has a strong predictive power. Although not formally part of the nuclear grading system, sarcomatoid change has a strongly negative effect, many of these patients dying in less than 12 months.

Histopathology
Clear cell RCC is architecturally diverse, with solid, alveolar and acinar patterns, the most common. The carcinomas typically contain a regular network of small thin-walled blood vessels, a diagnostically helpful characteristic of this tumour. No lumens are apparent in the alveolar pattern but a central, rounded luminal space filled with lightly acidophilic serous fluid or erythrocytes occurs in the

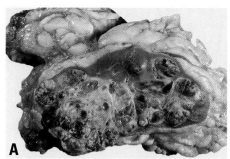
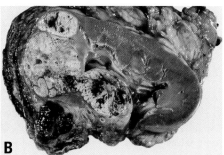
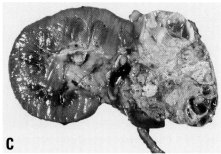

Fig. 1.16 Clear cell renal cell carcinoma. **A,B,C** Variable macroscopic appearances of the tumours.

acinar pattern. The alveolar and acinar structures may dilate, producing microcystic and macrocystic patterns. Infrequently, clear cell renal cell carcinoma has a distinct tubular pattern and rarely a pseudopapillary architecture is focally present.

The cytoplasm is commonly filled with lipids and glycogen, which are dissolved in routine histologic processing, creating a clear cytoplasm surrounded by a distinct cell membrane. Many tumours contain minority populations of cells with eosinophilic cytoplasm; this is particularly common in high grade tumours and adjacent to areas with necrosis or haemorrhage.

In well preserved preparations, the nuclei tend to be round and uniform with finely granular, evenly distributed chromatin. Depending upon the grade, nucleoli may be inconspicuous, small, or large and prominent. Very large nuclei lacking nucleoli or bizarre nuclei may occasionally occur. A host of unusual histologic findings are described in clear cell renal cell carcinoma. Sarcomatoid change occurs in 5% of tumours and is associated with worse prognosis. Some tumours have central areas of fibromyxoid stroma, areas of calcification or ossification {991}. Most clear cell RCCs have little associated inflammatory response; infrequently, an intense lymphocytic or neutrophilic infiltrate is present.

Immunoprofile

Clear cell RCCs frequently react with antibodies to brush border antigens, low molecular weight cytokeratins, CK8, CK18, CK19, AE1, Cam 5.2 and vimentin {1675,2086,2818,2880}. High molecular weight cytokeratins, including CK14 {464}, and 34βE12 are rarely detected. The majority of clear cell RCCs react positively for renal cell carcinoma marker {1675}, CD10 {140} and epithelial membrane antigen {776}. MUCl and MUC3 are consistently expressed {1479}.

Grading

Nuclear grade, after stage, is the most important prognostic feature of clear cell renal cell carcinoma {441,764, 815,949,2433,2473,2940}. The prognostic value of nuclear grade has been validated in numerous studies over the past 8 decades. Both 4-tiered and 3-tiered grading systems are in widespread use. The 4-tiered nuclear grading system {815} is as follows: Using the 10x objective, grade 1 cells have small hyperchromatic nuclei (resembling mature lymphocytes) with no visible nucleoli and little detail in the chromatin. Grade 2 cells have finely granular "open" chromatin but inconspicuous nucleoli at this magnification. For nuclear grade 3, the nucleoli must be easily unequivocally recognizable with the 10x objective. Nuclear grade 4 is characterized by nuclear pleomorphism, hyperchromasia and single to multiple macronucleoli. Grade is assigned based on the highest grade present. Scattered cells may be discounted but if several cells within a single high power focus have high grade characteristics, then the tumour should be graded accordingly.

Genetic susceptibility

Clear cell renal cell carcinoma constitutes a typical manifestation of von Hippel-Lindau disease (VHL) but may also occur in other familial renal cell cancer syndromes.

Somatic genetics

Although most clear cell RCCs are not related to von Hippel Lindau disease, 3p deletions have been described in the vast majority of sporadic clear cell renal cell carcinoma by conventional cytogenetic, FISH, LOH and CGH analyses {1372,1754,1760,1786,2109,2614,2690, 2691,2723,2925}. At least 3 separate regions on chromosome 3p have been implicated by LOH studies as relevant for sporadic renal cell carcinoma: one coincident with the von Hippel-Lindau (*VHL*) disease gene locus at 3p25-26 {1445,2400}, one at 3p21-22 {2689} and one at 3p13-14 {2721}, which includes the chromosomal translocation point in familial human renal cell carcinoma. These data suggest involvement of multiple loci on chromosome 3 in renal cancer development {474,2686}.

Mutations of the *VHL* gene have been described in 34-56% of sporadic clear cell RCC {307,792,897,2342,2400,2810}. DNA methylation was observed in 19% of clear cell renal cell carcinomas {1082}. Therefore, somatic inactivation of the *VHL* gene may occur by allelic deletion, mutation, or epigenetic silencing in 70% or more {897,1082,1445,2342}. These data suggest that the *VHL* gene is the most likely candidate for a tumour suppressor gene in sporadic clear cell RCC.

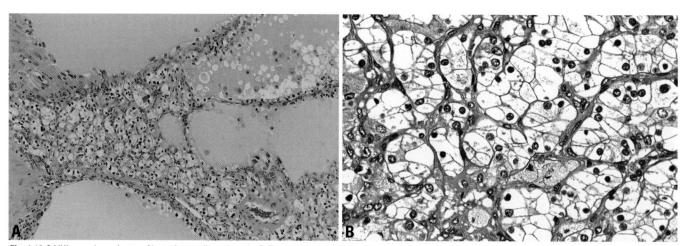

Fig. 1.18 A VHL, renal carcinoma. Note clear cells and cysts. **B** Clear cell renal cell carcinoma. Typical alveolar arrangement of cells.

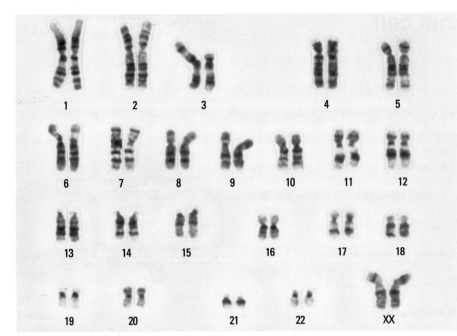

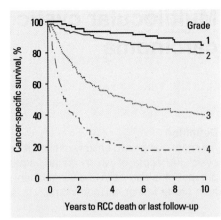

Fig. 1.20 Clear cell renal cell carcinoma. Survival curves by grade for patients with clear cell renal cell carcinoma. From C.M. Lohse et al. {1532}.

Fig. 1.19 Clear cell RCC. Note deletion of 3p as the only karyotype change.

However, recent data give evidence for other putative tumour suppressor genes at 3p, e.g. *RASSF1A* at 3p21 {1789} and *NRC-1* at 3p12 {1562}.

Chromosome 3p deletions have been observed in very small clear cell tumours of the kidney and are regarded as the initial event in clear cell cancer development {2107,2109,2925}. Inactivation of the *VHL* gene has consequences for VHL protein function. The VHL protein negatively regulates hypoxia-inducible factor, which activates genes involved in cell proliferation, neo-vascularization, and extracellular matrix formation {642,1310,1828}.

Clonal accumulation of additional genetic alterations at many chromosomal locations then occurs in renal cancer progression and metastasis {247,339,958, 1218,1754,2109,2179,2344,2345}. High level gene amplifications are rare in clear cell renal cell carcinoma {1754}. Individual chromosomal gains and losses have been analyzed for an association with patient prognosis. Chromosome 9p loss seems to be a sign of poor prognosis {1754,2341}. Losses of chromosome 14q were correlated with poorer patient outcome, high histologic grade and high pathologic stage {226,1080, 2344,2849}. LOH on chromosome 10q around the PTEN/MAC locus have been frequently detected and were related to poor prognosis {2722}.

Expression levels of many genes have been studied in clear cell RCC. The role of p53 expression in renal cell carcinoma is controversial. A few studies suggest that p53 overexpression is associated with poor prognosis and with sarcomatoid transformation {1932,1939,2164, 2659}. High expression levels of bFGF, VEGF, IL-8, MMP-2, MMP-9, vimentin, MHC class II and E-cadherin may be important for development and/or progression {320,1472,1892,2391,2437}. Expression of epidermal growth factor receptor (EGFR) is frequent in renal cell carcinoma and has been proposed as prognostic parameter {1755}. Whereas

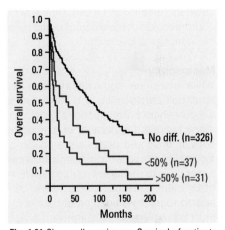

Fig. 1.21 Clear cell carcinoma. Survival of patients depends on the presence and extent of sarcomatoid differentiation, ranging from no differentiation (n=326), to sarcomatoid differentiation in <50% (n=37) and >50% (n=31) of tumour area. From H. Moch et al. {1753}. Copyright © 2000 American Cancer Society. Reprinted by permission of Wiley-Liss, Inc., a subsidiary of John Wiley & Sons, Inc.

amplification of the EGFR gene on chromosome 7p13 is a major cause for EGFR expression in brain tumours, this pathway is uncommon in renal cell carcinoma {1756}. HER2/neu amplifications are rare or absent in renal cell carcinoma {2339,2799}.

cDNA array analysis of clear cell renal carcinoma showed complex patterns of gene expression {1759,2887}. It has been shown that the integration of expression profile data with clinical data could serve to enhance the diagnosis and prognosis of clear cell RCC {2551}.

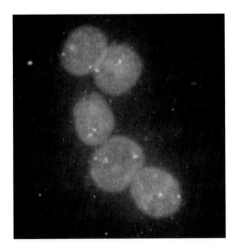

Fig. 1.22 Clear cell RCC. VHL deletion, there are two signals in red (chromosome 3), and one signal in green (*VHL* gene). FISH expression.

Multilocular cystic renal cell carcinoma

J.N. Eble

Definition
A tumour composed entirely of numerous cysts, the septa of which contain small groups of clear cells indistinguishable from grade I clear cell carcinoma.

ICD-O code   8310/3

Clinical features
There is a male:female predominance of 3:1. All have been adults (age range 20-76 years, mean = 51) {650}. No instance of progression of multilocular cystic renal cell carcinoma is known.

Macroscopy
While cysts are common in clear cell renal cell carcinomas, only rarely is the tumour entirely composed of cysts. In these tumours the number of carcinoma cells is small and diagnosis is challenging {1835}. In order to distinguish these tumours with excellent outcomes from other clear cell carcinomas, ones containing expansive nodules of carcinoma must be excluded and diagnosed simply as clear cell renal cell carcinoma {650}.
Multilocular cystic renal cell carcinoma consists of a well-circumscribed mass of small and large cysts filled with serous or haemorrhagic fluid and separated from the kidney by a fibrous capsule. Diameters have ranged from 25 mm to 130 mm. More than 20% have calcification in the septa and osseous metaplasia occasionally occurs.

Tumour spread and staging
No tumour with these features has ever recurred or metastasized.

Histopathology
The cysts are usually lined by a single layer of epithelial cells or lack an epithelial lining. The lining cells may be flat or plump and their cytoplasm ranges from clear to pale. Occasionally, the lining consists of several layers of cells or a few small papillae are present {2561}. The nuclei almost always are small, spherical, and have dense chromatin.
The septa consist of fibrous tissue, often densely collagenous. Within some of the septa there is a population of epithelial cells with clear cytoplasm. The epithelial cells resemble those lining the cysts and almost always have small dark nuclei. The clear cells form small collections but do not form expansile nodules. These epithelial cells often closely resemble histiocytes, or lymphocytes surrounded by retraction artefacts. Increased vascularity within the cell clusters is a clue to their nature.

Immunoprofile
The cells with clear cytoplasm in the septa frequently react strongly with antibodies to cytokeratins and epithelial membrane antigen and fail to react with antibodies to markers for histiocytes.

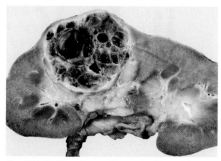

Fig. 1.23 Multilocular cystic renal cell carcinoma.

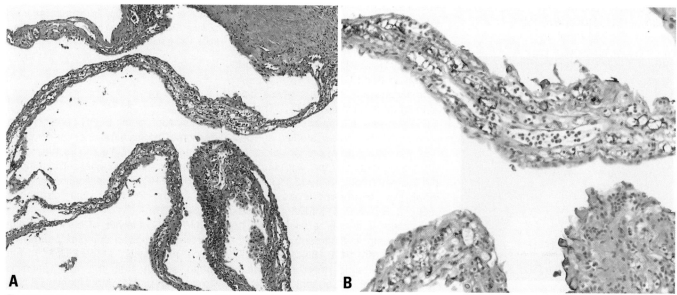

Fig. 1.24 Multilocular cystic renal cell carcinoma. **A** The septa of multilocular cystic renal cell carcinoma contain eptihelial cells which can be mistaken for lymphocytes. **B** The epithelial cells in the septa of multilocular cystic renal cell carcinoma react with antibodies to epithelial markers. EMA expression.

Papillary renal cell carcinoma

B. Delahunt
J.N. Eble

Definition
A malignant renal parenchymal tumour with a papillary or tubulopapillary architecture.

ICD-O code   8260/3

Epidemiology
Papillary renal cell carcinomas (PRCC) comprise approximately 10% of renal cell carcinoma in large surgical series {584,1860}. The age and sex distribution of PRCC is similar to clear cell renal cell carcinoma with reported mean age at presentation and sex ratio (M:F) for large series ranging from 52-66 years and 1.8:1 to 3.8:1, respectively {76,584,587, 1612}.

Clinical features
Signs and symptoms are similar to clear cell renal cell carcinoma {1612}. Radiological investigations are non-specific, although renal angiography studies have shown relative hypovascularity for PRCC {1860}.

Macroscopy
PRCC frequently contains areas of haemorrhage, necrosis and cystic degeneration, and in well-circumscribed tumours an investing pseudocapsule may be identified {76,1612}. Bilateral and multifocal tumours are more common in PRCC than in other renal parenchymal malignancies and in hereditary PRCC up to 3400 microscopic tumours per kidney have been described {1979,2169}.

Histopathology
PRCC is characterized by malignant epithelial cells forming varying proportions of papillae and tubules. Tumour lined cysts with papillary excrescences may also be seen {585,1612,1860}. The tumour papillae contain a delicate fibrovascular core and aggregates of foamy macrophages and cholesterol crystals may be present. Occasionally the papillary cores are expanded by oedema or hyalinized connective tissue {584,585}. Solid variants of PRCC consist of tubules or short papillae resembling glomeruli {585,2173}. Necrosis and haemorrhage is frequently seen and haemosiderin granules may be present in macrophages, stroma and tumour cell cytoplasm {1612}. Calcified concretions are common in papillary cores and adjacent desmoplastic stroma, while calcium oxalate crystals have been reported {587,641,1612}.

Two morphological types of PRCC have been described {585}:

Type 1 tumours have papillae covered by small cells with scanty cytoplasm, arranged in a single layer on the papillary basement membrane.

Type 2 tumour cells are often of higher nuclear grade with eosinophilic cytoplasm and pseudostratified nuclei on papillary cores. Type 1 tumours are more frequently multifocal.

Sarcomatoid dedifferentiation is seen in approximately 5% of PRCC and has been associated with both type 1 and type 2 tumours {585}.

Immunoprofile
Cytokeratin 7 (CK 7) expression has been reported for PRCC {831} however, this is more frequently observed in type 1 (87%) than type 2 (20%) tumours {585}. Ultrastructural findings are not diagnostic and are similar to clear cell renal cell carcinoma {1888,2609}.

Grading
There is no specific grading system for PRCC and the Fuhrman system {815} is accepted as applicable to both clear cell renal cell carcinoma and PRCC.

Table 1.04
Immunohistochemical profile of PRCC.

Antibody	Number of cases	% showing positive expression
AE1/AE3	36	100
CAM 5.2	11	100
EMA	11	45
Vimentin	116	51
S-100	11	55
Callus	36	92
34βE12	36	3
CEA	36	11
RCC	14	93
CD-10	14	93
Ulex europeaus	105	0

From {140,585,831,1693,2169}.

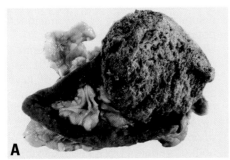
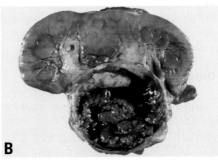
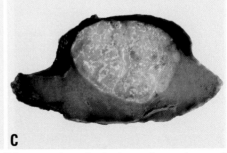

Fig. 1.25 Papillary renal cell carcinoma. **A** The papillary architecture is faintly visible in the friable tumour. **B** Gross specimen showing tumour haemorrhage and pseudoencapsulation. **C** Yellow streaks reflect the population of foamy macrophages.

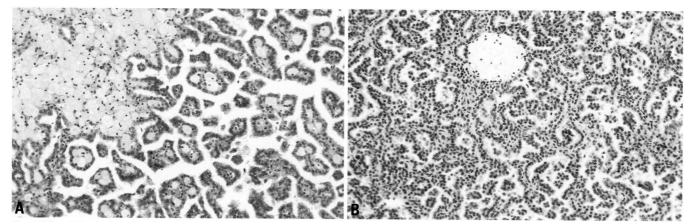

Fig. 1.26 Type 1 Papillary renal cell carcinoma. **A** Type 1 PRCC with foamy macrophages in papillary cores. **B** Type 1 PRCC showing a compact tubulopapillary pattern.

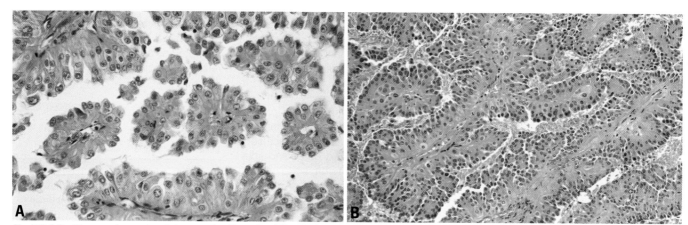

Fig. 1.27 A Papillary carcinoma, type 2. Large cells with eosinophilic cytoplasm in type 2 papillary RCC. **B** Type 2 Papillary renal cell carcinoma. Tumour cells show nuclear pseudostratification and eosinophilic cytoplasm.

Somatic genetics

Trisomy or tetrasomy 7, trisomy 17 and loss of chromosome Y are the common-

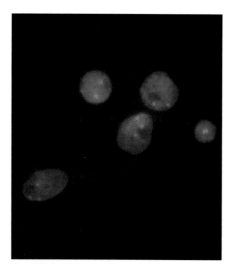

Fig. 1.28 Papillary carcinoma. Chromosome 17 trisomy, typical for papillary RCC. FISH technique.

est karyotypic changes in PRCC {1373}. High resolution studies have shown interstitial 3p loss of heterozygosity in some PRCC {1789,2723}. Trisomy of 12, 16 and 20 is also found in PRCC and may be related to tumour progression {618,1373}, while loss of heterozygosity at 9p13 is associated with shorter survival {2340}. Comparative genomic hybridization studies show more gains of chromosomes 7p and 17p in type 1 PRCC when compared to type 2 tumours {1219}, while more recently, differing patterns of allelic imbalance at 17q and 9p have been noted {2291}.

Prognosis and predictive factors

In series of PRCC containing both type 1 and 2 tumours, five year survivals for all stages range from 49% to 84% {584,1612}, with tumour grade {76, 675,1428,1753}, stage at presentation {76,1753} and the presence of sarcomatoid dedifferentiation {76,1753}

being correlated with outcome. Additionally the presence of extensive tumour necrosis and numerous foamy macrophages has been associated with a more favourable prognosis {76, 1612}, while on multivariate modelling only tumour stage retained a significant correlation with survival {76}.

While grade 1 tubulopapillary tumours between 0.5 and 2 cm are strictly defined as carcinomas, many pathologists prefer to report them as "papillary epithelial neoplasm of low malignant potential" for practical reasons.

Up to 70% of PRCC are intrarenal at diagnosis {76,1428,1612,1860} and type 1 tumours are usually of lower stage and grade than type 2 tumours {76,585,587,1753}. Longer survivals have been demonstrated for type 1 when compared with type 2 PRCC on both univariate {1753} and multivariate analysis that included both tumour stage and grade {587}.

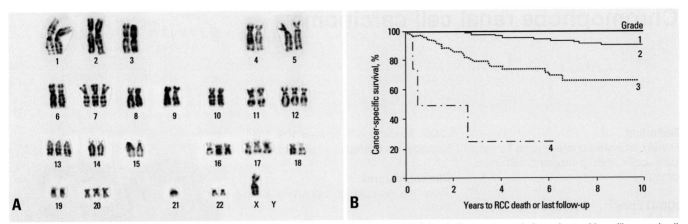

Fig. 1.29 Papillary renal cell carcinoma. **A** Trisomy 7, 12, 13, 16, 17 and 20 and deletion of 21 and Y. **B** Survival curves by grade for patients with papillary renal cell carcinoma. From C.M. Lohse et al. {1532}.

Chromophobe renal cell carcinoma

S. Störkel
G. Martignoni
E. van den Berg

Definition
Renal carcinoma characterized by large pale cells with prominent cell membranes.

ICD-O code   8317/3

Epidemiology
Chromophobe renal cell carcinoma (CRCC) accounts for approximately 5 per cent of surgically removed renal epithelial tumours. The mean age of incidence is in the sixth decade, with a range in age of 27-86 years, and the number of men and women is roughly equal. Mortality is less than 10% {512}. Sporadic and hereditary forms exist.

Clinical features
There are no specific signs and symptoms.

On imaging, these are mostly large masses without necrosis or calcifications.

Macroscopy
Chromophobe renal cell carcinomas are solid circumscribed tumours with slightly lobulated surfaces. In unfixed specimens the cut surface is homogeneously light

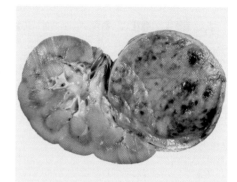

Fig. 1.30 Chromophobe renal cell carcinoma (RCC). Typical homogeneously tan coloured tumour of the lower pole of the kidney.

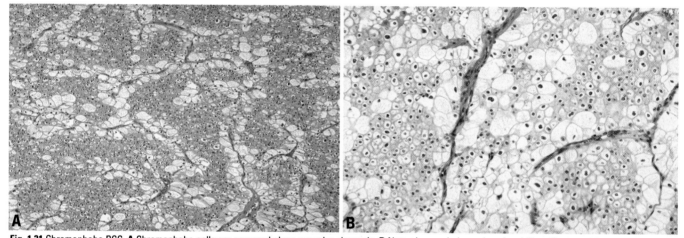

Fig. 1.31 Chromophobe RCC. **A** Chromophobe cells are arranged along vascular channels. **B** Note chromophobe and eosinophilic cells.

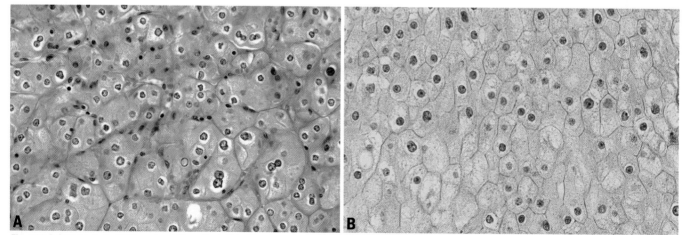

Fig. 1.32 A Chromophobe RCC, eosinophilic variant. Note binucleated cells, perinuclear halos and tight intercellular cohesion. **B** Chromophobe RCC. Note typical granular cytoplasm with perinuclear clearance.

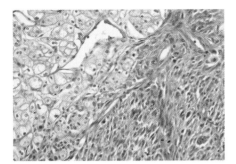

Fig. 1.33 Chromophobe RCC with sarcomatoid dedifferentiation.

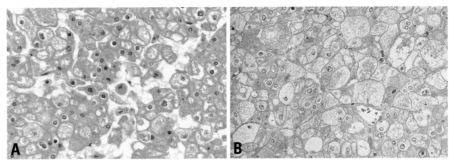

Fig. 1.34 Chromophobe RCC. **A** Hale's iron staining of eosinophilic variant. **B** Classic variant. Hale's colloidal iron stain positivity in the cytoplasm.

brown or tan turning light grey after formalin fixation.

Tumour spread and staging
The majority of CRCCs are stage T1 and T2 (86%) whereas only 10% show extension through the renal capsule into surrounding adipose tissue, only 4% show involvement of the renal vein (T3b) {512}. A few cases of lymph node and distant metastasis (lung, liver and pancreas) have been described {152,1635,2172}.

Histopathology
In general, the growth pattern is solid, sometimes glandular, with focal calcifications and broad fibrotic septa. In contrast to clear cell renal cell carcinoma, many of the blood vessels are thick-walled and eccentrically hyalinized. The perivascular cells are often enlarged. Chromophobe renal cell carcinoma is characterized by large polygonal cells

with transparent slightly reticulated cytoplasm with prominent cell membranes. These cells are commonly mixed with smaller cells with granular eosinophilic cytoplasm. The eosinophilic variant of chromophobe carcinoma is purely composed of intensively eosinophilic cells with prominent cell membranes {2610}. The cells have irregular, often wrinkled, nuclei. Some are binucleated. Nucleoli are usually small. Perinuclear halos are common. Sarcomatoid transformation occurs {2047}. Another diagnostic hallmark is a diffuse cytoplasmic staining reaction with Hale's colloidal iron stain {475,2608}.

Immunoprofile
Immunohistology presents the following antigen profile: pan-Cytokeratin+, vimentin-, EMA+ (diffuse), lectins+, parvalbumin+, RCC antigen-/+, CD10– {140,1635,1675,2513}.

Ultrastructure
Electron microscopically, the cytoplasm is crowded by loose glycogen deposits and numerous sometimes invaginated vesicles, 150-300 nm in diameter resembling those of the intercalated cells type b of the cortical collecting duct {722,2515}.

Somatic genetics
Chromophobe renal cell carcinomas are characterized by extensive chromosomal loss, most frequently -1,-2,-6,-10,-13,-17 and –21 {338,2464}.
The massive chromosomal losses lead to a hypodiploid DNA index {42}. Endoreduplication/polyploidization of the hypodiploid cells has been observed. Telomeric associations and telomere shortening have also been observed {1113,1375}.
At the molecular level, Contractor et al. {486} showed that there are mutations of

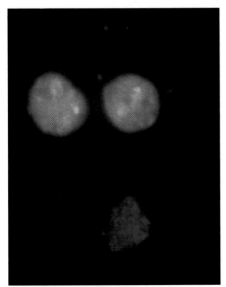

Fig. 1.35 Chromophobe RCC with typical monosomy (one signal for chromosome 17). FISH.

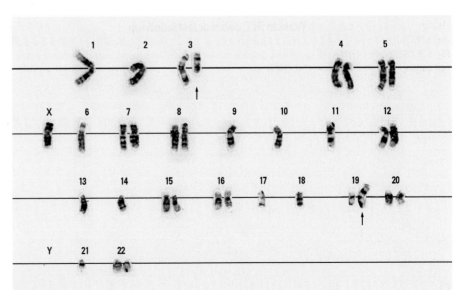

Fig. 1.36 Chromophobe renal cell carcinoma. A representative karyotype of a chromophobe RCC showing extensive loss of chromosomes.

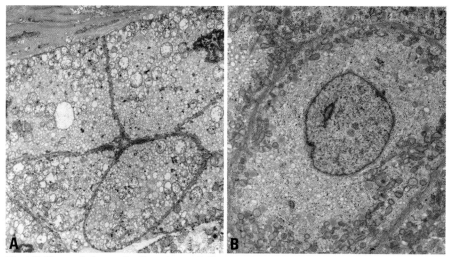

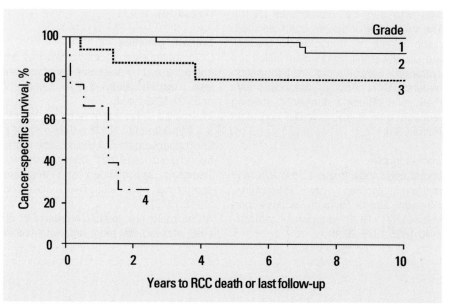

Fig. 1.37 Chromophobe renal cell carcinoma. **A** Electron micrograph showing the numerous cytoplasmic microvesicles and thick cytoplasmic membranes. **B** The perinuclear rarefaction and peripheral condensation of mitochondria responsible for the perinuclear halos.

Fig. 1.38 Chromophobe renal cell carcinoma. Survival curves by grade for patients with chromophobe renal cell carcinoma. From C.M. Lohse et al. {1532}.

TP53 tumour suppressor gene in 27% of the chromophobe RCCs. Sükösd et al. {2531} demonstrated loss of heterozygosity (LOH) around the *PTEN* gene at the 10q23.3 chromosomal region.

Prognosis and predictive factors
Sarcomatoid phenotype is associated with aggressive tumour growth and the development of metastasis.

Carcinoma of the collecting ducts of Bellini

J.R. Srigley
H. Moch

Definition
A malignant epithelial tumour thought to be derived from the principal cells of the collecting duct of Bellini.

ICD-O code   8319/3

Synonym
Collecting duct carcinoma, Bellini duct carcinoma.

Epidemiology
Collecting duct carcinoma is rare, accounting for <1% of renal malignancies. Over 100 cases have been described and there is a wide age range from 13-83 years (mean, about 55) with a male to female ratio of 2:1 {2470}.

Clinical features
Patients with collecting duct carcinoma usually present with abdominal pain, flank mass and haematuria. About one-third of patients have metastases at presentation. Metastases to bone are often osteoblastic. Upper tract imaging often suggests urothelial carcinoma and patients may occasionally present with positive urine cytology.

Macroscopy
Collecting duct carcinomas are usually located in the central region of the kidney. When small, origin within a medullary pyramid may be seen. Reported tumours range from 2.5 to 12 cm (mean, about 5 cm) and they typical-ly have a firm grey-white appearance with irregular borders {2470}. Some tumours grow as masses within the renal pelvis. Areas of necrosis and satellite nodules may be present.

Tumour spread and staging
Collecting duct carcinomas often display infiltration of perirenal and renal sinus fat. Metastases to regional lymph nodes, lung, liver, bone and adrenal gland are common. Sometimes gross renal vein invasion is seen.

Histopathology
The diagnosis of collecting duct carcinoma is often difficult and to some extent is one of exclusion. While most collecting duct carcinomas are located centrally in the medullary zone, other common forms of renal cell carcinoma (clear cell, papillary) may also arise centrally from cortical tissue of the columns of Bertin. Criteria for diagnosing collecting duct carcinoma have been proposed {2470}. The prototypic collecting duct carcinoma has a tubular or tubulopapillary growth pattern in which irregular angulated glands infiltrate renal parenchyma and are associated with a desmoplastic stroma {775,1298,2262,2470}. The edge of the tumour is often ill-defined and there is extensive permeation of renal parenchyma. Small papillary infoldings and micro-

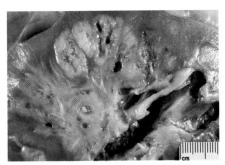

Fig. 1.39 Carcinoma of the collecting ducts of Bellini.

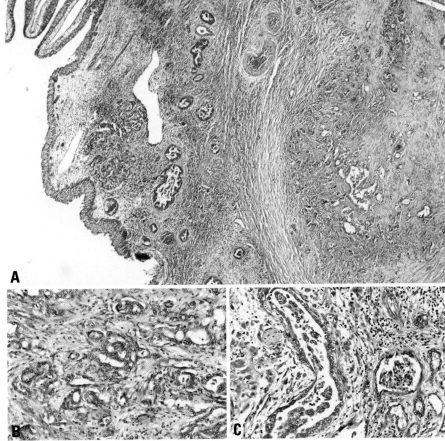

Fig. 1.40 Carcinoma of the collecting ducts of Bellini. **A** Medullary location of the tumour. **B** Tubular type of growth. **C** Higher magnification discloses small papillary infoldings to the tubular lumina.

cystic change may be seen. Solid, cord-like patterns and sarcomatoid features may be encountered. The sarcomatoid change is a pattern of dedifferentiation similar to that seen in other types of renal carcinoma {153}. The cells of collecting duct carcinoma usually display high grade (Fuhrman 3 and 4) nuclear features. The cells may have a hobnail pattern of growth and the cytoplasm is generally eosinophilic. Glycogen is usually inconspicuous in collecting duct carcinoma. Both intraluminal and intracytoplasmic mucin may be seen.

Some tumours with other morphologies have been proposed as collecting duct carcinomas. The most frequent ones have a predominantly papillary growth pattern but they differ from usual papillary carcinoma by a lack of circumscription, broad stalks containing inflamed fibrous stroma, desmoplasia, high nuclear grade and sometimes an association with more typical tubular patterns of collecting duct carcinoma elsewhere {2470}. The central location and associated tubular epithelial dysplasia (atypia) are helpful in supporting a diagnosis, although dysplasia may be seen in collecting ducts adjacent to other types of renal carcinoma.

Immunoprofile
Tumour cells usually display positivity for low molecular weight and broad spectrum keratins. High molecular weight keratins (34βE12, CK19) are commonly present and co-expression of vimentin may be seen {2470}. There is variable immunostaining for CD15 and epithelial membrane antigen. The CD10 and villin stains are negative. Lectin histochemistry, usual *Ulex europaeus* agglutinin-1 and peanut lectin are commonly positive.

Differential diagnosis
The main differential diagnoses of collecting duct carcinoma include papillary renal cell carcinoma, adenocarcinoma or urothelial carcinoma with glandular differentiation arising in renal pelvis and metastatic adenocarcinoma {2470}.

Somatic genetics
Molecular events that contribute to the development of collecting duct carcinomas (CDCs) are poorly understood because only few cases have been analyzed. LOH was identified on multiple chromosomal arms in CDC, including 1q, 6p, 8p, 13q, and 21q {2094}. Loss of chromosomal arm 3p can be found in CDC {674,990}. High density mapping of the entire long arm of chromosome 1 showed that the region of minimal deletion is located at 1q32.1-32.2 {2501}. One study suggested that 8p LOH might be associated with high tumour stage and poor patient prognosis {2335}. In contrast to clear cell RCC, HER2/neu amplifications have been described in CDCs {2357}.

Prognosis and predictive factors
The typical collecting duct carcinomas have a poor prognosis with many being metastatic at presentation. About two-thirds of patients die of their disease within two years of diagnosis {2470}.

Table 1.05
Diagnostic criteria for collecting duct carcinoma.

Major Criteria
- Location in a medullary pyramid (small tumours)
- Typical histology with irregular tubular architecture and high nuclear grade
- Inflammatory desmoplastic stroma with numerous granulocytes
- Reactive with antibodies to high molecular weight cytokeratin
- Reactive with *Ulex europaeus* agglutinin lectin
- Absence of urothelial carcinoma
Minor Criteria
- Central location (large tumours)
- Papillary architecture with wide, fibrous stalks and desmoplastic stroma
- Extensive renal, extrarenal, and lymphatic and venous infiltration
- Intra tubular epithelial atypia adjacent to the tumour

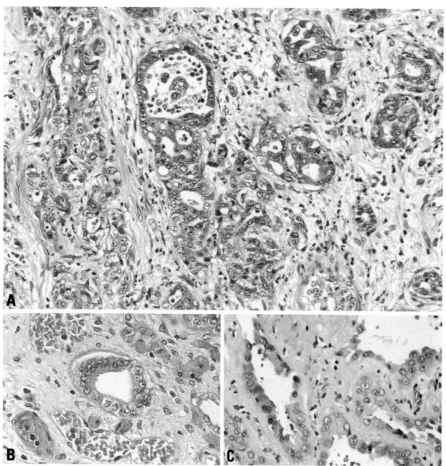

Fig. 1.41 Carcinoma of the collecting ducts of Bellini. **A** Tubulopapillary type of growth. **B,C** Note high grade cytological atypia.

Renal medullary carcinoma

C.J. Davis

Definition

A rapidly growing tumour of the renal medulla associated almost exclusively with sickle cell trait.

ICD-O code   8319/3

Epidemiology

This is a rare tumour. Over a period of 22 years the Armed Forces Institute of Pathology had collected only 34 cases {562} and over the next 5 years only 15 more had been described {1304}.

Clinical features

Signs and symptoms

With few exceptions these are seen in young people with sickle cell trait between ages 10 and 40 (mean age 22 years) and chiefly in males by 2:1. The common symptoms are gross haematuria and flank or abdominal pain. Weight loss and palpable mass are also common. Metastatic deposits such as cervical nodes or brain tumour may be the initial evidence of disease {2119}.

Imaging

In the clinical setting of a young person with sickle cell trait it is often possible to anticipate the correct diagnosis with imaging studies {557,1304}. Centrally located tumours with an infiltrative growth pattern, invading renal sinus, are typical. Caliectasis without pelviectasis and tumour encasing the pelvis are also described.

Macroscopy

These are poorly circumscribed tumours arising centrally in the kidney. Size ranges from 4 to 12 cm with a mean of 7 cm. Most show much haemorrhage and necrosis {562}.

Histopathology

Most cases have poorly differentiated areas consisting of sheets of cells. A reticular growth pattern and a more compact adenoid cystic morphology are the common features. The cells are eosinophilic with clear nuclei and usually with prominent nucleoli. The sheets of cells can have squamoid or rhabdoid quality. Neutrophils are often admixed with the tumour and the advancing margins often bounded by lymphocytes. Oedematous or collagenous stroma forms a considerable bulk of many

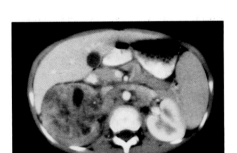

Fig. 1.42 Renal medullary carcinoma. Infiltrating tumour expanding renal contour.

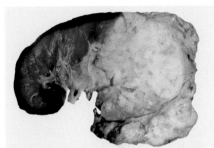

Fig. 1.43 Renal medullary carcinoma. Infiltrating tumour with perinephric extension at lower right.

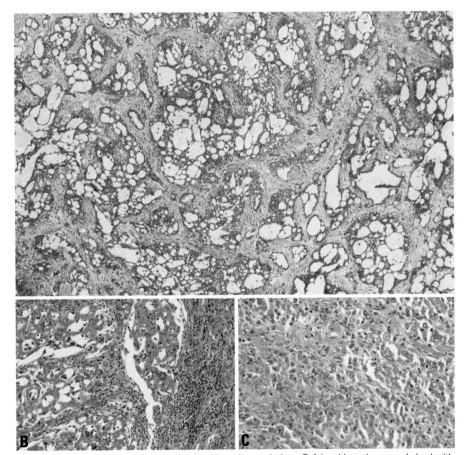

Fig. 1.44 Renal medullary carcinoma. **A** Adenoid cystic morphology. **B** Adenoid cystic area admixed with neutrophils. Note lymphocytes at advancing margin. **C** Poorly differentiated area. Note sickled red cells at lower left.

tumours. A majority of cases show droplets of cytoplasmic mucin and sickled erythrocytes {562}.

Immunoprofile
Keratin AE1/AE3 is nearly always positive as is EMA but typically less strongly so. CEA is usually positive. One study found strong expression of low molecular weight cytokeratin (CAM 5.2) but negative high molecular weight cytokeratin {2220}.

Prognosis and predictive factors
The prognosis is poor and the mean duration of life after surgery has been 15 weeks. Chemotherapy has been known to prolong survival by a few months {2084} but generally, this and radiotherapy has not altered the course of the disease {1304}. Metastases are both lymphatic and vascular with lymph nodes, liver and lungs most often involved. These tumours are now widely regarded as a more aggressive variant of the collecting duct carcinoma {648,2470}.

Renal carcinomas associated with Xp11.2 translocations / *TFE3* gene fusions

P. Argani
M. Ladanyi

Definition
These carcinomas are defined by several different translocations involving chromosome Xp11.2, all resulting in gene fusions involving the *TFE3* gene.

Clinical features
These carcinomas predominantly affect children and young adults, though a few older patients have been reported {108}. The *ASPL-TFE3* carcinomas characteristically present at advanced stage {109}.

Macroscopy
Renal carcinomas associated with Xp11.2 translocations are most commonly tan-yellow, and often necrotic and haemorrhagic.

Histopathology
The most distinctive histopathologic appearance is that of a carcinoma with papillary architecture comprised of clear cells; however, these tumours frequently have a more nested architecture, and often feature cells with granular eosinophilic cytoplasm. The *ASPL-TFE3* renal carcinomas are characterized by cells with voluminous clear to eosinophilic cytoplasm, discrete cell borders, vesicular chromatin and prominent nucleoli. Psammoma bodies are constant and sometimes extensive, often arising within characteristic hyaline nodules {109}. The *PRCC-TFE3* renal carcinomas generally feature less abundant cytoplasm, fewer psammoma bodies, fewer hyaline nodules, and a more nested, compact architecture {108}.

Immunoprofile
The most distinctive immunohistochemical feature of these tumours is nuclear immunoreactivity for TFE3 protein {113}. Only about 50% express epithelial markers such as cytokeratin and EMA by immunohistochemistry {108,109}, and the labeling is often focal. The tumours consistently label for the Renal Cell Carcinoma Marker antigen and CD10.

Ultrastructure
Ultrastructurally, Xp11.2-associated carcinomas most closely resemble clear cell renal carcinomas. Most of the *ASPL-TFE3* renal carcinomas also demonstrate membrane-bound cytoplasmic granules and a few contain membrane-bound rhomboidal crystals identical to those seen in soft tissue alveolar soft part sarcoma (ASPS) {109}. Occasional *PRCC-TFE3* renal carcinomas have demonstrated distinctive intracisternal microtubules identical to those seen in extraskeletal myxoid chondrosarcoma {108}.

Somatic genetics
These carcinomas are defined by several different translocations involving chromosome Xp11.2, all resulting in gene fusions involving the *TFE3* gene. These include the t(X;1)(p11.2;q21) {1710}, which results in fusion of the *PRCC* and *TFE3* genes, the t(X;17)(p11.2;q25)

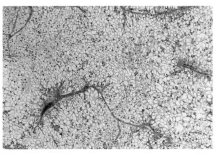

Fig. 1.45 t(X:17) renal carcinoma. Note sheet like growth pattern and clear cells.

{371,1055,1084,2626}, which results in fusion of the *ASPL* (also known as *RCC17* or *ASPSCR1*) and *TFE3* genes {109,1056,1424}, the t(X;1)(p11.2;p34), resulting in fusion of the *PSF* and *TFE3* genes, and the inv(X)(p11;q12), resulting in fusion of the *NonO* ($p54^{nrb}$) and *TFE3* genes {471}.

TFE3 is a member of the basic-helix-loop-helix family of transcription factors. Both the PRCC-TFE3 and ASPL-TFE3 fusion proteins retain the TFE3 DNA binding domain, localize to the nucleus, and can act as aberrant transcription factors {2432,2809}, and (M. Ladanyi, unpublished observations). The expression levels of TFE3 fusion proteins appear aberrantly high compared to native TFE3 {113}, perhaps because the fusion partners of *TFE3* are ubiquitously expressed and contribute their promoters to the fusion proteins.

Interestingly, while both the t(X;17) renal carcinomas and the soft tissue ASPS

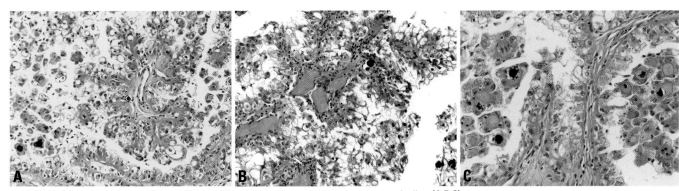

Fig. 1.46 t(X:17) renal carcinoma. Note papillary architecture, hyaline nodules and psammoma bodies. **(A,B,C)**

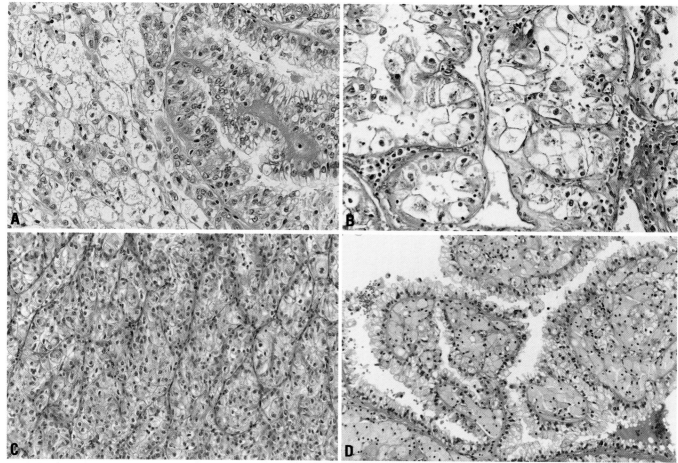

Fig. 1.47 A t(X:1) RCC. Note tubular and papillary architecture. **B** t(X:17) renal carcinoma. Note alveolar growth pattern and clear cells. **C** t(X:1) RCC. Note compact nested architecture. **D** t(X:1) RCC. Note papillary architecture with foam cells.

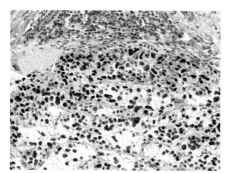

Fig. 1.48 Xp 11.2-translocation renal carcinoma. Note strong nuclear labeling of the tumour cells. TFE3 protein expression.

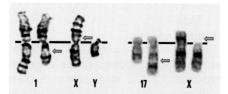

Fig. 1.49 Xp11 translocation carcinomas. Partial karyotypes showing t(X;1)(p11.2;q21) in a renal tumour from a male (courtesy of Dr. Suresh C. Jhanwar) and a t(X;17)(p11.2;q25.3) in a renal tumour from a female. The positions of the breakpoints are indicated by arrows (standard G-banding). Reprinted and adapted with permission from P. Argani et al. {109}.

contain identical *ASPL-TFE3* fusion transcripts, the t(X;17) translocation is consistently balanced (reciprocal) in the former but usually unbalanced in the latter (i.e. the derivative X chromosome is not seen in ASPS) {109}.

Prognosis and predictive factors

Very little is known about the clinical behaviour of these carcinomas. While the ASPL-TFE3 renal carcinomas usually present at advanced stage, their clinical course thus far appears to be indolent.

Renal cell carcinoma associated with neuroblastoma

L.J. Medeiros

Definition
Renal cell carcinoma associated with neuroblastoma occurs in long-term survivors of childhood neuroblastoma.

Etiology
Therapy for neuroblastoma may play a role in the pathogenesis of subsequent RCC. However, one patient was not treated for stage IVS neuroblastoma, and a second patient developed RCC and neuroblastoma simultaneously {1380,1694}. A familial genetic susceptibility syndrome may be involved.

Clinical features
Eighteen cases have been reported. Males and females are equally affected. {1281,1380,1394,1489,1694,2743}. Age was <2 years at time of diagnosis of neuroblastoma. Median age at time of diagnosis of RCC was 13.5 years (range, 2 to 35).

Macroscopy
Either kidney may be involved and four cases were bilateral. Median tumour size, in 12 cases, was 4 cm (range, 1.0-8 cm).

Tumour spread and staging
Five patients developed metastases involving the liver, lymph nodes, thyroid and adrenal glands, and bone {1394,1694,2743}.

Histopathology
These tumours are morphologically heterogeneous {1380}. Some tumours are characterized by solid and papillary architecture, cells with abundant eosinophilic cytoplasm with a lesser number of cells with reticular cytoplasm, and mild to moderate atypia {1281,1380, 1694}. In a second group, the tumours are small, clear cell renal cell carcinomas that were detected incidentally.

Immunoprofile
These tumours are usually positive for EMA, vimentin and keratins 8, 18, and 20 and are negative for keratins 7, 14, and 19.

Somatic genetics
Cytogenetic analysis of two tumours showed deletions of multiple chromosomal loci {2743}. Microsatellite analysis using polymorphic markers in three tumours showed allelic imbalances involving a number of loci, most often 20q13 {1281,1694,2743}.

Prognosis and predictive factors
Prognosis correlates with tumour stage and the presence of high grade nuclear atypia, similar to other histologic types of RCC.

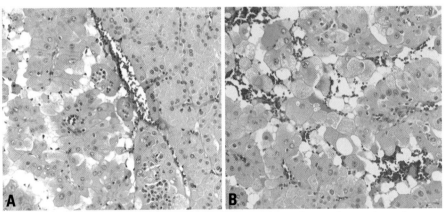

Fig. 1.50 Carcinoma associated with neuroblastoma. **A** Note a mixture of areas of compact growth resembling renal oncocytoma and areas of papillary growth. **B** Higher magnification showing nuclei of variable size, often with nucleoli of medium size. There is focal papillary architecture.

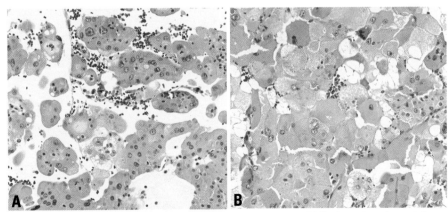

Fig. 1.51 Carcinoma associated with neuroblastoma. **A** Conspicuous variability in nuclear size and shape. The architecture is papillary and there is a psammoma body. **B** Tumour composed of large cells with finely and coarsely granular eosinophilic cytoplasm. Some are vacuolated.

Mucinous tubular and spindle cell carcinoma

J.R. Srigley

Definition
Low-grade polymorphic renal epithelial neoplasms with mucinous tubular and spindle cell features.

Epidemiology
There is a wide age range of 17-82 (mean 53) years and a male to female ratio of 1:4 {2024,2469}.

Clinical features
They usually present as asymptomatic masses, often found on ultrasound. Occasionally, they may present with flank pain or hematuria.

Macroscopy
Macroscopically, mucinous tubular and spindle cell carcinomas, are well circumscribed and have grey or light tan, uniform cut surfaces.

Histopathology
Histologically, they are composed of tightly packed, small, elongated tubules separated by pale mucinous stroma. The parallel tubular arrays often have a spindle cell configuration sometimes simulating leiomyoma or sarcoma. Many of these tumours had been previously diagnosed as unclassified or spindle cell (sarcomatoid) carcinomas.

Individual cells are small with cuboidal or oval shapes and low-grade nuclear features. Occasionally, areas of necrosis, foam cell deposits and chronic inflammation may be present. The mucinous stroma is highlighted with stains for acid mucins.

Immunoprofile
These tumours have a complex immunophenotype and stain for a wide variety of cytokeratins including low molecular weight keratins (CAM 5.2, MAK 6), CK7, CK18, CK19 and 34βE12 {2469}. Epithelial membrane antigen is commonly present, and vimentin and CD15 staining may be seen. Markers of proximal nephron such as CD10 and villin are generally absent. These tumours show extensive positivity for *Ulex europaeus*, peanut and soya bean agglutinins.

Ultrastructure
The spindle cells show epithelial features like tight junctions, desmosomes, microvillous borders, luminal borders and occasional tonofilaments {2469}.

Somatic genetics
Using comparative genomic hybridization and FISH, there is a characteristic combination of chromosome losses, generally involving chromosome 1, 4, 6, 8, 13 and 14 and gains of chromosome 7, 11, 16 and 17 {2137,2469}.

Prognosis and predictive factors
The prognosis sems to be favourable; only one example has been reported with metastasis and this tumour is best considered as a low-grade carcinoma {2471}.

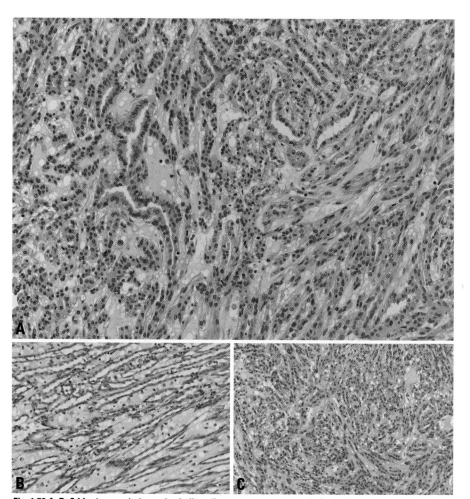

Fig. 1.52 A, B, C Mucinous tubular and spindle cell carconoma composed of spindle cells and cuboidal cells forming cords and tubules. Note basophilic extracellular mucin.

Papillary adenoma of the kidney

J.N. Eble
H. Moch

Definition
Papillary adenomas are tumours with papillary or tubular architecture of low nuclear grade and 5 mm in diameter or smaller.

ICD-O code   8260/0

Clinical features
Papillary adenomas are the most common neoplasms of the epithelium of the renal tubules. Autopsy studies have found papillary adenomas increase in frequency in adulthood from 10% of patients younger than 40 years to 40% in patients older than 70 years {653,2163, 2854}. Similar lesions frequently develop in patients on long-term hemodialysis and occur in 33% of patients with acquired renal cystic disease {1143}.

Macroscopy
Papillary adenomas are well circumscribed, yellow to greyish white nodules as small as less than 1 mm in diameter in the renal cortex. Most occur just below the renal capsule. The smallest ones usually are spherical, but larger ones sometimes are roughly conical with a wedge-shaped appearance in sections cut at right angles to the cortical surface. Usually, papillary adenomas are solitary, but occasionally they are multiple and bi-lateral. When they are very numerous, this has been called "renal adenomatosis".

Histopathology
Papillary adenomas have tubular, papillary, or tubulopapillary architectures corresponding closely to types 1 and 2 papillary renal cell carcinoma {585}. Some have thin fibrous pseudocapsules. The cells have round to oval nuclei with stippled to clumped chromatin and inconspicuous nucleoli; nuclear grooves may be present. Mitotic figures usually are absent. In most, the cytoplasm is scant and pale, amphophilic to basophilic. Less frequently, the cytoplasm is voluminous and eosinophilic, resembling type 2 papillary renal cell carcinoma. Psammoma bodies are common, as are foamy macrophages {2161}.

Somatic genetics
Loss of the Y chromosome and a combined trisomy of chromosome 7 and 17 are the first visible karyotype aberrations in papillary renal tumours. This combination of genetic alterations has been found as the sole karyotype change in small papillary renal tumours from 2 mm to 5 mm in diameter, all with nuclear grade 1 {1373}. Based on these findings, it has been suggested that papillary adenomas

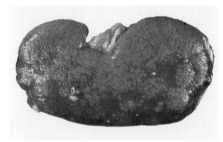

Fig. 1.53 Multiple renal papillary adenomas.

aquire additional genetic alterations during growth, which change their biological behaviour {1369}. One CGH analysis studied 6 papillary tumours less than 6 mm in diameter and observed gain of chromosome 7 in 4 specimens {2107}. These data suggest that initiating genetic events for papillary renal adenomas include gains of chromosome 7 and loss of a sex chromosome. Small renal tumours demonstrate similar, but less extensive genetic alterations than their papillary renal carcinoma counterparts. The clinically indolent course of small papillary tumours may, in part, be a result of the lower number of genetic alterations per tumour. However, it is not possible to distinguish adenomas and carcinomas by genetic changes, because many carcinomas show only few genetic alterations.

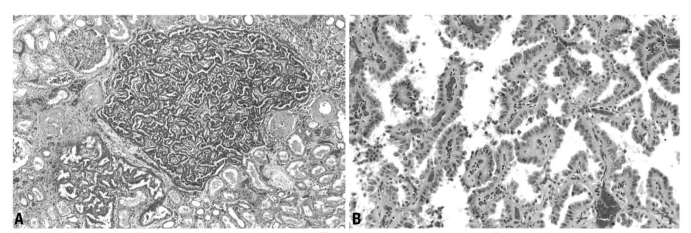

Fig. 1.54 Papillary adenoma. **A** Two papillary adenomas in the renal cortex. These type 1 adenomas have complex papillae covered by a single layer of small epithelial cells with inconspicuous cytoplasm. **B** Papillary adenoma composed of complex branching papillae on partially hyalinized stromal cores.

Oncocytoma

V.E. Reuter
C.J. Davis
H. Moch

Definition
Oncocytoma is a benign renal epithelial neoplasm composed of large cells with mitochondria-rich eosinophilic cytoplasm, thought to arise from intercalated cells.

ICD-O code   8290/0

Epidemiology
First described by Zippel in 1942 {2939} and later by Klein and Valensi {1335}, oncocytoma comprises approximately 5% of all neoplasms of renal tubular epithelium in surgical series {77,453,563, 607,812,1060,1174,1497,2050,2178, 2945}. Most series show a wide age distribution at presentation with a peak incidence in the seventh decade of life. Males are affected nearly twice as often as females. Most occur sporadically.

Clinical features
Signs and symptoms
The majority is asymptomatic at presentation with discovery occurring during radiographic work-up of unrelated conditions. Few patients present with hematuria, flank pain, or a palpable mass.

Imaging
The diagnosis of oncocytoma may be suggested by computed tomography or magnetic resonance imaging in tumours featuring a central scar {558,1094}.

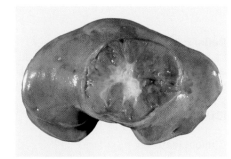

Fig. 1.55 Oncocytoma.

Macroscopy
Oncocytomas are well-circumscribed, nonencapsulated neoplasms that are classically mahogany-brown and less often tan to pale yellow. A central, stellate scar may be seen in up to 33% of cases but is more commonly seen in larger tumours. Haemorrhage is present in up to 20% of cases but grossly visible necrosis is extremely rare {77,563,2050}.

Histopathology
Characteristically, these tumours have solid compact nests, acini, tubules, or microcysts. Often there is a hypocellular-hyalinized stroma. The predominant cell type (so-called "oncocyte") is round-to-polygonal with densely granular eosinophilic cytoplasm, round and regular nuclei with evenly dispersed chromatin, and a centrally placed nucleolus. A smaller population of cells with scanty granular cytoplasm, a high nuclear: cytoplasmic ratio, and dark hyperchromatic nuclei may also be observed. If microcysts are present, they may be filled with red blood cells. Occasional clusters of cells with pleomorphic and hyperchromatic nuclei are common. A rare oncocytoma may have one or two mitotic figures in the sections examined. Atypical mitotic figures are not seen. A few small foci of necroses do not exclude an oncocytoma. Isolated foci of clear cell change may be present in areas of stromal hyalinizations. While small papillae may very rarely be seen focally, pure or extensive papillary architecture is not a feature

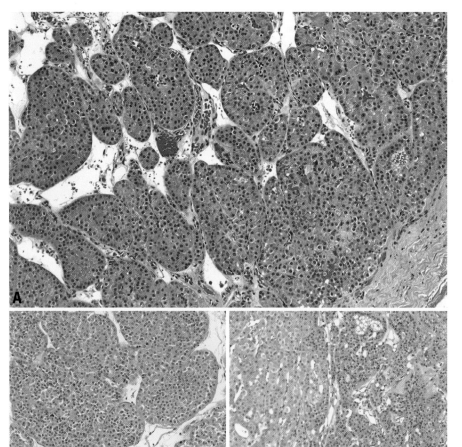

Fig. 1.56 A Oncocytoma. **B** Renal oncocytoma. Note rounded aggregates of small, eosinophilic cells. **C** Renal oncocytoma. Note clonal variation. Cells at left have more cytoplasm than on the right.

of this tumour. Microscopic extension into perinephric adipose tissue may be seen infrequently {1584} and vascular invasion has been described {77,563,2050}. Since oncocytomas are benign neoplasms, grading is not performed. There is no diffuse cytoplasmic Hale's colloidal iron staining in oncocytomas.

Oncocytosis (Oncocytomatosis)
Several cases have been reported in which the kidneys have contained a large number of oncocytic lesions with a spectrum of morphologic features, including oncocytic tumours, oncocytic change in benign tubules, microcysts lined by oncocytic cells and clusters of oncocytes within the renal interstitium {1181,2618,2782}. The oncocytic nodules usually have the morphologic and ultrastructural features of oncocytoma although some may have either chromophobe or hybrid features.

Ultrastructure
Through ultrastructural examination, renal oncocytoma is characterized by cells containing numerous mitochondria, the majority of which are of normal size and shape, though pleomorphic forms are rarely seen {722,2617}. Other cytoplasmic organelles are sparse and unremarkable. Notably absent are the microvesicles typical of chromophobe tumours.

Somatic genetics
Most renal oncocytomas display a mixed population of cells with normal and abnormal karyotypes {1376,1378}. In a few oncocytomas, translocation of t(5;11)(q35;q13) was detected {513,826,1376,2108,2687}. Some of the cases show loss of chromosome 1 and 14 {1079,2108}.

Prognosis and predictive factors
Renal oncocytomas are benign neoplasms. This conclusion is based largely on the data from several recent studies including rigorous pathologic review and adequate clinical follow-up in which not a single case of oncocytoma resulted in the death of a patient due to metastatic disease {77,563}.

Renal cell carcinoma, unclassified

J.N. Eble

ICD-O code   8312/3

Renal cell carcinoma, unclassified is a diagnostic category to which renal carcinomas should be assigned when they do not fit readily into one of the other categories {1370,2514}. In surgical series, this group often amounts to 4-5% of cases. Since this category must contain tumours with varied appearances and genetic lesions, it cannot be defined in a limiting way. However, examples of features, which might place a carcinoma in this category include: apparent composites of recognized types, sarcomatoid morphology without recognizable epithelial elements, mucin production, mixtures of epithelial and stromal elements, and unrecognizable cell types.
Sarcomatoid change has been found to arise in all of the types of carcinoma in the classification, as well as in urothelial carcinoma of the renal pelvic mucosa. Since there is no evidence that renal tumours arise de novo as sarcomatoid carcinomas, it is not viewed as a type of its own, but rather as a manifestation of high grade carcinoma of the type from which it arose. Occasionally, the sarcomatoid elements overgrow the antecedent carcinoma to the extent that it cannot be recognized; such tumours are appropriately assigned to renal cell carcinoma, unclassified.

Metanephric adenoma and metanephric adenofibroma

J.N. Eble
D.J. Grignon
H. Moch

Definition
Metanephric adenoma is a highly cellular epithelial tumour composed of small, uniform, embryonic-appearing cells.

ICD-O codes
Metanephric adenoma   8325/0
Metanephric adenofibroma   9013/0
Metanephric adenosarcoma   8933/3

Epidemiology
Metanephric adenoma occurs in children and adults, most commonly in the fifth and sixth decades. There is a 2:1 female preponderance {561}. Patients with *metanephric adenofibroma* have ranged from 5 months to 36 years (median = 30 months) {120}. There is a 2:1 ratio of males to females. A single case of high grade sarcoma arising in association with metanephric adenoma (*metanephric adenosarcoma*) has been reported {2072}.

Clinical features
Approximately 50% of metanephric adenoma are incidental findings with others presenting with polycythemia, abdominal or flank pain, mass, or hematuria. Presenting symptoms of metanephric adenofibroma have included polycythemia or hematuria; some have been incidental findings. Arroyo et al. {120} described several cases in which either Wilms tumour or carcinoma occurred in association with metanephric adenofibroma. Other than one patient with regional metastases from the carcinoma, these patients have had no progression.

Macroscopy
Metanephric adenomas range widely in size; most have been 30 to 60 mm in diameter {561}. Multifocality is uncommon. The tumours are typically well circumscribed but not encapsulated. The cut surfaces vary from grey to tan to yellow and may be soft or firm.
Foci of haemorrhage and necrosis are common; calcification is present in approximately 20%,and small cysts in 10% {561,1237}.
Metanephric adenofibromas are typically solitary tan partially cystic masses with indistinct borders {120}.

Histopathology
Metanephric adenoma is a highly cellular tumour composed of tightly packed small, uniform, round acini with an embryonal appearance. Since the acini and their lumens are small, at low magnification this pattern may be mistaken for a solid sheet of cells. Long branching and angulated tubular structures also are common. The stroma ranges from inconspicuous to a loose oedematous stroma.

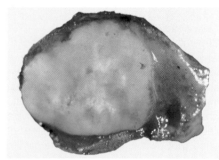

Fig. 1.57 Metanephric adenoma.

Hyalinized scar and focal osseous metaplasia of the stroma are present in 10-20% of tumours {561}. Approximately 50% of tumours contain papillary structures, usually consisting of tiny cysts into which protrude blunt papillae reminiscent of immature glomeruli. Psammoma bodies are common and sometimes numerous. The junction with the kidney is usually sharp and without a pseudocapsule. The cells of metanephric adenoma are monotonous, with small, uniform nuclei and absent or inconspicuous nucleoli. The nuclei are only a little larger than those of lymphocytes and are round or oval with delicate chromatin. The cytoplasm is scant and pale or light pink. Mitotic figures are absent or rare.
Metanephric adenofibroma is a compos-

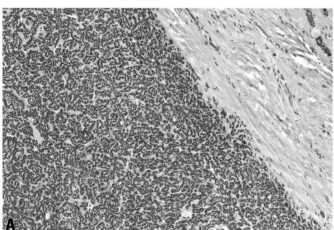
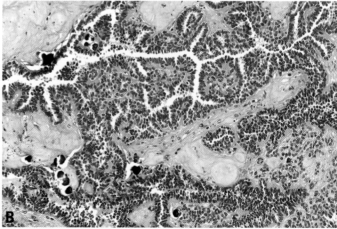

Fig. 1.58 Metanephric adenoma. **A** Well circumscribed tumour without encapsulation. **B** Complicated ductal architecture with psammoma bodies.

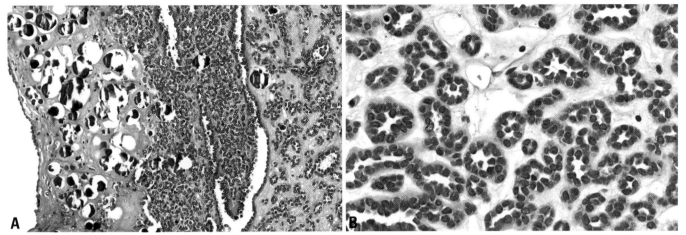

Fig. 1.59 Metanephric adenoma. **A** Metanephric adenoma with numerous psammoma bodies. **B** Multiple small tubules composed of a monotonous population of cuboidal cells.

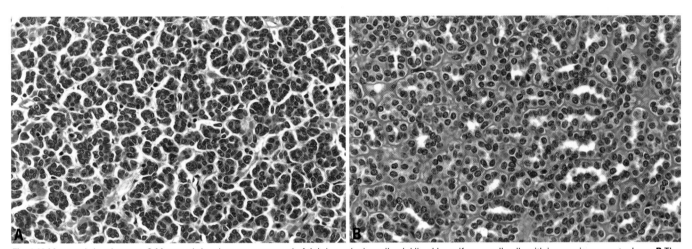

Fig. 1.60 Metanephric adenoma. **A** Metanephric adenoma composed of tightly packed small acini lined by uniform small cells with inconspicuous cytoplasm. **B** The nuclei are uniform, ovoid, and have inconspicuous nucleoli.

ite tumour in which nodules of epithelium identical to metanephric adenoma are embedded in sheets of moderately cellular spindle cells. The spindle cell component consists of fibroblast-like cells. Their cytoplasm is eosinophilic but pale and the nuclei are oval or fusiform. Nucleoli are inconspicuous and a few mitotic figures are present in a minority of cases. Variable amounts of hyalinization and myxoid change are present. Angiodysplasia and glial, cartilaginous, and adipose differentiation occur occasionally. The relative amounts of the spindle cell and epithelial components vary from predominance of spindle cells to a minor component of spindle cells. The border of the tumour with the kidney is typically irregular and the spindle cell component

may entrap renal structures as it advances. The epithelial component consists of small acini, tubules and papillary structures, as described above in metanephric adenoma. Psammoma bodies are common and may be numerous.

Immunoprofile
Immunohistochemical studies of *metanephric adenoma* have given variable results. Positive reactions with a variety of antibodies to cytokeratins have been reported, as have positive reactions with antibody to vimentin {951}. Positive intranuclear reactions with antibody to WT-1 are common in metanephric adenoma {1824}. Epithelial membrane antigen and cytokeratin 7 are frequently negative and CD57 is positive.

The stroma of *metanephric adenofibroma* frequently reacts with antibody to CD34 {120}. The reactions of the adenomatous elements are similar to those reported for metanephric adenoma.

Somatic genetics
Cytogenetic analysis of *metanephric adenoma* revealed normal karyotypes in 5 cases and normal copy numbers of chromosomes 7 and 17 were seen by FISH in 2 cases {840,926,1237,2171, 2652}. A deletion at chromosome 2p as the only genetic abnormality was described in 1 tumour {2522} and a tumour suppressor gene region on chromosome 2p13 was delineated {2058}.

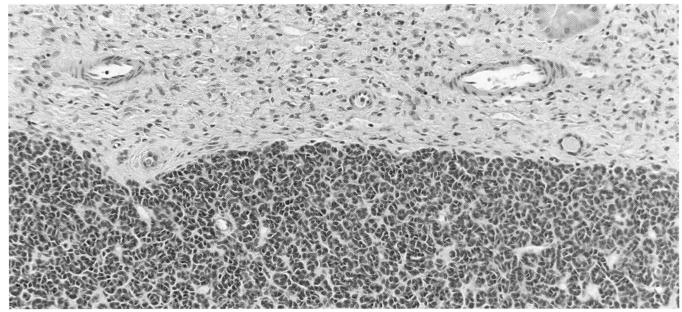

Fig. 1.61 Metanephric adenofibroma. Note epithelial area which is identical to metanephric adenoma (bottom), and stromal component which is identical to metanephric stromal tumour (top).

Metanephric stromal tumour

P. Argani

Definition
Metanephric stromal tumour is a rare benign paediatric renal neoplasm, which is identical to the stromal component of metanephric adenofibroma {110,1075}.

ICD-O code   8935/1

Clinical features
Metanephric stromal tumour (MST) is approximately one-tenth as common as congenital mesoblastic nephroma {110, 120}. The typical presentation is that of an abdominal mass, though haematuria is not uncommon and rare patients may present with manifestations of extra-renal vasculopathy such as hypertension or haemorrhage. Mean age at diagnosis is 24 months. A rare adult tumour has been identified {255}.

Macroscopy
MST is typically a tan, lobulated fibrous mass centred in the renal medulla. Mean diameter is 5 cm. Approximately one-half of cases are grossly cystic, while one-sixth are multifocal.

Histopathology
MST is an unencapsulated but subtly infiltrative tumour of spindled to stellate cells featuring thin, hyperchromatic nuclei, and thin, indistinct cytoplasmic extensions. Many of the characteristic features of MST result from its interaction with entrapped native renal elements. MST characteristically surrounds and entraps renal tubules and blood vessels to form concentric "onionskin" rings or collarettes around these structures in a myxoid background. More cellular, less myxoid spindle cell areas at the periphery of these collarettes yield nodular variations in cellularity. Most tumours induce angiodysplasia of entrapped arterioles, consisting of epithelioid transformation of medial smooth muscle and myxoid change. Rarely, such angiodysplasia

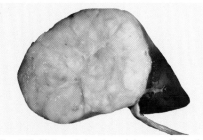

Fig. 1.62 Metanephric stromal tumour. Note the nodular appearance.

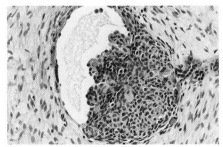

Fig. 1.63 Metanephric stromal tumour. Note juxtaglomerular cell hyperplasia.

results in intratumoral aneurysms. One-fourth of MSTs feature juxtaglomerular cell hyperplasia within entrapped glomeruli, which may occasionally lead to hypertension associated with hyperreninism. One-fifth of MSTs demonstrate heterologous differentiation in the form of glia or cartilage. Necrosis is unusual, and vascular invasion is absent in MST.

Immunoprofile
MSTs are typically immunoreactive for CD34, but labeling may be patchy. Desmin, cytokeratins, and S-100 protein are negative, though heterologous glial areas label for GFAP and S-100 protein.

Prognosis and predictive factors
All identified MSTs have had a benign course, with no reports of metastases or even local recurrence as of this writing. Excision is adequate therapy. Rare patients have suffered morbidity or mortality from the manifestations of extra renal angiodysplasia, apparently induced by MST.

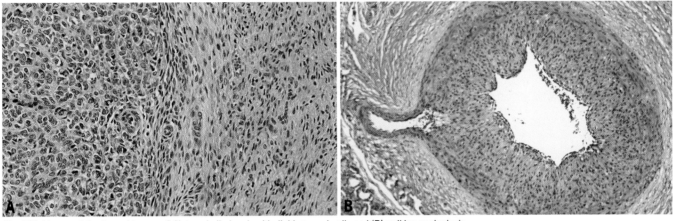

Fig. 1.64 Metanephric stromal tumour. **A** Note spindled and epithelioid stromal cells and (**B**) striking angioplasia.

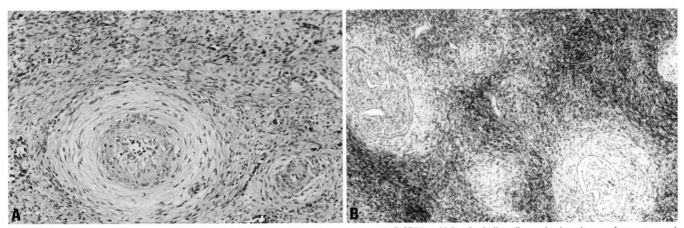

Fig. 1.65 Metanephric stromal tumour. **A** Angiodysplasia and concentric perivascular growth. **B** CD34 positivity of spindle cells, predominantly away from entrapped tubules.

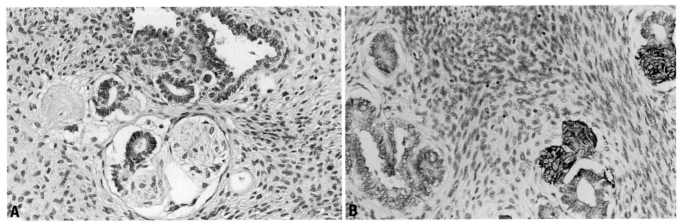

Fig. 1.66 Metanephric stromal tumour. **A** Glial-epithelial complexes. **B** Note positivity for GFAP in glial foci.

Nephroblastoma

E.J. Perlman
J.L. Grosfeld
K. Togashi
L. Boccon-Gibod

Definition

Nephroblastoma is a malignant embryonal neoplasm derived from nephrogenic blastemal cells that both replicates the histology of developing kidneys and often shows divergent patterns of differentiation.

ICD-O code   8960/3

Synonym

Wilms tumour.

Epidemiology

Nephroblastoma affects approximately one in every 8,000 children {317}. There is no striking sex predilection and tumours occur with equal frequency in both kidneys. The mean age at diagnosis is 37 and 43 months for males and females, respectively, and 98 percent of cases occur in individuals under 10 years of age, although presentation in adulthood has been reported {315,959, 1148}.

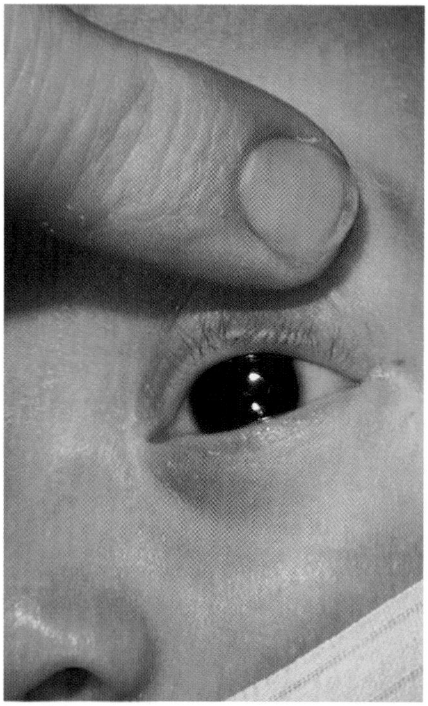

Fig. 1.67 Aniridia in a child, associated with nephroblastoma.

The stable incidence of nephroblastoma in all geographic regions suggests that environmental factors do not play a major role in its development. The variation in incidence among different racial groups, however, indicates a genetic predisposition for this tumour is likely: the general risk is higher among African-Americans and lower among Asians.

Clinical features

Nephroblastoma most commonly comes to clinical attention due to the detection of an abdominal mass by a parent when bathing or clothing a child.

Abdominal pain, hematuria, hypertension, and acute abdominal crisis secondary to traumatic rupture are also common. More rare presentations include anaemia, hypertension due to increased renin production, and polycythemia due to tumoural erythropoietin production {959,2087}.

The majority of nephroblastomas are treated using therapeutic protocols created by either the International Society of Paediatric Oncology (SIOP) or the Children's Oncology Group (COG). The SIOP protocols advocate preoperative therapy followed by surgical removal. This approach allows for tumour shrinkage prior to resection, yielding a greater frequency and ease of complete resectability. Continued therapy is then determined by the histologic evidence of responsiveness to therapy, as indicated by post-therapy classification. The COG (including the prior National Wilms Tumour Study Group) has long advocated primary resection of tumours, followed by therapy that is determined by stage and classification into "favourable" and "unfavourable" histology categories. This allows for greater diagnostic confidence and greater ability to stratify patients according to pathologic and biologic parameters. While the SIOP and COG protocols have intrinsically different philosophies regarding therapy, they have resulted in similar outcomes.

Imaging

Nephroblastoma typically manifests as a solid mass of heterogeneous appearance that distorts the renal parenchyma and collecting system. The lesion can be associated with foci of calcification. Isolated nephrogenic rests tend to appear as homogeneous nodules {1567}.

Macroscopy

Most nephroblastomas are unicentric. However, multicentric masses in a single kidney and bilateral primary lesions have been observed in 7 and 5 percent of cases, respectively {492,2381,2820}. Nephroblastomas are usually solitary rounded masses sharply demarcated from the adjacent renal parenchyma by a

Table 1.06
Revised SIOP Working Classification of Nephroblastoma.

A. For pretreated cases
I. Low risk tumours Cystic partially differentiated nephroblastoma Completely necrotic nephroblastoma
II. Intermediate risk tumours Nephroblastoma – epithelial type Nephroblastoma – stromal type Nephroblastoma – mixed type Nephroblastoma – regressive type Nephroblastoma – focal anaplasia
III. High risk tumours Nephroblastoma – blastemal type Nephroblastoma – diffuse anaplasia
B. For Primary nephrectomy cases
I. Low risk tumours Cystic partially differentiated nephroblastoma
II. Intermediate risk tumours Non-anaplastic nephroblastoma and its variants Nephroblastoma-focal anaplasia
III. High risk tumours Nephroblastoma – diffuse anaplasia

peritumoural fibrous pseudocapsule. Lesions most commonly have a uniform, pale grey or tan appearance and a soft consistency, although they may appear firm and whorled if a large fraction of the lesion is composed of mature stromal elements. Polypoid protrusions of tumour into the pelvicaliceal system may occur resulting in a "botryoid" appearance {1602}. Cysts may be prominent. Rarely, nephroblastoma occurs in extrarenal sites {28,1976}.

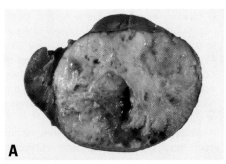 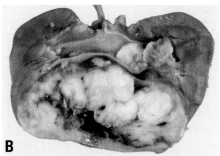

Fig. 1.68 Nephroblastoma. A circumscribed, encapsulated lesion with cyst formation. B Polypoid extension into renal pelvis.

Tumour spread and metastasis

Nephroblastomas generally have a restricted pattern of metastasis, most commonly regional lymph nodes, lungs, and liver {318}. Metastatic sites other than these (i.e., bone or brain) are unusual and should suggest alternative diagnoses.

Table 1.07
Staging of paediatric renal tumours: Children's Oncology Group (COG) and Societé International d'Oncology Paediatrique / International Society of Paediatric Oncology (SIOP).

Stage	Definition	
I	COG:	*Limited to kidney and completely resected. Renal capsule is intact.*
	SIOP:	*Limited to kidney or surrounded with fibrous pseudocapsule if outside the normal contours of the kidney.* Presence of necrotic tumour or chemotherapy-induced changes in the renal sinus or soft tissue outside the kidney does not upstage the tumour in the post-therapy kidney.
	COG & SIOP:	Renal sinus soft tissue may be minimally infiltrated, without any involvement of the sinus vessels. The tumour may protrude into the pelvic system without infiltrating the wall of the ureter. Intrarenal vessels may be involved. Fine needle aspiration does not upstage the tumour.
II	COG & SIOP:	*Tumour infiltrates beyond kidney, but is completely resected.* Tumour penetration of renal capsule or infiltration of vessels within the renal sinus (including the intrarenal extension of the sinus). Tumour infiltrates adjacent organs or vena cava but is completely resected. Includes tumours with prior open or large core needle biopsies. May include tumours with local tumour spillage confined to flank.
III	COG & SIOP:	*Gross or microscopic residual tumour confined to abdomen.* Includes cases with any of the following: a) Involvement of specimen margins grossly or microscopically; b) Tumour in abdominal lymph nodes; c) Diffuse peritoneal contamination by direct tumour growth, tumour implants, or spillage into peritoneum before or during surgery; d) Residual tumour in abdomen e) Tumour removed non-contiguously (piecemeal resection) f) Tumour was surgically biopsied prior to preoperative chemotherapy.
	SIOP:	The presence of necrotic tumour or chemotherapy-induced changes in a lymph node or at the resection margins should be regarded as stage III.
IV	COG & SIOP:	Hematogenous metastases or lymph node metastasis outside the abdominopelvic region.
V	COG & SIOP:	Bilateral renal involvement at diagnosis. The tumours in each kidney should be separately sub-staged in these cases.

Staging

The most widely accepted staging systems for nephroblastomas rely on the identification of penetration of the renal capsule, involvement of renal sinus vessels, positive surgical margins, and positive regional lymph nodes; there are minor differences between the staging systems utilized by the SIOP and COG. While bilateral nephroblastomas are designated as stage V, their prognosis is determined by the stage of the most advanced tumour and by the presence or absence of anaplasia.

Histopathology

Nephroblastomas contain undifferentiated blastemal cells and cells differentiating to various degrees and in different proportions toward epithelial and stromal lineages. Triphasic patterns are the most characteristic, but biphasic and monophasic lesions are often observed. While most of these components represent stages in normal or abnormal nephrogenesis, non renal elements, such as skeletal muscle and cartilage occur {193}.
The *blastemal* cells are small, closely packed, and mitotically active rounded or oval cells with scant cytoplasm, and overlapping nuclei containing evenly distributed, slightly coarse chromatin, and small nucleoli. Blastemal cells occur in several distinctive patterns. The *diffuse blastemal pattern* is characterized by a lack of cellular cohesiveness and an aggressive pattern of invasion into adjacent connective tissues and vessels, in contrast to the typical circumscribed, encapsulated, and "pushing" border characteristic of most nephroblastomas. Other blastemal patterns tend to be cohesive. The *nodular* and *serpentine blastemal patterns* are characterized by round or undulating, sharply defined cords or nests of blastemal cells set in a

Table 1.08
Histologic criteria for focal anaplasia.

- Anaplasia must be circumscribed and its perimeter completely examined
  (May require mapping of anaplastic foci that extend to the edge of tissue sections)

- Anaplasia must be confined to the renal parenchyma

- Anaplasia must not be present within vascular spaces

- Absence of severe nuclear pleomorphism and hyperchromasia (severe "nuclear unrest") in non-anaplastic tumour.

loose fibromyxoid stroma.

An *epithelial* component of differentiation is present in most nephroblastomas. This pattern may be manifested by primitive rosette-like structures that are barely recognizable as early tubular forms; other nephroblastomas are composed of easily recognizable tubular or papillary elements that recapitulate various stages of normal nephrogenesis. Heterologous epithelial differentiation may occur, the most common elements being mucinous and squamous epithelium.

A variety of *stromal patterns* may occur and may cause diagnostic difficulty when blastemal and epithelial differentiation, are absent. Smooth muscle, skeletal muscle and fibroblastic differentiation may be present. Skeletal muscle is the most common heterologous stromal cell type and large fields of the tumour often contain this pattern. Other types of heterologous stromal differentiation include adipose tissue, cartilage, bone, ganglion cells, and neuroglial tissue.

Post-chemotherapy changes
Chemotherapy induces necrosis, xanthomatous histiocytic foci, haemosiderin deposits and fibrosis. Other chemotherapy-induced changes include maturation of blastema, epithelial, and stromal components, with striated muscle being the most frequent. Remarkable responsiveness to chemotherapy has resulted in complete necrosis in some tumours; such cases are considered to be low risk and may receive minimal treatment after surgery {259}. In contrast, those tumours that do not show response to therapy have a reduced prognosis and increased requirement for therapy.

Anaplasia
Approximately 5% of nephroblastomas are associated with an adverse outcome and are recognized pathologically because of their "unfavourable" histology due to the presence of *nuclear anaplasia* {194,318,2952}. Anaplasia is rare during the first 2 years of life, and

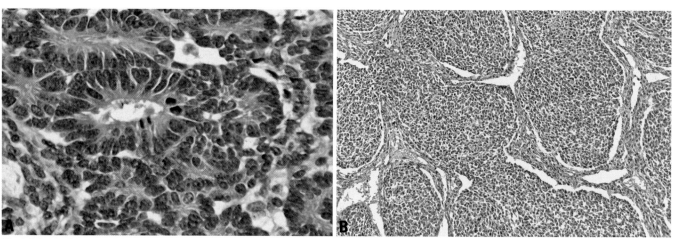

Fig. 1.69 Nephroblastoma. **A** Primitive epithelial differentiation. **B** Serpentine blastemal pattern.

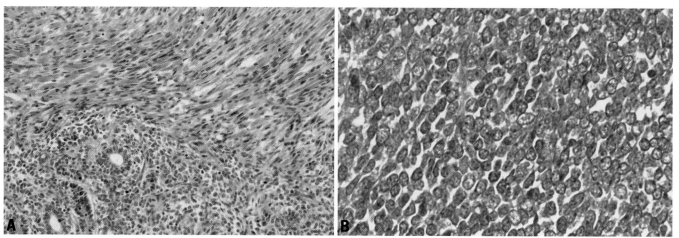

Fig. 1.70 Nephroblastoma. **A** Skeletal muscle differentiation. **B** Cytologic appearance of blastemal cells.

increases in prevalence to approximately 13 percent by 5 years of age {934}. Histologic diagnosis of anaplasia requires all of the following:

Presence of multipolar polyploid mitotic figures. In order to qualify for anaplasia each component of the abnormal metaphase, must be as large, or larger, than a normal metaphase.

Marked nuclear enlargement and hyperchromasia. The major dimensions of affected nuclei meeting the criteria are at least three times that of non-anaplastic nuclei in other areas of the specimen {2952}. Nuclear enlargement should involve all diameters of the nucleus and should not be confused with simple elongation. The enlarged nucleus must also be hyperchromatic.

Anaplasia has been demonstrated to correlate with responsiveness to therapy rather than to aggressiveness. Non-responsiveness of anaplasia to chemotherapy explains why it is not obliterated by preoperative treatment and therefore may be detected at a somewhat increase in frequency in post-therapy nephrectomy specimens {2759,2952}. Accordingly, anaplasia is most consistently associated with poor prognosis when it is diffusely distributed and when at advanced stages {742}. For these reasons, pathologic and therapeutic distinction, have been made between *focal anaplasia* and *diffuse anaplasia* {742}. Focal anaplasia is defined as the presence of one or a few sharply localized regions of anaplasia within a primary tumour, confined to

the kidney, with the majority of the tumour containing no nuclear atypia. The diagnosis of focal anaplasia has restrictive criteria. A tumour with anaplasia not meeting these requirements becomes classified as diffuse anaplasia.

Immunoprofile
The blastemal cells regularly express vimentin, and may also show focal expression of neuron specific enolase, desmin, and cytokeratin {690,786}. Expression of WT-1 is not present in all nephroblastomas, and may be present in various other tumours. In nephroblastomas, it is confined to the nucleus and correlates with tumour histology: areas of stromal differentiation and terminal epithelial differentiation show very low levels or no expression of WT-1, whereas areas of blastemal and early epithelial differentiation show high levels of WT-1 {415,965}.

Somatic genetics
Approximately 10% of nephroblastomas develop in association with one of several well-characterized dysmorphic syndromes {493,936}. The WAGR syndrome (Wilms tumour, aniridia, genitourinary malformation, mental retardation) carries a 30% risk of developing nephroblastoma. These patients have a consistent deletion of chromosome 11p13 in their somatic cells involving the *WT1* gene {362,860}. *WT1* encodes a zinc finger transcription factor that plays a major role in renal and gonadal development {981}. Abnormalities involving *WT1* are consistently found in the tumours of WAGR patients as well as in patients with

Table 1.09
Conditions associated with nephroblastoma.

Syndromes associated with highest risk of nephroblastoma
Wilms-Aniridia-Genital anomaly-Retardation (WAGR) syndrome
Beckwith-Wiedemann syndrome
Hemihypertrophy
Denys-Drash syndrome
Familial nephroblastoma

Conditions also associated with nephroblastoma
Frasier syndrome
Simpson-Golabi Behmel syndrome
Renal or genital malformations
Cutaneous nevi, angiomas
Trisomy 18
Klippel-Trenaunay syndrome
Neurofibromatosis
Bloom syndrome
Perlman syndrome
Sotos syndrome
Cerebral gigantism

Denys-Drash syndrome (a syndrome characterized by mesangial sclerosis, pseudohermaphroditism, and a 90% risk of nephroblastoma). Patients with WAGR have deletions of *WT1*, whereas patients with Denys-Drash syndrome have constitutional inactivating point mutations in one copy of *WT1* and their nephroblastomas show loss of the remaining normal

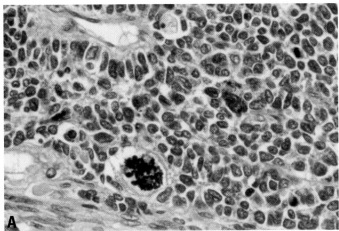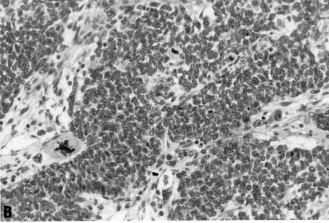

Fig. 1.71 Anaplastic nephroblastoma. **A** Blastemal tumour with multipolar mitotic figures and nuclear enlargement with hyperchromasia. **B** Anaplasia within the stromal component.

Table 1.10
Frequency of paediatric renal malignancies.

Neoplasm	Estimated relative frequency (%)
Nephroblastoma (nonanaplastic)	80
Nephroblastoma (anaplastic)	5
Mesoblastic nephroma	5
Clear cell sarcoma	4
Rhabdoid tumour	2

Miscellaneous
  Neuroblastoma
  Peripheral neuroectodermal tumour
  Synovial sarcoma
  Renal carcinoma
  Angiomyolipoma
  Lymphoma
  Other rare neoplasms
	4

WT1 allele {2043}. While WT1 alterations are strongly linked to the development of nephroblastoma in syndromic cases, their role in sporadic nephroblastoma is limited, with only one third of all nephroblastomas showing deletion at this locus and only 10% harbouring WT1 mutations. Beckwith-Wiedemann syndrome (characterized by hemihypertrophy, macroglossia, omphalocele, and visceromegaly) has been localized to chromosome 11p15, and designated WT2 although a specific gene has not been identified {747,1493,2077}. Attempts to determine the precise genetic event at this locus has revealed the presence of a cluster of imprinted genes; whether or not a single gene is responsible for the increased risk for nephroblastoma remains unclear {577}. The preferential loss of the maternal allele at this locus in cases of sporadic nephroblastoma suggests that genomic imprinting is involved in the pathogenesis of some tumours {2000}. Additional genetic loci are associated with familial nephroblastoma in patients with normal WT1 and WT2 {967, 1140,1141,1142,2134}. Approximately 1 percent of patients with nephroblastoma have a positive family history for the same neoplasm. Most pedigrees suggest autosomal dominant transmission with variable penetrance and expressivity.

Prognosis and predictive factors
Most nephroblastomas are of low stage, have a favourable histology, and are associated with an excellent prognosis. A favourable outcome can be expected even among most neoplasms with small foci of anaplasia. The most significant unfavourable factors are high stage, and the presence of anaplasia. The majority of blastemal tumours are exquisitely sensitive to therapy. However, tumours that demonstrate extensive blastemal cells following therapy are associated with poor response to therapy and reduced survival {197, 259}. In SIOP protocols, these blastemal chemoresistant tumours are classified as "high risk" and are treated like anaplastic tumours.

Nephrogenic rests and nephroblastomatosis

E.J. Perlman
L. Boccon-Gibod

Definition

Nephrogenic rests are abnormally persistent foci of embryonal cells that are capable of developing into nephroblastomas.

Nephroblastomatosis is defined as the presence of diffuse or multifocal nephrogenic rests.

Nephrogenic rests are classified into perilobar (PLNR) and intralobar (ILNR) types.

Epidemiology

Nephrogenic rests are encountered in 25% to 40% of patients with nephroblastoma, and in 1% of infant autopsies {190,192, 195,210,303}.

Histopathology

PLNRs and ILNRs have a number of distinguishing structural features.

Perilobar nephrogenic rests
PLNRs are sharply circumscribed and located at the periphery of the renal lobe. A PLNR may be *dormant* or may

Table 1.11
Features distinguishing perilobar from intralobar rests.

	Perilobar rests	Intralobar rests
Position in lobe	Peripheral	Random
Margins	Sharp, demarcated	Irregular, intermingling
Composition	Blastema, tubules Stroma scant or sclerotic	Stroma, blastema, tubules Stroma often predominates
Distribution	Usually multifocal	Often unifocal

have several other fates: most commonly the rest will regress with peritubular scarring resulting in an *obsolescent rest*. PLNR may also undergo active proliferative overgrowth, resulting in *hyperplastic nephrogenic rests*, which can be almost impossible to distinguish from nephroblastoma. Rarely, PLNRs form a band around the surface of the kidney resulting in massive renal enlargement, (*diffuse hyperplastic perilobar nephroblastomatosis*). Nephroblastoma developing within a PLNR is recognized by its propensity for spherical expansile growth and a peritumoural fibrous pseudocapsule separating

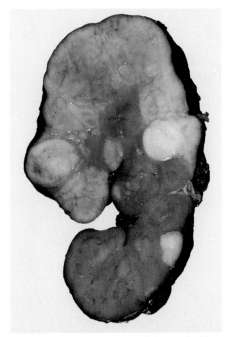

Fig. 1.72 Diffuse hyperplastic perilobar nephroblastomatosis (upper pole) with two spherical nephroblastomas and an separate perilobar nephrogenic rest in lower pole.

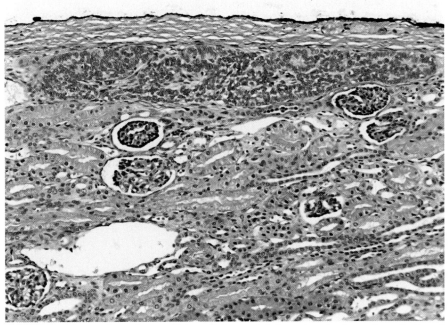

Fig. 1.73 Perilobar nephrogenic rest. Note well demarcated, lens shaped subcapsular collection of blastemal and tubular cells.

the neoplasm from the adjacent rest and normal kidney.

Intralobar nephrogenic rests
In contrast to PLNRs, ILNRs are typically located in the central areas of the lobe, are poorly circumscribed and composed of stromal elements as well as epithelial tubules. Like PLNRs, ILNRs may be dormant, regress, or undergo hyperplasia. Nephroblastoma developing with ILNRs are often separated from the underlying rest by a peritumoural fibrous pseudocapsule.

Prognosis and predictive factors
In diffuse hyperplastic nephroblastomatosis, the risk for the development of nephroblastoma is extraordinarily high. Chemotherapy is commonly utilized because it reduces the compressive burden of nephroblastic tissue, which enables normalization of renal function, and reduces the number of proliferating cells that may develop a clonal transformation. There is a high risk of developing multiple nephroblastomas as well as anaplastic nephroblastomas. Therefore, their tumours must be carefully watched and monitored for responsiveness to therapy.

In the management of patients with nephroblastomatosis, imaging screening by serial ultrasonography and CT scans enables an early detection of nephroblastoma {191}. Prompt therapy can minimize the amount of native kidney that requires surgical excision (nephron sparing approach), thereby maximizing the preservation of renal function.

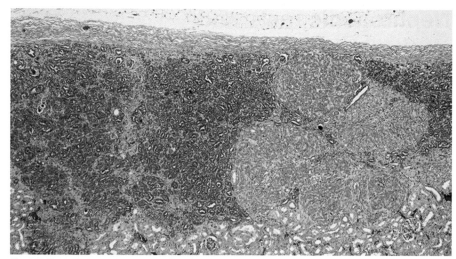

Fig. 1.74 Hyperplasia within a large perilobar nephrogenic rest.

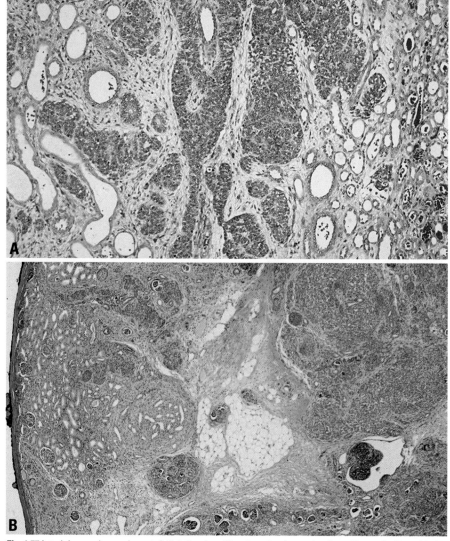

Fig. 1.75 Intralobar nephrogenic rest. **A** Ill defined proliferation of embryonal cells and intermingling with the native kidney. **B** Hyperplastic blastemal cells proliferating within the rest intermingling with the native kidney.

Cystic partially differentiated nephroblastoma

J.N. Eble

Definition

Cystic partially differentiated nephroblastoma is a multilocular cystic neoplasm of very young children, composed of epithelial and stromal elements, along with nephoblastomatous tissue.

ICD-O code   8959/1

Rarely, Wilms tumour may be composed entirely of cysts with delicate septa. Within the septa are small foci of blastema, immature-appearing stromal cells, and primitive or immature epithelium. Such tumours are called "cystic partially differentiated nephroblastoma" {329,1249}. When no nephroblastomatous elements are found, the term "cystic nephroma" has been applied although it is recognized that these lesions are not the same as the morphologically similar ones which occur in adults {646,650}.

Cystic partially differentiated nephroblastoma occurs with greater frequency in boys than in girls; almost all patients are less than 24 months old, and surgery is almost always curative {592, 1250,1251}. Joshi and Beckwith reported one recurrence, possibly a complication of incomplete resection {1250}.

The tumours often are large, particularly considering the patient's age, ranging up to 180 mm in diameter. Cystic partially differentiated nephroblastoma is well circumscribed from the remaining kidney by a fibrous pseudocapsule and consists entirely of cysts of variable size. The septa are thin and there are no expansile nodules to alter the rounded contour of the cysts.

The cysts in cystic partially differentiated nephroblastoma and are lined with flattened, cuboidal, or hobnail epithelium, or lack lining epithelium {1249}. The septa are variably cellular and contain undifferentiated and differentiated mesenchyme, blastema, and nephroblastomatous epithelial elements {1249}. Skeletal muscle and myxoid mesenchyme are present in the septa of most tumours. Cartilage and fat are present occasionally {1250,1251}. Focally, the septal elements may pro-

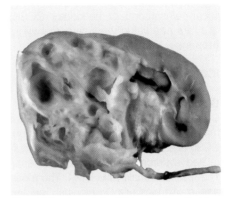

Fig. 1.76 Cystic partially differentiated nephroblastoma forms a well-circumscribed mass composed entirely of small and large cysts.

trude into the cysts in microscopic papillary folds, or gross polyps in the papillonodular variant of cystic partially differentiated nephroblastoma. The epithelial components consist mainly of mature and immature microscopic cysts resembling cross sections of tubules and stubby papillae resembling immature glomeruli.

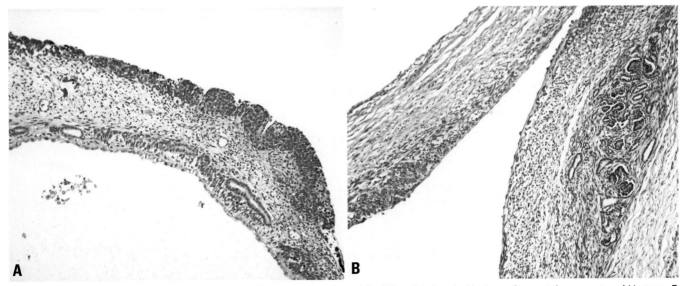

Fig. 1.77 Cystic partially differentiated nephroblastoma. **A** The septa of cystic partially differentiated nephroblastoma often contain aggregates of blastema. **B** Pericystic part of the tumour contains immature epithelial elements forming short papillae reminiscent of fetal glomeruli.

Clear cell sarcoma

P. Argani

Definition
Clear cell sarcoma of the kidney (CCSK) is a rare paediatric renal sarcoma with a propensity to metastasize to bone.

ICD-O code 9044/3

Clinical features
CCSK comprises approximately 3% of malignant paediatric renal tumours {114}. CCSK is not associated with Wilms tumour-related syndromes or nephrogenic rests. The male to female ratio is 2:1. The mean age at diagnosis is 36 months. The frequency of osseous metastases led to the proposed name "bone metastasizing renal tumour of childhood" {1630}.

Macroscopy
CCSKs are typically large (mean diameter 11 cm) and centred in the renal medulla, and always unicentric. CCSK are unencapsulated but circumscribed, tan, soft, and mucoid, and almost always focally cystic.

Histopathology
The classic pattern of CCSK features nests or cords of cells separated by regularly spaced, arborizing fibrovascular septa {114,196,1311,1628,1629,1630, 1783}. The cord cells may be epithelioid or spindled, and are loosely separated by extracellular myxoid material that mimics clear cytoplasm. Nuclei are round to oval shaped, have fine chromatin, and lack prominent nucleoli. The septa may be thin, regularly branching "chicken-wire" capillaries, or thickened sheaths of fibroblastic cells surrounding a central capillary. While CCSKs are grossly circumscribed, they characteristically have subtly infiltrative borders, entrapping isolated native nephrons. CCSK has varied histopathologic pat-

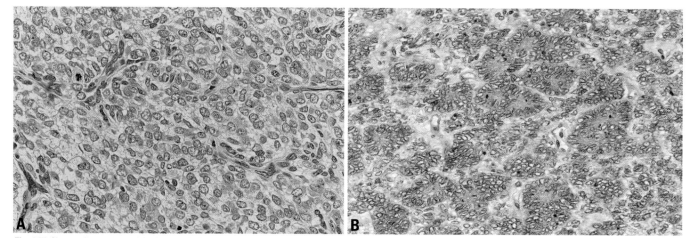

Fig. 1.78 Clear cell sarcoma of the kidney. **A** Classic pattern. **B** Acinar pattern mimicking nephroblastoma.

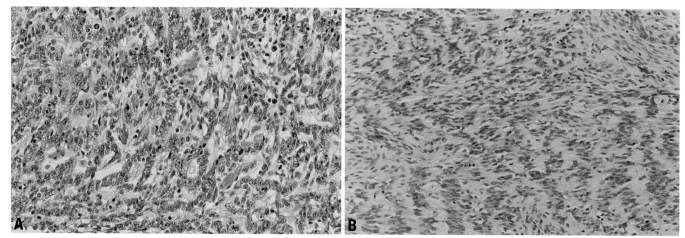

Fig. 1.79 Clear cell sarcoma of the kidney. **A** Trabecular pattern. **B** Palisading pattern mimicking schwannoma.

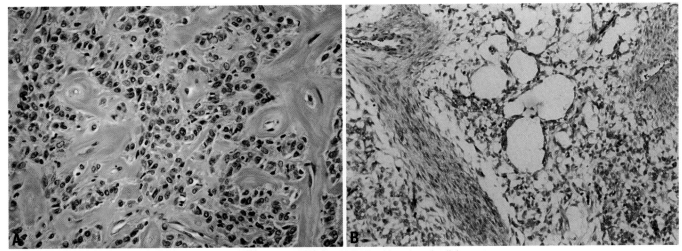

Fig. 1.80 Clear cell sarcoma of the kidney. **A** Sclerosing pattern mimicking osteoid. **B** Myxoid pools and cellular septa.

terns. Pools of acellular hyaluronic acid lead to the myxoid pattern {781}, while hyaline collagen simulating osteoid characterizes the sclerosing pattern. A cellular pattern mimics other paediatric small round blue cell tumours, whereas epithelioid (trabecular or pseudoacinar) patterns may mimic Wilms tumour. Prominent palisaded, spindled and storiform patterns mimic other sarcomas. Approximately 3% of CCSKs are anaplastic. Post-therapy recurrences may adopt deceptively-bland appearances simulating fibromatosis or myxoma {114,781}.

Immunoprofile / Ultrastructure
While vimentin and BCL2 are typically reactive, CCSK is uniformly negative with CD34, S100 protein, desmin, MIC2 (CD99), cytokeratin, and epithelial membrane antigen {114}.
The cord cells of CCSK have a high nucleus/cytoplasm ratio, with thin cytoplasmic extensions surrounding abundant extracellular matrix. The cytoplasm has scattered intermediate filaments {980}.

Prognosis and predictive factors
The survival of patients with CCSK has increased from only 20% up to 70% due in large part to the addition of adriamycin (doxorubicin) to chemotherapeutic protocols {114,935}. Nonetheless, metastases may occur as late as 10 years after initial diagnosis. While involvement of perirenal lymph nodes is common at diagnosis (29% of cases), bone metastases are the most common mode of recurrence {1628,1629}. CCSK is also distinguished from Wilms tumour by its proclivity to metastasize to unusual sites such as (in addition to bone) brain, soft tissue, and the orbit.

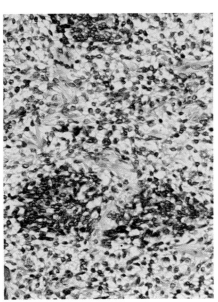

Fig. 1.81 Clear cell sarcoma of the kidney. Cellular pattern mimicking Wilms tumour.

Rhabdoid tumour

P. Argani

Definition
Rhabdoid tumour of the kidney (RTK) is a highly invasive and highly lethal neoplasm of young children composed of cells with vesicular chromatin, prominent nucleoli, and hyaline intracytoplasmic inclusions.

ICD-O code   8963/3

Epidemiology
Rhabdoid tumour comprises approximately 2% of all paediatric renal tumours. The mean age at diagnosis is approximately 1 year, and approximately 80% of patients are diagnosed in the first 2 years of life. The diagnosis is highly suspect over the age of 3, and virtually nonexistent over the age of 5. Most previously reported RTKs over the age of 5 have subsequently proven to be renal medullary carcinomas {2795}.

Clinical features
The most common presentation is that of haematuria. A significant number of patients present with disseminated disease. Approximately 15% of patients will develop a tumour of the posterior fossa of the brain that resembles PNET morphologically.

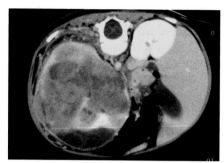

Fig. 1.82 Rhabdoid tumour. CT showing large focally cystic tumour (left).

Fig. 1.83 Rhabdoid tumour showing extensive tumour necrosis and haemorrhage.

Macroscopy
Tumours are typically large, haemorrhagic and necrotic, with ill defined borders that reflect its highly invasive nature.

Histopathology
These tumours are unencapsulated, and feature sheets of tumour cells that aggressively overrun native nephrons. Vascular invasion is usually extensive. Tumour cells characteristically display the cytologic triad of vesicular chromatin, prominent cherry-red nucleoli, and hyaline pink cytoplasmic inclusions. A subset of tumours may be composed predominantly of primitive undifferentiated small round cells, but on closer inspec-

tion small foci of cells with diagnostic cytologic features can be identified.

Immunoprofile
Nonspecific trapping of antibodies by the whorled cytoplasmic inclusions can give a wide range of false positive results. The most consistent and characteristic finding is that of strong vimentin labeling and focal but intense labeling for EMA.

Ultrastructure
The cytoplasmic inclusions correspond to whorls of intermediate filaments having a diameter of 8 to 10 nm.

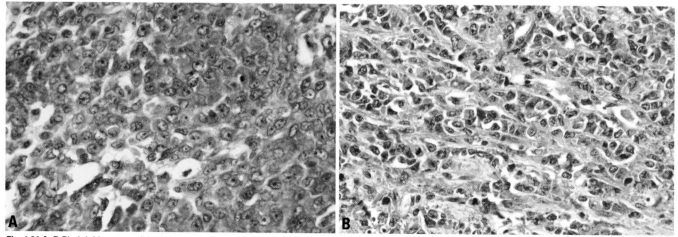

Fig. 1.84 A, B Rhabdoid tumour of the kidney. The nucleus is vesiculated. The cytoplasm contains eosinophilic inclusions.

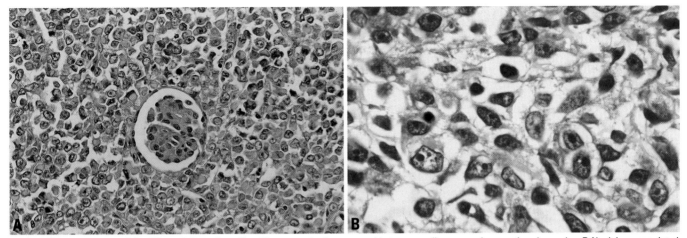

Fig. 1.85 Rhabdoid tumour of the kidney. **A** Note sheet-like diffuse growth of monomorphic tumour cells overrunning a native glomerulus. **B** Nuclei are angulated with prominent nucleoli.

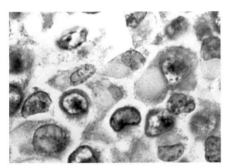

Fig. 1.86 Rhabdoid tumour of the kidney. Note characteristic vesicular chromatin, prominent nucleolus and hyalin intracytoplasmic inclusion.

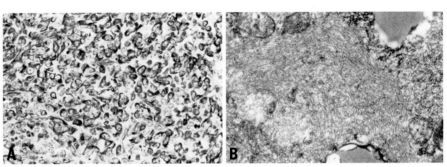

Fig. 1.87 Rhabdoid tumour of the kidney. **A** Strong cytoplasmic vimentin immunoexpression. **B** Transmission electron micrograph showing intracytoplasmic intermediate filiments.

Somatic genetics

Biallelic inactivation of the *hSNF5/INI1* tumour suppressor gene, which resides on the long arm of chromosome 22, is the molecular hallmark of RTK {242,2729}. Inactivation of this gene is also seen in morphologically similar rhabdoid tumours which occur in the soft tissue, brain, and occasionally other visceral sites. All of these tumours typically affect young children, and are usually lethal. The *hSNF5/INI1* gene encodes a protein involved in chromatin remodeling that is thought to regulate the accessibility of transcription factors to DNA, and its inactivation is thought to promote neoplasia by altering gene expression secondary to its effect upon chromatin structure. Inactivation occurs via mutation, deletion or whole chromosome loss, accounting for the frequent cytogenetic finding of monosomy 22 in these neoplasms. Children with concurrent RTK and PNET-like tumours of the posterior fossa of the CNS frequently harbour germline mutations in the *hSNF5/INI1* gene {241}. Inactivation of the second allele has been shown to occur by different mechanisms in these patients' two cancers, confirming the clinicopathologic impression that these are independent neoplasm {790,2311}. A familial "rhabdoid predisposition syndrome" encompassing renal and extrarenal rhabdoid tumours has been described in which affected family members harbour constitutional inactivation of *hSNF5/INI1* {2368,2588}.

Prognosis and predictive factors

Outcome is typically dismal, as over 80% of patients will die of tumour within 2 years of diagnosis. The rare patients who present with tumour confined to the kidney may have a slightly better prognosis.

Congenital mesoblastic nephroma

P. Argani
P.H.B. Sorensen

Definition
Congenital mesoblastic nephroma (CMN) is a low-grade fibroblastic sarcoma of the infantile kidney and renal sinus.

ICD-O code   8960/1

Clinical features
CMN comprises two percent of paediatric renal tumours {193,1845}. CMN is the most common congenital renal neoplasm, and ninety percent of cases occur in the first year of life. The typical presentation is that of an abdominal mass.

Macroscopy
Classic CMN has a firm, whorled texture, while cellular CMN are more typically soft, cystic and haemorrhagic.

Histopathology
Classic CMN (24% of cases) is morphologically identical to infantile fibromatosis of the renal sinus {265}. Tumours are composed of interlacing fascicles of fibroblastic cells with thin tapered nuclei, pink cytoplasm, low mitotic activity, and an abundant collagen deposition. The tumour dissects and entraps islands of renal parenchyma. Cellular CMN (66% of cases) is morphologically identical to infantile fibrosarcoma. These tumours have a pushing border, and are composed of poorly formed fascicles, which give way to sheet-like growth patterns. The tumour shows a high mitotic rate, and frequently features necrosis. Mixed CMN (10% of cases) has features of both classic and cellular CMN within the same tumour.

Immunoprofile
These tumours are immunoreactive for vimentin and often actin with desmin reactivity being rare and CD34 being absent. Ultrastructurally, tumours have features of myofibroblasts or fibroblasts.

Somatic genetics
While classic CMNs are typically diploid, cellular CMNs frequently feature aneuploidy of chromosomes 11, 8, and 17 {1377,2063,2338}. Cellular CMN but not classic CMN demonstrates a specific chromosome translocation, t(12;15)(p13;q25), which results in a fusion of the *ETV6* and *NTRK3* genes {1336,2255}. Interestingly, the same chromosome translocation and gene fusion present in cellular CMN was first identified in infantile fibrosarcoma, and is not present in infantile fibromatosis {1337}. Hence, the analogy between cellular CMN and infantile fibrosarcoma, and between classic CMN and infantile fibromatosis, appears appropriate.

The oncogenic mechanism of the *ETV6-NTRK3* gene fusion remains to be determined. *ETV6* is an ETS transcription factor previously implicated in translocations in paediatric B-cell acute lymphoblastic leukaemia. *NTRK3* is a tyrosine kinase receptor that responds to extracellular signals. ETV6-NTRK3 fusion transcripts encode a chimeric protein in which the sterile-alpha-motif (SAM) protein dimerization domain of the ETV6

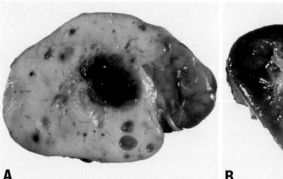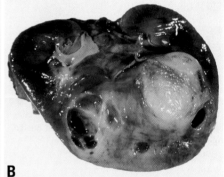

A   **B**

Fig. 1.88 A, B Congenital mesoblastic nephroma, cellular type.

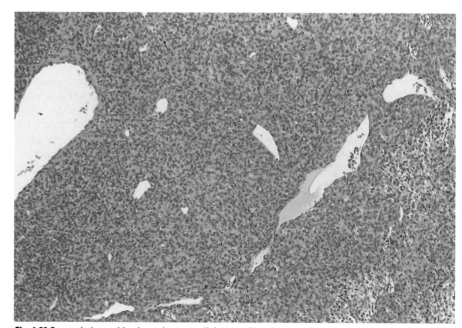

Fig. 1.89 Congenital mesoblastic nephroma, cellular type. Note haemangiopericytomatous vascular pattern, high cellularity and ill-defined fascicles.

transcription factor is fused to the protein tyrosine kinase (PTK) of NTRK3. ETV6-NTRK3 (EN) has potent transforming activity in murine fibroblasts, which is mediated by ligand-independent homod-imerization through the SAM domain and activation of the PTK domain. This in turn constitutively activates two major effector pathways of wild-type NTRK3, namely the Ras-MAP kinase (MAPK) mitogenic pathway and the phosphatidyl inositol-3-kinase (PI3K)-AKT pathway mediating cell survival, and both are required for EN transformation {1516,2621,2764}. Virtually all congenital fibrosarcoma and cellular CMN cases expressing *ETV6-NTRK3* also have trisomy 11 {1336,1337}. One intriguing possibility is that trisomy 11 provides cells with an additional copy of the 11p15.5 gene (*IGF2*) encoding the insulin-like growth factor (IGF)-2 anti-apoptotic factor {178}. IGF2 binds to the insulin-like growth factor 1 receptor, which was recently shown to be essential for EN transformation {1788}.

Prognosis and predictive factors

When completely excised, CMN is associated with an excellent prognosis. Five percent of patients develop recurrence, which is related to the incompleteness of resection and not to whether the tumour was of cellular or classic type. Only rare cases of hematogenous metastases and tumour related deaths have been reported {1051,2758}.

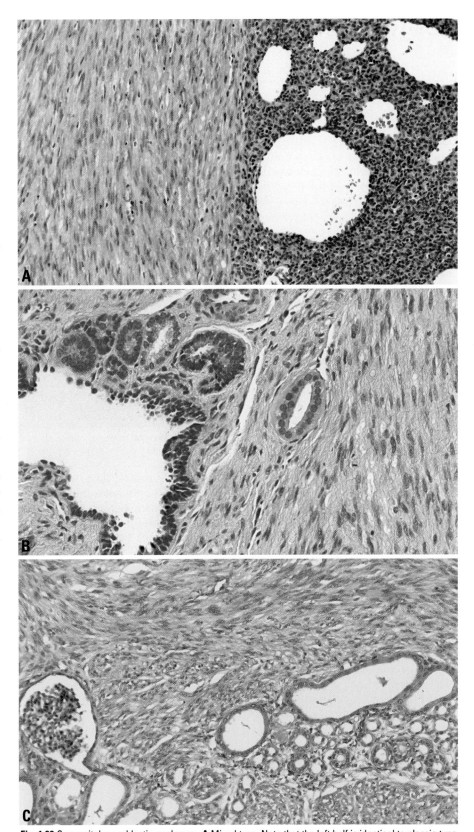

Fig. 1.90 Congenital mesoblastic nephroma. **A** Mixed type. Note that the left half is identical to classic type and the right half is identical to the cellular type. **B** Classic type. Note fascicles of fibroblastic cells adjacent to native renal tubules, which show embryonal hyperplasia. **C** Classic type. Note fascicles of fibroblastic cells resembling fibromatosis dissecting the native kidney.

Ossifying renal tumour of infancy

C.E. Keen

Definition

Ossifying renal tumour of infancy (ORTI) is an intracalyceal mass composed of osteoid trabeculae, osteoblast-like cells and a spindle cell component, arising from, and attached to the medullary pyramid.

ICD-O code   8967/0

ORTI is extremely rare, only 12 cases have been reported in the English literature {414,1184,2462,2715}. Males predominate (9/12). Age at presentation was 6 days to 17 months.

The exact nature of ORTI spindle cells is still uncertain. No cases have been reported in association with Wilms tumour or with WT1/WT2 gene syndromes on chromosome 11p.

All cases presented with gross haematuria except one which manifested as a palpable abdominal mass. Calcification of the tumour frequently suggests renal calculus.

ORTI is grossly well circumscribed and measures 1-6 cm in diameter.

Microscopically, there is a characteristic coarse trabecular osteoid meshwork

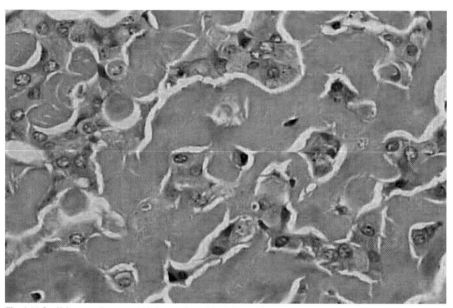

Fig. 1.91 Ossifying renal tumour of infancy. Osteoid meshwork interspersed with cuboidal cells.

with interspersed large cuboidal osteoblast-like cells that express EMA as well as vimentin, but not cytokeratin. Sheets of uniform spindle cells with ovoid nuclei may entrap renal tubules.

The outcome has been uniformly benign and conservative surgical management is recommended.

Haemangiopericytoma

A. Vieillefond
G. de Pinieux

ICD-O code   9150/1

Less than 30 primary renal haemangiopericytomas are reported in the literature `788,1715,1992}. Most of them arise in the renal sinus and the perirenal tissue. There are no specific radiological features. Paraneoplastic syndromes, like hypoglycemia or hypertension, may occur. These tumours are large, firm and histologically composed of a proliferation of fusiform pericytes separated by numerous capillaries presenting a staghorn configuration.

Immunohistochemically, the tumour cells are positive for CD34, negative for CD31, actin and CD99. Behaviour of haemangiopericytoma is difficult to predict. Late recurrence or metastases can never be excluded, especially when the tumour size is over 5 centimeters and mitotic rate over 4 per 10 HPF. Some haemangiopericytomas of the literature could be reevaluated as solitary fibrous tumours {1595}. These two entities share almost the same histological pattern and the same imprecise potential of malignancy.

Leiomyosarcoma

S.M. Bonsib

Definition
A leiomyosarcoma is a malignant neoplasm demonstrating smooth muscle differentiation.

ICD-O code
8890/3

Epidemiology
Although leiomyosarcoma is a rare primary renal neoplasm, it is the most common renal sarcoma accounting for 50-60% of cases {950,2742}. Most occur in adults, and men and women are equally affected.

Clinical features
Patients usually present with flank pain, haematuria and a mass. Leiomyosarcoma is aggressive with a 5-year survival rate of 29-36%; most patients die of disease within 1-year of diagnosis. It metastasizes to lung, liver, and bone. Irradiation and chemotherapy are ineffective, therefore, complete surgical extirpation is the only therapy. Small size (< 5 cm), low histological grade, and renal-limited disease are associated with the most favourable outcome.

Macroscopy
Leiomysarcoma may arise from the renal capsule, renal parenchyma, pelvic muscularis, or the main renal vein {273,274, 306,950,1816,1919,2742}. Tumours arising in the capsule or parenchyma cannot be distinguished from other renal cortical neoplasms by imaging studies. Pelvic leiomyosarcoma may be regarded as a transitional cell carcinoma until microscopic examination is performed.
Leiomyosarcomas are usually large solid grey-white, soft to firm, focally necrotic tumours. They may envelope the kidney if capsular in origin. If parenchymal in origin, they may replace large portions of the parenchyma, and extend through the renal capsule and into the renal sinus. Renal pelvic tumours fill the collecting system, and may invade the renal parenchyma or extend into the sinus or hilar perirenal fat.

Histopathology
Leiomyosarcomas are spindle cell lesions with a fascicular, plexiform, or haphazard growth pattern. Low grade lesions resemble smooth muscle cells,

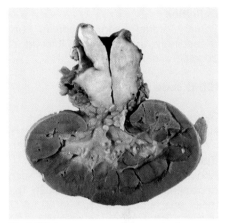

Fig. 1.92 Leiomyosarcoma of the renal vein.

but high grade lesions are pleomorphic and undifferentiated, requiring immunohistochemical stains to separate from other sarcomas, the more common sarcomatoid carcinomas, and from atypical forms of epithelioid angiomyolipoma {274}. Necrosis, nuclear pleomorphism, and more than a rare mitotic figure indicate malignancy.

Osteosarcoma

A. Vieillefond
G. de Pinieux

ICD-O code
9180/3

Primary osteosarcoma of the kidney is an exceedingly rare neoplasm with less than 20 cases reported in the literature {1716,2800,}. Pathogenesis of these tumours remains unclear and their relationship with carcinosarcoma may be suggested.
Compared to osteosarcoma of bone, it occurs in older patients, of over 40 years of age. The male/female ratio is roughly equal. Clinically, there are no specific symptoms. Nearly all the tumours exhibit a high stage (T3 or T4) at time of diagnosis. Early local recurrence and/or metastatic spread (especially pulmonary) are frequently observed. Histologically, primary renal osteosarcoma shows a pleomorphic pattern and consists of spindle and multinucleated giant tumour cells producing neoplastic osteoid and bone.
The prognosis of primary renal osteosarcoma is very poor despite aggressive therapeutic approach combinating radical surgery, radiotherapy and polychemotherapy.

Renal angiosarcoma

H. Arnholdt

Definition
Primary renal angiosarcomas are exceedingly rare aggressive tumours of endothelial cells.

ICD-O code   9120/3

Synonym
Haemangiosarcoma.

Epidemiology
About 23 cases of this tumour have been documented {396,1096,1447,1502}. The mean age is 58 years (range 30 to 77 years). The etiology is unknown. An androgen factor has been discussed because of a strong male predominance (ratio 19:4) and experimental data {420}.

Localization and clinical features
Primary renal angiosarcomas occur near the renal capsule. Clinical symptoms are flank pain, haematuria, palpable tumour and weight loss.

Macroscopy
Grossly, the tumours consist of ill-defined, haemorrhagic spongy masses.

Histopathology
Microscopically, they show the same changes that characterize other angiosarcomas. The tumour cells are spindle-shaped, rounded or irregular in outline with hyperchromatic and elongated or irregular nuclei. Bizarre nuclei and multinucleated cells may be seen. Mitotic figures are frequently identified. Poorly differentiated areas are composed of large sheets of spindled or epithelioid cells that are diffult to distinguish from other sarcomas or carcinomas. Some areas may reveal well-differentiated neoplastic capillary-size vessels comparable to haemangiomas or less well-differentiated vessels with rudimentary lumen formation and pleomorphic tumour cells.

Immunoprofile
Immunohistochemical confirmation of the diagnosis of angiosarcoma can be accomplished using antibodies directed against factor VIII, CD31 and CD34. CD31 seems to be the more sensitive and more specific antigen for endothelial differentiation. Some angiosarcomas produce cytokeratin.

Prognosis and predictive factors
Prognosis of renal angiosarcoma is poor with rapid development of haematogenous metastasis. The mean survival of the 19 documented cases is 7.7 months.

Malignant fibrous histiocytoma

A. Vieillefond
G. de Pinieux

ICD-O code   8830/3

Less than 50 renal MFH are documented in the literature {1269,2581}. Most of them have pararenal and retroperitonal extension and are considered to arise from the renal capsule. They are large fleshy tumours with haemorrhage and necrosis. They can extend into the renal and caval veins.

Diagnosis of MFH relies on morphologic criteria {1845}: pleomorphic cells (spindle, round histiocyte-like and multinucleated giant tumour cells) arranged haphazardly in sheets or in short fascicles in a storiform pattern (storiform-pleomorphic type). Myxoid and inflammatory MFH variants may occur in the kidney. The two main differential diagnoses are leiomyosarcoma, the most frequent renal (or capsular) sarcoma and sarcomatoid carcinoma, which are much more frequent than MFH. Epithelioid/pleomorphic angiomyolipoma and secondary intrarenal extension of a perirenal dedifferentiated liposarcoma may also be considered. This differential diagnosis relies on immunohistochemistry and extensive sampling of the tumour to exclude a tiny carcinomatous component.

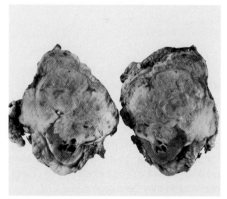

Fig. 1.93 Malignant fibrous histiocytoma.

Angiomyolipoma

G. Martignoni
M.B. Amin

Definition
Angiomyolipoma (AML) is a benign mesenchymal tumour composed of a variable proportion of adipose tissue, spindle and epithelioid smooth muscle cells, and abnormal thick-walled blood vessels.

ICD-O code   8860/0

Epidemiology
Age and sex distribution
In surgical series which are usually over-represented by non-tuberous sclerosis (TS) cases there is a 4:1 female predominance {1299,1825,2503,2628}, but there is no apparent sex predilection in TS patients with AML detected by imaging techniques {487}. The mean age at diagnosis in surgical series is between 45 and 55 for patients without TS and between 25 and 35 for those with TS {1299,1825,2503,2628}. It is possible that puberty influences the development of AML {487}.

Incidence
AMLs account for approximately 1% of surgically removed renal tumours. It has been considered an uncommon neoplasm, but its frequency is increasing because it is detected in ultrasonographic examinations performed to evaluate other conditions {816}. It can occur sporadically or in patients with TS, an inherited autosomal dominant syndrome {910}. Most surgical series report four times as many sporadic AMLs as AMLs associated with TS {1299, 1825,2503,2628}.

Etiology
AML is believed to belong to a family of lesions characterized by proliferation of perivascular epithelioid cells (PEC) {268, 269,785,917,1171,2707,2920}. Recent molecular studies have demonstrated its clonality {933,2008}, and immunohistochemical and ultrastructural studies support the idea of histogenesis from a single cell type {269,1103,2511,2570,2920}. The etiology and pathogenesis of the neoplasm are unknown. The different frequency of AML in females and males in the surgical series, the onset of AML after puberty and the frequent progesterone receptor immunoreactivity in AML {1077} suggest a hormonal influence.

Localization
AMLs may arise in the cortex or medulla of the kidney. Extrarenal growth in the retroperitoneal space with or without renal attachment can occur. Lesions may be multifocal {2570}. Multifocal AML in the kidney indicates a presumptive diagnosis of TS.

Clinical features
Signs and symptoms
Clinical features differ, depending on the presence or absence of TS. In TS, AMLs are usually asymptomatic and discovered by radiographic screening techniques. Patients without TS present with flank pain, haematuria, palpable mass, or a combination of these signs and symptoms. Retroperitoneal haemorrage may occur {2503}. Simultaneous occur-

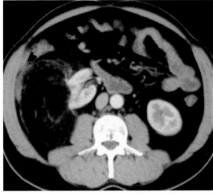

Fig. 1.94 Angiomyolipoma of the kidney. CT scan of angiomyolipoma characterized by high fat content.

rence of AML with renal cell carcinoma (RCC) and oncocytoma in the same kidney has also been reported {1224}. Another interesting aspect of AML is the association with lymphangioleiomyomatosis (LAM), a progressive disease which usually affects the lungs of young women and which is also related to TS. Histopathological and genetic studies have demonstrated that AML and LAM share numerous features {268,2909}.

Imaging
Computerized tomography (CT) and ultrasonography permit the preoperative diagnosis of AML in almost all cases. High fat content, which is present in most AMLs, is responsible for a distinctive pattern on a CT scan. Tumours composed predominantly of smooth muscle cells or with an admixture of all three compo-

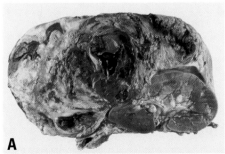

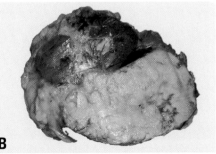

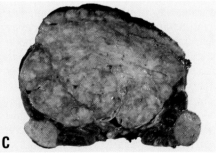

Fig. 1.95 A Angiomyolipoma. Large tumour with hemorrhagic component. **B** A large tumour with high lipid content, bulging into the perirenal fat is seen. Match with CT. **C** Multiple angiomyolipomas of the kidney.

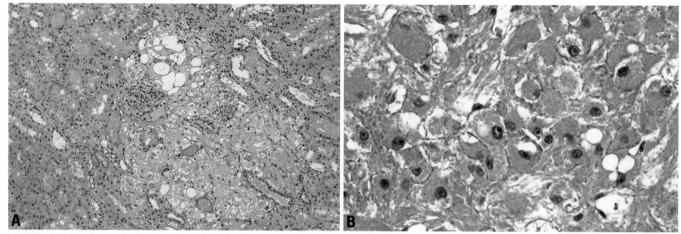

Fig. 1.96 Angiomyolipoma. **A** Microscopic angiomyolipoma composed of smooth muscle with a minority of fat cells, arising in the renal interstitium. **B** Rarely, angiomyolipoma may closely resemble renal oncocytoma.

nents or with prominent cystic change may be difficult to distinguish from an epithelial neoplasm preoperatively {2388}. In some of these cases the diagnosis is possible by fine-needle aspiration, supplemented if necessary by immunohistochemistry {275}.

Macroscopy

AMLs usually are well demarcated from the adjacent kidney, but not encapsulated. The colour varies from yellow to pink-tan, depending on the relative proportions of the various tissue components. Tumours composed of all three components may mimic a clear cell RCC whereas a smooth muscle predominant AML may mimic a leiomyoma. Although AMLs may grow to great size, they bulge into rather than infiltrate the perirenal fat. Most AMLs are solitary, but multiple tumours may be present; in such situations, a large dominant tumour associated with smaller lesions is typical.

Tumour spread and staging

Infrequently, AML extends into the intrarenal venous system, the renal vein or the vena cava. Vascular invasion and multifocality have occasionally been misinterpreted as evidence of malignancy and metastasis. Regional lymph node involvement can occur; it is considered to represent a multifocal growth pattern rather than metastasis {18,2570}.

Only three cases of sarcoma developing in sporadic AML have been reported; two patients had pulmonary metastases and one had hepatic metastases {466,757,1636}.

Histopathology

Most AMLs are composed of a variable mixture of mature fat, thick-walled poorly organized blood vessels and smooth muscle (classic triphasic histology). The border between AML and the kidney is typically sharp, although renal tubules may be entrapped at the periphery of some tumours. The smooth muscle cells appear to emanate from blood vessel walls in a radial fashion, and expansile growth thereafter may be fascicular. The smooth muscle cells are most frequently spindle cells but may appear as rounded epithelioid cells. Rarely, striking degrees of nuclear atypia (occasionally with mitotic activity and multinucleation) may be seen in these cells, raising the possibility of malignancy. Some AMLs that are often located subcapsularly and composed almost entirely of smooth muscle cells ("capsulomas") resemble leiomyomas. Cells associated with thin-walled, branching vessels with a pattern similar to lymphangioleiomyoma is another variation of the smooth muscle component.

The lipomatous component consists typically of mature adipose tissue but may contain vacuolated adipocytes suggesting lipoblasts, thus mimicking a liposarcoma when there is extensive adipocytic differentiation. The blood vessels are thick-walled and lack the normal elastic content of arteries. AMLs with a prominent vascular component may mimic a vascular malformation. Prominent cystic change may very rarely be present in AML.

Immunoprofile

AMLs are characterized by a coexpression of melanocytic markers (HMB45, HMB50, CD63, tyrosinase, Mart1/Melan A and microophthalmia transcription factor) and smooth muscle markers (smooth muscle actin, muscle-specific actin and calponin); CD68, neuron-specific enolase, S-100 protein, estrogen and progesterone receptors, and desmin may also be positive, whereas epithelial markers are always negative {125,762,1254, 1258,1419,2037,2922}. Coexpression of

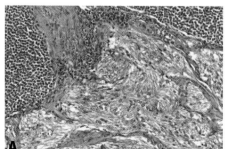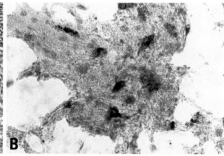

Fig. 1.97 Angiomyolipoma. **A** Deposit of angiomyolipoma in a para-aortic lymph node in the drainage basin of a kidney bearing an angiomyolipoma. **B** Cytologic specimen from renal angiomyolipoma. Scattered HMB45 positive cells within cytologic specimen.

melanocytic and smooth muscle markers in myoid-appearing and lipid-distended cells supports the unitary nature of AML being a neoplasm with ability for phenotypic and immunotypic modulation.

Ultrastructure
Ultrastructurally, AMLs show spindle cells with features of smooth muscle cells. Some spindle cells contain lipid droplets indicating transition forms between smooth muscle cells and adipocytes {1103}. Ultrastructural evidence of melanogenesis is reported, and intracytoplasmic membrane-bound dense bodies, crystals and granules (rhomboid and spherical) have been linked to renin and premelanosomes without conclusive or consistent evidence {1825,2796,2913}.

Precursor lesions
Small nodules with some features of AML are often present in the kidney bearing AMLs, suggesting that these lesions may be the source of AMLs. The smallest nodules are often composed predominantly of epithelioid smooth muscle cells, and the proportion of spindle cells and adipocytes increase as the lesions become larger {459}.
Intraglomerular lesions with features

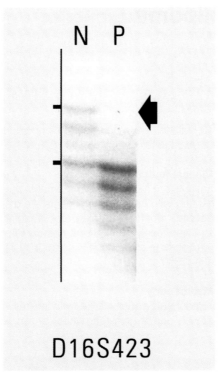

Fig. 1.98 Angiomyolipoma of the kidney. LOH of *TSC2* gene locus in both sporadic and tuberous sclerosis-associated tumours.

overlapping those of AML have been reported in patients with and without TS {1315,1632,1865}.

Somatic genetics
Two genes are known to cause TS. The *TSC1* gene is located on chromosome 9q34, consists of 23 exons and encodes hamartin, a 130 kDa protein {2704}. The *TSC2* gene is located on chromosome 16p13, consists of 41 exons and encodes tuberin, a 180 kDa GTPase-activating protein for RAP1 and RAB5 {2604}. Tuberin and hamartin interact with each other, forming a cytoplasmic complex {1878, 2088}. AML frequently shows loss of heterozygosity (LOH) of variable portions of *TSC2* gene locus in both sporadic and TS-associated tumours {370, 1078}. *TSC1* gene is involved occasionally in LOH.

Prognosis and predictive factors
The classic AMLs are benign. A very small minority are associated with complications and morbidity and mortality {1936}. Haemorrhage into the retroperitoneum, usually in tumours greater than 4.0 cm or in pregnant patients, may be life threatening. Renal cysts and multiple AMLs in TS patients can lead to renal failure {2321}.

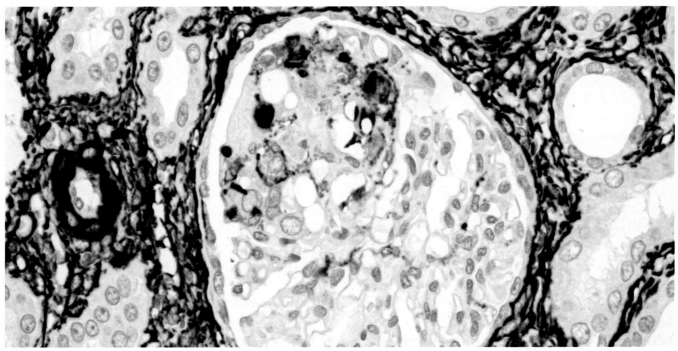

Fig. 1.99 Intraglomerular lesion associated with angiomyolipoma of the kidney. Focal positive immunoreactivity to actin in a glomerulus containing a group of smooth muscle epithelioid cells. SMA expression.

Epithelioid angiomyolipoma

M.B. Amin

Definition
Epithelioid angiomyolipoma (AML) is a potentially malignant mesenchymal neoplasm characterized by proliferation of predominantly epithelioid cells and is closely related to the triphasic (classic) AML.

Epidemiology
More than half of patients with epithelioid AML have a history of tuberous sclerosis (TS), which is a significantly higher association than classic AML has with TS {50,2036,1346}. Both sexes are equally affected similar to classic AML occurring in TS patients. The mean age of diagnosis is 38 years {649,50,463,466,593,1606,1634}.

Clinical features
Patients are frequently symptomatic, presenting with pain; some patients are discovered during TS follow-up. Imaging studies closely mimic renal cell carcinoma because of the paucity of adipose tissue {1289,463,224}.

Macroscopy
Tumours are usually large, with infiltrative growth and a grey-tan, white, brown or haemorrhagic appearance. Necrosis may be present. Extrarenal extension or involvement of the renal vein/vena cava may occur.

Histopathology
There is a proliferation of epithelioid cells with abundant granular cytoplasm arranged in sheets, often with perivascular cuffing of epithelioid cells. Many of the reported cases were initially misdiagnosed as a high grade carcinoma. Tumour cells are round to polygonal with enlarged vesicular nuclei often with prominent nucleoli.

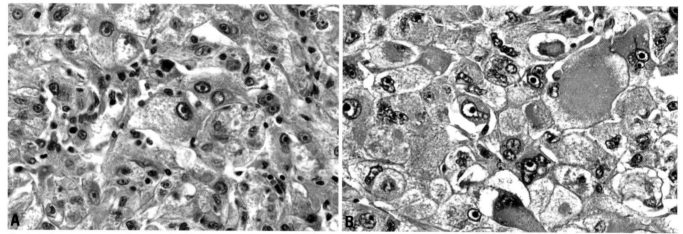

Fig. 1.100 Epithelioid angiomyolipoma. **A** Epithelioid angiomyolipoma is typically composed of a mixture of polygonal and spindle cells of variable size. Inflammatory cells often are mingled with the neoplastic cells. **B** Focally ganglion like and multinucleated cells are present.

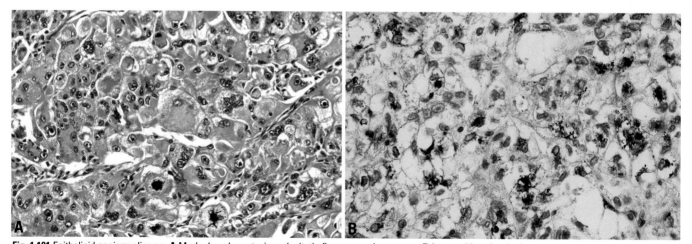

Fig. 1.101 Epithelioid angiomyolipoma. **A** Marked nuclear atypia and mitotic figures may be present. **B** Immunohistochemical reaction with HMB-45 shows numerous positive cells.

Multinucleated and enlarged ganglion-like cells may be present. A population of short spindle cells is present in many tumours. Tumours may display nuclear anaplasia, mitotic activity, vascular invasion, necrosis and infiltration of perinephric fat. Haemorrhage often is prominent. A few cases have focal classic AML areas {649,466}.

Variations in histology include variable admixture of clear cells, although occasionally they may predominate {2184,560}.

Immunoprofile
Epithelioid AML expresses melanocytic markers (HMB-45, HMB-50, Mart-1/Melan-A and microphthalmia transcription factor) with variable expression of smooth muscle markers (smooth muscle actin, muscle-specific actin) {125,1419, 2922,2511}.

Genetics
Allelic loss of chromosomal arm 16p (TS2 containing region) is noted in classic, epithelioid and sarcomatoid areas indicating clonality and relationship {2497}. *TP53* mutation is detected in epithelioid but not triphasic AML, suggesting a role in malignant transformation {1289}.

Prognostic and predictive factors
Approximately one-third of epithelioid AML have been reported to have metastasis to lymph nodes, liver, lungs or spine {1565,1636,757,2863}. Among adverse pathologic parameters, none correlate with outcome; however, tumours with necrosis, mitotic activity, nuclear anaplasia and extrarenal spread should raise significant concern for malignant outcome {463,466,2036,757,2863}.

Leiomyoma

S.M. Bonsib

Definition
Leiomyoma is a benign smooth muscle neoplasm.

ICD-O code   8890/0

Epidemiology and etiology
A leiomyoma may arise from the renal capsule (most common), muscularis of the renal pelvis, or from cortical vascular smooth muscle {273,624,1762,2502, 2585}. Most are encountered in adults as incidental small mm-sized capsular tumours at autopsy. They may on occasion be large (largest case reported 37 kg), resulting in surgery for a presumed carcinoma {273,624,2502}.

Macroscopy
Macroscopically, leiomyomas are firm well-demarcated solid lesions. Large examples have a trabeculated cut surface. Calcification and cystic change have been described, but necrosis should not be present.

Histopathology
Histologically, they are composed of spindled cells, usually arranged in intersecting fascicles with little nuclear pleomorphism and no mitotic activity. They have a smooth muscle immunophenotype, demonstrating a positive reaction on actin and desmin stains {273,508, 2585}. Some focally express HMB-45, suggesting a relationship to angiomyolipoma and other tumours of the perivascular epithelioid cell family of tumours {273}.

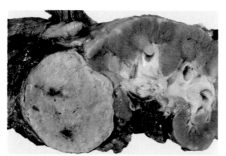

Fig. 1.102 Leiomyoma. A 5 cm leiomyoma with several mm-sized capsular leiomyomas.

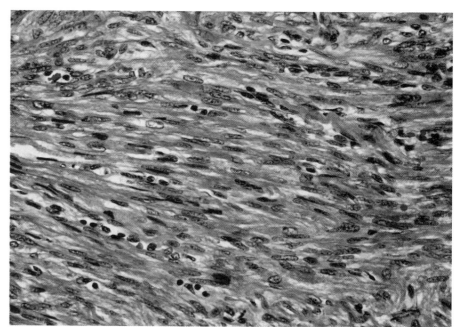

Fig. 1.103 A leiomyoma composed of uniform spindle cells arranged in fascicles without mitotic activity.

Haemangioma

P. Tamboli

Definition
Haemangioma is a benign vascular tumour that occasionally arises in the kidney.

ICD-O code 9120/0

Epidemiology
These tumours most commonly affect young to middle aged adults; however, the youngest reported patient was a newborn {2916}. There is no sex predilection. A number of these tumours are asymptomatic and are discovered incidentally at autopsy {1205}.

Clinical features
Symptomatic patients present with recurrent episodes of hematuria. Colicky pain may also be noted, caused by the passage of blood clots. In addition to sporadic tumours, haemangiomas may be part of a syndrome such as Sturge-Weber syndrome, Klippel-Trenaunay syndrome and systemic angiomatosis.

Macroscopy
Haemangiomas are generally unilateral and single, but may rarely be multifocal or bilateral {2573,2916}. The largest haemangioma reported to date was 18 cm in greatest diameter {2875}. Renal pyramids and renal pelvis are the most common sites of involvement, rarely these tumours may be found in the renal cortex or the renal capsule {2779}. On cut section they are unencapsulated, have a spongy red appearance, or may be apparent as a small red streak.

Histopathology
Both capillary and cavernous haemangiomas have been reported, the latter being more common. A case of intravascular capillary haemangioma, arising in a renal vein, and presenting as a renal mass has also been reported {1145}. They exhibit the typical histologic features of haemangiomas, i.e, irregular blood-filled vascular spaces lined by a single layer of endothelial cells. They may show an infiltrative growth pattern, but lack the mitosis and nuclear pleomorphism seen in angiosarcomas.

Lymphangioma

S.M. Bonsib

Definition
Lymphangioma is a rare benign renal tumour that may arise from the renal capsule, develop within the cortex, or most often, present as a peripelvic or renal sinus mass.

ICD-O code 9170/0

Epidemiology and etiology
These lesions are more common in adults. Children account for 1/3 of cases. Some cases may develop secondary to inflammatory lower urinary tract diseases, or represent a developmental abnormality in lymphatic formation. A bilateral presentation in children is referred to as lymphangiomatosis {1462}. Some cases appear neoplastic with karyotype abnormalities such as monosomy X, trisomy 7q, and defects in the von Hippel Lindau gene {358,578}. They are usually treated by nephrectomy because preoperative investigations cannot distinguish them from a malignant neoplasm.

Macroscopy
Lymphangiomas are encapsulated, diffusely cystic lesions ranging from small well-delineated tumours to large (19 cm) lesions that replace the entire renal parenchyma {89,1867,2921}.

Histopathology
The cysts communicate, contain clear fluid, and are composed of fibrous septae lined by flattened endothelium that is factor VIII and Ulex europaeus agglutinin positive but cytokeratin negative. The fibrous septa may contain small bland entrapped native tubules and lymphoid cells. Smooth muscle may be present as in lymphangiomas elsewhere.

Juxtaglomerular cell tumour

B. Têtu

Definition
Juxtaglomerular cell tumour is a benign renin-secreting tumour.

ICD-O code   8361/0

Epidemiology
Since the first description in 1967 {2213} over 60 JGCTs have been reported {1638}. JGCT usually occurs in younger individuals, averaging 27 years, and is twice as common in women. There is no reported recurrence or metastasis despite an interval of up to 17 years between the onset of hypertension and nephrectomy {1790} and a follow-up of up to 17 years after surgery {978}.

Localization
JGCT is unilateral, cortical and arises equally in both kidneys and in either pole.

Clinical features
The diagnosis of JGCT is usually suspected in patients with severe poorly controlled hypertension and marked

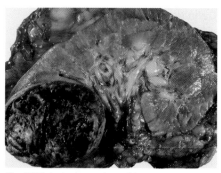
Fig. 1.104 Juxtaglomerular cell tumour.

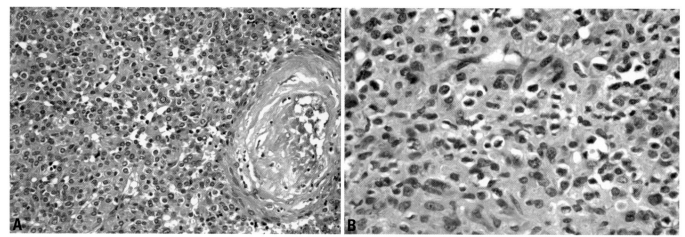
Fig. 1.105 Juxtaglomerular cell tumour. **A** Solid growth pattern of polygonal cells. **B** Higher magnification demonstrates pale halos about the nuclei.

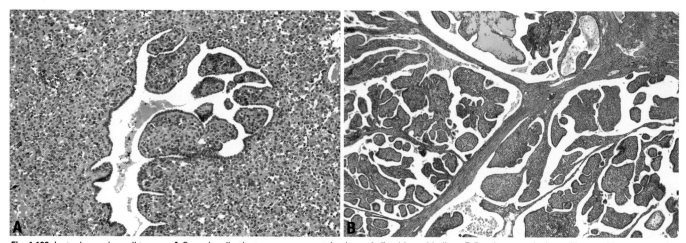
Fig. 1.106 Juxtaglomerular cell tumour. **A** Occasionally, the tumour may contain channels lined by epithelium. **B** Rarely, extensively papillary architecture may be seen.

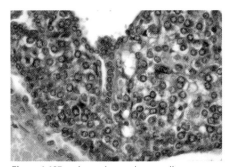

Fig. 1.107 Juxtaglomerular cell tumour. Immunohistochemistry with antibody to renin shows a diffusely positive reaction in juxtaglomerular cell tumour.

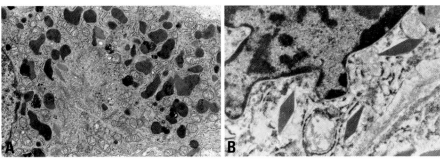

Fig. 1.108 Juxtaglomerular cell tumour. Electron micrograph showing irregular rounded renin-containing granules **(A)** and rhomboid crystalline renin granules **(B)**.

hypokalemia, although one patient presented with normal blood pressure {1044}. Investigation discloses high plasma renin activity, elevated secondary hyperaldosteronism and a renal mass. Hypertension and hypokalemia resolve after surgery.

Macroscopy and histopathology

JGCT is solid, well-circumscribed and yellow-tan. The tumour is usually smaller than 3 cm in diameter but cases ranging from 2 mm {1097} to 9 cm {1413} have been reported. JGCT is histologically made of sheets of polygonal or spindled tumour cells with central round regular nuclei, distinct cell borders and abundant granular eosinophilic cytoplasm staining for the Bowie stain, PAS and toluidine blue. Typically, tumours present with a complex vascular hemangiopericytic pattern. Mast cells and thick-walled hyalinized blood vessels are common and, in about one-half of reported cases, prominent tubular elements either neoplastic or entrapped are also present. Rarely, JGCT may be largely papillary {2602}. Tumour cells are immunoreactive for renin, actin,

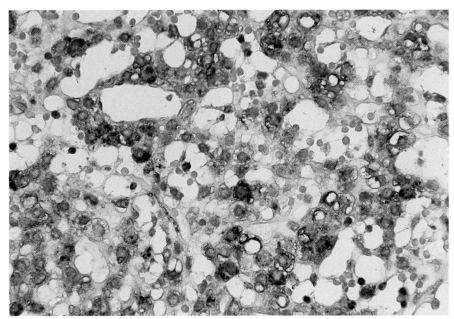

Fig. 1.109 Juxtaglomerular cell tumour. Renin expression in some cells.

vimentin and CD34 {1638}. Ultrastructural features include abundant rough endoplasmic reticulum, a well developed Golgi apparatus and numerous peripherally located sharply angulated rhomboid renin protogranules. A variable number of round electrondense mature renin-like granules are also found.

Renomedullary interstitial cell tumour

J.N. Eble

ICD-O code   8966/0

Renomedullary interstitial cell tumours are common autopsy findings in adults {2161,2163,2783}. They are present in nearly 50% of men and women. About half the patients who have one renomedullary interstitial cell tumour have more than one. They are asymptomatic and while renomedullary interstitial cells play a role in regulation of blood pressure, renomedullary interstitial cell tumours have no clear influence on blood pressure.

Almost all renomedullary interstitial cell tumours are 1-5 mm in diameter and appear as white or pale grey nodules within a renal medullary pyramid. Rarely, they are larger {1604} and can form polypoid masses protruding into the renal pelvic cavity {896}.

Microscopically, renomedullary interstitial cell tumours are seen to contain only small amounts of collagen. The renomedullary interstitial cells are small stellate or polygonal cells in a background of loose faintly basophilic stroma reminiscent of renal medullary stroma. At the periphery, renal medullary tubules often are entrapped in the matrix. Interlacing bundles of delicate fibers usually are present. Some renomedullary interstitial cell tumours contain deposits of amyloid. In these, the delicacy of the stroma is lost and irregular eosinophilic deposits of amyloid are present within the nodule.

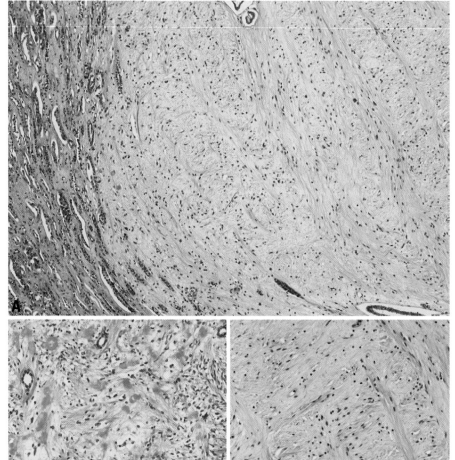

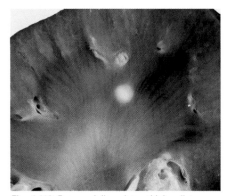

Fig. 1.110 Renomedullary interstitial cell tumour forms a white nodule in a medullary pyramid.

Fig. 1.111 Renomedullary interstitial cell tumour. **A** Well circumscribed tumour composed of spindle cells in a basophilic matrix. **B** Note deposits of amyloid. **C** This example is sparsely cellular and composed of interlacing bands of nondescript spindle cells.

Intrarenal schwannoma

I. Alvarado-Cabrero

ICD-O code   9560/0

Schwannoma is a common, benign tumour of peripheral and auditory nerves {723}. Its occurrence in the kidney is very rare, with only eighteen reported cases {73,2424}. Distribution of the 18 renal schwannomas was as follows: parenchyma, 33%; hilum 28%; pelvis 28%; capsule 11% {73,1585, 2424}.

Patients have nonspecific symptoms and signs. Malaise, weight loss, fever, and abdominal or flank pain are common findings. A palpable abdominal mass is frequently present. Hematuria may also be present {73,2424,2460}.

Tumours are well circumscribed, sometimes lobulated, rounded masses, 4 to 16cm (mean 9.7cm) in diameter and vary in colour from tan to yellow {1167,2653}.

Microscopically, renal schwannoma is composed of spindle cells often arranged in a palisading fashion (Antoni A pattern) and less cellular loosely textured tumour areas (Antoni B) {2424}. Some tumours display the histologic features of cellular schwannomas, with hypercellular areas composed exclusively or predominantly of Antoni A tissue, and devoid of Verocay bodies {2839}.

Solitary fibrous tumour

T. Hasegawa

ICD-O code   8815/0

The lesion may be clinically confused with renal cell carcinoma or sarcoma because of its large size by physical examination and radiographic studies as well as the frequent presence of painless hematuria {1595,2778}. The tumours are grossly well-circumscribed masses arising in the renal parenchyma. They are variable in cellularity, consisting of a mixture of haphazard, storiform, or short fascicular arrangements of bland spindle cells and less cellular dense collagenous bands. A haemangiopericytoma-like growth pattern is typically seen. Immunostaining for CD34, bcl-2 and CD99 confirms the diagnosis.

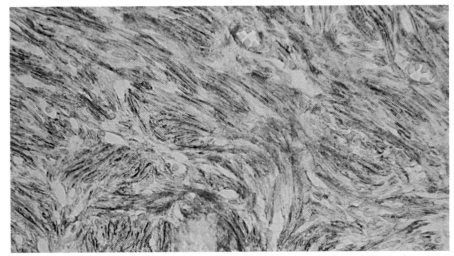

Fig. 1.112 Solitary fibrous tumour. Haphazard proliferation of uniform spindle cells with strong immunoreactvity for CD34.

Cystic nephroma

S.M. Bonsib

Definition
Cystic nephroma is a benign cystic neoplasm composed of epithelial and stromal elements.

ICD-O code   8959/0

Epidemiology
Typically, cystic nephroma presents after age 30 and has an 8:1 female to male ratio.

Clinical features
Cystic nephroma presents as a mass and cannot be distinguished radiographically from other cystic neoplasms. Pleuropulmonary blastoma is a very rare paediatric tumour associated with cystic nephroma in the same patient and in other family members {1175}.

Macroscopy
Cystic nephroma is an encapsulated well-demarcated tumour composed entirely of cysts and cyst septa. No solid areas or necrosis is present. The cysts contain serosanginous fluid that can occasionally appear haemorrhagic. The

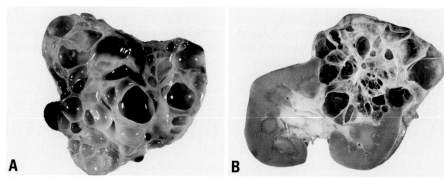

Fig. 1.113 Cystic nephroma. **A** The tumour consists of small and large cysts. **B** The tumour is sharply demarcated from an otherwise normal kidney.

lesion may be focal or replace the entire kidney. Rarely, a predominantly intrapelvic presentation occurs {1411}.

Histopathology
The cysts are lined by a single layer of flattened, low cuboidal, or hobnail epithelium. The cytoplasm may be eosinophilic or clear. The fibrous septa may be paucicellular or cellular resembling ovarian stroma. The septa may contain clusters of mature tubules.

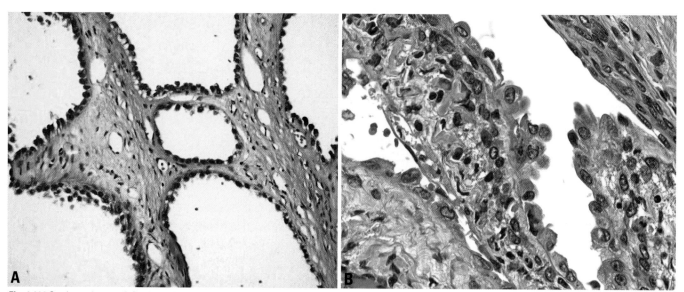

Fig. 1.114 Cystic nephroma. **A** Cystic nephroma composed entirely of cysts and septae. **B** Cellular details of single cell layer composed of hobnail epithelium.

Mixed epithelial and stromal tumour

J.N. Eble

Definition
Mixed epithelial and stromal tumour is a complex renal neoplasm composed of a mixture of stromal and epithelial elements.

Synonyms
Some authors have applied other names (cystic hamartoma of renal pelvis or adult mesoblastic nephroma) but the name "mixed epithelial and stromal tumour" best captures its nature {2035}.

Clinical features
There is a 6:1 predominance of women over men {35}. All have been adults and the mean age is perimenopausal (46 years). Presenting symptoms include flank pain, haematuria or symptoms of urinary tract infection; 25% are incidental findings. Histories of estrogen therapy are common. Surgery has been curative in all cases.

Macroscopy
The tumours often arise centrally in the kidney and grow as expansile masses, frequently herniating into the renal pelvic cavity. The tumours are typically composed of multiple cysts and solid areas.

Histopathology
These are complex tumours composed of large cysts, microcysts, and tubules. The largest cysts are lined by columnar and cuboidal epithelium, which sometimes forms small papillary tufts. Urothelium, which may be hyperplastic, may also line some portion of the cysts. The microcysts and tubules are lined by flattened, cuboidal, or columnar cells. Their cytoplasm ranges from clear to pale, eosinophilic, or vacuolated. Epithelium with müllerian characteristics has also been described {205}. The architecture of the microcysts is varied and ranges from simple microcysts with abundant stroma between them, to densely packed clusters of microcysts,

to complex branching channels which may be dilated. These varied elements often are present intermingled in the same area of the tumour. The stroma consists of a variably cellular population of spindle cells with plump nuclei and abundant cytoplasm. Areas of myxoid stroma and fascicles of smooth muscle cells may be prominent. Densely collagenous stroma is common and fat is occasionally present. Mitotic figures and atypical nuclei have not been reported.

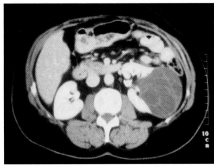

Fig. 1.115 Mixed epithelial and stromal tumour. Large tumour attached to the renal pelvis.

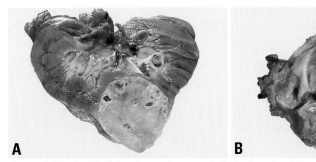

Fig. 1.116 Mixed epithelial and stromal tumour. **A** Predominantly solid mass with scattered cysts. **B** Note glancing inner surface of the cystic tumour.

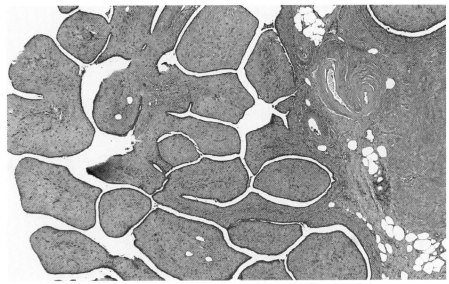

Fig. 1.117 Mixed epithelial and stromal tumour forming spatulate papillae. Note fat cells in stroma.

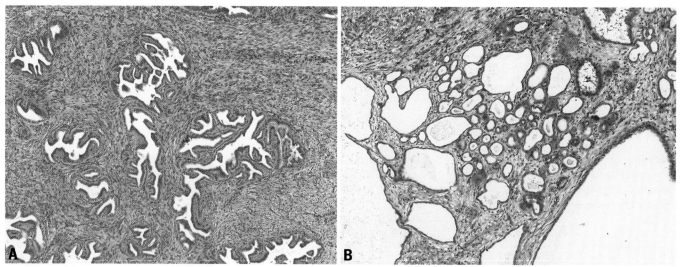

Fig. 1.118 Mixed epithelial and stromal tumour. **A** Complex branching tubules in a spindle cell stroma with smooth muscle differentiation. **B** Cysts and small tubular structures resembling nephrogenic adenoma.

Immunoprofile

Immunohistochemistry shows that the spindle cells, which look like smooth muscle have strong reactions with antibodies to actins and to desmin. The nuclei of the spindle cells also frequently react with antibodies to estrogen and progesterone receptors {35}. The epithelial elements react with antibodies to a variety of cytokeratins and often vimentin. They occasionally react with antibody to estrogen receptor.

Genetics

Little is known of the genetics of these tumours except that they lack the translocation characteristic of cellular congenital mesoblastic nephroma {2073}.

Synovial sarcoma of the kidney

J.Y. Ro
K.R. Kim
P. Argani
M. Ladanyi

Definition
Synovial sarcoma (SS) of the kidney is a spindle cell neoplasm that infrequently displays epithelial differentiation and is characterized by a specific translocation, t(X;18)(p11.2;q11).

ICD-O code   9040/3

Synonyms and historical annotation
A subset of previously described embryonal sarcoma of the kidney is now recognized to be primary renal SS {112}.

Epidemiology
Age and sex distribution
Renal synovial sarcoma occurs in an age range 12-59 years, with a mean of 35 years and shows a slight male predilection (1.6:1).

Localization
Tumour equally involves either kidney, but no bilateral tumours were identified.

Clinical features
Symptoms and signs
Flank or abdominal pain with or without abdominal distension is the presenting

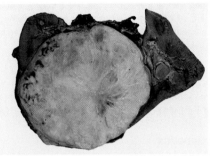

Fig. 1.119 Synovial sarcoma of the kidney.

symptom in more than half of cases.

Macroscopy
Most of the tumours are solid, but multiple areas of haemorrhage, necrosis and cyst formation can be observed on gross examination.

Histopathology
Tumours are typically mitotically active, with monomorphic plump spindle cells and indistinct cell borders growing in short, intersecting fascicles or in solid sheets. Cysts are lined by mitotically inactive polygonal eosinophilic cells with apically located nuclei ("hobnailed epithelium"), and appear to be entrapped native renal tubules, which may be extensively dilated. Areas of solid aggregation or fascicles of the tumour cells alternating with hypocellular myxoid tissues, together with areas displaying a prominent haemangiopericytoma-like pattern, may be found. Rhabdoid cells in the tumour have been recently described {1253}.

Immunoprofile
The tumour cells are consistently immunoreactive with vimentin and BCL2, frequently reactive for CD99 but desmin and muscle specific actin are negative. The tumour cells are often negative or only focally positive for cytokeratins (AE1/AE3, or CAM 5.2) and epithelial membrane antigen, but the epithelial lin-

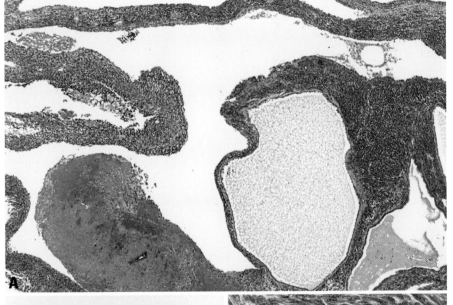

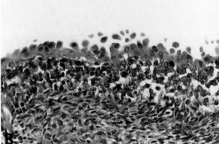

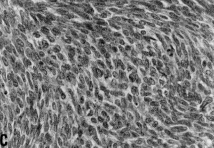

Fig. 1.120 Renal synovial sarcoma. **A** Note prominent cystic change. **B** The cysts are lined by hobnail epithelium with abundant eosinophilic cytoplasm representing entrapped dilated tubules. **C** Higher magnification shows monomorphic small spindle cells.

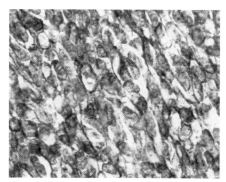

Fig. 1.121 Synovial sarcoma of the kidney. Immunoexpression of CD99 in the synovial sarcoma of the kidney.

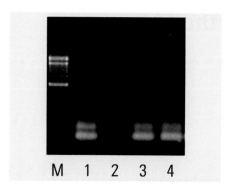

Fig. 1.122 Synovial sarcoma of the kidney. SYT-SSX fusion transcripts demonstrated by RT-PCR. M, molecular size marker;1, positive control; 2,negative control; 3 and 4, synovial sarcomas.

ing cells of the cysts are consistently highlighted by these markers {112,1316}.

Genetics
Synovial sarcoma is cytogenetically char-acterized by the translocation t(X;18) (p11.2/q11.2) generating a fusion between the *SYT* gene on chromosome 18 and one member of the *SSX* family gene(*SSX1;SS X2;SSX4*) on chromosome X.

Molecularly confirmed primary renal synovial sarcomas have demonstrated the characteristic *SYT-SSX* gene fusion {112, 1316,1379}. In contrast to soft tissue synovial sarcoma where the *SYT-SSX1* gene fusion is more common than the alternative *SYT-SSX2* form {1422}, the majority of renal synovial sarcomas have so far demonstrated the *SYT-SSX2* gene fusion {112,1316,1379}. In soft tissue synovial sarcomas, the *SYT-SSX2* form of the gene fusion is strongly correlated with monophasic histology {1422}; this tendency is also consistent with the predominance of monophasic spindled morphology of these tumours in the kidney and the rarity of biphasic histology.

Prognosis and predictive factors
Prognostic data are limited, some have responded to chemotherapy, however recurrence is common.

Renal carcinoid tumour

L.R. Bégin

Definition
A well differentiated neuroendocrine neoplasm arising within the kidney.

ICD-O code   8240/3

Epidemiology
Primary renal carcinoid is very rare, only about 50 cases having been reported and there appears to be an association with horseshoe kidney {202,1180,1662, 1690,2463,2878}. There is no sex predilection. Presentation is most common in the fourth to seventh decades, including a range from 13-79 years (mean, 49 years; median, 51 years).

Clinical features
The most common mode of presentation is abdominal pain, mass, or haematuria. Carcinoid syndrome symptoms are uncommon (<10%) {1006,1819, 2150,2174}. Computed tomography usually reveals a circumscribed and solid mass with an occasional cystic component or calcification. Somatostatin receptor scintigraphy (pentetreotide scan) is of adjunct value in staging and surveillance for the development of recurrent or metastatic disease {1662}.

Macroscopy
Renal carcinoid is a solitary tumour with a well circumscribed, lobulated and bulging appearance. The tumour is yellow-tan, beige-white or red-brown, and has a soft to moderately firm consistency. The appearance is homogeneous or may depict focal haemorrhage, calcification and cystic changes, whereas necrosis is uncommon {203,903,1764,2150}.

Tumour spread and staging
Capsular invasion and/or renal vein involvement (pT3) has been reported.

Histopathology
Renal carcinoid displays the typical histologic features of carcinoids in other organs of the body.

Immunoprofile
The immunohistochemical profile is similar to that of carcinoid tumours elsewhere.   {202,203,759,903,1764,2150, 2688}. Immunoreactivity for prostatic acid phosphatase (PAP) has been documented in at least five tumours {202,203, 677,903,2560}.

Somatic genetics
Only a few tumours have been studied by genetic methods {677,2688}.

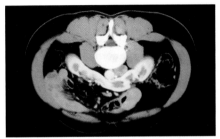

Fig. 1.123 Renal carcinoid arising in a horseshoe kidney, CT scan. Horseshoe renal malformation.

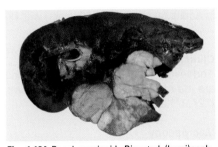

Fig. 1.124 Renal carcinoid. Bisected (hemi)nephrectomy specimen (from a horseshoe kidney) reveals a well circumscribed, lobulated tumour bulging from the central region close to the isthmus. Cut surface is homogeneous and yellow-tan.

Prognosis
The clinical outcome is difficult to predict and a significant proportion of patients with metastatic disease have a protracted clinical course.

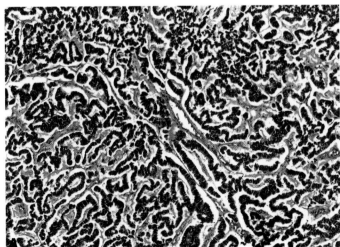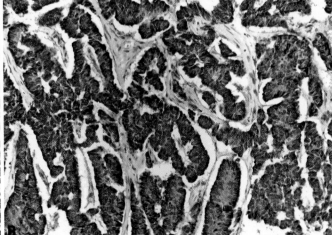

Fig. 1.125 Renal carcinoid. **A** Trabecular pattern. **B** Tumour cell expression of synaptophysin.

Neuroendocrine carcinoma of the kidney

L. Guillou

Definition
A poorly-differentiated epithelial neoplasm showing neuroendocrine differentiation.

ICD-O code   8246/3

Epidemiology
Accounts for much less than 1% of all epithelial renal malignancies, neuroendocrine carcinoma of the kidney occurs in adults (average age: 60 years) with no sex predilection.

Clinical features
Abdominal pain and gross haematuria are the most frequent clinical symptoms {727,971,2601}.

Macroscopy
Most neuroendocrine carcinomas of the kidney are located close to the renal pelvis, often surrounding the pelvicaliceal cavities. The tumour presents as a soft, whitish, gritty and necrotic renal mass, often extending into renal sinus adipose tissue. Tumours range in size from 2.5 to 23 cm (median: 8 cm) {368, 727,971,1326,1658,1735,2601}.

Histopathology
Morphologically, the tumour is composed of sheets, nests and trabecula of apparently poorly-differentiated small, round to fusiform cells separated by sparse intervening stroma. These cells show characteristic hyperchromatic nuclei with stippled chromatin and inconspicuous nucleoli. Their cytoplasm is hardly visible on HE sections. Mitoses are numerous, vascular tumour emboli common, and tumour necrosis often extensive and accompanied with perivascular DNA deposition (Azzopardi phenomenon). A concomitant urothelial carcinoma is common {727,971,1326,1658}.

Immunoprofile
Immunohistochemically, tumour cells show dot-like cytoplasmic staining with cytokeratins and are variably positive for neuroendocrine markers including chromogranin A, synaptophysin, CD56 (N-Cam), and neurone specific enolase {727,971,1658,1735}.

Prognosis and predictive factors
The prognosis is poor and stage dependent. Most patients present with large and locally aggressive tumours, often extending into perirenal adipose tissue at diagnosis {368,727,971,1658}. Regional lymph nodes and distant metastases are common {368,971,1658, 1735,2601}. At least, 75% of patients die of their disease within one year {727, 971,1326,1658,1735,2601} regardless of treatment.

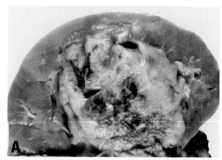

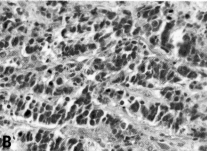

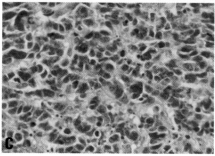

Fig. 1.126 Small cell carcinoma of the kidney. **A** Large, centrally located, necrotic tumour with renal pelvis invasion. Adapted from L. Guillou et al. {971}, with permission. **B,C** Tumour cells show scant cytoplasm and granular chromatin with inconspicuous nucleoli. Note nuclear molding and numerous mitoses.

Primitive neuroectodermal tumour (Ewing sarcoma)

L.P. Dehner

Definition

A malignant tumour composed of small uniform round cells, characterized by a translocation resulting in a fusion transcript of the EWS gene and ETS-related family of oncogenes.

ICD-O codes

Ewing sarcoma   9260/3
Peripheral neuroectodermal
tumour   9364/3

Epidemiology

This neoplasm is rare {2009,2124}. A review of 35 cases of renal PNET-EWS revealed an age range from 4-69 years which is somewhat wider than that recorded for this tumour in the bone and soft tissues. The mean age was 27 years with a median age of 21 years. There was a predilection for males (21 males, 14 females).

Clinical features

Signs and symptoms

Abdominal pain of recent (weeks) or sudden onset, flank pain and gross hematuria were the most common presenting symptoms. Fever, weight loss and bone pain were other less frequent manifestations. A palpable abdominal or flank mass was detected in less than 25% of cases. Pulmonary, hepatic and bony metastases were noted at presentation in 10% of patients {385}.

Imaging

A sizable, inhomogeneous mass often replacing almost the entire kidney was the common computed tomographic appearance {630}. Areas of high and low intensity reflected the common presence of haemorrhage and necrosis in resected specimen.

Macroscopy

A mass measuring in excess of 10 cm in diameter with replacement of the kidney and weighing 1 kg or more in some cases served to characterize these neoplasms as a group {1225}. Cross-sectional features included a greyish-tan to white lobulated surface with interspersed areas of haemorrhage and necrosis. A capsule or pseudocapsule was described in a minority of tumours.

Histopathology

The tumour in the kidney is no different than the more common counterpart in soft tissues. The cells are relatively monotonous polygonal cells whose appearance is dominated by a hyperchromatic rounded nucleus. A finely dispersed chromatin and a micronucleolus in some cases are the nuclear characteristics. Interspersed smaller "dark" cells

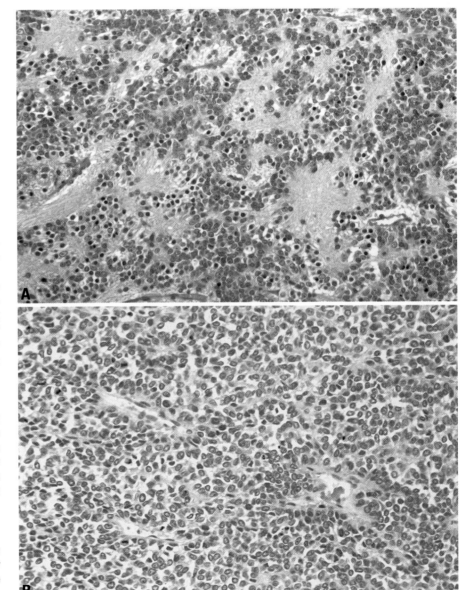

Fig. 1.127 A PNET of the kidney. **B** Renal PNET. Note sheet-like growth pattern and rosettes.

representing tumour cells undergoing pyknosis are prominent in some cases. Mitotic figures may be numerous. Though the nuclear to cytoplasmic ratio is high, a rim of clear cytoplasm and discrete cell membranes are often apparent in well-fixed tumours without extensive degenerative changes. The presence of clear cytoplasm is often associated with abundant glycogen as demonstrated by diastase sensitive PAS-positivity.

Immunoprofile
The basic immunophenotype of PNET-EWS, regardless of the primary site, is the expression of vimentin and the surface antigen of the MIC2 gene, CD99 (O13) or HBA-71. Approximately 20% of cases also express pan-cytokeratin. The staining pattern for vimentin and cytokeratin may be perinuclear or Golgi zone punctate reactivity.

Somatic genetics
Virtually all of the recently reported PNET-EWSs have had the t(11;22)(q24;q12) translocation with the fusion transcript between the EWS gene (22q12) and the ETS-related oncogene, FLI1 (11q24) {1627,2124}. Variant translocations with EWS are those with other ETS-related oncogenes: (21q22), (7p22), (17q12) and (2q33).

Prognosis
Pathologic stage is the major determinant in the prognosis of PNET-EWS regardless of the primary site. Aggressive multidrug chemotherapy has resulted in an improvement in the clinical outcome {525}.

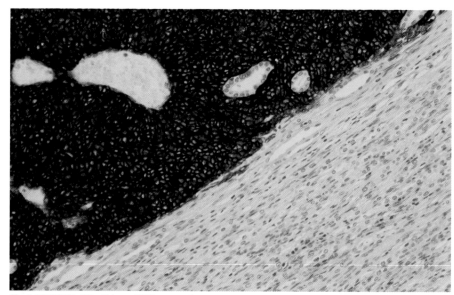
Fig. 1.128 PNET of the kidney. CD99 expression.

Table 1.12
Immunohistochemical differentiation of neuroectodermal tumours from other tumours with similar microscopic features.

	VIM	CK	CHR	SYN	NSE	CD99	CD45	WT-1	CD117
PNET-EWS	+	+/–	+/–	+/–	+	+	–	–	+
NB	–	–	+	+	+	–	–	–	+
Carcinoid	–	+	+	+	+	–	–	–	–
NEC	–	+	+	+	+	–	–	–	–
NHL	+	–	–	–	–	+*	+	–	–
Blastemal WT	+	+	–	–	+/–	–	–	+	+

Abbreviations: PNET-EWS = primitive neuroectodermal tumour / Ewing sarcoma, NB= neuroblastoma, NEC= neuroendocrine carcinoma, NHL= non-Hodgkin lymphoma, WT = Wilms tumour, VIM = vimentin, CK = cytokeratin, CHR = chromogranin, SYN = synaptophysin, NSE - neuron specific enolase.
* CD99 is expressed by lymphoblastic lymphoma.

Neuroblastoma

D.M. Parham

ICD-O code   9500/3

Neuroblastomas arising as a true intrarenal mass are extremely rare; only six cases were identified in the National Wilms Tumour Study Pathology Centre in 1993 {2225}. Pure intrarenal lesions hypothetically arise from either adrenal rests or intrarenal sympathetic tissue {2385}. Far more frequently, adrenal neuroblastomas invade the adjacent kidney; this occurs in approximately five per cent of cases {2375}. Because most neuroblastomas arise from the adrenal, those affecting the kidney predominate in the superior pole. Extensive renal sinus invasion may simulate a pelvic tumour. Preoperative determination of urine catecholamine excretion is helpful in diagnosis of neuroblastoma but may not exclude nephroblastomas with neural elements {2273}. The presence of primitive neural tissue defines neuroblastomas, which contain Homer Wright rosettes, neurofibrillary stroma, and embryonal cells with round nuclei containing granular, "salt and pepper" chromatin. Important positive indicators of neuronal differentiation include neuron-specific enolase, synaptophysin, S100 protein, and chromogranin.

Paraganglioma / Phaeochromocytoma

Ph.U. Heitz

ICD-O codes
Paraganglioma   8680/1
Pheochromocytoma   8700/0

A very small number of tumours have been described in the kidney {595,1426}. Most tumours are small. The cut surface is grey, often well vascularized. The colour of the parenchyma often rapidly turns brown when exposed to air. This is due to oxidation of chromaffin substances, including catecholamines. The architecture is characterized by cell clusters ("Zellballen") surrounded by a network of fine collagenous septa, containing blood vessels and sustentacular cells. The immunoreactions for synaptophysin, chromogranin A, and CD56 are consistently strong in virtually all tumour cells. Protein S-100 highlights tumour cells and sustentacular cells.

Lymphomas

A. Marx
S.M. Bonsib

Definition
Primary renal lymphoma is a lymphoma without evidence of systemic involvement.

Epidemiology
Less than 100 cases of primary renal lymphomas, both Hodgkin disease and non-Hodgkin lymphoma, have been described. However, post-transplant lymphoproliferative disorders are the most frequently encountered disorder today. In the non-transplant patients, primary lymphomas may present as a mass lesion and regarded clinically as a renal epithelial neoplasm and treated by nephrectomy. The diagnosis requires renal and bone marrow biopsy and thoraco-abdominal CT {2477}. Dissemination following the diagnosis of PRL is common.
Secondary renal lymphomas (SRL) affect the kidney as the second most common site for metastasis {2284}. It is 30x more common than PRL {374,537}. Most present (48%) in advanced stage lymphoma {1267}.

Etiology
PRL arising in transplanted kidneys are usually EBV-associated monomorphic or polymorphic B-cell lymphoproliferations of donor origin and related to iatrogenic immunosuppression {439,839,1695,2833}.

Clinical features
Common symptoms are flank or abdominal pain, haematuria, fever, weight loss, hypertension, renal insufficiency, or acute renal failure {448,537,626,1354, 2097,2382}. Complications are renal failure {750} and paraneoplastic hypercalcemia {2676}.

Macroscopy
Nephrectomy specimens in primary or secondary lymphoma show single or multifocal nodules (eventually associated with hydronephrosis) or diffuse renal enlargment. In secondary lymphoma, bilateral involvement is frequent (10% to 30%) {13,1881,2097,2408,2647,2696}. The cut surface is usually homogeneous, firm and pale, but necrosis, haemorrhage, cystic changes, calcifications and tumoral thrombus formation in the renal vein may occur {2677,2760}. Intravascular large B-cell lymphoma almost always affects the kidneys but may cause no macroscopic change {2819}.

Histopathology
There are three patterns of renal involvement. The most common is diffuse involvement with lymphoma cells permeating between the native nephron structures resulting in marked organ enlargement. The second pattern is formation of one or more tumour masses. The least common pattern is the intravascular form where lymphoma cells fill all vascular components. Almost every histological lymphoma subtype may be encountered. Diffuse large B-cell lymphoma, including its variants, constitutes the single most frequent type of PRL and SRL {448,750, 755,2097,2647}.

Prognosis and predictive factors
Secondary renal lymphoma usually indicates stage IV disease with dismal prognosis {327,622,1267,2097}. In PRL, dissemination to extrarenal sites is common and confers a bad prognosis as well {622}. Modern radiochemotherapy has improved survival and renal functional compromise {2097,2696}.

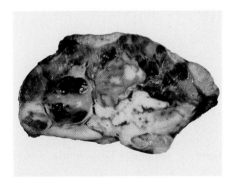

Fig. 1.129 Lymphoma.

Plasmacytoma

A. Orazi

Plasmacytoma (PC) of the kidney most often occurs as a manifestation of disseminated multiple myeloma. The kidney, however, may rarely be the site of origin of a solitary (primary) extraosseous PC {1266,2933}. PC of the kidney is histologically indistinguishable from plasmacytoma occurring elsewhere. To qualify as a primary PC, a complete radiologic work-up must show no evidence of other lesions. The bone marrow must show no evidence of plasmacytosis and/or plasma cell monoclonality. The other myeloma associated criteria are also absent.

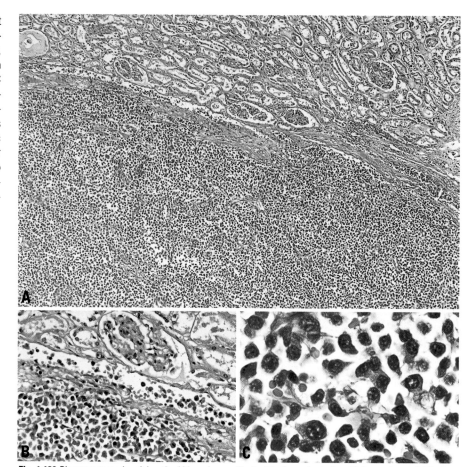

Fig. 1.130 Plasmacytoma involving the kidney in a patient with disseminated multiple myeloma. **A** The low power photomicrograph shows a well demarked nodular lesion surrounded by unremarkable kidney parenchyma. **B** High magnification illustrating the plasma cell proliferation which is characterized by a mixture of both mature and immature plasma cells.

Leukaemia

A. Orazi

Interstitial infiltration of leukaemic cells without a nodular mass is best referred to as extramedullary leukaemia in kidney. Diffuse infiltration of the kidney secondary to acute myeloid and lymphoblastic leukaemias, megakaryoblastic leukaemia, or chronic lymphocytic leukaemia has rarely been reported in the literature {989}. Myeloid sarcoma (MS) is a neoplastic proliferation of myeloblasts or immature myeloid cells forming a mass in an extramedullary site. MS may occur "de novo" or simultaneously with acute myeloid leukemia, myeloproliferative disorder, or myelodysplastic syndrome {154,989}. It may represent the first manifestation of leukaemia relapse in a previously treated patient. The commonest type of myeloid sarcoma occurring in the kidney is known as granulocytic sarcoma, a tumour composed of myeloblasts and promyelocytes {154}.

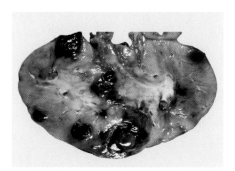

Fig. 1.131 Myeloid sarcoma in the kidney showing multiple haemorrhagic fleshy nodules.

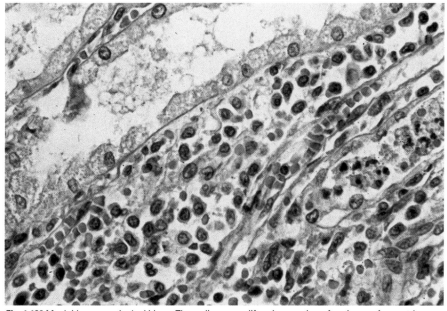

Fig. 1.132 Myeloid sarcoma in the kidney. The malignant proliferation consists of a mixture of promyelocytes and myeloblasts.

Germ cell tumours

I.A. Sesterhenn

Primary renal choriocarcinomas have rarely been reported and are difficult to distinguish from high grade urothelial carcinomas with syncytiotrophoblasts. Most of the cases in the literature {1019, 1135} are metastases from testicular germ cell tumours {1168,1728,1804}. The wide range of differentiation in nephroblastoma can resemble teratoma. Reports of teratomas of the kidney are very rare. Reported cases have involved the renal parenchyma or the renal hilus and have been indistinguishable from teratomas of the gonads. {6,138,580, 916,1986,2878}.

CHAPTER 2

Tumours of the Urinary System

With approximately 260,000 new cases per year worldwide, tumours of the urinary system contribute significantly to the overall human cancer burden. Progress in the early detection and treatment of bladder cancer has improved the prognosis, with five-year survival rates of 60 - 80%.

The origin of bladder cancer is multifactorial, with tobacco smoking as the principal cause in most countries. Other etiological factors include analgesic abuse, occupational exposure and chronic *Schistosoma* cystitis.

Urothelial carcinomas are the most frequent and important tumour type. Improvements in early detection have made reproducible grading and staging important criteria for clinical management and prognosis.

WHO histological classification of tumours of the urinary tract

Urothelial tumours

Infiltrating urothelial carcinoma	8120/3[1]
with squamous differentiation	
with glandular differentiation	
with trophoblastic differentiation	
Nested	
Microcystic	
Micropapillary	8131/3
Lymphoepithelioma-like	8082/3
Lymphoma-like	
Plasmacytoid	
Sarcomatoid	8122/3
Giant cell	8031/3
Undifferentiated	8020/3
Non-invasive urothelial neoplasias	
Urothelial carcinoma in situ	8120/2
Non-invasive papillary urothelial carcinoma, high grade	8130/23
Non-invasive papillary urothelial carcinoma, low grade	8130/21
Non-invasive papillary urothelial neoplasm of low malignant potential	8130/1
Urothelial papilloma	8120/0
Inverted urothelial papilloma	8121/0

Squamous neoplasms

Squamous cell carcinoma	8070/3
Verrucous carcinoma	8051/3
Squamous cell papilloma	8052/0

Glandular neoplasms

Adenocarcinoma	8140/3
Enteric	
Mucinous	8480/3
Signet-ring cell	8490/3
Clear cell	8310/3
Villous adenoma	8261/0

Neuroendocrine tumours

Small cell carcinoma	8041/3
Carcinoid	8240/3
Paraganglioma	8680/1

Melanocytic tumours

Malignant melanoma	8720/3
Nevus	

Mesenchymal tumours

Rhabdomyosarcoma	8900/3
Leiomyosarcoma	8890/3
Angiosarcoma	9120/3
Osteosarcoma	9180/3
Malignant fibrous histiocytoma	8830/3
Leiomyoma	8890/0
Haemangioma	9120/0
Other	

Haematopoietic and lymphoid tumours

Lymphoma	
Plasmacytoma	9731/3

Miscellaneous tumours

Carcinoma of Skene, Cowper and Littre glands
Metastatic tumours and tumours extending from other organs

---

[1] Morphology code of the International Classification of Diseases for Oncology (ICD-O) {808} and the Systematized Nomenclature of Medicine (http://snomed.org). Behaviour is coded /0 for benign tumours, /2 for in situ carcinomas and grade III intraepithelial neoplasia, /3 for malignant tumours, and /1 for borderline or uncertain behaviour.

TNM classification of carcinomas of the urinary bladder

TNM classification [1,2]

T – Primary tumour

TX   Primary tumour cannot be assessed
T0   No evidence of primary tumour
Ta   Non-invasive papillary carcinoma
Tis   Carcinoma in situ: "flat tumour"
T1   Tumour invades subepithelial connective tissue
T2   Tumour invades muscle
T2a   Tumour invades superficial muscle (inner half)
T2b   Tumour invades deep muscle (outer half)
T3   Tumour invades perivesical tissue:
T3a   Microscopically
T3b   Macroscopically (extravesical mass)
T4   Tumour invades any of the following: prostate, uterus, vagina, pelvic wall, abdominal wall
T4a   Tumour invades prostate, uterus or vagina
T4b   Tumour invades pelvic wall or abdominal wall

N – Regional lymph nodes

NX   Regional lymph nodes cannot be assessed
N0   No regional lymph node metastasis
N1   Metastasis in a single lymph node 2 cm or less in greatest dimension
N2   Metastasis in a single lymph node more than 2 cm but not more than 5 cm in greatest dimension, or multiple lymph nodes, none more than 5 cm in greatest dimension
N3   Metastasis in a lymph node more than 5 cm in greatest dimension

M – Distant metastasis

MX   Distant metastasis cannot be assessed
M0   No distant metastasis
M1   Distant metastasis

Stage Grouping

Stage	T	N	M
Stage 0a	Ta	N0	M0
Stage 0is	Tis	N0	M0
Stage I	T1	N0	M0
Stage II	T2a, b	N0	M0
Stage III	T3a, b	N0	M0
	T4a	N0	M0
Stage IV	T4b	N0	M0
	Any T	N1, N2, N3	M0
	Any T	Any N	M1

[1] {944,2662}.
[2] A help desk for specific questions about the TNM classification is available at http://www.uicc.org/tnm/

TNM classification of carcinomas of the renal pelvis and ureter

TNM classification [1,2]

T – Primary tumour

TX   Primary tumour cannot be assessed
T0   No evidence of primary tumour
Ta   Non-invasive papillary carcinoma
Tis   Carcinoma in situ

T1   Tumour invades subepithelial connective tissue
T2   Tumour invades muscularis
T3   *(Renal pelvis)* Tumour invades beyond muscularis into peripelvic fat or renal parenchyma
      (Ureter) Tumour invades beyond muscularis into periureteric fat
T4   Tumour invades adjacent organs or through the kidney into perinephric fat

N – Regional lymph nodes

NX   Regional lymph nodes cannot be assessed
N0   No regional lymph node metastasis
N1   Metastasis in a single lymph node 2 cm or less in greatest dimension
N2   Metastasis in a single lymph node more than 2 cm but not more than 5 cm in greatest dimension, or multiple lymph nodes, none more than 5 cm in greatest dimension
N3   Metastasis in a lymph node more than 5 cm in greatest dimension

M – Distant metastasis

MX   Distant metastasis cannot be assessed
M0   No distant metastasis
M1   Distant metastasis

Stage Grouping

Stage	T	N	M
Stage 0a	Ta	N0	M0
Stage 0is	Tis	N0	M0
Stage I	T1	N0	M0
Stage II	T2	N0	M0
Stage III	T3	N0	M0
Stage IV	T4	N0	M0
	Any T	N1, N2, N3	M0
	Any T	Any N	M1

[1] {944,2662}.
[2] A help desk for specific questions about the TNM classification is available at http://www.uicc.org/tnm/

TNM classification of carcinomas of the urethra

TNM classification [1,2]

T – Primary tumour

TX	Primary tumour cannot be assessed
T0	No evidence of primary tumour

Urethra (male and female)

Ta	Non-invasive papillary, polypoid, or verrucous carcinoma
Tis	Carcinoma in situ
T1	Tumour invades subepithelial connective tissue
T2	Tumour invades any of the following: corpus spongiosum, prostate, periurethral muscle
T3	Tumour invades any of the following: corpus cavernosum, beyond prostatic capsule, anterior vagina, bladder neck
T4	Tumour invades other adjacent organs

Urothelial carcinoma of prostate (prostatic urethra)

Tis pu	Carcinoma in situ, involvement of prostatic urethra
Tis pd	Carcinoma in situ, involvement of prostatic ducts
T1	Tumour invades subepithelial connective tissue
T2	Tumour invades any of the following: prostatic stroma, corpus spongiosum, periurethral muscle
T3	Tumour invades any of the following: corpus cavernosum, beyond prostatic capsule, bladder neck (extra- prostatic extension)
T4	Tumour invades other adjacent organs (invasion of bladder)

N – Regional lymph nodes

NX	Regional lymph nodes cannot be assessed
N0	No regional lymph node metastasis
N1	Metastasis in a single lymph node 2 cm or less in greatest dimension
N2	Metastasis in a single lymph node more than 2 cm in greatest dimension, or multiple lymph nodes

M – Distant metastasis

MX	Distant metastasis cannot be assessed
M0	No distant metastasis
M1	Distant metastasis

Stage Grouping

Stage 0a	Ta	N0	M0
Stage 0is	Tis	N0	M0
	Tis pu	N0	M0
	Tis pd	N0	M0
Stage I	T1	N0	M0
Stage II	T2	N0	M0
Stage III	T1, T2	N1	M0
	T3	N0, N1	M0
Stage IV	T4	N0, N1	M0
	Any T	N2	M0
	Any T	Any N	M1

---

[1] {944,2662}.
[2] A help desk for specific questions about the TNM classification is available at http://www.uicc.org/tnm/

Infiltrating urothelial carcinoma

A. Lopez-Beltran
G. Sauter
T. Gasser
A. Hartmann
B.J. Schmitz-Dräger
B. Helpap
A.G. Ayala
P. Tamboli

M.A. Knowles
D. Sidransky
C. Cordon-Cardo
P.A. Jones
P. Cairns
R. Simon
M.B. Amin
J.E. Tyczynski

Definition

Infiltrating urothelial carcinoma is defined as a urothelial tumour that invades beyond the basement membrane.

ICD-O code   8120/3

Synonym

Transitional cell carcinoma.

Epidemiology of urothelial bladder cancer

Bladder cancer is the 7th most common cancer worldwide, with an estimated 260,000 new cases occurring each year in men and 76,000 in women {749}.

Cancer of the urinary bladder accounts for about 3.2% of all cancers worldwide and is considerably more common in males than in females (ratio worldwide is about 3.5:1) {2014}. In both sexes, the highest incidence rates of bladder cancer are observed in Western Europe, North America and Australia {2016}.

The highest incidence rates of bladder cancer in males in 1990s were observed in the following registries: Limburg (Belgium) – 42.5/105, Genoa Province (Italy) – 41.1/105, and Mallorca (Spain) – 39.5/105 {2016}. The highest rates in females were noted in Harare (Zimbabwe) – 8.3/105, Scotland (UK) – 8.1/105, North Western England (UK) – 8.0/105, and white population of Connecticut (USA) – 8.0/105. The highest prevalence of bladder cancers in both males and females is observed in North America and in countries of the European Union {2084}. In general, the prevalence of bladder tumours in developed countries in approximately 6-times higher compared with that in developing countires.

The most common type of bladder cancer in developed countries is urothelial carcinoma, derived from the uroepithelium, which constitutes more than 90% of bladder cancer cases in USA, France or Italy. However, in other regions (e.g.

Eastern and Northern Europe, Africa, Asia) the relative frequency of urothelial carcinoma of the bladder is lower. In general, among all registries included into the 8th volume of "Cancer Incidence in Five Continents" {2016} urothelial carcinoma constitutes 84% of bladder cancer in males and 79% in females. Other types of bladder cancer, i.e. squamous cell carcinoma and adenocarcinoma have much lower relative frequency. In all "Cancer Incidence in Five Continents" {2016} registries squamous cell carcinoma accounts for 1.1% and 2.8% of all bladder cancers in men and women respectively. Adenocarcinoma of the bladder constitutes respectively 1.5% and 1.9% of all bladder tumours worldwide {2016}. It is estimated that approximately 70-80% of patients with newly diagnosed bladder cancer present with non-invasive or early invasive (i.e. stage Ta, Tis, or T1).

Etiology of urothelial bladder cancer

Risk factors

There are several known and potential risk factors of bladder cancer. Cigarette smoking and occupational exposure to aromatic amines are the most important among them {1877}.

Tobacco smoking

Tobacco smoking is the major established risk factor of bladder cancer. It is estimated that the risk of bladder cancer attributed to tobacco smoking is 66% for men and 30% for women {1158}.

The risk of bladder cancer in smokers is 2-6 fold that of non-smokers {313,391, 1877}. The risk increases with increasing duration of smoking, and for those with the longest history of smoking (60 years or more) reaches approximately 6 in men and 5 in women {313}. The excess of risk is observed also with increasing intensity of smoking (number of cigarettes per day), reaching maximum of about 3 for those smoking 40 or more cigarettes per day {313}. The increase of risk with the increasing duration and intensity of smoking is similar in both sexes {1158} but, some studies indicate higher risk in women than in men at the equivalent level of exposure {391}.

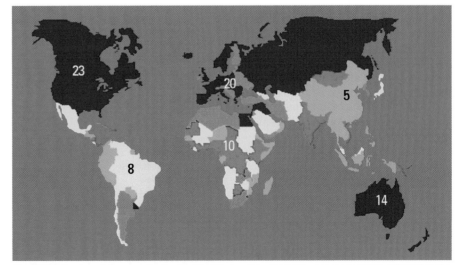

Fig. 2.01 Estimates of the age-standardized incidence rates of bladder cancer in males, adjusted to the world standard age distribution (ASR). From Globocan 2000 {749}.

The risk of bladder cancer goes down after stopping smoking, and 15 years cessation tends to be approximately that of non-smokers {1158}. The decrease of risk after cessation is similar in both sexes {391}.
Glutathione S-transferase M1 (GSTM1) null status is associated with a modest increase in the risk of bladder cancer {700}.

Occupational exposure
Bladder cancer is associated with a number of occupations or occupational exposures. The first such association was observed in 1895 by Rehn, who reported high rates of bladder cancer among men employed in the aniline dye industry {617}. Subsequent research among dyestuffs workers identified the aromatic amines benzidine and 2-naphthylamine, and possibly 1-naphthylamine, as bladder carcinogens {1150}. It has been estimated that contact with occupational carcinogens causes up to 25% of all bladder tumours {2025}.

Phenacetin
Several epidemiological studies indicate that chronic abuse of analgesics containing phenacetin greatly enhance the risk of developing urothelial cancer of the renal pelvis, ureter and bladder. The relative risk has been estimated in the range of 2.4 to more than 6 {1150}. Early cases have been reported from Scandanavia {253,460}, Switzerland {1729} and Australia {1668}.

Medicinal drugs
The cytostatic agent, cyclophosphamide, has long been associated with the development of leukemia and lymphoma. In addition, treatment with cyclophosphamide has been reported to be associated with an increased risk of squamous cell carcinomas and sarcomas, especially leiomyosarcomas {1150, 2577}. Similarly, chlornaphazine is associated with the development of bladder cancer {2606}.

Chronic infections
Chronic cystitis caused by *Schistosoma haematobium* is an established cause of bladder cancer. The resultant bladder tumours are usually squamous cells carcinomas.
Some authors suggested association between bladder cancer and urinary tract infections and urinary tract stones.

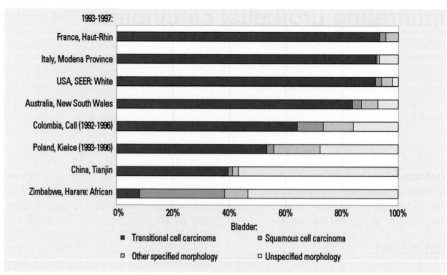

Fig. 2.02 Relative frequency of major histological types of bladder tumours in females. From D.M. Parkin et al. {2016}.

The underlying mechanism may lead to chronic irritation of the bladder epithelium, which may increase bladder cancer risk.

Arsenic
Several studies showed that use of drinking water containing chlorination by-products or contaminated by arsenic may increase risk of bladder cancer {367,1117,1150,2444}. An IARC Monographs Working Group reviewed in 2004 the relevant epidemiological studies and concluded that arsenic in drinking-water is carcinogenic to humans (Group 1) and that there is sufficient evidence that it

Table 2.01
Alphabetical list of agents, mixtures or exposure circumstances associated with bladder cancer.

Aluminium production
4-Aminobiphenyl
Analgesic mixtures containing phenacetin
Arsenic in drinking water
Auramine manufacture
Benzidine
Chlornaphazine
Coal gasification
Coal-tar pitch
Cyclophosphamide
Magenta manufacture
2-Naphthylamine
Rubber industry
Schistosoma haematobium (infection)
Tobacco smoke

Compiled from the IARC Monographs on the Evaluation of Carcinogenic Risks to Humans. The above exposures have been classified into IARC Group-1 (carcinogenic to humans).

causes urinary bladder cancer. Key evidence came from ecological studies in Chile and Taiwan (China) where large populations were exposed {1157}.

Coffee
There is no clear evidence of carcinogenic effect of coffee or caffeine in experimental animals {1151}, but some epidemiological studies in humans showed elevated risk in coffee drinkers as compared with non-coffee drinkers. {1027}. A recent study showed increased risk of bladder cancer caused by coffee drinking only in never smokers, while no increase of risk was observed in ever smokers {2840}.

Artificial sweeteners
There is no convincing evidence that artificial sweeteners (such as saccharin) play a role in the etiology of bladder cancer {1877}. The IARC currently classifies saccharin in group 3, i.e. not classifiable as to its carcinogenicity to humans {1155}.

Clinical features
Signs and symptoms
The type and severity of clinical signs and symptoms of infiltrating urothelial carcinoma depends on the extent and location of the tumour. Most patients with urothelial tumours present with at least microscopic hematuria {1718}.
The most common presenting symptom of *bladder* cancer is painless gross hematuria which occurs in 85% of patients {2713}. Subsequent clotting and

painful micturition may occur. In case of large tumours bladder capacity may be reduced resulting in frequency. Tumours located at the bladder neck or covering a large area of the bladder may lead to irritative symptoms, i.e. dysuria, urgency and frequency. Similar symptoms may be present in the case of extensive carcinoma in situ. Tumours infiltrating the ureteral orifice may lead to hydronephrosis, which is considered a poor prognostic sign {999}. Rarely, patients with extensive disease present with a palpable pelvic mass or lower extremity oedema. In case of advanced disease weight loss or abdominal or bone pain may be present due to metastases.

Although diagnosis of a bladder neoplasm may sometimes be suspected on ultrasound or computed tomography scan, it is confirmed on cystoscopy. Histological diagnosis is secured by resecting the tumour deep into the muscular layer of the bladder wall. A fraction of patients with T1 disease may be treated by repeat transurethral resection alone. However, in case of extensive disease most patients are candidates for potentially curative treatment.

Upper tract tumours occur in less than 10% of patients with bladder tumours. Microscopic hematuria may be the first clinical signs of infiltrating tumours of the renal pelvis and ureter and roughly half of the patients present with gross hematuria {94}. In case of blood clotting obstruction may be acute and lead to painful ureteral flank colic and can be mistaken for ureterolithiasis. Hydronephrosis may result but may go clinically unnoticed if obstruction develops slowly. In case of a single kidney or bilateral obstruction anuria and renal insufficiency result.

In case of suspected upper urinary tract tumour radiological imaging (intravenous urogram or computed tomography) or endoscopic examination is advised {1405}. Approximately two thirds of the tumours are located in the distal ureter {146}. Standard treatment for upper tract tumours is nephroureterectomy including the ureteral orifice {25}, which recently is also performed laparoscopically {879}.

Primary infiltrating urothelial tumours of the urethra are rare. Conversely, approximately 15 % of patients with carcinoma in situ of the bladder present with prostatic urethral involvement {1907}. Occasionally, recurrent tumour is found in the urethral stump after cystectomy. Bloody discharge from the urethra requires endoscopic examination and surgical resection if tumour is found.

Imaging

Various imaging modalities are used not only for detection but also for staging of infiltrating urothelial carcinoma. They include ultrasound, intravenous urography (IVU), computed tomography (CT) and magnetic resonance imaging (MRI). Transabdominal ultrasonography of the bladder is quick, non-invasive, inexpensive and available in most institutions. However, staging accuracy is less than 70% for infiltrating bladder tumours {598}. Sensitivity reaches only 63%, yet with a specificity of 99% {554}. There is a high false negative rate for ultrasound examination because of tumour location, obesity of the patient or postoperative changes. Transurethral ultrasonography may increase accuracy to >95% for T2 and T3 bladder tumours {1357}. Endoureteric sonographic evaluation of ureteral and renal pelvic neoplasms is technically feasible {1515}. However, as endoluminal sonography is invasive and examiner dependent it is not routinely used. Iliac lymph nodes cannot be assessed reliably on ultrasound.

While IVU is reliable in diagnosing intraluminal processes in ureter, pelvis and – with lesser accuracy – in bladder, it fails to detect the extent of extramural tumour. In addition IVU misses many extraluminal pathologic processes (such as renal mass) and, therefore, has increasingly been replaced by CT and MRI {96}. In most institutions CT is used as a primary staging tool as it is more accessible and more cost effective than MRI. However, both CT and MRI scanning often fail to differentiate between post-transurethral resection oedema and tumour {168}. Staging accuracy of CT has been described in the range of 55% for urothelial carcinoma in the urinary bladder {1997}. Understaging of lymph node metastases in up to 40% and overstaging 6% of the cases are the major causes of error. Spiral CT has increased accuracy as breathing artefacts are diminished. Enhanced computing methods bear the potential to improve accuracy by transforming data into three dimensional images allowing for "virtual" endoscopy {765}. MRI appears to be somewhat better to assess the depth of intramural invasion and extravesical tumour growth but does not exceed 83% {2454}.

Unlike in other tumours diagnostic accuracy of positron emission tomography (PET) in patients with invasive carcinoma of the bladder is poor {1481}.

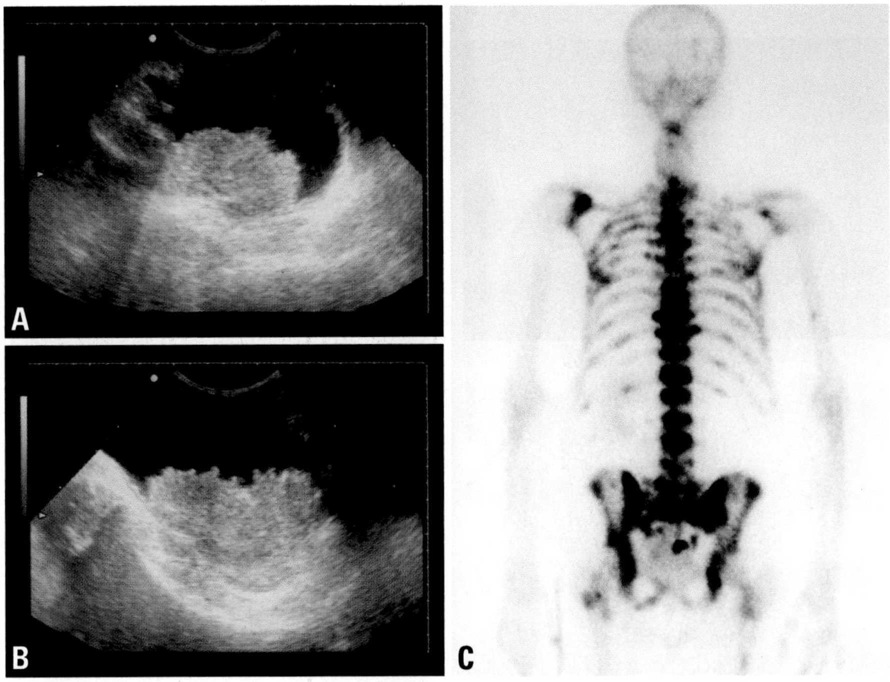

Fig. 2.03 Infiltrative urothelial carcinoma. **A,B** Ultrasound images of a solid bladder tumour. Bladder (black) with tumour (white) protruding into the lumen. **C** Multiple metastases (hot spots) of the bone.

Tumour spread and staging
Urinary bladder

T category

Cystoscopy provides a limited role in the staging process {468,1085,2302}. Transurethral resection (TURB) of all visible lesions down to the base is required for accurate assessment of depth of tumour invasion. pT categorization in TURB allows for recognition of pT1 and pT2 disease but the definitive categorization requires examination of the cystectomy specimen. Tumour infiltrating muscle is not equivalent to muscularis propria invasion as small slender fascicles of muscle are frequently present in lamina propria (muscularis mucosae) {2203}. Tumour infiltrating the adipose tissue is not always indicative of extravesical extension as fat may be normally present in all layers of the bladder wall {2069}.

The impact of additional random biopsies remains unclear {751}. In case of positive urine cytology without a visible lesion or evidence of upper urinary tract tumours random biopsies from different areas of the bladder wall are taken to detect Tis bladder cancer.

Re-biopsy 1-6 weeks after the primary resection is most often performed in large pTa and all pT1 tumours {411,540, 645,1332,2323}.

The role of intravenous pyelography for detecting simultaneous tumours of the upper urinary tract (UUT) and/or ureteral obstruction is controversial {63,901}. The accuracy of imaging techniques (CT, MRI, PET) for determining the T-category is limited {234,394,1050,1997,2402, 2651,2864}. Bimanual palpation to diagnose organ-exceeding tumours has lost its impact.

N category

The impact of CT and MRI {352,2740, 2746} has been investigated in numerous studies, however, sensitivity and specificity of these techniques remains limited. Nevertheless, lymph node enlargement is highly predictive of metastatic disease. The use of CT-guided needle biopsy of lymph nodes has been reported {239}.

Pelvic lymph node dissection up to the aortic bifurcation represents the state-of-art procedure. Furthermore, a potential therapeutic impact has been assigned to this procedure {2102,2732,2733}. Modifications, i.e. sentinel lymph node resection or laparascopic lymph node dissection for N-staging are considered experimental {686,2387}.

M category

In muscle-invasive tumours lung X-ray and exclusion of liver metastases by imaging (ultrasound, CT, MRI) are required. Skeletal scintigraphy for the detection of bone metastases should be performed in symptomatic patients. In T1 disease, M-staging is recommended before cystectomy.

Upper urinary tract tumours

T category

T-staging of tumours of the upper urinary tract tumours is performed after radical surgery in the vast majority of cases or after endoscopical tumour resection. Imaging procedures (CT, MRI) may be of value {838,2089}.

To identify simultaneous bladder tumours cystoscopy of these patients is mandatory {99,319}.

N category

N-staging is performed by imaging techniques (CT, MRI) and by lymph node dissection {1349,1747,1750}.

M category

Because of similarities with bladder tumours {552,1137}, M-staging in upper urinary tract tumours follows the same rules.

Prostatic and urethral urothelial tumours

T category

T-staging of urothelial tumours of the prostate ducts or urethra is performed after biopsy or after radical surgery. Imaging procedures (CT, MRI) may be helpful {771}.

Because of the coincidence of simultaneous bladder tumours cystoscopy of these patients is mandatory {99,119}.

N category

N-staging is performed by imaging techniques (CT, MRI) or by lymph node dissection {542}. Specifically for meatal or distal urethral tumours the inguinal region must be considered.

M category

In general, M-staging in urothelial tumours of the prostate or urethra follows the same rules as in bladder tumours.

Macroscopy

Infiltrative carcinomas grossly span a range from papillary, polypoid, nodular, solid, ulcerative or transmural diffuse growth. They may be solitary or multifocal. The remaining mucosa may be nor-

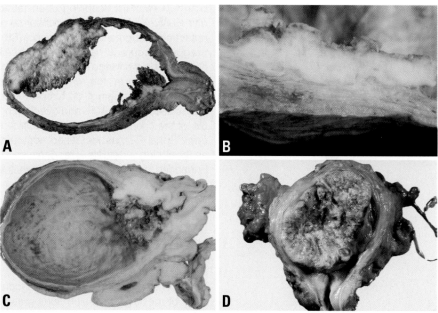

Fig. 2.04 Invasive urothelial carcinoma. **A** Papillary and invasive bladder carcinoma. **B** Invasive urothelial carcinoma with infiltration of the muscular bladder wall. **C** Invasive urothelial carcinoma with deep infiltration of the bladder wall. **D** Ulcerative carcinoma. Cystectomy specimen, ulcerative gross type of carcinoma.

mal or erythematous which sometimes represents the microscopic areas of carcinoma in situ.

Histopathology

The histology of infiltrating urothelial carcinomas is variable {80,293,944}. Most of pT1 cancers are papillary, low or high grade, whereas most pT2-T4 carcinomas are non-papillary and high grade.

These carcinomas are graded as low grade and high grade depending upon the degree of nuclear anaplasia and some architectural abnormalities {706, 1548,1798}. Some cases may show relatively bland cytology {2896}.

The most important element in pathologic evaluation of urothelial cancer is recognition of the presence and extent of invasion {293}. In early invasive urothelial carcinomas (pT1), foci of invasion are characterized by nests, clusters, or single cells within the papillary cores and/or lamina propria. It is recommended that the extent of lamina propria invasion in pT1 tumours should be stated {706}. The depth of lamina propria invasion is regarded as a prognostic parameter in pT1 cancer. Morphologic criteria useful in assessing of lamina propria invasion include the presence of desmoplastic stromal response, tumour cells within the retraction spaces, and paradoxical differentiation (invasive nests of cells with abundant eosinophilic cytoplasm at the advancing edge of infiltration {2117}). Recognition of invasion may be problematic because of tangential sectioning, thermal and mechanical injury, marked inflammatory infiltrate obscuring neoplastic cells and inverted or broad front growth {78}. Thermal artefact can also hamper the interpretation of muscularis propria invasion.

The histology of infiltrative urothelial carcinoma has no specific features and shows infiltrating cohesive nests of cells with moderate to abundant amphophilic cytoplasm and large hyperchromatic nuclei. In larger nests, palisading of nuclei may be seen at the edges of the nests. The nucleus is typically pleomorphic and often has irregular contours with angular profiles. Nucleoli are highly variable in number and appearance with some cells containing single or multiple small nucleoli and others having large eosinophilic nucleoli. Foci of marked pleomorphism may be seen, with bizarre and multinuclear tumour cells {293}. Mitotic figures are common, with numerous abnormal forms. The invasive nests usually induce a desmoplastic stromal reaction which is occasionally pronounced and may mimic a malignant spindle cell component, a feature known as pseudosarcomatous stromal reaction {1555}. In most cases, the stroma contains a lymphocytic infiltrate with a variable number of plasma cells. The inflammation is usually mild to moderate and focal, although it may be severe, dense, and widespread. Neutrophils and eosinophils are rarely prominent. Retraction clefts are often present around the nests of carcinoma cells, mimicking vascular invasion. It is important to be aware of this feature in order to avoid misinterpretation as vascular invasion. Foci of squamous and glandular differentiation are common, and should be reported {1554,2177,2276}. Intraepithelial neoplasia including carcinoma in situ is common in the adjacent urothelium {1547,1552}. Occasionally, mucoid cytoplasmic inclusions may be present.

Histologic variants

Urothelial carcinoma has a propensity for divergent differentiation with the most common being squamous followed by glandular. Virtually the whole spectrum of bladder cancer variants may be seen in variable proportions accompanying otherwise typical urothelial carcinoma. Divergent differentiation frequently parallels high grade and high stage urothelial cancer. When small cell differentiation is present, even focally, it portends a poor prognosis and has different therapeutic ramifications, and hence should be diagnosed as small cell carcinoma.

Infiltrating urothelial carcinoma with squamous differentiation

Squamous differentiation, defined by the presence of intercellular bridges or keratinization, occurs in 21% of urothelial carcinomas of the bladder, and in 44% of tumours of the renal pelvis {1554,1637}. Its frequency increases with grade and stage {1554}. Detailed histologic maps of urothelial carcinoma with squamous differentiation have shown that the proportion of the squamous component may vary considerably, with some cases having urothelial carcinoma in situ as the only urothelial component {2276}. The diagnosis of squamous cell carcinoma is reserved for pure lesions without any associated urothelial component, including urothelial carcinoma in situ {2177}. Tumours with any identifiable urothelial element are classified as urothelial carcinoma with squamous differentiation {1554,2177} and an estimate of the percentage of squamous component should be provided. Squamous differentiation may show basaloid or clear cell features. Cytokeratin 14 and L1 antigen have been reported as immunohistochemical markers of squamous differentiation {1025, 2655}. Uroplakins, are expressed in urothelial carcinoma and not in squamous differentiation {2848}.

The clinical significance of squamous differentiation remains uncertain, but seems to be an unfavourable prognostic

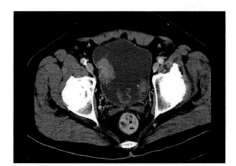

Fig. 2.05 Infiltrative urothelial carcinoma. CT image of a solid bladder tumour protruding into the lumen.

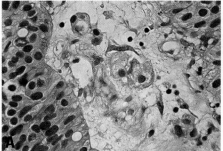
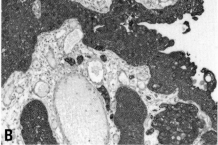

Fig. 2.06 Infiltrative urothelial carcinoma (stage T1). **A** Early tumour invasion into papillary stalk (H&E). **B** Immunohistochemistry with anticytokeratin may aid in establishing early tumour invasion.

feature in such patients undergoing radical cystectomy, possibly, because of its association with high grade tumours {336}. Squamous differentiation was predictive of a poor response to radiation therapy and possibly also to systemic chemotherapy {336,1637,2276}.

Infiltrating urothelial carcinoma with glandular differentiation

Glandular differentiation is less common than squamous differentiation and may be present in about 6% of urothelial carcinomas of the bladder {1554}. Glandular differentiation is defined as the presence of true glandular spaces within the tumour. These may be tubular or enteric glands with mucin secretion. A colloid-mucinous pattern characterized by nests of cells "floating" in extracellular mucin occasionally with signet ring cells may be present {1554}. Pseudoglandular spaces caused by necrosis or artefact should not be considered evidence of glandular differentiation. Cytoplasmic mucin containing cells are present in 14-63% of typical urothelial carcinoma and are not considered to represent glandular differentiation {633}. The diagnosis of adenocarcinoma is reserved for pure tumours {2177}. A tumour with mixed glandular and urothelial differentiation is classified as urothelial carcinoma with glandular differentiation {923} and an estimate of the percentage of glandular component should be provided. The expression of MUC5AC-apomucin may be useful as immunohistochemical marker of glandular differentiation in urothelial tumours {1408}.

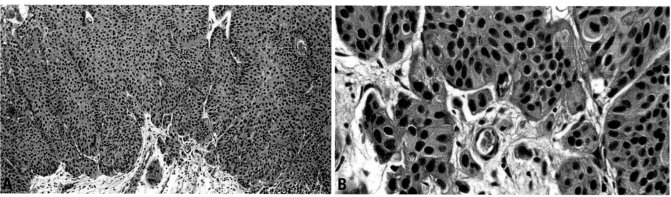

Fig. 2.07 A,B Infiltrative urothelial carcinoma. Early invasion not reaching muscularis mucosae (pT1a).

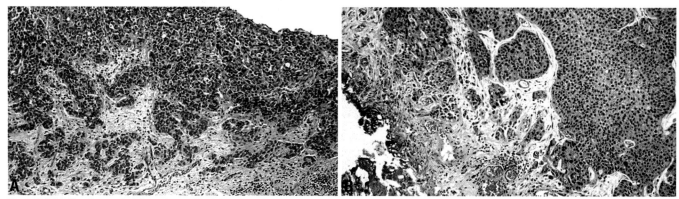

Fig. 2.08 A,B Infiltrative urothelial carcinoma. The infiltration of lamina propria goes beyond the muscularis mucosae (pT1b).

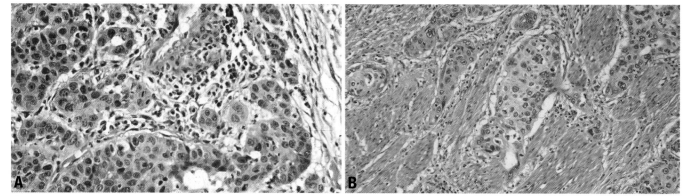

Fig. 2.09 Infiltrative urothelial carcinoma. **A** Invasive urothelial carcinoma grade 3. **B** Islands of high grade urothelial carcinoma extending through the muscularis propria (detrusor muscle).

The clinical significance of glandular differentiation and mucin positivity in urothelial carcinoma remains uncertain {1528}.

Nested variant

The nested variant of urothelial carcinoma is an aggressive neoplasm with less than 50 reported cases {639,1109,1848, 2562,2896}. There is a marked male predominance {639}, and 70% of patients died 4-40 months after diagnosis, in spite of therapy {1109}. This rare pattern of urothelial carcinoma was first described as a tumour with a "deceptively benign" appearance that closely resembles Brunn nests infiltrating the lamina propria. Some nests have small tubular lumens {2562,2896}. Nuclei generally show little or no atypia, but invariably the tumour contains foci of unequivocal anaplastic cells exhibiting enlarged nucleoli and coarse nuclear chromatin {639,1848}. This feature is most apparent in deeper aspects of the tumour {1848}.

Useful features in recognizing this lesion as malignant are the tendency for increasing cellular anaplasia in the deeper aspects of the lesion, its infiltrative nature, and the frequent presence of muscle invasion. The differential diagnosis of the nested variant of urothelial carcinoma includes prominent Brunn nests, cystitis cystica and glandularis, inverted papilloma, nephrogenic metaplasia, carcinoid tumour, paraganglionic tissue and paraganglioma {639,1109,1848,2562, 2896}. The presence of deep invasion is most useful in distinguishing carcinoma from benign proliferations, and the nuclear atypia, which is occasionally present is also of value. Closely packed and irregularly distributed small tumour cells favour carcinoma. Inverted papilloma lacks a nested architecture. Nephrogenic metaplasia typically has a mixed pattern, including tubular, papillary, and other components, and only rarely has deep muscle invasion {639}.

The nested variant of carcinoma may mimic paraganglioma, but the prominent vascular network of paraganglioma, which surrounds individual nests, is not usually present in nested carcinoma.

Microcystic variant

Occasionally urothelial carcinomas show a striking cystic pattern with cysts ranging from microscopic up to 1-2 mm in diameter. The cysts are round to oval, sometimes elongated and may contain necrotic material or pale pink secretions. The cyst lining may be absent, flattened or urothelial and may show the differentiation towards mucinous cells. The differential diagnosis therefore includes urothelial carcinoma with gland like lumina, as well as benign processes like cystitis cystica, cystitis glandularis or even nephrogenic adenoma. The pattern should be separated from the nested variant of urothelial carcinoma with tubular differentiation. Urothelial carcinoma

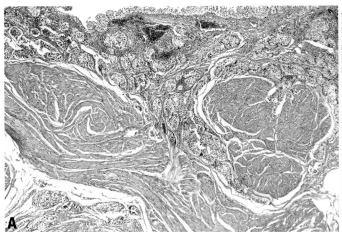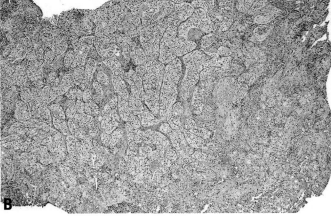

Fig. 2.10 A,B Nested cell variant of urothelial carcinoma of the urinary bladder.

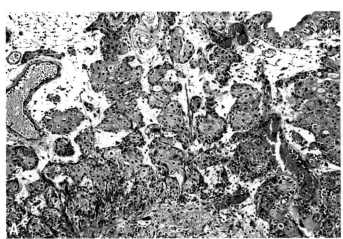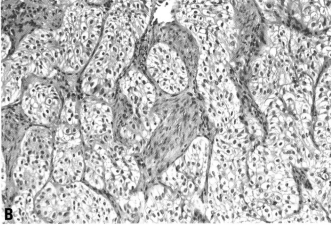

Fig. 2.11 A, B Infiltrative urothelial carcinoma. Nested variant.

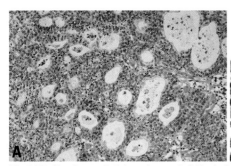
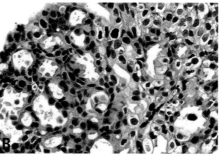

Fig. 2.12 Infiltrative urothelial carcinoma. **A, B** Urothelial carcinoma of the bladder, microcystic variant characterized by the formation of microcysts, macrocysts, or tubular structures containing cellular debris and/or mucin (H&E).

with microcystic pattern is unrelated to primary adenocarcinoma of the urinary bladder {656,1480,2891}.

Micropapillary variant
Micropapillary bladder carcinoma is a distinct variant of urothelial carcinoma that resembles papillary serous carcinoma of the ovary, and approximately 60 cases were reported in the literature {81,1228,1558,1622,1941,2876}. There is a male predominance and patients age range from fifth to the ninth decade with a mean age of 66 years. The most common presenting symptom is hematuria.
Histologically, micropapillary growth pattern is almost always associated with conventional urothelial carcinoma or rarely with adenocarcinoma. The micropapillary pattern exhibits two distinct morphologic features. Slender-delicate fine papillary and filiform processes, often with a central vascular core, are observed on the surface of the tumours: on cross sections they exhibit a glomeruloid appearance. In contrast, the invasive portion is characterized by tiny nests of cells or slender papillae, which are contained within tissue retraction spaces that simulate lymphatic spaces. However, in most cases vascular/lymphatic invasion is present. The individual cells of micropapillary carcinoma show nuclei with prominent nucleoli and irregular distribution of the chromatin. Also, the cytoplasm is abundant, eosinophilic or clear, and mitotic figures range from few to numerous. Although the nuclear grade is frequently high, a few micropapillary carcinomas may appear deceptively low grade {81}.
Immunohistochemical studies in one large series disclosed immunoreactivity of the micropapillary carcinoma in 20 of 20 cases for EMA, cytokeratin (CK) 7, CK

20, and Leu M1. CEA was positive in 13 of 20 cases {1228}. Other markers including CA-125 antigen, B72.3, BerEp4, placental alkaline phosphatase immunoreacted in less than one third of the cases {1228}. Psammoma bodies are infrequent. The tumours are invariably muscle invasive and this histology is often retained in the histology of metastases. Image analysis shows aneuploidy. Micropapillary carcinoma is a high grade, high stage variant of urothelial

cancer with high incidence of metastases and morbidity. The presence of a micropapillary surface component or lamina propria invasive tumour without muscularis propria in the specimen should prompt suggestion for rebiopsy because of the high association of muscularis propria invasion. Awareness of the micropapillary histology is important when dealing with metastases of unknown primary. Urothelial carcinoma with micropapillary component must be considered as a primary especially in males and women with normal gynecologic examination {81,1228}.

Lymphoepithelioma-like carcinoma
Carcinoma that histologically resembles lymphoepithelioma of the nasopharynx has recently been described in the urinary bladder, with fewer than 40 cases reported {1106,1553}. These tumours are more common in men than in women (10:3, ratio) and occur in late adulthood (range: 52-81 years, mean 69 years). Most patients present with hematuria and are stage T2-T3 at diagnosis {1106,

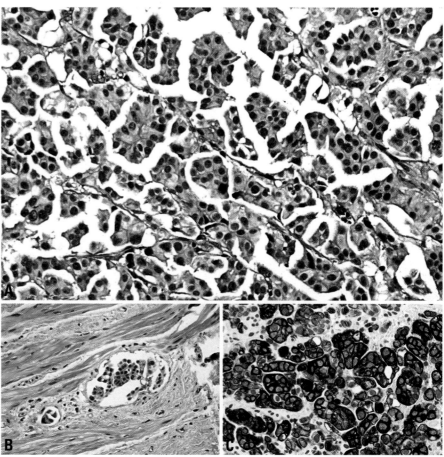

Fig. 2.13 A, B, C Micropapillary urothelial carcinoma. Papillary tumours. **C** CK 7 expression.

1553}. The etiopathogenesis of this tumour is unknown, although it is suspected that it originates from modified urothelial cells, that are possibly derived from basal (stem) cells {1106}. Hybridization with Epstein-Barr virus encoded RNA has been reported to be consistently negative in different series {82,973,1106,1553}. The tumour is solitary and usually involves the dome, posterior wall, or trigone, often with a sessile growth pattern.

Lymphoepithelioma-like carcinoma may be pure, predominant or focally admixed with typical urothelial carcinoma, or in some cases with squamous cell carcinoma or adenocarcinoma {1106,1553}. The proportion of lymphoepithelioma-like carcinoma histology should be provided in tumours with mixed histology. Histologically, the tumour is composed of nests, sheets, and cords of undifferentiated cells with large pleomorphic nuclei and prominent nucleoli. The cytoplasmic borders are poorly defined imparting a syncytial appearance. The background consists of a prominent lymphoid stroma that includes T and B lymphocytes, plasma cells, histiocytes, and occasional neutrophils or eosinophils, the latter being prominent in rare cases. Carcinoma in situ elsewhere in the bladder is rarely present.

The epithelial cells of this tumour stain with several cytokeratin (CK) markers as follows: AE1/AE3, CK8, CK 7, and they are rarely positive for CK20 {1106,1553}. In some cases, it is possible to overlook the malignant cells in the background of inflamed bladder wall and misdiagnose the condition as florid chronic cystitis {1553}.

The major differential diagnostic considerations are poorly differentiated urothelial carcinoma with lymphoid stroma; poorly differentiated squamous cell carcinoma, and lymphoma {1553}. The presence of recognizable urothelial or squamous cell carcinoma does not exclude lymphoepithelioma-like carcinoma; rather, the diagnosis is based on finding areas typical of lymphoepithelioma-like carcinoma reminiscent of that in the nasopharynx. Differentiation from lymphoma may be difficult, but the presence of a syncytial pattern of large malignant cells with a dense polymorphous lymphoid background is an important clue {1553}.

Most reported cases of the urinary bladder had a relatively favourable prognosis

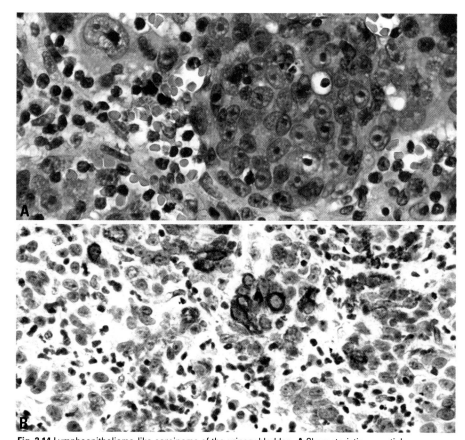

Fig. 2.14 Lymphoepithelioma-like carcinoma of the urinary bladder. **A** Characteristic syncytial appearance of neoplastic cells (H&E). **B** Note the characteristic immunostaining with CK.

when pure or predominant, but when lymphoepithelioma-like carcinoma is focally present in an otherwise typical urothelial carcinoma, these patients behave like patients with conventional urothelial carcinoma alone of the same grade and stage {1106,1553}. Some examples of lymphoepithelioma-like carcinoma have been described in the ureter and the renal pelvis {820,2224}.

This tumour, thus far has been found to be responsive to chemotherapy when it is encountered in its pure form {82,623}. Experience at one institution has shown a complete response to chemotherapy and transurethral resection of the bladder {82,623}. Another series of nine patients treated with a combination of transurethral resection, partial or complete cystectomy, and radiotherapy disclosed four patients without evidence of disease, three who died of their disease and two who died of other causes {1106}.

Lymphoma-like and plasmacytoid variants

The lymphoma-like and plasmacytoid variants of urothelial carcinoma are those

in which the malignant cells resemble those of malignant lymphoma or plasmacytoma {1618,2272,2571,2933,2949}.

Less than 10 cases have been reported. The histologic features of the lymphoma-like and plasmacytoid variants of urothelial carcinoma are characterized by the presence of single malignant cells in a loose or myxoid stroma. The tumour cells have clear or eosinophilic cytoplasm and eccentrically placed, enlarged hyperchromatic nuclei with small nucleoli. Almost all of the reported cases have had a component of high grade urothelial carcinoma in addition to the single malignant cells. In some of the cases, the single-cell component was predominant on the initial biopsy, leading to the differential diagnosis of lymphoma/plasmacytoma. The tumour cells stain with cytokeratin (CK) cocktail, CK 7 and (in some cases) CK 20 {2571}. Immunohistochemical stains for lymphoid markers have consistently been reported as negative.

Each of these variants of urothelial carcinoma may cause a significant differential diagnostic dilemma, especially in cases in which it constitutes the predominant or

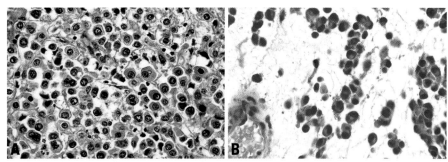

Fig. 2.15 A Infiltrating urothelial carcinoma of the bladder, plasmocytoid variant. **B** Plasmacytoid variant of urothelial carcinoma of the urinary bladder.

exclusive component in a small biopsy sample. The importance of recognizing these variants lies in not mistaking them as a lymphoma or plasmacytoma. Limited information is available about the outcome of patients with these variants of urothelial carcinoma. Of 6 cases reported by Tamboli et al. {2571} 4 died of their disease, one died post-operatively and one is alive without evidence of disease.

Sarcomatoid variant
(with/without heterologous elements)

The term sarcomatoid variant of urothelial carcinoma should be used for all biphasic malignant neoplasms exhibiting morphologic and/or immunohistochemical evidence of epithelial and mesenchymal differentiation (with the presence or absence of heterologous elements acknowledged in the diagnosis). There is considerable confusion and disagreement in the literature regarding nomenclature and histogenesis of these tumours. In some series, both carcinosarcoma and sarcomatoid carcinoma are included as "sarcomatoid carcinoma" {2175}. In others they are regarded as separate entities.

The mean age is 66 years (range, 50-77 years old) and most patients present with hematuria {1555,2175}. A previous history of carcinoma treated by radiation or the exposition to cyclophosphamide therapy is common {1551}. Rare examples of carcinosarcoma and sarcomatoid carcinomas have been described in the ureter and the renal pelvis {1549}.

The gross appearance is characteristically "sarcoma-like", dull grey with infiltrative margins. The tumours are often polypoid with large intraluminal masses. Microscopically, sarcomatoid carcinoma is composed of urothelial, glandular or small cell component showing variable degrees of differentiation {1555}. A small

subset of sarcomatoid carcinoma may have a prominent myxoid stroma {1238}. The mesenchymal component most frequently observed is an undifferentiated high grade spindle cell neoplasm. The most common heterologous element is osteosarcoma followed by chondrosarcoma, rhabdomyosarcoma, leiomyosarcoma, liposarcoma angiosarcoma or multiple types of heterologous differentiation may be present {957,1238,1549, 1555,2175}. By immunohistochemistry, epithelial elements react with cytokeratins, whereas stromal elements react with vimentin or specific markers corresponding to the mesenchymal differentiation. The sarcomatoid phenotype retains the epithelial nature of the cells by immunohistochemistry or electronmi-

croscopy {1549,1555}. Recent molecular studies, strongly argue for a monoclonal origin of both components {957}.

The cytological atypia of sarcomatoid carcinoma excludes non-neoplastic lesions such as the postoperative spindle cell nodule and inflammatory pseudotumour {1161,1550}. Sarcomatoid carcinoma should be distinguished from the rare carcinoma with metaplastic, benign-appearing bone or cartilage in the stroma or those showing other pseudosarcomatous stromal reactions.

Nodal and distant organ metastases at diagnosis are common {957,1555,1960, 2175} and 70% of patients died of cancer at 1 to 48 months (mean 17 months) {1555}

Urothelial carcinoma with giant cells

High grade urothelial carcinoma may contain epithelial tumour giant cells or the tumour may appear undifferentiated resembling giant cell carcinoma of the lung. This variant is very infrequent. It must be distinguished from occasional cases showing giant cells (osteoclastic or foreign body type) in the stroma or urothelial carcinoma showing trophoblastic differentiation. In some cases the giant cell reaction is so extensive that it may mimic giant cell tumour of the bone {2948}.

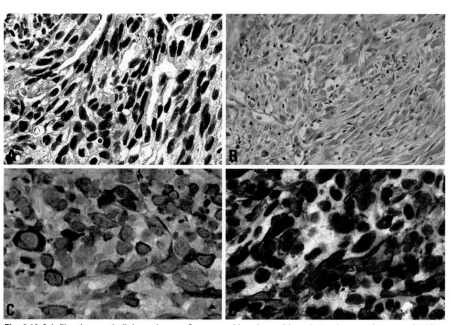

Fig. 2.16 A Infiltrative urothelial carcinoma. Sarcomatoid variant without heterologous elements showing spindle cell morphology. **B** Infiltrating urothelial carcinoma of the bladder. Sarcomatoid variant with heterologous smooth muscle elements. **C** Immunohistochemical expression of cytokeratin AE1/AE3 in a case of sarcomatoid carcinoma of the urinary bladder (same case as in panel A). **D** Immunohistochemical expression of smooth muscle actin of the sarcomatoid carcinoma shown in panel B.

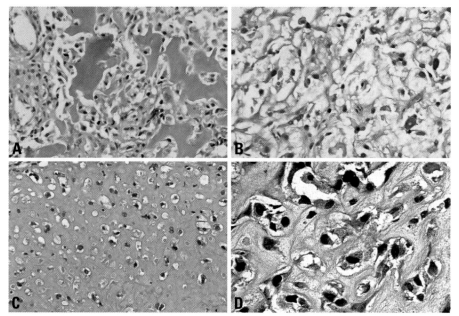

Fig. 2.17 A, B Infiltrating urothelial carcinoma of the bladder. Sarcomatoid variant with heterologous elements of osteosarcoma and myxoid sarcoma. **C, D** Infiltrating urothelial carcinoma of the bladder. Sarcomatoid variant with heterologous elements of chondrosarcoma showing binucleation and atypical chondrocytes within lacunae.

Urothelial carcinoma with trophoblastic differentiation

Trophoblastic differentiation in urothelial carcinoma occurs at different levels. High grade invasive urothelial carcinomas may express ectopic human chorionic gonadotropin (HCG) and other placental glycoproteins at the immunohistochemical level only or may contain numerous syncytiotrophoblastic giant cells {365,656,925,2891}. Very rarely, choriocarcinomatous differentiation has been reported.

Clear cell variant

The clear cell variant of urothelial carcinoma is defined by a clear cell pattern with glycogen-rich cytoplasm {1365, 1954}. The clear cell pattern may be focal or extensive and awarness of this pattern is important in differential diagnosis with clear cell adenocarcinoma of the urinary bladder and metastatic carcinoma from the kidney and prostate. The pattern may be seen in typical papillary or in situ lesions, but is relatively more common in poorly differentiated urothelial carcinomas.

Lipid-cell variant

Very infrequently urothelial carcinomas contain abundant lipid in which lipid distended cells mimic signet ring cell adenocarcinoma {1798}. The differential diagnosis is typical liposarcoma and signet ring cell carcinoma.

Undifferentiated carcinoma

This category contains tumours that cannot be otherwise classified. In our experience, they are extremely rare. Earlier the literature has included small cell carcinoma, giant cell carcinoma, and lymphoepithelioma-like carcinoma in this category, but these tumours are now recognized as specific tumour variants {656,1553}. Large cell undifferentiated carcinoma as in the lung is rare in the urinary tract, and those with neuroendocrine features should be recognized as a specific tumour variant {2816}.

Genetic susceptibility

Urothelial carcinoma is not considered to be a familial disease. However numerous reports have described families with multiple cases {1313,1669}. There is strong evidence for an increased risk of ureteral and renal pelvic urothelial carcinomas, but not bladder cancers, in families with hereditary nonpolyposis colon cancer {2411,2789}. In addition several epidemiological studies showed that urothelial carcinomas have a familial component with a 1.5 to 2-fold increased risk among first-degree relatives of patients {23,905, 1312,1387}. The only constitutional genetic aberration demonstrated so far in a family with urothelial carcinomas in two generation was a t(5;20)(p15;q11) balanced translocation {2336}. No chro-

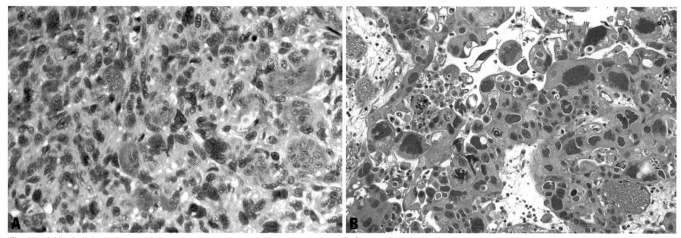

Fig. 2.18 A Urothelial carcinoma, high grade with giant cells of osteoclastic type. **B** Giant cells in Infiltrating urothelial carcinoma of the bladder.

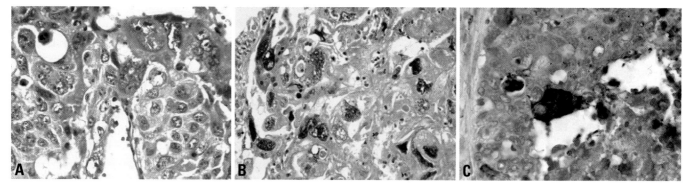

Fig. 2.19 A Infiltrative urothelial carcinoma. Urothelial carcinoma with trophoblastic differentiation. **B** Trophoblastic differentiation of urothelial cell carcinoma. Syncytiotrophoblastic malignant cells with high grade urothelial cancer. **C** Infiltrative urothelial carcinoma. Urothelial carcinoma with trophoblastic differentiation, HCG immunostaining.

mosomal alterations were found in 30 additional families with at least 2 affected individuals {22}. Interestingly, patients with sporadic urothelial carcinomas revealed a higher mutagen sensitivity than controls whereas patients with hereditary bladder cancer demonstrated no increased mutagen sensitivity {21}. A small increase in bladder cancer risk was demonstrated for polymorphic variants of several detoxifying enzymes, like NAT2 and GSTM1 {700,1624}.

Somatic genetics

The genetic studies to date have used tumours classified according to WHO Tumours Classification (1973) and further studies are underway to link available genetic information to the current classification. It is assumed that invasive urothelial cancers are mostly derived from either non-invasive high grade papillary urothelial carcinoma (pTaG3) or urothelial carcinoma in situ. On the genetic level invasively growing urothelial cancer (stage pT1-4) is highly different from low grade non-invasive papillary tumours (Papillary Urothelial Neoplasm of Low Malignant Potential, Non-Invasive Low Grade Papillary Urothelial Carcinoma).

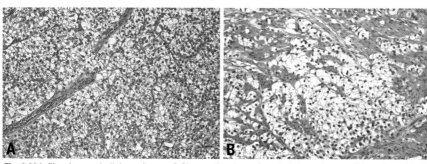

Fig. 2.20 Infiltrative urothelial carcinoma. **A** Clear cell variant of urothelial carcinoma of the urinary bladder. **B** Clear cell variant of urothelial carcinoma of the urinary bladder.

Chromosomal abnormalities

Invasively growing urothelial bladder cancer is characterized by presence of a high number of genetic alterations involving multiple different chromosomal regions. Studies using comparative genomic hybridization (CGH) have described an average of 7-10 alterations in invasive bladder cancer {2188,2189, 2191,2418,2419}. The most frequently observed gains and losses of chromosomal regions are separately summarized for cytogenetic, CGH, and LOH (loss of heterozygosity). Taken together, the data highlight losses of 2q, 5q, 8p, 9p, 9q, 10q, 11p, 18q and the Y chromosome as well as gains of 1q, 5p, 8q, and 17q as most consistent cytogenetic changes in these tumours.

The large size of most aberrations detected by CGH or cytogenetics makes

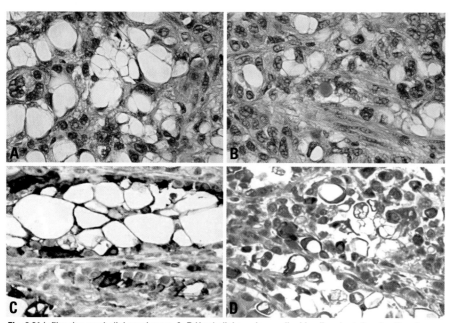

Fig. 2.21 Infiltrative urothelial carcinoma. **A, B** Urothelial carcinoma, lipoid cell variant showing the characteristic lipoblast-like features of proliferating cells (H&E). **C** Urothelial carcinoma, lipoid cell variant with immunohistochemical expression of cytokeratin 7 in most proliferating cells. **D** Urothelial carcinoma, lipoid cell variant with immunohistochemical expression of epithelial membrane antigen.

it difficult to identify genes leading to a selective growth advantage. The most important genes for bladder cancer development and progression remain to be discovered. Importantly, co-amplification and simultaneous overexpression of multiple adjacent oncogenes is often seen. For example, amplification of CCND1 at 11q13 can be accompanied by amplification of FGF4/FGF3 in 88% (R. Simon, personal communication), MDM2 amplification at 12q15 is accompanied by CDK4 amplification in 11% {2422}, and HER2 amplification at 17q23 includes TOP2A in 15%. Simultaneous overexpression of two or more adjacent genes may provide cells with a significant growth advantage.

Oncogenes

Her2/neu is a transmembrane receptor tyrosine kinase without a known ligand. Its activation occurs through interaction with other members of the *EGFR* gene family. HER2 has regained considerable interest as the protein is the molecular target of trastuzumab (Herceptin®) therapy in breast cancer. HER2 is amplified in 10-20% and overexpressed in 10-50% of invasively growing bladder cancers {225,489,836,914,1509,1527,1708,1974, 2152,2309}. This makes bladder cancer the tumour entity with the highest frequency of HER2 overexpression. In contrast to breast cancer, where HER2 overexpression is almost always due to gene amplification, the majority of HER2 positive bladder cancers are not amplified. The reason for Her2 overexpression is unknown in these tumours. Amplifications or deletions of the adjacent topoisomerase 2 alpha (TOP2A) are present in about 23% of HER2 amplified cases {2417}. TOP2A is the target of anthracyclines. Thus, the anatomy of the 17q23 amplicon may also influence the response to cytotoxic therapy regimens.

H-*ras* is the only member of the ras gene family with known importance in urinary bladder cancer {279,1397}. H-*ras* mutations are almost always confined to specific alterations within the codons 12, 13, and 61 {1484}. Depending on the method of detection, H-*ras* mutations have been reported in up to 45% of bladder cancers, without clear cut associations to tumour stage or grade {395,533, 772,1339,1341,1980}.

Table 2.02
Cytogenetic changes in pT1-4 urothelial carcinoma of the urinary bladder.

Chromosomal location	Frequency of alteration by		
	Karyo-typing [1]	CGH [2]	LOH
1p-	18%	n.a.	20%
1q+	11%	37-54%	
2p+	2%	8-30%	
2q-	13%	17-30%	58%
3p-	4%	2-9%	23%
3q+	7%	7-24%	
4p-	7%	8-21%	22%
4q-	4%	10-30%	26%
5p+	20%	24-25%	
5q-	9%	16-30%	6-50%
6p+	7%	16-24%	
6q-	18%	19%	27%
7p+	13%	20-23%	
8p-	16%	29%	18-83%
8q+	11%	37-54%	
9p-	22%	31-47%	33-82%
9q-	27%	23-47%	43-90%
10p+	4%	13-19%	
10q-	11%	18-28%	39-45%
11p-	11%	24-43%	9-72%
11q-	9%	22-34%	17-30%
12p+	4%	4-30%	
12q+	9%	14-30%	
13q-	18%	19-29%	15-32%
17p-	2%	19-24%	32-57%
17q+	4%	29-49%	
18q-	4%	13-30%	36-51%
20q+	7%	22-28%	
Y	11%	15-37%	

[1] Average frequency from 45 bladder cancers from references {131,132,148,216,868,869,1368,1731,2030,2289,2441,263 9,2709,2710}.
[2] Only large studies on invasive tumours (pT1-pT4; >50 analyzed tumours) included.
n.a. = not analyzed.

The *epidermal growth factor receptor* (EGFR) is another member of the class II receptor family. EGFR is a transmembrane tyrosine kinase acting as a receptor for several ligands including epidermal growth factor (EGF) and transforming growth factor alpha. EGFR also serves as a therapeutic target for several drugs including small inhibitory molecules and antibodies. *EGFR* is amplified in 3-5% and overexpressed in 30-50% of invasively growing bladder cancers {217, 457,914,1510,1890,2305,2844}.

Cyclin dependent kinases (CDKs) and their regulatory subunits, the cyclins, are important promoters of the cell cycle. The cyclin D1 gene (CCND1) located at 11q13 is one of the most frequently amplified and overexpressed oncogenes in bladder cancer. About 10-20% of bladder cancers show gene amplification {322,983,2114,2308}, and overexpression has been reported in 30-50% of tumours {1464,1991,2371,2394,2762}. Some investigators found associations between CCND1 expression and tumour recurrence and progression or patient survival {1984,2371,2394}, but these data were not confirmed by others {1517, 2540,2762}.

The *MDM2* gene, located at 12q14.3-q15, codes for more than 40 different splice variants, only two of which interact with TP53 and thereby inhibit its ability to activate transcription {173}. Conversely, the transcription of MDM2 is induced by wild type TP53. In normal cells this autoregulatory feedback loop regulates TP53 activity and MDM2 expression. MDM2 also promotes TP53 protein degradation, making *MDM2* overexpression an alternate mechanism for TP53 inactivation. *MDM2* amplification is frequent in human sarcomas {1270}, but it occurs in only 4-6% of invasively growing bladder cancers {983,2422}. *MDM2* amplification was unrelated to patient prognosis in one study {2422}. Detectable MDM2 protein expression has been reported in 10-40% of bladder cancers, but there is disagreement about associations to tumour stage and grade between the studies {1172,1206, 1358,1495,2067, 2068,2330, 2390}.

Tumour suppressor genes

Genes that provide a growth advantage to affected cells in case of reduced

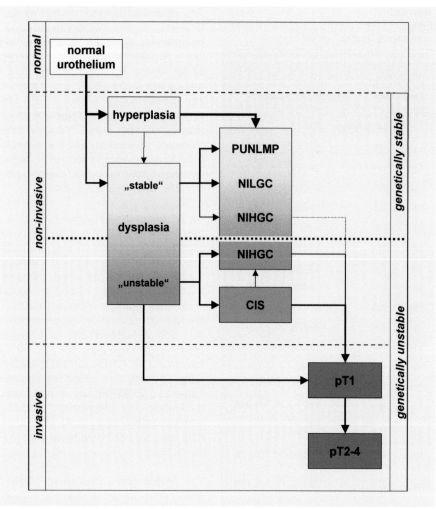

Fig. 2.22 Putative model of bladder cancer development and progression based on genetic findings. Thick arrows indicate the most frequent pathways, dotted lines the most rare events. The typical genetic alterations in genetically stable and unstable tumours are described in the text.

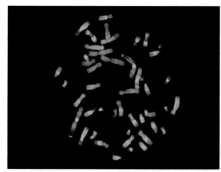

Fig. 2.23 Infiltrative urothelial carcinoma. FISH analysis of a human metaphase chromosome spread showing locus specific hybridization signals for the telomeric (green signals) and the centromeric (red signals) regions of chromosome 1. The chromosomes have been counterstained with 4,6-Diamidino-2-phenylindol (DAPI).

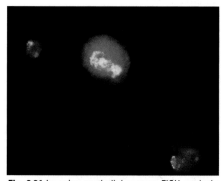

Fig. 2.24 Invasive urothelial cancer. FISH analysis shows two copies if centromere 17 (red) and more than 30 copies of the HER2 gene (green) reflecting HER2 gene amplification.

expression or inactivation are summarized below.

The *TP53* gene, located at 17q23 encodes a 53kDa protein which plays a role in several cellular processes including cell cycle, response to DNA damage, cell death, and neovascularization {1089}. Its gene product regulates the expression of multiple different genes {2757}. Mutations of the *TP53* gene, mostly located in the central, DNA binding portion of the gene, are a hallmark of invasively growing bladder cancers. An online query of the International Agency for Research on Cancer (IARC) database (R7 version, september 2002) at www.iarc.fr/P53/ {1957} revealed TP53 mutations in 40-60% {1569,2619} of invasive bladder cancers (in studies investigating at least 30 tumours). Although there are no specific mutational hotspots, more than 90% of mutations have been found in exons 4-9. Often TP53 mutations can be detected immunohistochemically

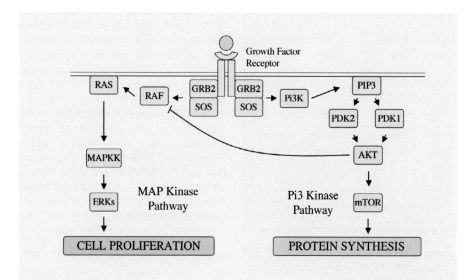

Fig. 2.25 Infiltrative urothelial carcinoma. Contribution of several oncogenes in cellular signalling pathways.

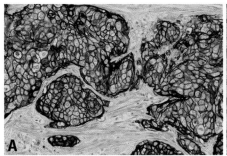
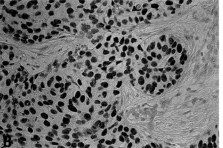

Fig. 2.26 A Invasive urothelial cancer. Strong membranous expression of EGFR in a case of invasive urothelial carcinoma. **B** Infiltrative urothelial carcinoma. Strong nuclear TP53 immunoreactivity in invasive urothelial carcinoma.

since many *TP53* mutations lead to protein stabilization resulting in nuclear TP53 accumulation. Immunohistochemical TP53 analysis has practical utility in surgical pathology. In addition to a postulated role as a prognostic marker, immunohistochemical TP53 positivity is a strong argument for the presence of genetically instable neoplasia in cases with questionable morphology.

The *PTEN* (phosphatase and tensin homology) gene also known as *MMAC1* (mutated in multiple advanced cancers) and *TEP1* (TGFbeta regulated and epithelial cell enriched phosphatase) is a candidate tumour suppressor gene located at chromosome 10q23.3. The relative high frequency (20-30%) of LOH at 10q23 in muscle invasive bladder cancer {1256} would make *PTEN* a good tumour suppressor candidate. However, the frequency of *PTEN* mutations is not clear at present. In three technically well performed studies including 35, 63, and 345 tumour samples, mutations were detected in 0%, 0.6%, and 17% of cases {141, 359,2776}. These results leave the question for the predominant mechanism of inactivation of the second allele open, or indicate that *PTEN* is not the (only) target gene at 10q23.

The *retinoblastoma* (*RB1*) gene product was the first tumour suppressor gene to be identified in human cancer. *RB1* which is localized at 13q14, plays a crucial role in the regulation of the cell cycle. Inactivation of *RB1* occurs in 30-80% of muscle invasive bladder cancers {360,1172,1530,2845}, most frequently as a consequence of heterozygous 13q deletions in combination with mutation of the remaining allele {497}. A strong association has been found between *RB1*

inactivation and muscle invasion {360, 1177,2110,2112}. Some investigators have reported an association between altered Rb expression and reduced patient survival {498,1530}.

Alterations of DNA repair genes are important for many cancer types. In invasive bladder cancer, alterations of mismatch repair genes (mutator phenotype) are rare. A metaanalysis of 7 studies revealed that microsatellite instability (MSI) was found only in 12 of 524 (2.2%) of cases suggesting that MSI does not significantly contribute to bladder cancer development {1032}.

The genes encoding *p16* (CDKN2A) and *p15* (CDKN2B) map to chromosome 9p21, a site that is frequently involved in heterozygous and homozygous deletions in urinary bladder cancer of all types.

Alterations of 9p21 and *p15/p16* belong to the few genetic alterations that are equally frequent or even more frequent in non-invasive low grade neoplasms than in invasively growing/high grade tumours.

Prognostic and predictive factors
Clinical factors

In general, individual prognosis of infiltrating bladder tumours can be poorly predicted based on clinical factors alone. Tumour multifocality, tumour size of >3 cm, and concurrent carcinoma in situ have been identified as risk factors for recurrence and progression {2215}. Tumour extension beyond the bladder on bimanual examination, infiltration of the ureteral orifice {999}, lymph node metastases and presence of systemic dissemination are associated with a poor prognosis.

Morphologic factors

Morphologic prognostic factors include grade, stage, as well as other specific morphologic features.

Histologic grade probably has prognostic importance for pT1 tumours. As most pT2 and higher stage tumours are high grade, its value as an independent prognostic marker remains questionable.

Depth of invasion, which forms the basis of pT categorization is the most important prognostic factor. In efforts to stratify category pT1 tumours further, sub-stag-

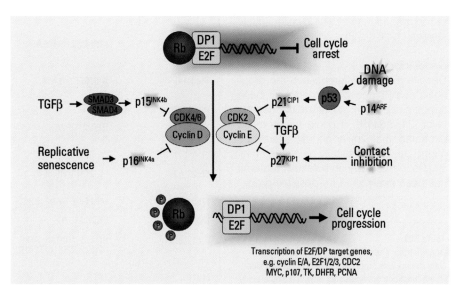

Fig. 2.27 Infiltrative urothelial carcinoma. Tumour suppressor genes and cell cycle control at the G1/S checkpoint. Progression of the cell cycle depends on the release of pRb from transcription factors including DP1 and E2Fs. For this purpose, pRb needs to be phosphorylated by cyclin dependent kinases (CDKs) which are, in turn, actived by D and E cyclins. Cell cycle control may get lost if pRb or inhibitors of cyclin/CDK complexes are inactivated, e.g. by mutation, deletion or methylation.

ing systems have been proposed on the basis of the level of invasion into the lamina propria. Tumours that infiltrate beyond the muscularis mucosae have a higher progression rate {1039,2886}. An alternative is to stratify patients according to the level of invasion into lamina propria measured by a micrometer attached to the microscope {435,2562}. Stage T1 is frequently found in tumours of high grade, and stage T1 tumours that are high grade {1798} have a recurrence rate of 80%, 60% progression, and 35% 10-year survival rate.

Carcinoma in situ is more frequent with increasing grade and stage of the associated tumour, and carcinoma in situ with micro-invasion seems to increase the probability of aggressive behaviour {1547}. Lymphatic and/or vascular invasion is associated with decreased survival in pT1 tumours (44% 5-year survival). Because vascular invasion is frequently overdiagnosed the prognostic significance of that factor remains uncertain {1436}. Specific subtypes or histologic variants of urothelial carcinomas such as small cell carcinoma, sarcomatoid carcinoma, nested variant, micropapillary carcinoma, and lymphoepithelioma-like carcinoma may be clinically relevant in patient's prognosis. Margin status after cystectomy is also an important predictor of prognosis.

The pattern of tumour growth has been suggested to be important; a pushing front of invasion had a more favourable prognosis than tentacular invasion in few studies {1226,1798}.

Genetic factors

Despite marked differences in the prognosis of pT1 and pT2-4 cancers, these tumours are highly similar on the genetic level {2188,2419}. It could therefore be expected, that similar genetic alterations might be prognostically relevant in all stages. A multitude of molecular features has been analyzed for a possible prog-

Table 2.03
Amplification sites in invasive bladder cancer.
Only studies with more than 20 patients are included. If one amplicon was detected only in a single study with less than 20 tumours, the number of amplified cases is given in relation to the total number of analyzed tumours. Capital letters in brackets indicate the method of analysis: (C) = CGH; (F) = FISH; (S) = Southern blotting; (P) = PCR; (K) = Karyotyping.

Amplicon	Putative target gene(s)	Amplification frequency *	
1p22-p32	JUN, TAL1	2 of 10	(C)
1q21-q24	TRK, SKI, MUC1, CKS1, COAS2	3-11% 2%	(C) (K)
2q13	RABL2A	2%	(K)
3pter-p23	RAF1	1-3% 4%	(C) (F)
3p11	EPHA3	1-2%	(C)
3q26	PIK3CA, MDS1, SKIL	1 of 10	(C)
5p11-p13		1%	(C)
5p15	TRIO, SKP2	1-2%	(C)
5q21	EFNA5	1%	(C)
6p22	E2F3	3-6% 2%	(C) (K)
7p12-p11	EGFR	case report	(K)
7q21-q31	MET, WNT2	1%	(C)
7q36		2%	(C)
8p12-p11	FGFR1	2% 1-3% 2%	(C) (F) (K)
8q21-q22	MYBL1	4-7%	(C)
8q24	MYC	1-2% 3-8% 33%	(C) (F) (S)
9p24	JAK2	1%	(C)
9p21		4%	(F)
10p11-p12	MAP3K8	2%	(C)
10p13-p15	STAM, IL15RA	1-2%	(C)
10q22-q23		33%	(C)
10q25	CSPG6, FACL5	1%	(C)
11q13	CCND1, EMS1, TAOS1	4-9% 30% 21%	(C) (F) (S)
12q13-q21	MDM2, CDK4, SAS	3% 5% 4%	(C) (F) (S)
13q3414	ARHGEF7, GAS6, TFDP1, FGF14	1%	(C)
16q21-q22		1 of 2	(C)
17q11-q21	HER2, TOP2A, KSR, WNT3	2-24% 3%-7% 4-14% 11%	(C) (F) (S) (P)
17q22-q23	FLJ21316, HS.6649, RPS6KB1, PPM1D	1 of 14	(C)
17q24-q25	MAP2K6, GRB2, BIRC5	3%	(C)}
18p11	YES1, MC2R	1-3%	
20q12-q13	BCAS1, NCOA3, STK6, MYBL2, CSE1L, TFAP2C	35% 50% 2-9%	(S) (F) (C)
21p11	TPTE	2%	(K)
22q11-q13	MAPK1, CECR1, ECGF1	1 of 14	(C)
Xp21		2%	
Xq21	RPS6KA6	1%	

nostic role in invasively growing bladder cancer {1287,2496,2620}. Despite all this extensive research, there is currently no molecular parameter that is sufficiently validated and has sufficient predictive power to have accepted clinical value in these tumours.

TP53 Alterations of the *TP53* tumour suppressor gene have been by far the most intensively studied potential prognostic marker {2329}. Early studies suggested a strong prognostic importance of immunohistochemically detectable nuclear TP53 protein accumulation in both pT1 {963,2295} and pT2-4 cancers {725}, and TP53 analysis was close to routine application in urinary bladder cancer {1980}. However, many subsequent studies could not confirm these data {777, 1494,2064}. It is possible that part of these discrepancies are due to different response rates to specific therapy regimens for tumours with and without TP53 alterrations {505,1421,2293}. A recent metaanalysis of more than 3700 tumours found a weak but significant association between TP53 positivity and poor prognosis {2329}. An independent prognostic role of TP53 alterations was only found in 2 out of 7 trials investigating pT2-4 cancer. TP53 alterations may be clinically more important in pT1 cancer, since more than 50% of these studies found independent prognostic significance. However, it cannot be excluded that a fraction of overstaged TP53 negative pTa tumours with good prognosis has contributed to some of these results {2306}. Overall, it appears that 1) TP53 alterations do not sufficiently well discriminate good and poor prognosis groups in properly staged bladder cancers to have clinical utility, and 2) currently used methods for immunohistochemical TP53 analysis are not reliable enough for clinically useful measurement of TP53 alterations.

Cell cycle regulation p21 and p27 inhibit or stimulate cyclin dependent kinases. Stein et al. {2495} showed in a series of 242 invasive cancers treated by cystectomy that TP53+/p21- tumours were associated with worst prognosis compared to those with TP53+/p21+ phenotype. A similar result was obtained by Qureshi et al. {2126} in a series of 68 muscle invasive non-metastatic tumours treated with radical radiotherapy. The expression of p27 protein was a striking predictor of prognosis in a set of patients treated by cystectomy and adjuvant chemotherapy {2620}. A 60% long term survival was observed in 25 patients with p27+ tumours as compared to 0% of patients with p27- tumours. No survival difference between p27 positive and negative tumours was observed in the same study in patients that had not received adjuvant chemotherapy {2620}. Inactivation of the retinoblastoma (RB) gene occurs in 30-80% of bladder cancers {360,1172,1530,2845}, most frequently as a consequence of heterozygous 13q deletions in combination with mutation of the remaining allele {497}. Several investigators reported an association between altered Rb expression and reduced patient survival in muscle invasive cancers {498,504,1530} and with tumour progression in pT1 carcinomas {963}. Others could not confirm these results {1207,1359,2095}.

HER2 overexpression occurs in 30-70% of invasive bladder cancers. Some studies suggested that Her2 expression is a predictor for patient survival or metastatic growth {1358,1534,1787,2301} but these associations were not confirmed by others {1509,1708,2675}. Gandour-Edwards et al. recently described an intriguing link between Her2 expression and improved survival after paclitaxel-based chemotherapy {832}. Co-amplification and co-expression of the adjacent topoisomerase 2 alpha (TOP2A) may also play a role for an altered chemosensitivity of HER-2 amplified tumours {1209, 1210}.

EGFR is overexpressed in 30-50% of invasively growing bladder cancers {217,457,914,1510,1890,2305,2844}. Early reports linked EGFR expression to an increased risk for tumour recurrence and progression, as well as to reduced survival {1717,1875,1876}. In one study with 212 patients, EGFR expression was even found to be an independent predictor of progression and survival {1709}, but later studies could not confirm these results {2152,2475,2611,2748}.

Angiogenesis The extent of angiogenesis can be quantitated by immunostaining microvessels using antibodies against factor VIII or CD34. At least one study has suggested microvessel density as an independent prognostic factor in muscle invasive bladder cancer {260}. However, this finding was not confirmed in a subsequent study {1494}. Thrombospondin (TSP-1) is an inhibitor of angiogenesis that is enhanced by interaction with TP53 protein {961}. In one study, a reduced TSP-1 expression was significantly associated with disease recurrence and decreased overall survival {960}.

Cyclooxygenase (COX) is an enzyme that converts arachidonic acid into prostaglandin H2. COX-2 is one enzyme subtype that is induced by various stimuli including inflammation and occurs at elevated levels in many tumour types. A high COX-2 expression was related to good prognosis in a series of 172 patients treated by radical cystectomy {2620}. In another study, however, low COX-2 expression was significantly associated with good prognosis in pT1 cancers {1320}.

Non-invasive urothelial tumours

G. Sauter
F. Algaba
M.B. Amin
C. Busch
J. Cheville

T. Gasser
D.J. Grignon
F. Hofstädter
A. Lopez-Beltran
J.I. Epstein

The aim of classification of tumours has always been to define groups with differences in clinical outcomes that are significant enough to be clinically relevant. Also classifications need to be sufficiently reproducible and comprehensive to be uniformly applied by all pathologists and urologists. Further, patients having a benign disease should not be threatened by an unnecessary diagnosis of cancer. And lastly, as molecular pathology research progresses, classification should reflect genetic differences between tumour categories. The presently recommended nomenclature is similar to the WHO-ISUP classification of 1998, but the diagnostic criteria are further defined for practice. the terms non-invasive have been added to low and high grade papillary carcinoma to emphasize biologic differences between these tumours and infiltrating urothelial cancer. The strong points of the current system are:

1. It includes three distinct categories and avoids use of ambiguous grading such as Grade I/II or II/III. The description of the categories has been expanded in the current version of the classification to further improve their recognition.

2. One group (PUNLMP) with particularly good prognosis does not carry the label of 'cancer'.

3. The group of non-invasive high grade carcinomas is large enough to contain virtually all of those tumours that have similar biological properties (high level of genetic instability) as invasive urothelial carcinomas.

The current classification reflects work in progress. Genetic studies are suggesting two major subtypes of urothelial neoplasms which might have a distinctly different clinical course. As the group of genetically stable tumours appears to include most of the non-invasive low grade carcinomas, it is likely that the group that does not deserve the designation of cancer will increase in the future. If further refinements or modifications to this classification are made, they must be on the basis of studies that show superior prediction of prognosis as well as a high degree of reproducibility of morphological or molecular criteria for any newly proposed tumour categories.

The previously used classifications are not recommended for use. It is believed that the consistent use of the current classification will result in the uniform diagnosis of tumours between institutions which will facilitate comparative clinical and pathological studies, incorporation of molecular data and identification of biologically aggressive, genetically instable, non-invasive papillary

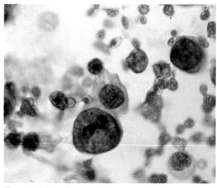

Fig. 2.28 Non-invasive urothelial neoplasm. High grade urothelial carcinoma showing atypical urothelial cells that vary in size and shape. The nuclei are enlarged, with coarsely granular chromatin, hyperchromasia, abnormal nuclear contours and prominent nucleoli. (Papanicolaou staining).

neoplasms. The potential for this objective to be met also depends on accurate diagnosis and consistent separation of pTa from pT1 tumours in such studies.

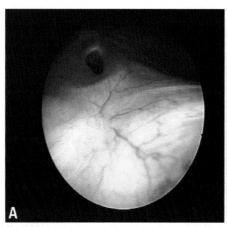
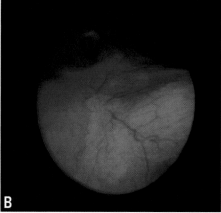
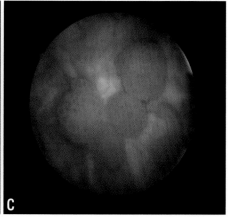

Fig. 2.29 Non-invasive urothelial neoplasm. **A, B** Photodynamic diagnostic image of normal bladder and carcinoma in situ. Tumour red, normal urothelium blue and carcinoma in situ. Tumour red, normal urothelium blue. **C** Endoscopy, pTa tumour.

Urothelial hyperplasia

J.I. Epstein

Urothelial hyperplasia is defined as markedly thickened mucosa without cytological atypia. It may be seen in the flat mucosa adjacent to low grade papillary urothelial lesions. When seen by itself there is no evidence suggesting that it has any premalignant potential. However, molecular analyses have shown that at least the lesions in bladder cancer patients may be clonally related to the papillary tumours {1930}. Within the spectrum of hyperplasia a papillary architecture may be present; most of these patients have concomitant papillary tumours {2545,2587}.

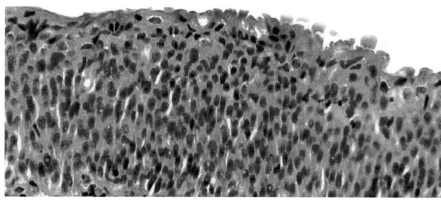

Fig. 2.30 Non-invasive urothelial neoplasm. Flat urothelial hyperplasia consisting of an increase in number of cell layers, with few or no significant cytological abnormalities (H&E).

Urothelial dysplasia

M.B. Amin

Since dysplasia may be mimicked by reactive inflammatory atypia and even by normal urothelium, the spectrum of atypical changes in the urothelium that fall short of carcinoma in situ are described here together.

Definition
Dysplasia (low grade intraurothelial neoplasia) has appreciable cytologic and architectural changes felt to be preneoplastic but which fall short of carcinoma in situ (CIS) {79,84,706}.

Epidemiology
Reliable data is unavailable, as most registries record dysplasia along with CIS or consider bladder cancer as a single entity. Since dysplasia is conceptually thought of as precursor lesion of bladder cancer, similar etiopathogenetic factors may apply in dysplasia.

Clinical features
In most cases the diagnosis of bladder cancer precedes dysplasia, and in this setting dysplasia is usually clinically and

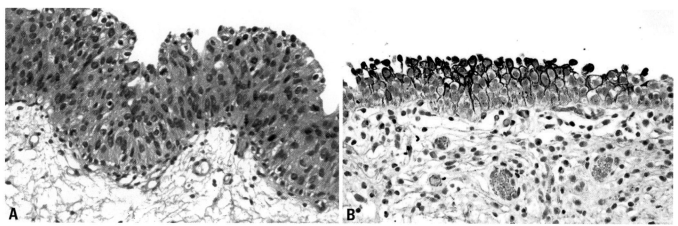

Fig. 2.31 A Urothelial dysplasia with loss of polarity, nuclear atypia and increased cellularity. **B** Aberrant immunohistochemical expression of cytokeratin 20 in urothelial dysplasia.

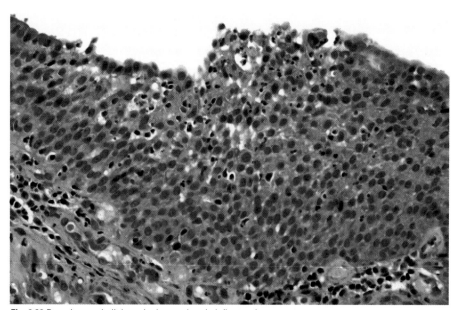

Fig. 2.32 Reactive urothelial atypia due to chronic inflammation.

cystoscopically silent. Primary (de novo) dysplasia may present with irritative bladder symptoms with or without hematuria {423,1849,2947}. A clinical history of stones, infection, instrumentation or intravesical therapy is often available in reactive cases.

Macroscopy
Lesions may be inapparent or associated with erythema, erosion or, rarely, ulceration.

Histopathology
Normal urothelium
Normal urothelium is urothelium without cytologic atypia and overall maintenance of polarity, or mild architectural alteration {706}. It is three to six layers thick, depending on the state of distention, and is composed of basal cells, intermediate cells and superficial cells. Minimal crowding and nuclear overlap without any cytologic abnormality is within the range of normal {79,84,706}.

Dysplasia
Lesions show variable often appreciable loss of polarity with nuclear rounding and crowding and cytologic atypia that is not severe enough to merit a diagnosis of CIS. The cells may have increased cytoplasmic eosinophilia and the nuclei have irregular nuclear borders, mildly altered chromatin distribution, inconspicuous nucleoli and rare mitoses. Pleomorphism, prominent nucleoli throughout the urothelium and upper level mitoses argue for a CIS diagnosis {79,84,424,706,1851}. Cytokeratin 20 may be of value in its recognition {261,1023}.

Reactive atypia
Reactive atypia occurs in acutely or chronically inflamed urothelium and has nuclear changes clearly ascribable to a reactive/regenerative process. Cells are uniformly enlarged with a single prominent nucleolus and evenly distributed vesicular chromatin. Mitotic activity may be brisk but without atypical forms. Inflammation may be present in the urothelium or lamina propria {79,424}.

Urothelial atypia of unknown significance
Atypia of unknown significance is not a diagnostic entity, but a descriptive category for cases with inflammation in which the severity of atypia appears out of proportion to the extent of inflammation such that dysplasia cannot be confidently excluded {424,706}. Alterations vary significantly. This is not meant to be a "waste basket" term but should be used for lesions with atypia that defy categorization but which the observer feels would benefit from clinical follow-up {424,706}.

Somatic genetics
Alterations of chromosome 9 and p53 and allelic losses have been demonstrated {534,1031}.

Prognostic and predictive factors
Dysplasia is most relevant in non-invasive papillary neoplasms, where its presence indicates urothelial instability and a marker for progression or recurrence (true risk remains to be established) {71,1361,1802,1866,2450}. It is frequently present with invasive cancer, whose attributes determine outcome {1361, 1846}. De novo dysplasia progresses to bladder neoplasia in 5-19% of cases; in most cases, however progressive lesions do not arise from dysplastic regions {79, 423,424,1849,1851,2947}.

Urothelial papilloma

C. Busch
S.L. Johansson

Definition
Exophytic urothelial papilloma is composed a delicate fibrovascular core covered by urothelium indistinguishable from that of the normal urothelium.

ICD-O code   8120/0

Epidemiology
The incidence is low, usually 1-4% of bladder tumour materials reported given the above strict definition, but it may be more rare, since in a prospective study of all bladder tumour cases diagnosed during a two year period in Western Sweden no case of urothelial papilloma was idenfied among 713 patients. The male-to-female ratio is 1.9:1 {432}. Papillomas tend to occur in younger patients, and are seen in children.

Localization
The posterior or lateral walls close to the ureteric orifices and the urethra are the most common locations.

Clinical features
Gross or microscopic hematuria is the main symptom. The endoscopic appearance is essentially identical to that of PUNLMP or Low Grade Papillary Urothelial Carcinoma. Almost all patients have a single tumour. Complete transurethral resection is the treatment of choice. Urothelial papillomas rarely recur (around 8%) {432,1678}.

Histopathology
The lesion is characterized by discrete papillary fronds, with occasional branching in some cases, but without fusion. The stroma may show oedema and or scattered inflammatory cells, the epithelium lacks atypia and superficial (umbrella) cells are often prominent. Mitoses are absent to rare and, if present are basal in location and not abnormal. The lesions are often small and occasionaly show concomitant inverted growth pattern. Rarely, papilloma may show extensive involvement of the mucosa. This is referred to as diffuse papillomatosis.

There has been significant consensus in previous classification systems with regard to the definition and criteria for exophytic urothelial papilloma.

The lesions are diploid, mitoses rare and proliferation rates low as deemed by immunohistochemical assessment of e.g. Ki-67 expression {469}. Cytokeratin 20 expression is identical to that in normal urothelium i.e. in the superficial (umbrella) cells only {600,1024}. Recent studies claim frequent FGFR3 mutations in urothelial papilloma (75%) {2701} with comparable percentage of mutations in PUNLMP (85%) and Low Grade Papillary Urothelial carcinoma (88%). Alteration of p53 is not seen {469}.

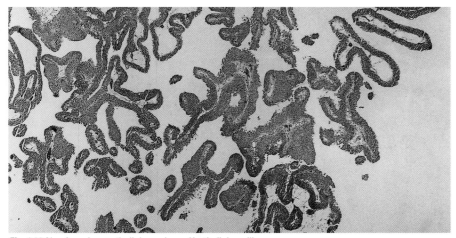

Fig. 2.33 Non-invasive urothelial neoplasm. Urothelial papilloma.

Inverted papilloma

G. Sauter

Definition

Benign urothelial tumour that has an inverted growth pattern with normal to minimal cytologic atypia of the neoplastic cells.

Epidemiology

The lesion occurs mostly solitary and comprises less than 1% of urothelial neoplasms {1843}. The male: female ratio is about 4-5:1. Ages of affected patients range from 10 years {2861} to 94 years {1309} with a peak frequency in the 6th and 7th decades.

Etiology

The etiology of inverted papilloma is unknown. Hyperplasia of Brunn nests and chronic urothelial inflammation have been suggested as possible causes.

Localization

More than 70% of the reported cases were located in the bladder but inverted papillomas can also be found in ureter, renal pelvis, and urethra in order of decreasing frequency. The trigone is the most common location in the urinary bladder {363,596,1037,1049,1071,1190, 2416,2494}.

Clinical features

Hematuria is the most common symptom. Some cases have produced signs of obstruction because of their location in the low bladder neck or the ureter {503}. Dysuria and frequency have been recorded but are uncommon {376}.

Macroscopy

Inverted papillomas appear as smooth-surfaced pedunculated or sessile polypoid lesions. Most are smaller than 3 cm in greatest dimension, but rare lesions have grown to as large as 8 cm {363,596,1071,1190,2101}.

Histopathology

Inverted papilloma has a relatively smooth surface covered by histologically and cytologically normal urothelium. Randomly scattered endophytic cords of urothelial cells invaginate extensively from the surface urothelium into the subadjacent lamina propria but not into the muscular bladder wall. The base of the lesion is well circumscribed. Anastomosing islands and cords of uniform width distribution appear as if a papillary lesion had invaginated into the lamina propria. In contrast to conventional papillary urothelial neoplasms, the central portions of the cords contain urothelial cells and the periphery contains palisades of basal cells. The relative proportion of the stromal component is mostly minimal but varies from case to case, and within the same lesions.

A trabecular and a glandular subtype of inverted papilloma have been described {1409}. The trabecular type is composed of interanastomosing sheets of urothelium sometimes including cystic areas. The glandular subtype contains urothelium with pseudoglandular or glandular differentiation.

Foci of mostly non-keratinizing squamous metaplasia are often seen in inverted papillomas. Neuroendocrine differentiation has also been reported {2534}. Urothelial cells have predominantly benign cytological features but focal minor cytologic atypia is often seen {363,1409,1843}. Mitotic figures are rare or absent {363,1409}.

It is important to not extend the diagnosis to other polypoid lesions with predominantly subsurface growth pattern such as florid proliferation of Brunn nests or areas of inverted growth in non-invasive papillary tumours.

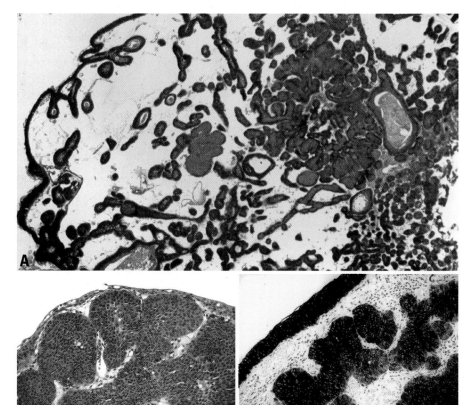

Fig. 2.34 Noninvasive urothelial neoplasm. **A, B** Inverted papilloma. **C** Most urothelial cells in this example of inverted papilloma are immunohistochemically reactive with antibodies anti-cytokeratin 7.

Somatic genetics

Ultrastructure, antigenic composition, and DNA- content of inverted papilloma cells have been non-contributory to the diagnosis in the few evaluated cases {68,447,1190,1406}.

Prognosis

If the diagnosis of inverted papilloma is strictly confined to the criteria described above, these tumours are benign. Recurrent lesions have been observed in less than 1% of the reported cases {376} and progression from pure inverted papilloma to carcinoma is extremely rare. An initial diagnosis of inverted papilloma should be challenged if progression is observed as many recurring or progressing cases have exophytic papillary structures in their initial biopsy {78}.

Papillary urothelial neoplasm of low malignant potential

S.L. Johansson
C. Busch

Definition

Papillary Urothelial Neoplasm of Low Malignant Potential (PUNLMP) is a papillary urothelial tumour which resembles the exophytic urothelial papilloma, but shows increased cellular proliferation exceeding the thickness of normal urothelium.

ICD-O code   8130/1

Epidemiology

The incidence is three cases per 100,000 individuals per year. The male to female ratio is 5:1 and the mean age at diagnosis (+/- standard deviation) is 64.6 years +/-13.9 years (range 29-94) {1107}. The latter is virtually identical to that of 112 patients treated at the Mayo Clinic {432}.

Localization

The lateral and posterior walls close to the ureteric orifices are the preferred sites for these tumours.

Clinical features

Most patients present with gross or microscopic hematuria. Urine cytology is negative in most cases. Cystoscopy reveals, in general, a 1-2 cm regular tumour with a appearance reminiscent of "seaweed in the ocean". Complete transurethral resection is the treatment of choice.

Histopathology

The papillae of PUNLMP are discrete, slender and non fused and are lined by multilayered urothelium with minimal to absent cytologic atypia. The cell density appears to be increased compare to normal. The polarity is preserved and there is an impression of predominant order with absent to minimal variation in architectural and nuclear features. The nuclei are slightly enlarged compare to normal. The basal layers show palisading and the umbrella cell layer is often preserved. Mitoses are rare and have a basal location. These architectural and cytological features should be evaluated in well oriented, non tangentional cut areas of the neoplasm. The tumours are predominantly diploid.

Prognosis

The prognosis for patients with PUNLMP is excellent. Recurrences occur, but at a significantly lower frequency than in non-invasive papillary carcinomas {1610}. Rarely, these patients may present with another tumour of higher grade and/or stage, usually years after the initial diagnosis. In a series of 95 cases, 35% had recurrence but no tumour progressed. If the patients were tumour free at the first follow-up cystoscopy, 68% remained tumour free during a follow-up period of at least 5 years {1104,1110}. In another study, 47% of the patients developed local recurrence but none of the 19 PUNLMP patients progressed {2071}. In contrast, in a retrospective study of 112 patients with long term follow up, four patients progressed in stage, two to

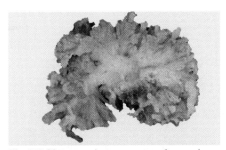

Fig. 2.35 Macroscopic appearance of a non-invasive low grade urothelial carcinoma with delicate papillae obtained at time of transurethral resection.

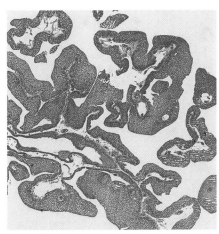

Fig. 2.36 Non-invasive urothelial neoplasm. Papillary urothelial neoplasm of low malignant potential.

muscle invasive disease, but there was only a 25% recurrence rate {432}.

Non-invasive papillary urothelial carcinoma, low grade

Definition
A neoplasm of urothelium lining papillary fronds which shows an orderly appearance, but easily recognizable variations in architecture and cytologic features.

ICD-O code   8130/21

Epidemiology
The incidence is five cases per 100,000 individuals per year. The male-to-female ratio is 2.9:1. The mean age (+/- standard deviation) is 69.2 years, +/- 11.7 (range 28-90 years) {1107}.

Localization
The posterior or lateral walls close to the ureteric orifices is the site of approximately 70% of the cases.

Clinical symptoms
Gross or microscopic hematuria is the main symptom. The endoscopic appearance is similar to that of PUNLMP. In 78% of the cases the patients have a single tumour and in 22% there are two or more tumours {1108}.

Histopathology
The tumour is characterized by slender, papillary stalks which show frequent branching and minimal fusion. It shows an orderly appearance with easily recognizable variations in architectural and cytologic features even at scanning power. In contrast to PUNLMP, it is easy to recognize variations in nuclear polarity, size, shape and chromatin pattern. The nuclei are uniformly enlarged with mild differences in shape, contour and chromatin distribution. Nucleoli may be

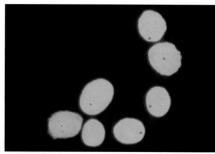

Fig. 2.39 Non-invasive low grade papillary urothelial cancer. FISH analysis shows monosomy of Chromosome 9 (red dot).

present but inconspicuous. Mitoses are infrequent and may occur at any level but are more frequent basally. The papillary fronds should be evaluated where sectioned lengthwise through the core or perpendicular to the long axis of the papillary frond. If not, there may be a false impression of increased cellularity, loss of polarity and increased mitotic activity.

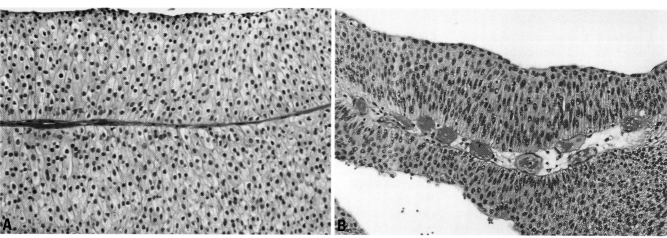

Fig. 2.37 Non-invasive urothelial neoplasm. **A,B** Papillary urothelial neoplasm of low malignant potential (PUNLMP).

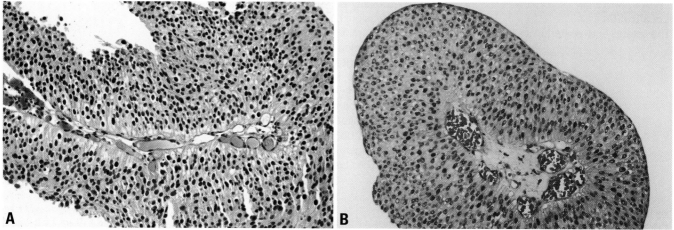

Fig. 2.38 Non-invasive urothelial neoplasm. **A,B** Non-invasive low grade urothelial carcinoma.

In spite of the overall orderly appearance, there are tumours that show focal high grade areas and in these cases the tumour should be classified as a high grade tumour.

Expression of cytokeratin 20, CD44, p53 and p63 immunostaining is intermediate between that of PUNLMP and non-invasive high grade papillary urothelial carcinoma {600,2678}. The tumours are usually diploid {2071}.

Prognosis

Progression to invasion and cancer death occurs in less than 5% of cases. In contrast, recurrence is common and occurs in 48-71% of the patients {69, 1104,1110}.

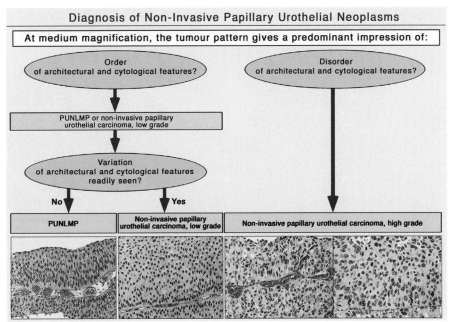

Fig. 2.40 Flow chart of the differential diagnosis of non-invasive papillary urothelial tumours.

Non-invasive papillary urothelial carcinoma, high grade

V.E. Reuter

Definition

A neoplasm of urothelium lining papillary fronds which shows a predominant pattern of disorder with moderate-to-marked architectural and cytologic atypia.

ICD-O code   8130/23

Clinical symptoms

Gross or microscopic hematuria is the main symptom. The endoscopic appearance varies from papillary to nodular/solid sessile lesions. Patients may have single or multiple tumours.

Histopathology

The tumour is characterized by a papillary architecture in which the papillae are frequently fused and branching, although some may be delicate. It shows a predominant pattern of disorder with easily recognizable variations in archi-

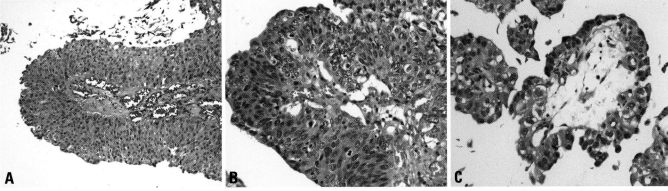

Fig. 2.41 Non-invasive papillary urothelial carcinoma, high grade. **A** The papillary fronds are partially fused and lined by markedly atypical and pleomorphic urothelial cells, some of which have exfoliated. **B** The architecture is disordered and there is marked nuclear pleomorphism and hyperchromasia. Mitotic figures are readily visible away from the basement membrane. **C** The nuclei have open chromatin, irregular nuclear contours and variably prominent nucleoli. There is total lack of polarization and maturation.

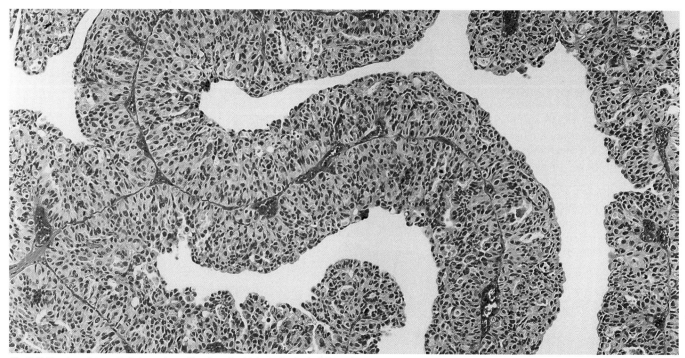

Fig. 2.42 Non-invasive urothelial neoplasm. Non-invasive high grade urothelial carcinoma.

tectural and cytologic features even at scanning power. In contrast to non-invasive low grade papillary urothelial carcinoma, it is easy to recognize more marked variations in nuclear polarity, size, shape and chromatin pattern. The nuclei often show pleomorphism with moderate-to-marked variation in size and irregular chromatin distribution. Nucleoli are prominent. Mitoses are frequent, may be atypical, and occur at any level, including the surface. The thickness of the urothelium may vary considerably and often with cell dyscohesion. Within this category of these tumours there is a spectrum of atypia, the highest of which show marked and diffuse nuclear pleomorphism. Pathologists have the option of recording the presence or absence of diffuse anaplasia in a comment. The papillary fronds should be evaluated where sectioned lengthwise through the core or perpendicular to the long axis of the papillary frond. Due to the likelihood of associated invasion, including that of papillary cores, these features should be closely looked for.

Detection of cytokeratin 20, p53 and p63 is more frequent than in low grade tumours {600,2678}. The tumours are usually aneuploid {2071}.

Urothelial carcinoma in situ

I.A. Sesterhenn

Definition
A non-papillary, i.e. flat, lesion in which the surface epithelium contains cells that are cytologically malignant.

ICD-O code   8120/2

Synonym
High grade intraurothelial neoplasia.

Incidence
De novo (primary) carcinoma in situ accounts for less than 1-3% of urothelial neoplasms, but is seen in 45–65% of invasive urothelial carcinoma. It is present in 7-15% of papillary neoplasms {744,1362,1850,2315,2836}.

Site of involvement
Urothelial carcinoma in situ is most commonly seen in the urinary bladder. In 6 - 60%, the distal ureters are involved. Involvement of the prostatic urethra has been reported in 20-67% and in the prostate, involving ducts and acini, in up to 40%. It may be seen in the renal pelvis and proximal ureters {744,798,921,1362, 1596,2187,2319,2679}.

Clinical features
CIS patients are usually in the 5th to 6th decade of life. They may be asymptomatic or symptomatic with dysuria, frequency, urgency or even hematuria. In patients with associated urothelial carcinoma, the symptoms are usually those of the associated carcinoma.

Macroscopy
The mucosa may be unremarkable or erythematous and oedematous. Mucosal erosion may be present.

Histopathology
Urothelial carcinoma in situ shows nuclear anaplasia identical to high grade urothelial carcinoma. The enlarged nuclei are frequently pleomorphic, hyperchromatic, and have a coarse or condensed chromatin distribution; they may show large nucleoli. Mitoses including atypical ones are common and can extend into the upper cell layers. The cytoplasm is often eosinophilic or amphophilic. There is loss of cell polarity with irregular nuclear crowding {425,706, 743,1547,1798,1844,1845,1982}. The neoplastic change may or may not involve the entire thickness of the epithelial layer and umbrella cells may be present. It may be seen at the basal layer only or may overlay benign appearing epithelium. Individual cells or clones of neoplastic cells may be seen scattered amidst apparently normal urothelial cells and this is referred to as pagetoid spread {425,1547,1552,1678,1982}. Loss of

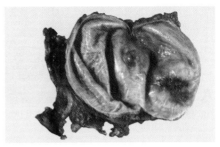

Fig. 2.43 Carcinoma in situ.

intercellular cohesion may result in a denuded surface ("denuding cystitis") {688} or in residual individual neoplastic

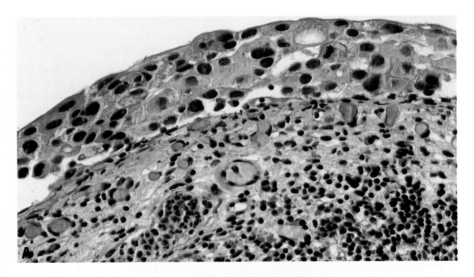

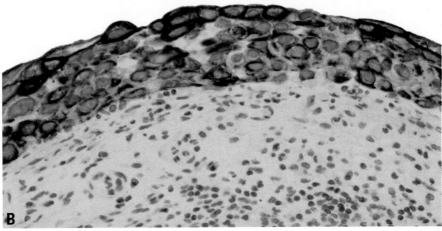

Fig. 2.44 Nonvasive urothelial neoplasm. **A, B** Urothelial carcinoma in situ.

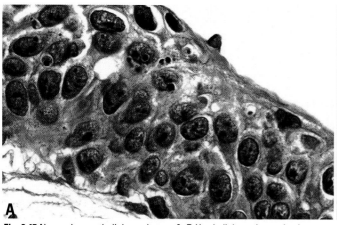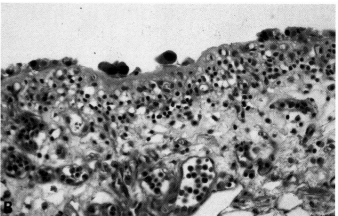

Fig. 2.45 Nonvasive urothelial neoplasms. **A, B** Urothelial carcinoma in situ.

cells attached to the surface referred to as "clinging" CIS. In such cases cytology is very helpful. Von Brunn nests and cystitis cystica may be completely or partially replaced by the cytologically malignant cells. CIS may consist of predominantly small cells referred to as small cell variant or of rather large cells. CIS commonly is multifocal and may be diffuse. It can involve several sites in the urinary tract synchronously or metachronously. The degree of cellular atypia may vary from site to site. The lamina propria usually shows an inflammatory infiltrate, some degree of oedema and vascular congestion.

Immunoprofile
Markers, which are abnormally expressed in invasive and papillary urothelial neoplasm have also been evaluated in CIS {494,964}. Cytokeratin 20 is abnormally expressed in CIS {1023}. Abnormal expression of p53 and RB protein may correlate with progression of CIS {498,725,1530,2294,2331,2364, 2457}. The nuclear matrix protein NMP22 is present in CIS {2484}.

Ploidy
The DNA analysis shows an aneuploid cell population, in some patients several aneuploid cell populations are present in the same lesion {977,1918,2060,2641}.

Prognosis
Data suggest that de novo (primary) CIS is less likely to progress to invasive disease than secondary CIS {1981,2115, 2237,2803}. Patients with CIS and concomitant invasive tumours die in 45-65% of cases compared to 7-15% of patients with CIS and concomitant non-invasive papillary tumour {1846}. CIS with multiple aneuploid cell lines appears to be at high risk of progression {1918}. Extensive lesions associated with marked symptoms have a guarded prognosis.

Genetics and predictive factors of non-invasive urothelial neoplasias

R. Simon
P.A. Jones
D. Sidransky
C. Cordon-Cardo

P. Cairns
M.B. Amin
T. Gasser
M.A. Knowles

Genetics of urinary bladder cancer development and progression
The genetic studies to date have used tumours classified according to the 1973 WHO Tumours Classification; studies are underway to link available genetic information to the current classification.

Urinary bladder cancer has earlier been categorized into "superficial" (pTa, pT1, CIS) and "invasive" (pT2-4) cancer depending on whether or not tumour infiltration extended to the muscular bladder wall {2133}. The available genetic data now suggest another subdivision of uri-

nary bladder neoplasia. Two genetic subtypes with marked difference in their degree of genetic instability correspond to morphologically defined entities. The genetically stable category includes low grade non-invasive papillary tumours (pTa). The genetically unstable category contains high grade (including pTa G3 and CIS) and invasively growing carcinomas (stage pT1-4).

Non-invasive low grade papillary bladder neoplasms (pTa, G1-2) have only few genomic alterations and are therefore viewed as "genetically stable" {2189,

2418,2552,2934}. Losses of chromosome 9, often involving the entire chromosome, and mutations of *FGFR3* are the most frequent known genetic alterations in these tumours. Gene amplifications and *TP53* mutations are rare {818,1748,2066,2190,2421,2422}. DNA aneuploidy occurs in less than 50% {2304,2599,2931}.

Invasively growing and high grade neoplasias are markedly different from non-invasive papillary low grade tumours. They appear to be genetically unstable and have many different chromosomal aberrations, often including high level amplifications and p53 mutations {495,1415,1920,2468}. DNA aneuploidy is seen in >90% {2304,2931}. Genetic differences between minimally invasive (pT1) and extensively invasive (pT2-4) carcinomas are only minimal {2188, 2419}. Some reports have suggested a possible role of 5p+, 5q-, and 6q- for further progression from pT1 to pT2-4 cancers {263,1101,2191,2316}. Only few studies have investigated non-invasive high grade precursor lesions (pTaG3, CIS) {1031,2241}. These data suggest a strong similarity between these tumours and invasively growing cancers, which is consistent with their assumed role as precursors of invasive bladder cancer. The high number of individual genetic alterations that are much more frequent in high grade or invasive tumours than in pTaG1-G2 neoplasias makes it unlikely that a relevant fraction of invasive cancers derives from non-invasive papillary low grade tumours. This is also consistent with the clinical observation that the vast majority of invasive bladder cancer was not preceded by a pTa G1/G2 tumour {1363}. Combining pT1 cancers and pTa tumours into one group as "superficial bladder cancer" should be rigorously avoided {2188,2419}.

Precursor lesions of either invasive or non-invasive urothelial tumours include hyperplasia since significant chromosomal aberrations can be found in these lesions, also in absence of dysplasia {1029}. Chromosomal aberrations can also be seen in histologically "normal appearing urothelium" in bladders from cancer patients. This suggests that genetic analysis may be superior to histology for diagnosis of early neoplasia {2492}. Only few studies have analyzed genetic changes in dysplasia {1031, 1488,2397,2492}. They showed, that alterations that are typical for CIS can be also be found in some dysplasias suggesting that at least a fraction of them can be considered CIS precursors.

Multifocal bladder neoplasms
Neoplasias of the urothelium are typically not limited to one single tumour. Multifocality, frequent recurrence, and presence of barely visible flat accompanying lesions such as hyperplasia or dysplasia are characteristic for these tumours. Morphological, cytogenetic and immunohistochemical mapping studies of cystectomy specimens have demonstrated areas of abnormal cells adjacent to grossly visible tumours {1164,1362} (cytogenetic). The majority (80-90%) of multicentric bladder neoplasias are of monoclonal origin {437,541,733,986, 1030,1492,1564,1751,2405,2420,2552,2 553,2859}. It is assumed that neoplastic cells that have originated in one area later spread out to other regions either by active migration through the urothelium or through the urine by desquamation and reimplantation {992}. However, there are also reports of polyclonal cancers, mainly in early stage tumours or in premalignant lesions {915,993,1030,1751, 2059,2467,2883}. These observations have given rise to the 'field defect' hypothesis suggesting that environmental mutagens may cause fields of genetically altered cells that become the source of polyclonal multifocal tumours {1362}. It appears possible that selection and overgrowth of the most rapidly growing clone from an initially polyclonal neoplasia might lead to pseudoclonality in some cases of multiple bladder cancer. Presence or absence of monoclonality may have an impact on the clinical treatment modalities.

Chromosomal abnormalities
Non-invasive papillary low grade neoplasms (pTa, G1-2) have only few cytogenetic changes suggesting that these tumours are genetically stable neoplasms {2189,2418,2552,2934}. Total or partial losses of chromosome 9 is by far the most frequent cytogenetic alteration in these tumours, occuring in about 50% of bladder cancers of all grades and stages {2189,2307,2418}. Chromosome 9 loss can also be found in hyperplasia and even in morphologically normal appearing urothelium {1029,2492}. Losses of the Y chromosome represent the next most frequent cytogenetic alteration in low grade tumours {2310,2934}. The biologic significance of this alteration is unclear since Y losses can also be found in normal urothelium from patients without a bladder cancer history {2310}. High grade non-invasive precursor lesions (pTaG3, CIS) are very different from low grade neoplasias. Cytogenetically, they resemble invasively growing tumours and have many different genomic alterations {2241,2656, 2934}. A CGH study showed predominant deletions at 2q, 5q, 10q, and 18q as well as gains at 5p and 20q in 18 pTaG3 tumours {2934}. A high frequency of LOH at different loci was also observed in 31 CIS samples. Predominant alterations were LOH at 3p, 4q, 5q, 8p, 9p, 9q, 11p, 13q, 14q, 17p and18q in this study {2241}. Alterations in the cellular DNA content occur frequently in bladder cancer {1120,2059,2304}. Aneuploidy is strongly associated to stage and grade, and differences are most striking between pTa and pT1 tumours {2304}. Aneuploidy detection (e.g. by FISH or by cytometry) may be a suitable tool for the early detection of bladder cancer and recurrences. It has been shown that a panel of 4 FISH probes is sufficient to detect chromosomal alterations in bladder tumours and tumour cells in voided urines {334,2304, 2492}.

Chromosome 9
The similar frequency of chromosome 9 losses in non-invasive papillary low grade tumours and in high grade invasive cancers triggered extensive research to find the suggested one or several tumour suppressor genes on chromosome 9 that appear to play an important role in bladder cancer initiation {361,985,2648}. Mapping studies using microsatellite analysis identified multiple common regions of loss of heterozygosity (LOH) {361,982,1291,2423}. Two of them have been identified at 9p21, the loci of the cell cycle control genes CDKN2A (p16/p14^{ARF}) and CDKN2B (p15) {1291}. Another three putative suppressor gene loci have been mapped to 9q13-q31, 9q32-q33 and 9q34, containing the PTCH, DBCCR1 and TSC1 genes {988}. Because homozygous deletions are slightly more frequent for CDKN2A than for CDKN2B it has been postulated that p16/p14^{ARF} might be the primary target of 9p21 deletions {1975}. On 9q, the putative cell cycle regulator DBCCR1 (deleted in bladder cancer chromosome region candidate 1), which might be involved in cell cycle regulation {984, 1898}, seems to be a promising candidate tumour suppressor. Loss of DBCCR1 expression has been found in 50% of bladder tumours {984}, and FISH analysis revealed deletions of 9q33 in 73% of samples {2476}. Mutations of DBCCR1 have not been reported yet. Although hemizygous deletions have been seen in rare cases it is believed that promoter hypermethylation and homozygous deletions are the main mechanisms

for DBCCR1 silencing {984,2476}. The role of the sonic hedgehog receptor PTCH and the tuberous sclerosis gene TSC1 in bladder cancer is only poorly investigated to date.

FGF receptor 3 (FGFR3)
Mutations of the gene, located at chromosome 4p16.3, have only recently been identified as a molecular alteration that is characteristic for pTa tumours. In the largest study reported to date, 74% of pTa tumours had FGFR3 mutation as compared to 16% of T2-4 tumours {243}. All mutations described are missense mutations located in exons 7, 10 or 15 that have been previously described as germline mutations in skeletal dysplasia syndromes {369,2403}. These mutations are predicted to cause constitutive activation of the receptor. In one study, mutations have been linked to a lower risk of recurrence indicating that this genetic event may identify a group of patients with favourable disease course {2700}. In a recent study {2701}, comparable FGFR3 mutation frequencies were reported in 9 of 12 papillomas (75%), 53 of 62 tumours of low malignant potential (85%), and 15 of 17 low grade papillary carcinomas (88%). These data support the idea that these categories represent variations of one tumour entity (non-invasive low grade papillary tumours; genetically stable).

TP53 and RB
Alterations of TP53 {818,1748,2066}, and the retinoblastoma gene (RB) {1749, 2112} occur in a fraction of non-invasive papillary low grade tumours that is much smaller than in invasive cancer.

HER2 & EGFR
Overexpression of HER2 or EGFR have been described in a variable fraction of pTaG1/G2 tumours depending on the analytical methodology {914,1757,1758}. Few studies have examined gene alterations in CIS or pTaG3 tumours; they showed comparable frequencies of p53 alterations (50-70%) {1031,1119}, HER2 overexpression (50-75%) {489,2761}, or EGFR overexpression (45-75%) {373, 2761}, and loss of p21 (50-70%) {472, 797} or p27 (50%) {797} as described in invasive cancers. Increased expression of Ras protein has been described in CIS and high grade tumours but not in hyperplasia or low grade tumours in an early

study {2736}. However, the role of RAS especially in non-invasive bladder cancer needs further clarification {2395}.

Prognosis and predictive factors
Clinical factors
There are no specific urinary symptoms of non-invasive bladder tumours. Microscopic or gross hematuria are the most common findings {1719}. Irritative bladder symptoms such as dysuria, urgency and frequency occur if the tumour is localized in the trigone, in case of large tumour volume due to reduction of bladder capacity, or in case of carcinoma in situ.
At the time of first diagnosis approximately 70% of the tumours are non-invasive and of these only 5 to 10% will progress to infiltrating tumours {544}. However, half of all the tumours will recur at some time. Large tumours, multifocal tumours and those with diffuse appearance have a higher risk of recurrence {773}. In case of recurrent tumour, the probability of future recurrences, increase to approximately 80%. Short disease-free interval is also an indication for future recurrence. In case of carcinoma in situ, irritative symptoms and extensive disease are associated with poor prognosis {71}.
As discrimination between non-invasive and invasive tumours is not reliably possible on cystoscopy alone, complete transurethral resection of any visible lesion of the bladder including deep muscle layers is usually performed.
Regular cystoscopic follow-up is recommended at intervals for all patients with non-invasive tumours to detect recurrent tumour at an early stage. The risk of recurrence decreases with each normal cystoscopy and is less than 10% at 5 years and extremely low at 10 years if all interval cystoscopies had been normal.

Morphological factors
Histologic grade is a powerful prognostic factor for recurrence and progression in non-invasive urothelial tumours {706,1440,1610}. Urothelial papilloma has the lowest risk for either recurrence or progression {426,654,1678}, while PUNLMP has a higher risk for recurrence (up to 35%) and a very low risk for progression in stage {432,1104,1107, 1247,1460}. Patients with papilloma and PUNLMP have essentially a normal age-related life expectancy. Non-invasive low

Table 2.04
Overview of cytogenetic changes in non-invasive urothelial of the urinary bladder.

Chromosome	Frequency of alteration in		
	pTa G1/2	pTa G3	CIS
1p-	3%(K)		1 of 2 (F)
1q+	13%(C)	17%(C)	
2p+		5%(C)	
2q-	4-5%(C)	39%(C)	
3p-	1%(C) 6%(K)	5%(C)	31%(L)
3q+	1%(C)	5%(C)	
4p-	2-5%(C)	22%(C)	32%(L)
4q-	1-10%(C)	17%(C)	52%(L)
5p+	2%(C) 3%(K)	28%(C)	
5q-	4-20%(C) 3%(K)	33%(C)	20%(L)
6p+	1-5%(C)	11%(C)	
6q-	1-10%(C) 16%(K)	33%(C)	
7p+	5-10%(C) 19%(K)	5%(C)	
8p-	5-15%(C) 19%(K)	28%(C)	1 of 2 (F) 65%(L)
8q+	5-10%(C) 3%(K)	22%(C)	
9p-	36-45%(C) 28%(K) 15-33%(L)	45%(C)	40-77%(F) 61-76%(L)
9q-	45%(C) 31%(K) 2 of 7 (L)	38%(C)	74%(F) 52-61%(L)
10p+	3%(K)	5%(C)	
10q-	5%(C) 9%(K)	28%(C)	
11p-	10%(C) 16%(K) 1 of 3 (L)	17%(C)	54%(L)
11q-	6%(C) 3%(K)	23%(C)	36%(L)
11q+	5-25%(C)		1 of 2 (F)
12p+	1%(C)	5%(C)	
12q+	1-15%(C) 3%(K)	5%(C)	
13q-	0-20%(C) 19%(L)	17%(C)	56%(L)
14q-	1%(C) 9%(L)		70%(L)
17p-	1-5%(C) 6%(K)	11%(C)	81%(F) 60-64%(L)
17q+	10-30%(C)	33%(C)	
18q-	7-10%(C) 3%(K)	39%(C)	29%(L)
20q+	7-15%(C)	33%(C)	
Y	10-20%(C) 6%(K)	28%(C)	29%(K)

(C) = CGH; (K) = karyotyping/classical cytogenetics (average of 32 cases from references {131,132,134,148,867,868,869,2029,2442,2639,2710,2766}; (L) = LOH; (F) = FISH (FISH analyses of ICGNU have been included because of the lack of CGH data in this tumour type).

grade carcinomas recur frequently (up to 70%), but only up to 12% of patients progress in stage {433,600,1104, 1107,1460}. The prognosis for non-invasive high grade carcinomas is strikingly different. Tumours frequently progress in stage, and death due to disease can be as high as 65% {1247,1461}.

Patients with multifocal tumours in the bladder or involving other regions of the urothelial tract (ureter, urethra, renal pelvis) are at increased risk for recurrence, progression or death due to disease {531,1314,1579,2019}.

The presence of dysplasia and CIS in the nonpapillary urothelium is associated with increased risk for progression in stage and death due to disease {71,425, 726,1981,2450}. CIS is a stronger adverse factor {425,726,1981}.

Large tumours (>5 cm) are at an increased risk for recurrence and progression {1072}.

Genetic factors

Hundreds of studies have analyzed the prognostic significance of molecular features in non-invasive urinary bladder cancer {1340,2496,2725,2827}. Overall, there is no thoroughly evaluated molecular marker that has sufficient predictive power to be of clinical value in these tumours. There is circumstantial evidence that in some studies the substantial biological differences between non-invasive (pTa) and invasively growing (pT1) neoplasias were not taken into account {2189,2306,2418,2421}. Since the risk of progression is much higher in pT1 than in pTa tumours, and the frequency of most molecular changes is highly different between pTa and pT1 tumours, it must be assumed that interobserver variability in the distinction of pTa and pT1 tumours may markedly influence the results {19,2633,2835}. A systematic review of large series of pT1 tumours resulted in a downstaging to stage pTa in 25-34% of tumours {19,2633,2835}. Accordingly, the percentage of pT1 cancers varies between 20% and 70% in consecutive series of "superficial bladder cancers" {249,2065, 2066,2322}. A too large fraction of overstaged "false" pT1 tumours can even suggest independent prognostic impact of molecular features in combined pTa/pT1 studies.

Risk of recurrence

Non-invasive urothelial neoplasia often involves invisible flat neoplastic lesions in addition to a visible papillary tumour {285,1362}. After complete resection of a tumour, the risk of recurrence is determined by the amount and biologic properties of neoplastic cells remaining in the bladder. Multicentric neoplastic lesions in the bladder are clonally related in about 80-90% of cases {992}. Only in these cases, the molecular characteristics of the removed tumour may be representative of the "entire" disease. The best candidates for predicting early recurrence include molecular changes that are related to an increased tumour cell proliferation or an improved potential for multicentric tumour extension. Indeed, several studies showed that rapid tumour cell proliferation as measured by flow cytometry, mitotic index, PCNA labeling, or Ki67 labeling index predicts an increased risk of or recurrence in these tumours {573,1452,1512, 1518,2942}. Cytokeratin 20 expression and *FGFR* mutations are examples of markers that may be representative for a clinically distinct tumour subtype without having a direct role for the development of early recurrence. Cytokeratin 20 is normally expressed in the superficial and upper intermediate urothelial cells. In a study of 51 non-invasive papillary tumours, none of 10 tumours with a normal cytokeratin 20 staining pattern recurred {1024}. Mutations of the FGF receptor 3 (*FGFR3*) have recently been identified to occur in more than two thirds of non-invasive low grade urothelial carcinoma {243}. Early studies suggest that mutations are linked to a decreased risk of recurrence {2700}. Other molecular features that were proposed to predict tumour recurrence in non-invasive papillary low grade tumours include overexpression of proline-directed protein kinase F {1132}, *p14^{ARF}* promoter hypermethylation {632}, clusterin overexpression {1746}, expression of the imprinted *H19* gene {115}, and reduced expression of E-cadherin {1511}.

Early tumour recurrence could also be predicted by the analysis of urine cells after surgical removal of all visible tumours. Studies using fluorescence in situ hybridization (FISH) have indeed shown a strong prognostic significance of genetically abnormal cells for early recurrence in cystoscopically and cytologically normal bladders {801,1179, 2298}.

Risk of progression

Data on the prognostic importance of genetic changes for progression of non-invasive low grade neoplasias are largely missing because of the rarity of progression in these patients. In theory, molecular changes that decrease genetic stability are expected to herald poor prognosis in these patients, because an acquisition of multiple additional molecular changes may be required to transform non-invasive low grade neoplasia to invasive cancer. In fact, p53 alterations, known to decrease genomic stability, have been suggested as a prognostic marker in pTa tumours {2296}.

Molecular parameters that were suggested to herald a particularly high risk of progression include p53 accumulation {2294}, reduced thrombospondin expression {898}, loss of p63 expression {2678}, loss of E-cadherin expression {1210}, abnormal expression of pRb {963}, LOH at chromosome 16p13 {2879}, as well as alterations of chromosomes 3p, 4p, 5p, 5q, 6q, 10q, and 18q {2191}.

Squamous cell carcinoma

D.J. Grignon
M.N. El-Bolkainy
B.J. Schmitz-Dräger
R. Simon
J.E. Tyczynski

Definition

A malignant neoplasm derived from the urothelium showing histologically pure squamous cell phenotype.

ICD-O code   8070/3

Epidemiology

The most common histological type of bladder cancer is urothelial carcinoma, which comprises 90-95% of bladder cancers in Western countries {2016}. Squamous cell carcinoma (SSC) of the bladder is much less frequent. Worldwide, it constitutes about 1.3% of bladder tumours in males, and 3.4% in females.

In the United States, the differences in histology by race are small, with, whites having 94.5% urothelial and 1.3% squamous cell carcinomas (SCCs), while the proportions are 87.8% and 3.2%, respectively, in Blacks. In Africa, the majority of bladder cancers in Algeria and Tunisia (high incidence countries) are urothelial carcinomas, with SCCs comprising less than 5%. In some West African countries (Mali, Niger), and in east and south-east Africa (Zimbabwe, Malawi, Tanzania), SCC predominates, as it does in Egypt. In South Africa, there are marked differences in histology between Blacks (36% SCC, 41% urothelial) and Whites (2% SCC, 94% urothelial) {2013}. Similar findings with respect to black–white differences in proportions of the different histological types of bladder cancer have been reported from clinical series, for example in the Durban hospitals {955}. These observations (as well as clinical features such as sex ratio, mean age at diagnosis and stage) relate to the prevalence of infection with *Schistosoma haematobium*.

Etiology

Tobacco smoking

Tobacco smoking is the major established risk factor of bladder cancer. The risk of bladder cancer in smokers is 2-6 fold that of non-smokers {1158}. The risk increases with increasing duration of smoking, as well as with increasing intensity of smoking {313}.

Tobacco smoking is also an important risk factor for SCC of the bladder. It has been estimated that the relative risk for current smokers is about 5-fold of that in non-smokers {791}. The risk increases with the increasing lifetime consumption, and for those with the highest consumption (more than 40 pack-years) is about 11 {791}, as well as with increasing intensity of smoking {1271}.

Occupational exposures

As described earlier, bladder cancer risk is increased in various occupational groups, but the effect of occupational exposures has not been quantified for different histological types.

Schistosomiasis

Schistosomes are trematode worms that live in the bloodstream of humans and animals. Three species (*Schistosoma haematobium*, *S. mansoni* and *S. japonicum*) account for the majority of human infections. The evidence linking infection with *Schistosoma haematobium* with bladder cancer has been extensively reviewed {419,1152,1791}). There are essentially three lines of evidence:

Clinical observations that the two diseases appear to frequently co-exist in the same individual, and that the bladder cancers tend to be of squamous cell origin, rather than urothelial carcinomas.

Descriptive studies showing a correlation between the two diseases in different populations.

Case-control studies, comparing infection with *S. haematobium* in bladder cancer cases and control subjects. Several studies investigated this relationship, taking as a measure of infection the presence of *S. haematobium* eggs in a urine sample, presence of calcified eggs identified by X-ray or information from a questionnaire {199,687,846,1859,2739}. The

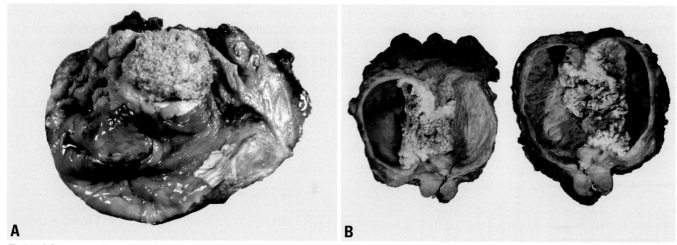

Fig. 2.46 A Squamous cell carcinoma. Cystectomy specimen, nodular squamous cell carcinoma associated with leukoplakia. **B** Bladder squamous carcinoma in diverticulum.

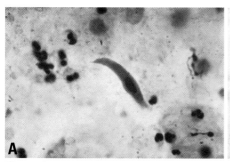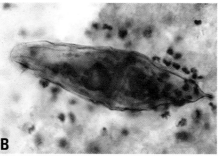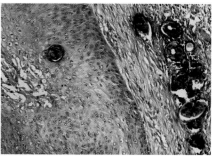

Fig. 2.47 Squamous cell carcinoma. **A** Urine cytology, spindle cells of squamous carcinoma. **B** Urine cytology, *S. haematobium* egg with terminal spine.

Fig. 2.48 Low grade squamous cell carcinoma of the bladder with calcifed schistosomal eggs (H&E).

estimated relative risk varied from 2 to 15 compared with non-infected subjects.

Pathogenesis

Numerous explanations have been offered for the proposed association between schistosomiasis and human cancers:

Chronic irritation and inflammation with increased cell turnover provide opportunities for mutagenic events, genotoxic effects and activation of carcinogens through several mechanisms, including the production of nitric oxide by inflammatory cells (activated macrophages and neutrophils) {2240,2242}.

Altered metabolism of mutagens may be responsible for genotoxic effects {851,852,853}. Quantitatively altered tryptophan metabolism in *S. haematobium*-infected patients results in higher concentrations of certain metabolites (e.g. indican, anthranilic acid glu-curonide, 3-hydroxyanthranilic acid, L-kynurenine, 3-hydroxy-L-kynurenine and acetyl-L-kynurenine) in pooled urine {11,12,806}. Some of these metabolites have been reported to be carcinogenic to the urinary bladder {332}.

Immunological changes have been suggested as playing a role {854,2156, 2157,2158}.

Secondary bacterial infection of *Schistosoma*-infected bladders is a well documented event {678,1091,1093,1449, 1468} and may play an intermediary role in the genesis of squamous-cell carcinoma via a variety of metabolic effects. Nitrate, nitrite and N-nitroso compounds are detected in the urine of *S. haematobium*-infected patients {14,1090,1091, 1092,2642,2643}. Nitrosamines are formed by nitrosation of secondary amines with nitrites by bacterial catalysis (or via urinary phenol catalysis); they may be carcinogenic to bladder mucosa.

Elevated β-glucuronidase levels in schistosome-infected subjects could increase the release of carcinogenic metabolites from their glucuronides. No data are available at present to confirm this association, although schistosome-infected humans are known to have elevated β-glucuronidase activity in urine {9,10,15, 679,683,805,1916}, for reasons that are unknown.

Genetic damage in the form of slightly increased sister chromatid exchange and micronucleus frequencies were seen in peripheral blood lymphocytes harvested from schistosomiasis patients {104, 2399}, and micronuclei were more frequent in urothelial cells from chronic schistosomiasis patients than in controls {2239}.

Macroscopy

Most squamous cell carcinomas are bulky, polypoid, solid, necrotic masses, often filling the bladder lumen {2297}, although some are predominantly flat and irregularly bordered {1884} or ulcerated and infiltrating {1233}. The presence of necrotic material and keratin debris on the surface is relatively constant.

Histopathology

The diagnosis of squamous cell carcinoma is restricted to pure tumours {232,745,2297}. If an identifiable urothelial element including urothelial carcinoma in situ is found, the tumour should be classified as urothelial carcinoma with squamous differentiation {2276}. The presence of keratinizing squamous metaplasia in the adjacent flat epithelium, especially if associated with dysplasia, supports a diagnosis of squamous cell carcinoma. Squamous metaplasia is identifiable in the adjacent epithelium in 17-60% of cases from Europe and North America {232}.

The invasive tumours may be well differ-

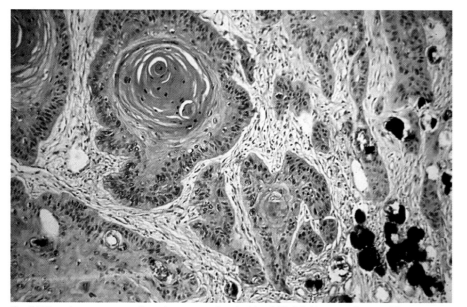

Fig. 2.49 Invasive squamous cell carcinoma associated with calcified Schistosoma haematobium eggs.

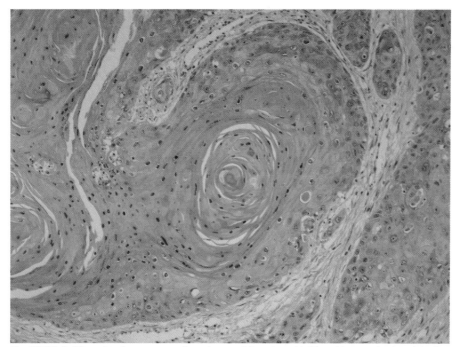

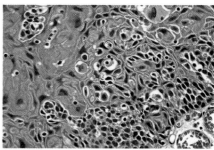
Fig. 2.51 Squamous cell carcinoma.

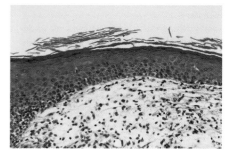
Fig. 2.52 Keratinizing squamous metaplasia.

Fig. 2.50 Well differentiated squamous cell carcinoma of the urinary bladder with extensive keratinization (H&E).

entiated with well defined islands of squamous cells with keratinization, prominent intercellular bridges, and minimal nuclear pleomorphism. They may also be poorly differentiated, with marked nuclear pleomorphism and only focal evidence of squamous differentiation. A basaloid pattern has been reported {2682}.

Somatic genetics
Genetic analyses of squamous cell carcinomas (SQCC) of the urinary bladder focused on Schistosoma associated tumours. Cytogenetic and classic molecular analyses showed overrepresentation of chromosomal material predominantly at 5p, 6p, 7p, 8q, 11q, 17q, and 20q, while deletions were most frequent at 3p, 4q, 5q, 8p, 13q, 17p, and 18q {74,681, 735,912,1858,2118,2380}. Several studies suggested differences in the frequency and type of p53 alterations between urothelial carcinoma and Schistosoma associated SQCC {987,2141,2784}. However, the rate of p53 positive tumours ranged between 30-90% in all studies (average 40%; n=135) {987, 2141,2784}, which is not significantly different from the findings in urothelial cancer. In one study, TP53 mutations in Schistosoma associated SQCC included more base transitions at CpG dinucleotiodes than seen in urothelial carcinomas

{2784}. Other molecular alterations known to occur in urothelial carcinomas such as HRAS mutations (6-84%) {2117,2127}, EGFR overexpression (30-70%) {337,1921}, and HER2 expression (10-50%) {225,489,836,914,1509,1527, 1708,1974,2152,2309} were also found at comparable frequencies in Schistosoma associated SQCC {2141}. Only few non Schistosoma associated "sporadic" SQCC have been molecularly analyzed. Four cases of SQCC had been investigated by classical cytogenetics {731,1573,2710} and another eleven by comparative genomic hybridization (CGH) {681}. The predominant changes in the CGH study were losses of 3p (2/11), 9p (2/11), and 13q (5/11) as well as gains of 1q (3/11), 8q (4/11), and 20q (4/11) {681}. Circumscribed high level amplifications were reported at 8q24 (2 cases) and 11q13 (one case) in this study. No significant genetic differences have been found between Schistosoma associated and non Schistosoma associated urothelial carcinoma with or without squamous cell differentiation {225,489, 836,914,1509,1527,1708,1974,2152,230 9}. Methylation of DNA as shown by detection of O⁶-methyldeoxyguanosine has been found in a high percentage of patients with schistosomiasis-associated cancers in Egypt {149,150}.

Prognosis and predictive factors
Clinical criteria
Patient-related factors, e.g. sex and age are not prognostic in squamous cell bladder cancer {692}. In contrast, T-stage, lymph node involvement and tumour grade have been shown to be of independent prognostic value {2118, 2373}. Patients undergoing radical surgery appear to have an improved survival as compared to radiation therapy and/or chemotherapy, while neoadjuvant radiation improves the outcome in locally advance tumours {866}.

Morphologic factors
Pathologic stage is the most important prognostic parameter for squamous cell carcinoma {692}. The tumours are staged using the AJCC/TNM system as for urothelial carcinoma {944}. In a series of 154 patients, overall 5-year survival was 56%; for those patients with organ-confined tumour (pT1,2) it was 67% and for non organ-confined (pT3,4) it was only 19% {692}.
There are no uniformly accepted criteria for grading of squamous cell carcinoma. Squamous cell carcinoma of the bladder has been graded according to the amount of keratinization and the degree of nuclear pleomorphism {745,1884}. Several studies have demonstrated

grading to be a significant morphologic parameter {692,745,1884}. In one series, 5-year survivals for Grade 1, 2 and 3 squamous cell carcinoma was 62%, 52% and 35%, respectively {692}. This has not been a uniform finding however {2263}.

One recent study analyzing 154 patients that underwent cystectomy suggested that a higher number of newly formed blood vessels predicts unfavourable disease outcome {692}.

Genetic predictive factors
Nothing is known on the impact of genetic changes on the prognosis of SQCC of the urinary bladder.

Verrucous squamous cell carcinoma

D.J. Grignon
M.N. El-Bolkainy

ICD-O code   8051/3

Verrucous carcinoma is an uncommon variant of squamous cell carcinoma that occurs almost exclusively in patients with *schistosomiasis*, accounting for 3% to 4.6% of bladder cancers in such a setting {680,682}. Isolated cases of verrucous carcinoma of the urinary bladder have been described in the literature from non-endemic areas {691,1102, 2772,2851}. This cancer appears as an exophytic, papillary, or "warty" mass with epithelial acanthosis and papillomatosis, minimal nuclear and architectural atypia and rounded, pushing, deep borders. Cases having typical verrucous carcinoma with an infiltrative component are described and should not be included in the verrucous carcinoma category {1603}. In other organs, verrucous carcinoma has a good prognosis, but results

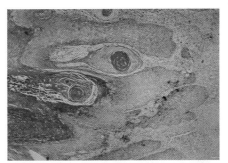
Fig. 2.53 Verrucous squamous cell carcinoma of the urinary bladder showing typical exophytic papillary growth and high degree of differentiation.

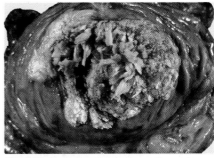
Fig. 2.54 Verrucous squamous cell carcinoma associated with schistosoma infection.

in the bladder are limited. Cases of classic verrucous carcinoma are associated with minimal risk of progression whether associated with *schistosomiasis* or without {680,691,1102,2772,2851}. Tumours developing in patients with longstanding

anogenital condyloma acuminata and condyloma acuminatum of the urinary bladder are reported suggesting a possible link to HPV infection {186,2772}.

Squamous cell papilloma

B. Helpap

ICD-O code   8052/0

Squamous cell papilloma of the urinary bladder is a very rare benign, proliferative squamous lesion. It occurs in elderly

women without specific clinical symptoms {428}. In most cases the cystoscopy shows a solitary papillary lesion {428}. It is not associated with human papillomavirus (HPV) infection.

Histologically, the tumour is composed of papillary cores covered by benign squamous epithelium without koilocytic atypia.

Adenocarcinoma

A.G. Ayala
P. Tamboli
M.N. El-Bolkainy
M.P. Schoenberg

E. Oliva
D. Sidransky
P. Cairns
R. Simon

Definition
A malignant neoplasm derived from the urothelium showing histologically pure glandular phenotype.

Epidemiology
Bladder adenocarcinoma is an uncommon malignant tumour accounting for less than 2% of all the malignant urinary bladder tumours {1192,2612}. It includes primary bladder adenocarcinoma and urachal carcinoma.

Clinical features
Adenocarcinoma of the urinary bladder occurs more commonly in males than in females at about 2.6:1, and affects adults with a peak incidence in the sixth decade of life {24,878,953,1192,1245,1263,1388, 1813,2832}. Haematuria is the most common symptom followed by dysuria, but mucusuria is rarely seen {953}.

Macroscopy
Grossly, this tumour may be exophytic, papillary, sessile, ulcerating, or infiltrating and may exhibit a gelatinous appearance.

Histopathology
Histologically, pure adenocarcinoma of the bladder may show different patterns of growth {953}. These include: enteric (colonic) type, {953} adenocarcinoma not otherwise specified (NOS) {953}, signet ring cell {257,952}, mucinous (colloid) {953}, clear cell {456,2901}, hepatoid {344}, and mixed {953}. The NOS

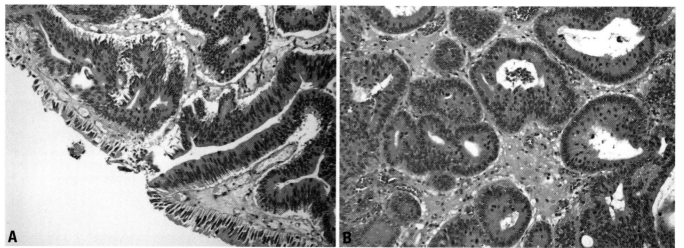

Fig. 2.55 Adenocarcinoma of bladder, colonic type. **A** In this view, the surface shows intestinal metaplastic changes that merge with the invaginating glandular elements. **B** In this illustration there are multiple glands embedded in a loose stroma.

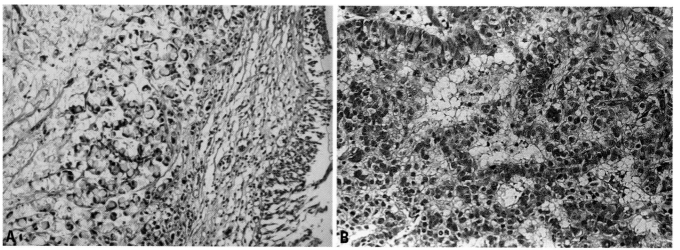

Fig. 2.56 A Signet ring cell carcinoma of bladder. The lamina propria exhibits diffuse infiltration of signet ring cells. **B** Adenocarcinoma. Hepatoid adenocarcinoma of the urinary bladder showing irregular areas of conventional adenocarcinoma (H&E).

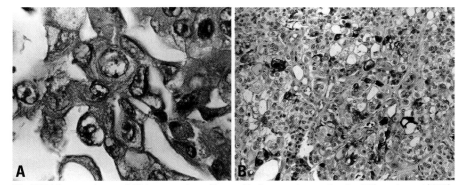

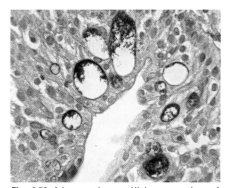

Fig. 2.57 Adenocarcinoma. **A** High power view of hepatoid adenocarcinoma showing billiary pigment (H&E). **B** Immunohistochemical detection of alpha-fetoprotein in hepatoid adenocarcinoma with so-called medullary pattern.

Fig. 2.58 Adenocarcinoma. High power view of intracytoplasmic lumina with mucin in a low grade urothelial carcinoma (Alcian blue pH 2.5, staining).

type consists of an adenocarcinoma with a non-specific glandular growth. The enteric type closely resembles adeno-carcinoma of the colon. Tumours that show abundant mucin with tumour cells floating within the mucin are classified as mucinous or colloid type. The signet ring cell variant may be diffuse or mixed, can have a monocytoid or plasmacytoid phe-notype, and an accompanying in situ component with numerous signet ring cells may be present {456}. An extreme-ly rare variant of adenocarcinoma is the clear cell type (mesonephric), which consists of papillary structures with cyto-plasmic cells that characteristically exhibit a HOBNAIL appearance {456}. The hepatoid type is also rare and con-sists of large cells with eosinophilic cyto-plasm {344}. Finally, it is not uncommon to find a mixture of these growth patterns. Adenocarcinoma in situ may be found in the urinary bladder alone or in combina-tion with an invasive adenocarcinoma. The mucosa is replaced by glandular structures with definitive nuclear atypia. Three patterns are described and these are, papillary, cribriform and flat. A pure

pattern is rarely seen, but various combi-nations of these are the rule {405}.
There is no generally accepted grading system ascribed to adenocarcinoma of the bladder.

Immunoprofile

The immunohistochemical profile of these tumours that has been reported in the literature is variable and closely matches that of colonic adenocarcino-mas {2572,2629,2777}. Reports of cytok-eratin (CK) 7 positivity are variable rang-ing from 0-82%, while CK-20 is reported to be positive in most bladder adenocar-cinomas. Villin has recently been report-ed to be positive in enteric type adeno-carcinomas of the urinary bladder {2572}. Another marker of interest is β-catenin, which has been reported to be of help in distinguishing primary adeno-carcinoma of the bladder from metastat-ic colonic adenocarcinoma {2777}.

Differential diagnosis

The differential diagnosis includes metastatic disease or direct extension, most commonly from colorectum and

prostate. Secondary involvement is much more common than the primary adenocarcinoma of the bladder.

Precursor lesions

Most cases of adenocarcinoma of the urinary bladder are associated with longstanding intestinal metaplasia of the urothelium, such as may be seen in a non-functioning bladder {341,660,1504, 2898}, obstruction {2379}, chronic irrita-tion {660,1928,2538} and cystocele. Adenocarcinoma arising in extrophy is felt to be secondary to the long-standing intestinal metaplasia common to this dis-ease {919, 1677,2521,2791}. The risk of development of adenocarcinoma in extrophy is in the range of 4.1-7.1% {1677,2791}. Although traditionally investigators have felt that intestinal metaplasia is a strong risk factor for the development of adenocarcinoma in extrophy {341,660,919,1327,1504,1677, 2379,2396,2521,2538,2791,2898}, a recent study is challenging this theory {499}. Fifty-three patients with extrophy of the bladder were followed for more than 10 years, and none developed car-

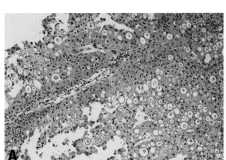

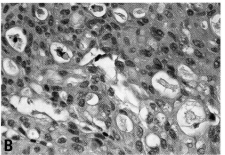

Fig. 2.59 Adenocarcinoma. **A** Low grade papillary urothelial carcinoma with intracytoplasmic lumina. This is not considered to be glandular differentiation (H&E). **B** Pseudoglandular arrangement of urothelial cells in a low grade urothelial carcinoma (H&E).

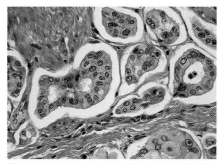

Fig. 2.60 Adenocarcinoma of the urinary bladder with squamous area.

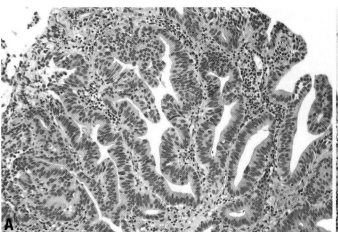 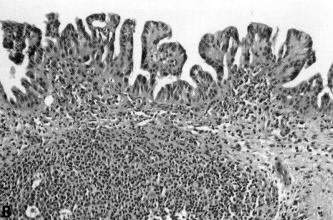

Fig. 2.61 A Adenocarcinoma in situ of urinary bladder. **B** Adenocarcinoma in situ. Note columnar epithelium with nuclear anaplasia involving mucosal surface.

cinoma {499}.

Cystitis glandularis is present in invasive adenocarcinoma ranging from 14- 67% of cases {24,2612}, but its role in the pathogenesis of invasive adenocarcinoma is not clear. However, in patients with pelvic lipomatosis, which harbors cystitis glandularis, adenocarcinoma may occur {1088,2862}. Adenocarcinoma may also arise in conjunction with villous adenomas, S. haematobium infestation, and endometriosis of the bladder {2885}.

Somatic genetics

To date, few studies have examined the genetic alterations underlying adenocarcinoma of the bladder. A partial allelotype reported loss of chromosomal arm 9p (50%), 9q (17%), 17p (50%), 8p (50%) and 11p (43%) in 8 schistosomiasis-associated adenocarcinomas. Chromosomal arms 3p, 4p and 4q, 14q and 18q also showed LOH but no loss of 13q was seen {2380}. With the exceptions of a lower frequency of loss of 9q and 13q, this spectrum of chromosomal loss is similar to urothelial and squamous cell carcinoma of the bladder. LOH of 9p likely targets the p16/p14 tumour suppressor genes. The 17p LOH targets the p53 gene as a separate study reported 4/13 adenocarcinomas to have p53 point mutation {2784}. Further support for the observation of 18q loss is provided by a study that detected LOH of the D18S61 microsatellite marker in a patient's adenocarcinoma and urine DNA {628}.

Predictive factors

Clinical factors

Management of invasive adenocarcinoma of the bladder includes partial or radical cystectomy followed by consideration of chemotherapy or radiotherapy according to the extent of the lesion. Partial cystectomy is usually associated with a relatively high recurrence rate {2853}.

Poor prognosis of this variant is associated with advanced stage at diagnosis. These tumours typically arise in the bladder base or dome, but can occur anywhere in the bladder. Primary vesical adenocarcinoma represents the most common type of cancer in patients with bladder extrophy. Signet-ring carcinoma is a rare variant of mucus-producing adenocarcinoma and will often produce linitis plastica of the bladder {454}.

Morphologic factors

Stage is the most important prognostic factors for this disease {953}. However, the prognosis is poor since most adenocarcinomas present at advanced stage with muscle invasive disease and beyond (T2/T3). Survival at 5 years is 31% {953} -35% {551}.

It is important to distinguish between urachal and non-urachal adenocarcinomas especially for treatment purposes. Some studies have suggested that non-urachal adenocarcinomas carry a worse prognosis {95,953,2612}, but this was not confirmed.

Among histologic types of adenocarci-

noma, pure signet ring cell carcinoma carries the worst prognosis, otherwise histologic type has no prognostic significance {953}.

Immunohistochemical markers

Little is known about genetic factors associated with prognosis of adenocarcinoma of the bladder. Proliferation indices of markers such as the nucleolar organizer region (AgNOR), Ki-67, and proliferating cell nuclear antigen (PCNA) are associated with grade and stage of nonurachal bladder adenocarcinomas {1994}. There is an increased incidence of local recurrence and distant metastasis in patients with a high Ki-67, PCNA, and AgNOR proliferation index.

Table 2.05
Variants of adenocarcinomas of the bladder.

Variant	Reference
Adenocarcinomas, NOS	{953}
Enteric (colonictype)	{953}
Signet ring cell	{257,952}
Mucinous	{953}
Clear cell	{456,2901}
Hepatoid	{344}
Mixed	{953}

Urachal carcinoma

A.G. Ayala
P. Tamboli

Definition
Primary carcinoma derived from urachal remnants. The vast majority of urachal carcinomas are adenocarcinomas; urothelial, squamous and other carcinomas may also occur.

ICD-O code   8010/3

Epidemiology
Urachal adenocarcinoma is far less common than non-urachal adenocarcinoma of the bladder. Most cases of urachal carcinoma occur in the fifth and sixth decades of life; the mean patient age is 50.6 years, which is about 10 years less than that for bladder adenocarcinoma. This disease occurs slightly more in men than in women, with a ratio, of about 1.8:1 {878,953,1230,1261,1263,1526, 1813,2383,2832}.

Localization
Urachal carcinomas arise from the urachus. Urachal remnants are reported to occur predominantly in the vertex or dome and the anterior wall, less frequently in the posterior wall, and they extend to the umbilicus {2343}.

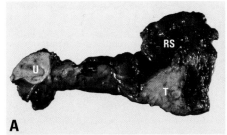 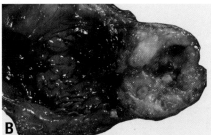

Fig. 2.62 Urachal adenocarcinoma of bladder. **A** Partial cystectomy including the dome of the bladder with the Retzious space (RS), tumour (T), and connective tissue between bladder and anterior abdominal wall at umbilicus (U). **B** Total cystectomy specimen. The urachal carcinoma is located within the wall of the bladder in the dome of the bladder, and the cut surface is glistening demonstrating its mucinoid appearance.

Clinical features
Hematuria is the most common symptom (71%), followed by pain (42%), irritative symptoms (40%), and umbilical discharge (2%) {878,953,1230,1261,1263, 1526,1813,2383,2832}. The patient may present with the suprapubic mass. Mucusuria occurs in about 25% of the cases {953}, and its presence should raise the question of urachal mucous carcinoma.

Macroscopy
Urachal carcinoma usually involves the muscular wall of the bladder dome, and it may or may not destroy the overlying mucosa. The mass may be discrete, but it may involve the route of the urachal remnants, forming a relatively large mass that may invade the Retzius space and reach the anterior abdominal wall. Mucinous lesions tend to calcify, and these calcifications may be detected on plain X-ray films of the abdomen. The mucosa of the urinary bladder is not destroyed in early stages of the disease, but it eventually becomes ulcerated as the tumour reaches the bladder cavity. The cut surface of this tumour exhibits a glistening, light-tan appearance, reflecting its mucinous contents.

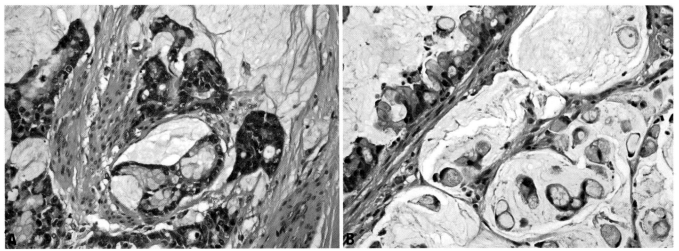

Fig. 2.63 Urachal adenocarcinoma of bladder. **A** Moderately differentiated mucinous adenocarcinoma. **B** In this illustrations of mucinous adenocarcinoma there is a row of mucin producing cells lining a fibrovascular septae. On the other side there are signet ring cells floating within the mucinous material. The presence of a mucinous adenocarcinoma containing signet ring cells floating within mucin is a very common occurrence in urachal carcinoma.

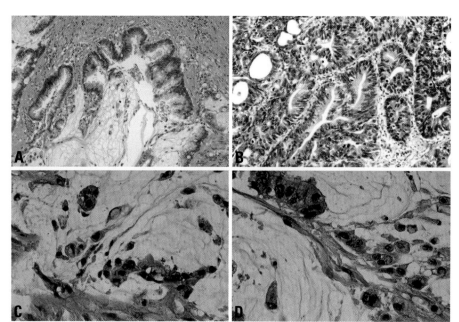

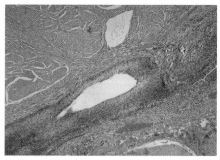

Fig. 2.65 Intramural urachal canal without complexity, covered by urothelium.

Fig. 2.64 Adenocarcinoma. **A** Mucinous (colloid) pattern of adenocarcinoma of the urachus with its characteristic mucin pool. **B** Primary urachal adenocarcinoma, intestinal type with complex atypical glands infiltrating the bladder wall. **C** Malignant cells floating in a mucin pool, a characteristic finding in mucinous (colloid) adenocarcinoma of the urachus. **D** Mucinous (colloid) pattern of adenocarcinoma of the urachus with malignat cells floating in a mucin pool.

Staging

Although urachal adenocarcinoma has been staged as a bladder carcinoma using the TNM staging system which is difficult to apply because the majority of urachal adenocarcinomas are "muscle invasive". Hence, a specific staging system for this neoplasm has been proposed {2383}.

Histopathology

This discussion pertains mainly to adenocarcinomas as the most common. Urachal adenocarcinomas are subdivided into mucinous, enteric, not otherwise specified, signet ring-cell, and mixed types; these subtypes are similar to those

Table 2.06
Staging system of the urachal carcinoma.

I. Confined to urachal mucosa
II. Invasive but confined to urachus
III. Local extension to:
A. Bladder muscle
B. Abdominal wall
C. Peritoneum
D. Other viscera
IV. Metastases to:
A. Regional lymph nodes
B. Distant sites

From Sheldon et al. {2383}.

of adenocarcinoma of the urinary bladder. In one study with 24 cases of urachal carcinoma, 12 (50%) tumours were mucinous, seven (29%) were enteric, four (17%) were mixed, and one (4%) was a signet ring-cell carcinoma {953}.

Mucinous carcinomas are characterized by pools or lakes of extracellular mucin with single cells or nests of columnar or signet ring-cells floating in it. The enteric type closely resembles a colonic type of adenocarcinoma and may be difficult to differentiate from it. Pure signet ring-cell carcinoma rarely occurs in the urachus; most commonly, signet ring-cell differentiation is present within a mucinous carcinoma.

The cells of urachal adenocarcinoma stain for carcinoembryonic antigen {24,953}, and Leu-M1 {24,953}.

Criteria to classify a tumour as urachal in origin were initially established by Wheeler and Hill in 1954 {2811} and consisted of the following: (1) tumour in the dome of the bladder, (2) absence of cystitis cystica and cystitis glandularis, (3) invasion of muscle or deeper structures and either intact or ulcerated epithelium, (4) presence of urachal remnants, (5) presence of a suprapubic mass, (6) a sharp demarcation between the tumour and the normal surface epithelium, and (7) tumour growth in the bladder wall,

branching into the Retzius space. These criteria, believed to be very restrictive, were modified by Johnson et al. {1230}, who proposed the following criteria: (1) tumour in the bladder (dome), (2) a sharp demarcation between the tumour and the surface epithelium, and (3) exclusion of primary adenocarcinoma located elsewhere that has spread secondarily to the bladder. Bladder adenocarcinoma may be very difficult to rule out because it has the same histologic and immunohistochemical features as urachal adenocarcinoma does. Urachal adenocarcinoma may be associated with cystitis cystica and cystitis glandularis; the cystitis cystica or cystitis glandularis must show no dysplastic changes, however, because dysplastic changes of the mucosa or presence of dysplastic intestinal metaplasia would tend to exclude an urachal origin.

Precursor lesion

The pathogenesis of urachal adenocarcinoma is unknown. Although a urachal adenocarcinoma may arise from a villous adenoma of the urachus {1571}, intestinal metaplasia of the urachal epithelium is believed to be the favoured predisposing factor {201}.

Prognosis

Management of urachal adenocarcinoma consists of complete eradication of the disease. Partial or radical cystectomy, including the resection of the umbilicus, is the treatment of choice. Recurrences, are common, however, especially in cases in which a partial cystectomy is done {878,2853}. Examination of the surgical margins with frozen section has been advocated {878}. The 5 year survival rate has been reported to range from 25% {2813} to 61% {953}.

Clear cell adenocarcinoma

E. Oliva

Definition
Clear cell adenocarcinoma is a distinct variant of urinary bladder carcinoma that resembles its Müllerian counterpart in the female genital tract.

ICD-O code   8310/3

Synonym
Mesonephric carcinoma {2901}.

Epidemiology
Clear cell adenocarcinomas of the urinary bladder are rare. Patients are typically females that range in age from 22 to 83 (mean 57 years), commonly presenting with hematuria and/or dysuria {640,876,1954,2901}.

Macroscopy
Although the gross appearance is non-specific, frequently they grow as polypoid to papillary masses.

Tumour spread and stage
Clear cell adenocarcinomas may infiltrate the bladder wall and metastasize to lymph nodes and distant organs similarly to urothelial carcinomas. They should be staged using the TNM system for bladder cancer.

Histopathology
Clear cell adenocarcinomas have a characteristic morphology, showing one or more of the typical three morphologic patterns, tubulo-cystic, papillary and/or diffuse, the former being the most common. The tubules vary in size and may contain either basophilic and/or eosinophilic secretions. The papillae are generally small and their fibrovascular cores may be extensively hyalinized. When present, diffuse sheets of tumour cells are a minor component in most cases. The tumour cells range from flat to cuboidal to columnar and they may have either clear or eosinophilic cytoplasm or an admixture thereof. Hobnail cells are frequently seen but are only rarely conspicuous. Cytologic atypia is usually moderate to severe, frequently associat-

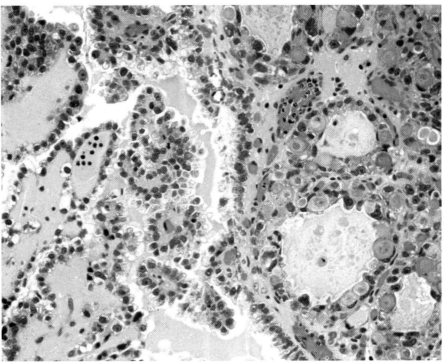

Fig. 2.66 Clear cell adenocarcinoma variant of the urinary bladder.

ed with a brisk mitotic activity {876,1954,2901}. In some cases, clear cell adenocarcinomas may be associated with urothelial carcinoma or even rarely with adenocarcinoma non-special type (NOS) {876,1954}.

The differential diagnosis of clear cell adenocarcinoma includes most frequently nephrogenic adenoma, a benign reactive process, but also malignant tumours such as urothelial carcinoma with clear cells, metastatic clear cell renal carcinoma, cervical or vaginal clear cell adenocarcinoma or rarely adenocarcinoma of the prostate secondarily involving the bladder {1954}.

Immunohistochemical studies have shown that clear cell adenocarcinomas are positive for CK7, CK20, CEA, CA125, LeuM-1 and negative for prostate specific antigen, prostate-specific acid phosphatase, estrogen and progesterone receptors. These tumours show high MIB-1 activity and are often positive for p53 {876,2708}.

Precursor lesions
Occasional clear cell adenocarcinomas have been associated with endometriosis or a Müllerian duct remmant, rare cases coexisted with urothelial dysplasia, and some clear cell adenocarcinomas arise in a diverticulum. Although exceptional cases have been reported to arise from malignant transformation of nephrogenic adenoma, this is a highly controversial area.

Histogenesis
In the past, bladder clear cell adenocarcinomas were thought to be of mesonephric origin, and were designated as mesonephric adenocarcinomas despite lack of convincing evidence for a mesonephric origin. As these tumours occur more frequently in women, they are histologically very similar to clear cell adenocarcinomas of the female genital tract, and they are occasionally associated with benign Müllerian epithelium, a

Müllerian origin is postulated for some of them {640,876,1954}. However, most clear cell adenocarcinomas probably originate from peculiar glandular differentiation in urothelial neoplasms as most bladder clear cell adenocarcinomas have not been associated with endometriosis, they have been diagnosed in patients with a previous history of urothelial carcinoma, and their immunohistochemical profile overlaps with that of urothelial carcinoma. In this setting it is presumed that aberrant differentiation which frequently occurs in high grade bladder cancer has an unusual morphology of clear cell adenocarcinoma in a small subset of patients {876,1954}.

Prognosis and predictive factors

No long follow-up is available in many of these tumours. Cumulative experience from the literature indicates that clear cell adenocarcinoma may not be as aggressive as initially believed {85,640}. Many of these tumours have an exophytic growth pattern, they may be diagnosed at an early stage and have a relative better prognosis. High stage tumours have a poor prognosis.

Villous adenoma

L. Cheng
A.G. Ayala

Definition

Villous adenomas is a benign glandular neoplasm of the urinary bladder which histologically mimics its enteric counterpart.

ICD-O code   8261/0

Epidemiology

Villous adenomas of the urinary bladder are rare with fewer than 60 cases reported. There is no apparent gender predominance. The tumour usually occurs in elderly patients (mean age, 65 years; range, 23-94 years).

Localization

It shows a predilection for the urachus, dome, and trigone of the urinary bladder.

Clinical symptoms

The patients often present with hematuria and/or irritative symptoms {430,2356}. Cystoscopic examination often identifies an exophytic tumour.

Macroscopy

On gross examination the lesion is a papillary tumour that is indistinguishable from a papillary urothelial carcinoma.

Histopathology

Microscopically, the tumour is characterized by a papillary architecture with central fibrovascular cores, consisting of pointed or blunt finger-like processes lined by pseudostratified columnar epithelium. The epithelial cells display nuclear stratification, nuclear crowding, nuclear hyperchromasia, and occasional prominent nucleoli. The overall morphology of this lesion is similar to the colonic counterpart.

Villous adenomas of the bladder often coexist with in situ and invasive adenocarcinoma. On limited biopsy specimens there may be only changes of villous adenoma. Therefore, the entire specimen should be processed to exclude invasive disease.

Immunoprofile

Villous adenomas of the bladder are positive for cytokeratin 20 (100% of cases), cytokeratin 7 (56%), carcinoembryonic antigen (89%), epithelial membrane antigen (22%), and acid mucin with alcian blue periodic acid-Schiff stain (78%) {430}.

Prognosis

Patients with an isolated villous adenoma have an excellent prognosis. Progression to adenocarcinoma is rare.

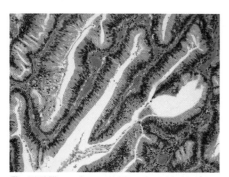

Fig. 2.67 Villous adenoma of the urinary bladder (urachus) showing papillary fronds covered by columnar mucus-secreting epithelium and its characteristic nuclear crowding and pseudostratification (H&E).

Small cell carcinoma

F. Algaba
G. Sauter
M.P. Schoenberg

Definition
Small cell carcinoma is a malignant neuroendocrine neoplasm derived from the urothelium which histologically mimics its pulmonary counterpart.

ICD-O code   8041/3

Clinical features
Gross haematuria is the most common presenting symptom in patients with small cell carcinoma (SCC) of the bladder. Other symptoms include dysuria or localized abdominal/pelvic pain {1531}. Approximately 56% of patients will present with metastatic disease at the time of diagnosis. The most common locations for disease spread include: regional lymph nodes, 56%; bone, 44%; liver, 33%; and lung, 20% {2640}. Peripheral (sensory) neuropathy may also be a clinical sign of metastatic disease and is attributed to the paraneoplastic syndrome associated with tumour production of antineuronal autoantibodies. The presence of antiHU autoantibodies (IgG) is a specific marker of the paraneoplastic syndrome and should prompt careful evaluation for SCC (particularly in the lung) in a patient without a history of cancer {93}. Electrolyte abnormalities such as hypercalcemia or hypophosphatemia, and ectopic secretion of ACTH have also

been reported as part of the paraneoplastic syndrome associated with primary SCC of the bladder {2021,2182}.

Localization and macroscopy
Almost all the small cell carcinomas of the urinary tract arise in the urinary bladder {2640}. The tumour may appear as a large solid, isolated, polypoid, nodular mass with or without ulceration, and may extensively infiltrate the bladder wall. The vesical lateral walls and the dome are the most frequent topographies, in 4.7% they arise in a diverticulum {100}.

Histopathology
All tumours are invasive at presentation {2640}. They consist of small, rather uniform cells, with nuclear molding, scant cytoplasm and nuclei containing finely stippled chromatin and inconspicuous nucleoli. Mitoses are present and may be frequent. Necrosis is common and there may be DNA encrustation of blood vessels walls (Azzopardi phenomenon).
Roughly 50% of cases have areas of urothelial carcinoma {1934} and exceptionally, squamous cell carcinoma and/or adenocarcinoma. This is important, because the presence of these differentiated areas does not contradict the diagnosis of small cell carcinoma.
The neuroendocrine expression of this

tumour is identified by many methods. In some papers, neuroendocrine granules are found with electron microscopy or histochemical methods, but in the majority of them, the immunohistochemical method is used. The neuronal-specific enolase is expressed in 87% of cases, and Chromogranin A only in a third of cases {2640}. The diagnosis of small cell carcinoma can be made on morphologic grounds alone, even if neuroendocrine differentiation cannot be demonstrated.
The differential diagnosis is metastasis of a small cell carcinoma from another site (very infrequent) {608}, malignant lymphoma, lymphoepithelioma-like carcinoma, plasmacytoid carcinoma and a poorly differentiated urothelial carcinoma.

Histogenesis
In the spite of the low frequency of associated flat carcinoma "in situ" referred in the literature (14%) {2640}, the high frequency of cytokeratin (CAM5.2 in 64%) expression in the small cell component supports the hypothesis of urothelial origin {60}. Other hypotheses are the malignant transformation of neuroendocrine cells demonstrated in normal bladder {60}, and the stem cell theory {254}.

Somatic genetics
Data obtained by comparative genomic

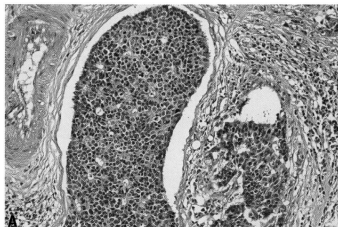
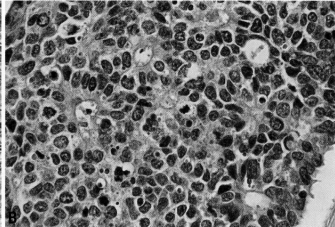

Fig. 2.68 Neuroendocrine carcinoma of the urinary bladder. **A** Low power view of a neuroendocrine carcinoma showing both atypical carcinoid and undifferentiated small cell features. **B** Well differentiated neuroendocrine carcinoma characterized by cell pleomorphism and high mitotic rate.

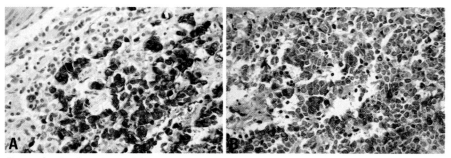

Fig. 2.69 Small cell carcinoma. A Cytoplasmatic expression of cytokeratin 5.2. B Chromogranin A expression.

hybridization suggest that urinary bladder small cell carcinoma is a genetically unstable tumour, typically exhibiting a high number of cytogenetic changes {2596}. The most frequent changes included deletions of 10q, 4q, 5q, and 13q as well as gains of 8q, 5p, 6p, and 20q. High level amplifications, potentially pinpointing the location of activated oncogenes were found at 1p22-32, 3q26.3, 8q24 (including CMYC), and 12q14-21 (including MDM2) {2596}. Only one tumour was analyzed by cytogenetics {133}. Complex and heterogeneous cytogenetic alterations were found in this tumour including rearrangements of the chromosomes 6, 9, 11, 13, and 18. The same tumour also showed a nuclear p53 accumulation.

Prognosis and predictive factors
Clinical factors
This tumour type is characterized by an aggressive clinical course with early vascular and muscle invasion. The overall 5-year survival rate for patients with small cell carcinoma of the bladder with local disease has been reported as low as 8% {8,2640}. Overall prognosis has been shown to be related to the stage of disease at presentation; however, it has also been suggested that clinical stage is not independently associated with survival {1105,1587}. The latter observation is based upon the theory that micrometastases are already present at the time of diagnosis in patients with clinically localized disease {1587}. Age greater than 65, high TNM stage and metastatic disease at presentation are predictors of poor survival. Administration of systemic chemotherapy and cystectomy or radiotherapy, have variable success {182, 1062,1587}.

Morphological factors
No difference has been shown between tumours with pure or mixed histology. Tumour confined to the bladder wall may have a better prognosis {100,2640}.

Genetic factors
The prognostic or predictive significance of cytogenetic or other molecular changes in small cell carcinoma of the urinary bladder is unknown. The immunohistochemical detection of p53 (77%) failed to mark cases with a poorer prognosis {2640}.

Paragraglioma

C.J. Davis

Definition
Paraganglioma of the bladder is a neoplasm derived from paraganglion cells in the bladder wall. They are histologically identical to paragangliomas at other sites.

ICD-O code   8680/1

Synonym
Phaeochromocytoma.

Incidence
These are rare tumours and by 1997 only about 200 cases had been reported {948}. In the AFIP experience there were 77 bladder paragangliomas out of 16.236 bladder tumours (0.47%), but the commonly cited incidence is 0.06-0.10% {1420,1508,1845,2081}.

Clinical features
These occur over a wide age range of 10-88 years with a mean in the forties {429,1845}. They are a little more com-

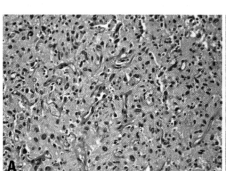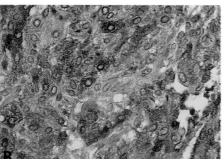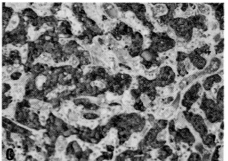

Fig. 2.70 A Paraganglioma. Cell clusters surrounded by network of fine collagenous septa containing blood vessels and sustentacular cells in a paravesicular paraganglioma. B Paraganglioma. Intense chromogranin reaction in the tumour cells of a paraganglioma localized within the wall of the urinary bladder. C Paraganglioma. Chromogranin expression.

mon in females by 1.4:1 {1845}. The clinical triad of sustained or paroxysmal hypertension, intermittent gross hematuria and "micturition attacks" is the characteristic feature {1420,1845}. These attacks consist of bursting headache, anxiety, tremulousness, pounding sensation, blurred vision, sweating and even syncope related to increased levels of catecholamines or their metabolites which can be found in serum or urine {1845}. Some cases have been familial.

Macroscopy

An autopsy study has shown that paraganglia were present in 52% of cases {1115}. They were present in any part of the bladder and at any level of the bladder wall. Most were in the muscularis propria and this is where most of the tumours are located. In 45 cases where the location was known, we found 38% in the dome, 20% in the trigone, 18% posterior wall, 13% anterior wall and the others in the bladder neck and lateral walls. Most of these are circumscribed or multinodular tumours, usually less then 4.0 cm in size. In one study there was an average diameter of 1.9 cm {1420}.

Histopathology

Microscopically, the cells are arranged in discrete nests, the "Zellballen" pattern, separated by a prominent vascular network. Cells are round with clear, amphophilic or acidophilic cytoplasm and ovoid nuclei. Scattered larger or even bizarre nuclei are often present {1845}. Mitoses are rare, and usually absent {1466}. In some cases there may be striking resemblance to urothelial carcinoma. In about 10% of the cases, small neuroblast-like cells are present, usually immediately beneath the urothelium. By immunohistochemistry, bladder paragangliomas react as they do at other sites – negative for epithelial markers

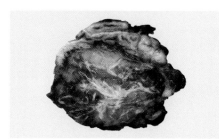

Fig. 2.72 Paraganglioma of the urinary bladder. Large paraganglioma adjacent to the wall of the urinary bladder.

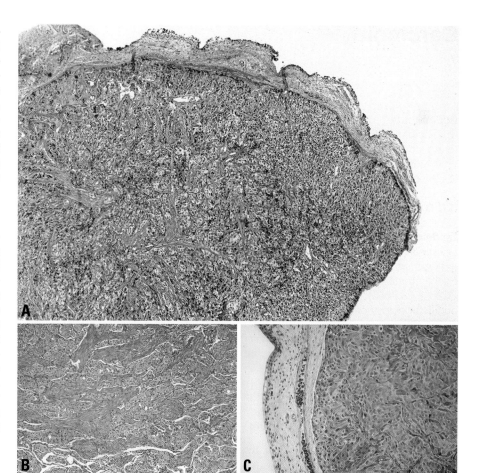

Fig. 2.71 Paraganglioma. **A** Paraganglioma with circumscribed growth pattern. **B** Paraganglioma with dissection through the muscularis propria. **C** Paraganglioma with circumscribed growth pattern.

and positive for the neuroendocrine markers – chromogranin, synaptophysin and others. Flattened sustentacular cells can sometimes be highlighted in the periphery of the cell nests with S-100 protein. Ultrastructural features include dense core neurosecretory granules, usually having the typical morphology of catecholamine–secreting tumours with eccentric dense cores {948,1280}.

Prognosis and predictive factors

The criteria for diagnosing malignant paraganglioma are metastasis and/or "extensive local disease" {1508}. Long-term follow-up is always indicated because metastases have been known to occur many years later {948,1280, 1508}. A recent study found that those tumours staged as T1 or T2 did not show any recurrences or metastases while those that were stage T3 or higher were at risk for both {429}. A review of 72 AFIP cases accumulated since the initial 58 cases reported in 1971 {1466} has

recently been done (unpublished data). Twelve of the 72 (16.7%) were judged to be malignant based upon the presence of metastasis or extension beyond the bladder. Four features appear to indicate an increased potential for malignant behaviour:

1. Younger age: there were 8 cases in the second decade of life and 5 of these were malignant.
2. Hypertension: this was seen in 50% of malignant cases and 12% of the benign ones.
3. Micturition attacks: these were also seen in 50% of malignant cases and 12% of benign ones.
4. Invasive dispersion through the bladder wall. The malignant tumours usually demonstrated widespread dispersion through the bladder wall, sometimes with fragmentation of muscle fascicles by tumour nests. This was rarely seen in those that proved to be benign.

Carcinoid

L. Cheng

Definition
Carcinoid is a potentially malignant neuroendocrine neoplasm derived from the urothelium which histologically is similar to carcinoid tumours at other locations.

ICD-O code   8240/3

Epidemiology
Less than two-dozen cases of carcinoid tumours of the urinary bladder have been reported {343,449,480,1068,2485, 2527,2768,2865}. The tumour usually occurs in elderly patients (mean age, 56 years; range, 29-75 years), with slight male predominance (the male-to-female ratio, 1.8:1).

Clinical features
Hematuria is the most common clinical presentation, followed by irritative voiding symptoms. Association with carcinoid syndrome has not been reported.

Macroscopy
The tumours are submucosal with a predilection for the trigone of the bladder, and range in size from 3 mm-3 cm in the largest dimension. The tumour often presents as a polypoid lesion upon cystoscopic examination. One case arose in an ileal neobladder {803}. Coexistence of carcinoid with other urothelial neoplasia, such as inverted papilloma {2485} and adenocarcinoma {449}, has been reported.

Histopathology
Carcinoid tumours of the bladder are histologically similar to their counterparts in other organ sites. The tumour cells have abundant amphophilic cytoplasm and arranged in an insular, acini, trabecular, or pseudoglandular pattern in a vascular stroma. An organoid growth pattern, resembling that seen in paraganglioma, can be appreciated. The nuclei have finely stippled chromatin and inconspicuous nucleoli. Mitotic figures are infrequent, and tumour necrosis is absent. The tumours show immunoreactivity for neuroendocrine markers (neuron-specific enolase, chromogranin, serotonin, and synaptophysin) and cytokeratin (AE1 and 3). The tumours are positive for the argyrophil reaction by Grimelius silver stains and argentaffin reaction by Fontana-Masson stains. Ultrastructural examinations demonstrate characteristic uniform, round, membrane-bound, electron-dense neurosecretory granules. Flow cytometric studies revealed an aneuploid cell population in one case {2768}.

Differential diagnosis
This includes paraganglioma, nested variant of urothelial carcinoma and metastastic prostatic carcinoma.

Prognosis and predictive factors
More than 25% of patients will have regional lymph node or distant metastasis {2527} but majority are cured by excision.

Rhabdomyosarcoma

I. Leuschner

Definition
Rhabdomyosarcoma is a sarcoma occurring in the urinary bladder that recapitulates morphologic and molecular features of skeletal muscle.

ICD-O code   8900/3

Epidemiology
They are the most common urinary bladder tumours in childhood and adolescence. Almost all bladder rhabdomyosarcomas are of embryonal subtype, whereas the genetically distinct alveolar subtype is extremely rare in this site {1887}. In adults rhabdomyosarcoma is rare and usually of the pleomorphic type.

Macroscopy
Growth pattern of embryonal rhabdomyosarcoma in urinary bladder has two basic forms with prognostic impact: polypoid, mostly intraluminal tumours associated with a favourable prognosis (botryoid subtype) and deeply invasive growing tumours involving the entire bladder wall and usually adjacent organs showing a worse prognosis.

Histopathology
Tumour cells of embryonal rhabdomyosarcoma are usually small, round cells, often set in a myxoid stroma. Some cells may have classic rhabdomyoblastic appearance with abundant eosinophilic cytoplasm and cross striations. Botryoid subtype of embryonal rhabdomyosarcoma has a condensation of tumour cells beneath the covering surface epithelium, called the cambium layer. Deeper parts of the tumours are often hypocellular. The

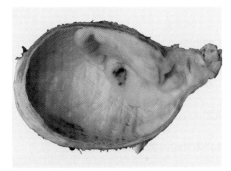

Fig. 2.73 Embryonal rhabdomyosarcoma.

botryoid subtype of embryonal rhabdomyosarcoma is the end of a spectrum of polypoid growing embryonal rhabdomyosarcomas sharing a similar favourable prognosis {1482}. Primarily deep invasive growing tumours of the urinary bladder wall have usually a low degree of differentiation and are associated to a similar worse prognosis as seen for embryonal rhabdomyosarcoma of prostate.

Immunohistochemically, the tumour cells express myogenin (myf4) and MyoD1 in the nucleus {612,1404}. This is assumed to be specific for a skeletal muscle differentiation. Highly differentiated tumour cells can lack myogenin expression. Desmin and pan-actin (HHF35) can also be detected in almost all rhabdomyosarcomas but it is not specific. Staining for myosin and myoglobin can be negative because it is usually found only in well differentiated tumour cells. Recurrences of embryonal rhabdomyosarcoma can show a very high degree of differentiation forming round myoblasts.

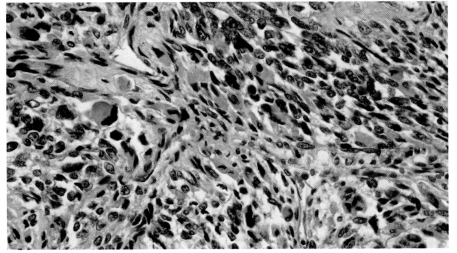

Fig. 2.74 Rhabdomyosarcoma of the bladder.

Leiomyosarcoma

J. Cheville

Definition
Leiomyosarcoma is a rare malignant mesenchymal tumour that arises from urinary bladder smooth muscle.

ICD-O code   8890/3

Epidemiology and etiology
Although leiomyosarcoma is the most common sarcoma of the urinary bladder it accounts for much less than 1% of all bladder malignancies. Males are more frequently affected than females by over 2:1 {1639,1734,2543}. This sarcoma occurs primarily in adults in their 6th to 8th decade. Several cases of leiomyosarcoma of the bladder have occurred years after cyclophosphamide therapy {2039,2253}.

Localization
Leiomyosarcoma can occur anywhere within the bladder, and very rarely can involve the ureter or renal pelvis {947, 1816}.

Clinical features
The vast majority of patients present with haematuria, and on occasion, a palpable pelvic mass, abdominal pain or urinary tract obstruction may be present.

Macroscopy
Leiomyosarcoma of the urinary bladder is typically a large, infiltrating mass with a mean size of 7 cm. High grade leiomyosarcoma frequently exhibits gross and microscopic necrosis.

Histopathology
Histopathologic examination reveals a tumour composed of infiltrative interlacing fascicles of spindle cells. Grading of leiomyosarcoma is based on the degree of cytologic atypia. Low grade leiomyosarcoma exhibits mild to moderate cytologic atypia, and has mitotic activity less than 5 mitoses per 10 HPF. In contrast, high grade leiomyosarcoma shows marked cytologic atypia, and most cases have greater than 5 mitoses per 10 HPF. Immunohistochemically, leiomyosarcoma stains with antibodies directed against actin, desmin and vimentin, and are negative for epithelial markers {1410,1639, 1734,2817}.

Leiomyoma can be morphologically separated from leiomyosarcoma based on its small size, low cellularity, circumscription, and lack of cytologic atypia {1639}. Reactive spindle cell proliferations such as inflammatory pseudotumour or postoperative spindle cell nodule/tumour can be difficult to distinguish from leiomyosarcoma {1572,2889}. Leiomyosarcoma exhibits greater cytologic atypia, abnormal mitoses, and an arrangement in compact cellular fascicles in contrast to reactive spindle cell proliferations, which have a loose vascular myxoid background. However, myxoid change can occur in leiomyosarcoma {2899}. Sarcomatoid carcinoma can resemble leiomyosarcoma but is usually associated with a malignant epithelial component or exhibits cytokeratin positivity.

Prognosis
Although previous reports suggest that 5-year survival after partial or radical cystectomy approaches 70%, the largest recent study indicates that 70% of patients with leiomyosarcoma developed recurrent or metastatic disease, resulting in death in nearly half {1639}.

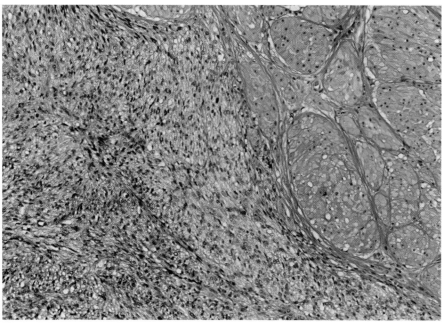

Fig. 2.75 Leiomyosarcoma of the bladder.

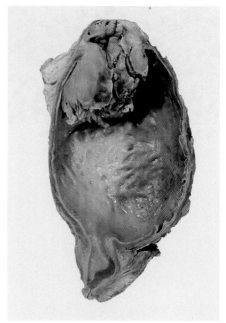

Fig. 2.76 Bladder leiomyosarcoma.

Angiosarcoma

J. Cheville

Definition

Angiosarcoma of the urinary bladder is a very rare sarcoma that arises from the endothelium of blood vessels.

ICD-O code   9120/3

Clinical features

Only 10 cases of urinary bladder angiosarcoma have been reported, all as case reports {699}. Males are more frequently affected than females, and tumours occur in adults with a mean age at diagnosis of 55 years. Patients present with hematuria, and approximately a third of cases are associated with prior radiation to the pelvis, either for gynecologic malignancies or prostate cancer {699,1874}.

Macroscopy

Angiosarcoma of the bladder is typically a large tumour but can be as small as 1 cm. Most tumours exhibit local or distant extension beyond the bladder at the time of diagnosis.

Histopathology

Histopathologic features consist of anastomosing blood-filled channels lined by cytologically atypical endothelial cells. Some angiosarcomas have solid areas, and epithelioid features can be present {2322}. Urinary bladder angiosarcoma stains positively with the immunohistochemical markers of endothelium including CD31 and CD34. The only epithelioid angiosarcoma of the urinary bladder reported to date was negative for cytokeratin, but some epithelioid angiosarcomas at other sites can be cytokeratin positive. Angiosarcoma must be distinguished from haemangioma of the bladder. Haemangioma of the bladder is typically small (usually less than 1 cm), and nearly 80% are of the cavernous type {431}. Urinary haemangioma lacks cytologic atypia and the anastomosing and solid areas of angiosarcoma. Pyogenic granuloma is another benign vascular proliferation that very rarely occurs in the bladder, and is composed of closely spaced capillaries lined by bland endothelium which may show mitotic activity {90}. Kaposi sarcoma may involve the urinary bladder and should be considered in the differential diagnosis, especially in immunocompromised patients {2183,2866}. Rarely, high grade urothelial carcinoma can mimic angiosarcoma but the identification of a clearly epithelial component as well as immunohistochemistry can be diagnostic {2085}.

Prognosis

Urinary bladder angiosarcoma is a very aggressive neoplasm, and approximately 70% of patients die within 24 months of diagnosis {699}.

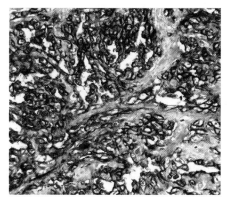

Fig. 2.77 Angiosarcoma of urinary bladder. CD31 expression.

Osteosarcoma

L. Guillou

Definition
A malignant mesenchymal tumour showing osteoid production.

ICD-O code   9180/3

Epidemiology
Most osteosarcomas of the urinary bladder occurred in male patients (male to female ratio: 4:1), with an average age of 60-65 years {215,863,2900}.

Etiology
One case of bladder osteosarcoma occurred 27 years after radiation therapy for urothelial carcinoma {754}. A few patients had concurrent urinary schistosomiasis {2900}.

Localization
Most osteosarcomas occurred in the urinary bladder, especially in the trigone region {2900}. Anecdotal cases have been reported in the renal pelvis {655}.

Clinical features
Haematuria, dysuria, urinary frequency, and recurrent urinary tract infections are the most common presenting symptoms. Pelvic pain and/or palpable abdominal mass are less frequent.

Macroscopy
Osteosarcoma of the urinary bladder typically presents as a solitary, large, polypoid, gritty, often deeply invasive, variably haemorrhagic mass. Tumour size varies between 2 and 15 cm (median: 6.5 cm) {215,863,2900}.

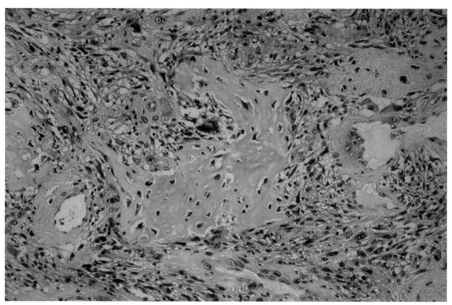

Fig. 2.78 Osteosarcoma of the urinary bladder. Abundant trabeculae of neoplastic bone surrounded by a malignant spindle cell component.

Histopathology
Histologically, the tumour is a high grade, bone-producing sarcoma. Foci of chondrosarcomatous differentiation and/or spindle cell areas may also be observed {215,2900}. Variably calcified, woven bone lamellae are rimmed by malignant cells showing obvious cytologic atypia (as opposed to stromal osseous metaplasia occurring in some urothelial carcinomas {655}). A recognizable malignant epithelial component should be absent, allowing discrimination from sarcomatoid carcinoma {2057}, which is the most important differential diagnosis.

Prognosis
Osteosarcoma of the urinary tract is an aggressive tumour with poor prognosis. A majority of patients have advanced stage (pT2 or higher) disease at presentation and die of tumour within 6 months, most from the effects of local spread (urinary obstruction, uremia, secondary infection, etc.) {863,2900}. Metastases often occurred late in the course of the disease, mainly in lungs {215,2900}. The stage of the disease at diagnosis is the best predictor of survival.

Malignant fibrous histiocytoma

J. Cheville

Definition
Malignant fibrous histiocytoma (MFH) is a malignant mesenchymal neoplasm occurring in the urinary bladder composed of fibroblasts and pleomorphic cells with a prominent storiform pattern.

ICD-O code   8830/3

Synonym
Undifferentiated high grade pleomorphic sarcoma.

Epidemiology
Malignant fibrous histiocytoma is one of the most frequent soft tissue sarcomas, and in some series, the second most frequent sarcoma of the urinary tract in adults {1410}. It is difficult to determine the incidence of urinary bladder malignant fibrous histiocytoma as it is likely that several tumours previously reported as malignant fibrous histiocytoma are sarcomatoid urothelial carcinoma.
Malignant fibrous histiocytoma more frequently affects men, and is most common in patients in their 5th to 8th decade.

Clinical features
Patients present with haematuria.

Macroscopy
Similar to other sarcomas of the urinary bladder, most malignant fibrous histiocytomas are large but tumours as small as 1 cm have been reported.

Histopathology
All subtypes of malignant fibrous histiocytoma have been described involving the bladder including myxoid, inflammatory, storiform-fascicular, and pleomorphic {809,1410,1935}. Malignant fibrous histiocytoma must be separated from sarcomatoid urothelial carcinoma as well as reactive spindle cell proliferations of the bladder. The much more commonly encountered sarcomatoid urothelial carcinoma can be associated with a malignant epithelial component, and stains positively for the immunohistochemical markers of epithelial differentiation such as cytokeratin {1038,1555,2038}. In contrast, malignant fibrous histiocytoma is negative for cytokeratin, and can stain for alpha-1-antichymotrypsin, and CD68. Reactive spindle cell proliferations lack the cytologic atypia of malignant fibrous histiocytoma.

Prognosis
The rarity of malignant fibrous histiocytoma makes it difficult to assess the biologic behaviour of these tumours. However, from the limited reports, malignant fibrous histiocytoma of the bladder appears aggressive with high local recurrence rates and metastases similar to malignant fibrous histiocytoma at other sites {809}. Treatment consists of resection, systemic chemotherapy and external beam radiation. The only patient with myxoid malignant fibrous histiocytoma of the bladder has been free to tumour following surgical resection, local radiation and systemic chemotherapy for 3 years {809}.

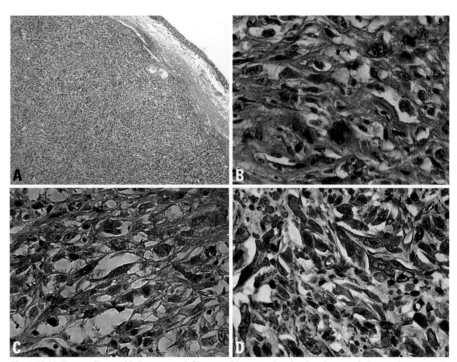

Fig. 2.79 Malignant fibrous histiocytoma. **A** Pleomorphic type, showing its characteristic storiform growth pattern and histologically normal urothelium (right bottom). **B** Pleomorphic giant cells are a common finding in this high grade, pleomorphic type, malignant fibrous histiocytoma. **C** Some pleomorphic cells proliferating in this malignant fibrous histiocytoma were immunorreactive with Anti-Alpha-1-Antitrypsin antibody. **D** Virtually all proliferating cells in this case of malignant fibrous histiocytoma displayed immunorreactivity with anti-vimentin antibody.

Leiomyoma

J. Cheville

Definition
A benign mesenchymal tumour occurring in the bladder wall showing smooth muscle differentiation.

ICD-O code   8890/0

Epidemiology
Leiomyoma of the urinary bladder is the most common benign mesenchymal neoplasm of the urinary bladder {908, 1255,1338}. Unlike sarcomas of the bladder, there is a predominance of females {908}. There is a wide age range from children to the elderly, but the vast majority of patients are middle-aged to older adults.

Clinical features
Patients present most frequently with obstructive or irritative voiding symptoms, and occasionally haematuria.

Macroscopy
Most leiomyomas are small with a mean

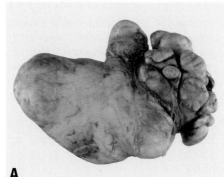 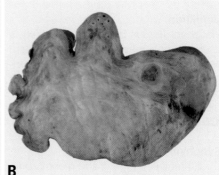

Fig. 2.80 A, B Lobulated giant leiomyoma.

size less than 2 cm {1338}. Tumours up to 25 cm have been reported {908}. Grossly, the tumours are circumscribed, firm, and lack necrosis.

Histopathology
Histopathological features include well formed fascicles of smooth muscle. Leiomyoma of the bladder is circumscribed with low cellularity, lack of mitotic activity and bland cytologic features {1639}. They are immunoreactive to smooth muscle actin and desmin.

Prognosis
Patients are treated by transurethral resection for small tumours, and open segmental resection for larger tumours. Surgical removal is curative in all cases.

Other non-epithelial tumours

J. Cheville

Malignant mesenchymal neoplasms such as *malignant peripheral nerve sheath tumour*, *liposarcoma*, *chondrosarcoma* and *Kaposi sarcoma* can very rarely involve the bladder {1410}. The diagnosis of primary liposarcoma and malignant peripheral nerve sheath tumour of the bladder requires that bladder involvement by direct extension from another site be excluded. In the case of primary bladder osteosarcoma and chondrosarcoma, sarcomatoid carcinoma must be excluded. *Solitary fibrous tumour* of the bladder of the urinary bladder has recently been recognized {159,502,2808}. Solitary fibrous tumour

of the bladder occurs in older patients who present with pain or haematuria. Two of the seven cases that have been reported were incidental findings {2808}. The tumour is typically a polypoid submucosal mass. Histopathologic features include spindle cells arranged haphazardly in a variably collagenous stroma. Dilated vessels reminiscent of haemangiopericytoma are present. Solitary fibrous tumour at other sites can act in an aggressive manner, but all solitary fibrous tumours of the bladder have had a benign course, although the number of cases is small, and follow-up has been short term in several cases.

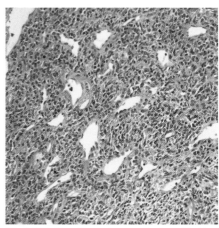

Fig. 2.81 Solitary fibrous tumour of urinary bladder.

Granular cell tumour

I.A. Sesterhenn

Definition
A circumscribed tumour consisting of nests of large cells with granular eosinophilic cytoplasm due to abundant cytoplasmic lysosomes.

ICD-O code   9580/0

Epidemiology
This tumour is rarely seen in the urinary bladder. The 11 cases reported in the literature and the 2 cases in the Bladder Tumour Registry of the Armed Forces Institute of Pathology occurred in adult patients from 23-70 years of age {88,779,1631,1752,1821,1949, 2351,2881}. There is no gender predilection.

Macroscopy
The tumours are usually solitary, well circumscribed and vary in size up to 12 cm.

Histopathology
Microscopically, the cells have abundant granular eosinophilic cytoplasm and vesicular nuclei. S-100 protein can be identified in the tumour cells {2490}. A congenital granular cell tumour of the gingiva with systemic involvement including urinary bladder has been reported {2011}.

Prognosis
To date, only one malignant granular cell tumour of the bladder has been described {2153}.

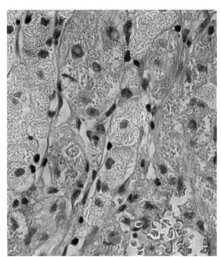

Fig. 2.82 Granular cell tumour of the urinary bladder.

Neurofibroma

L. Cheng

Definition
A benign mesenchymal tumour occurring in a urinary bladder wall consisting of a mixture of cell types including Schwann cell, perineurial like cells and fibroblasts.

ICD-O code   9540/0

Epidemiology
Neurofibromas of the urinary bladder occur infrequently; fewer than 60 cases have been reported. The tumours typically occur in young patients with neurofibromatosis type 1. The mean age at diagnosis is 17 years, and the male-to-female ratio is 2.3:1 {434}.

Clinical features
Patients typically exhibit physical stigmata of neurofibromatosis type 1. The urinary bladder is the most common site of genitourinary involvement in neurofibromatosis, and involvement of the bladder is often extensive, necessitating cystectomy in approximately one-third of cases. Clinical signs include hematuria, irritative voiding symptoms, and pelvic mass.

Macroscopy
The tumours frequently are transmural, showing a diffuse or plexiform pattern of growth.

Histopathology
Histologically, the tumours are usually of the plexiform and diffuse type. Neurofibroma of the bladder is characterized by a proliferation of spindle cells with ovoid or elongate nuclei in an Alcian blue positive, variably collagenized matrix. Cytoplasmic processings of tumour cells are highlighted on immunostaining for S-100 protein. Differential diagnostic considerations include low grade malignant peripheral nerve sheath tumour, leiomyoma, postoperative spindle nodule, inflammatory pseudotumour, leiomyosarcoma, and rhabdomyosarcoma. It is critical to distinguish neurofibrooma of atypical or cellular type from malignant peripheral nerve sheath tumour. Atypical neurofibromas lack mitotic figures or appreciable MIB-1 labeling. Cellular neurofibromas lack significant cytologic atypia or mitotic figures. The finding of rare mitotic figures in a cellular neurofibroma is not sufficient for a diagnosis of malignancy {434}. Adequate sampling is critical when increased cellularity is noted in superficial biopsies.

Prognosis
Long-term urinary complications include bladder atony, neurogenic bladder, and recurrent urinary tract infection with hematuria. Only 4 tumours (7%) underwent malignant transformation, none of these occurred in children {434,1737}.

Haemangioma

L. Cheng

Definition
Haemangioma of the urinary bladder is a rare benign tumour that arises from the endothelium of blood vessels.

ICD-O code   9120/0

Epidemiology
It may be associated with the Klipel-Trenaunnay-Weber or Sturge-Weber syndromes {1000,1098,1474}. The mean age at presentation is 58 years (range, 17-76 years); the male/female ratio of is 3.7:1 {431}.

Clinical features
Patients often present with macroscopic hematuria and cystoscopic findings are usually non-specific. However, cystoscopic findings of a sessile, blue, multiloculated mass are highly suggestive of haemangioma; the cystoscopic differential diagnostic considerations for pigmented raised lesions include endometriosis, melanoma, and sarcoma. Accurate diagnosis requires biopsy confirmation.

Macroscopy
The tumour has a predilection for the posterior and lateral walls, the lesion is non descript but may be haemorrhagic.

Histopathology
Three histologic types of haemangiomas are reported. Cavernous haemangioma is more common than capillary and arteriovenous haemangiomas. These tumours are morphologically identical to their counterparts in other organ sites, and the same criteria should be used for the diagnosis. Haemangioma is distinguished from angiosarcoma and Kaposi sarcoma by its lack of cytologic atypia and well circumscribed growth. Exuberant vascular proliferation may be observed in papillary cystitis and granulation tissue; but these lesions contain prominent inflammation cells, which is not seen or is less pronounced in haemangioma.

Histogenesis
Haemangioma of the urinary bladder arises from embryonic angioblastic stem cells {431,1000,1098,1474}.

Malignant melanoma

J.N. Eble

Definition
Malignant melanoma is a malignant melanocytic neoplasm which may occur in the urinary bladder as a primary or, more frequently, as metastatic tumour.

ICD-O code   8720/3

Epidemiology
Melanoma primary in the bladder has been reported in less than twenty patients {1303}. All have been adults and men and women have been equally affected.

Clinical features
Gross hematuria is the most frequent presenting symptom but some have presented with symptoms from metastases {2550}. The generally accepted criteria for determining that melanoma is primary in the bladder are: lack of history of a cutaneous lesion, failure to find a regressed melanoma of the skin with a Woods lamp examination, failure to find a different visceral primary, and pattern of spread consistent with bladder primary.

Macroscopy
Almost all of the tumours have appeared darkly pigmented at cystoscopy and on gross pathologic examination. Their sizes ranged from less than 1 cm to 8 cm.

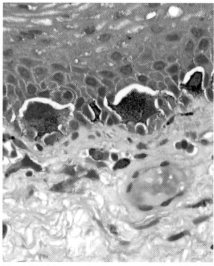

Fig. 2.83 Melanoma in situ extending into bladder from vagina.

Histopathology
Microscopically, the great majority of tumours have shown classic features of malignant melanoma: pleomorphic nuclei, spindle and polygonal cytoplasmic contours, and melanin pigment. Pigment production is variable and may be absent; one example of clear cell melanoma has been reported. A few of the tumours have been associated with melanosis of the vesical epithelium {1300}. One arose in a bladder diverticulum.

Immunohistochemical procedures have shown positive reactions with antibodies to S-100 protein and with HMB-45. Electron microscopy has shown melanosomes in several of the tumours.

Prognosis
Two-thirds of the patients have died of metastatic melanoma within 3 years of diagnosis; follow up of those alive at the time of the report has been less than 2 years.

Lymphomas

A. Marx

Definition
Malignant lymphoma is a malignant lymphoid neoplasm which may occur in the urinary bladder as a primary or part of a systemic disease.

Epidemiology
Lymphomas constitute about 5% of non-urothelial tumours of the urinary tract. More than 90% affect the bladder {1730}, constituting less than 1% of bladder neoplasms {86,106,530}. Secondary lymphoma of the bladder is common (12-20%) in advanced stage systemic lymphoma, shows a slight male predominance and may occur in children {885, 1297}. Primary lymphomas of the bladder {1297,1946,2793} and urethra {127, 398,1040,1414} are rare, affect mainly females (65-85%) and occur at an age of 12 - 85 (median 60) years. In one series only 20% of cases were primary lymphomas {1297}.

Etiology
The etiology of urinary tract lymphomas is unclear. Chronic cystitis is regularly encountered in MALT lymphoma of the bladder {1297,1402,2034}, but less frequently (20%) in other lymphomas {1946}. EBV and HIV infection have been reported in rare high grade urinary tract lymphoma (UTL) {1257,1692,1947}. Schistosomiasis was associated with a T-cell lymphoma of the bladder {1820}. Posttransplant lymphoproliferative disease restricted to the ureter allograft may occur after renal transplantation {591,2360}.

Clinical features
The most frequent symptom of urinary tract lymphomas is gross hematuria, followed by dysuria, urinary frequency, nocturia and abdominal or back pain {1297,1946}. Fever, night sweats, and weight loss or ureteral obstruction with hydronephrosis and renal failure occur almost only in patients with secondary urinary tract lymphomas due to retroperitoneal disease. Antecedent or concurrent MALT lymphomas in the orbit {1297} and stomach {1396}, and papillary urothelial tumours rarely occur {2034}.

Urinary tract lymphomas affect the renal pelvis, ureter, bladder and urethra. Primary urinary tract lymphomas are confined to the urinary tract, while secondary lymphoma results from disseminated lymphoma/leukaemia. Secondary bladder lymphoma as the *first* sign of disseminated disease is termed "nonlocalized lymphoma" with a much better prognosis than "secondary [recurrent] lymphoma" in patients with a history of lymphoma {1297}.

Macroscopy
Bladder lympomas may form solitary (70%) or multiple (20%) masses or diffuse thickening (10%) of the bladder wall. Ulceration is rare (<20%) in primary, but common in secondary urinary tract lymphomas. Frankly haemorrhagic changes have been observed {637}. Lymphoma of the ureter may form nodules or a diffuse wall thickening. In the urethra, lymphomas often present as a caruncle {127}.

Histopathology
Among primary urinary tract lymphomas, low grade MALT lymphoma is the most frequent in the bladder {27,47,1297, 1402,2034,2793}. Reactive germinal centers are consistently present while lymphoepithelial lesions occur in only 20% of cases associated with cystitis cystica or cystitis glandularis. Other bladder lymphomas, like Burkitt lymphoma {1692}, T-cell lymphoma {1820}, Hodgkin lymphoma {1243,1623} and plasmacytomas {398,1730} are very rare. In the ureter and renal pelvis, primary MALT lymphoma {1018}, diffuse large B-cell lymphoma {238,1035} and post-transplant lymphoproliferative disease {591,2360} have been reported.
In the urethra, several diffuse large B-cell lymphomas {1040} and single mantle cell {1259} and T-cell NOS lymphomas {1257} and plasmacytoma {1473} were described.
Among secondary urinary tract lymphomas, diffuse large B-cell lymphoma is the single most frequent histological subtype, followed by follicular, small cell,

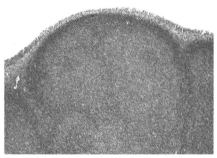

Fig. 2.84 Follicular lymphoma of urinary bladder.

low grade MALT, mantle cell {1297,1946} Burkitt {1946} and Hodgkin lymphoma {1702,1946,2635}.

Histogenesis (postulated cell of origin)
The histogenesis of urinary tract lymphomas is probably not different from that of other extranodal lymphomas.

Somatic genetics and genetic susceptibility
Genetic findings specific to urinary tract lymphomas have not been reported

Prognosis and predictive factors
Primary MALT of the urinary tract has an excellent prognosis after local therapy with virtually no tumour-related deaths {127,1040,1297,2034,2793}. "Nonlocalized lymphomas" and secondary [recurrent] lymphomas of the bladder have a worse prognosis (median survival 9 years and 0.6 year, respectively) {1297}, comparable to patients with advanced lymphomas of respective histological type elsewhere.

Metastatic tumours and secondary extension in urinary bladder

B. Helpap
A.G. Ayala
D.J. Grignon
E. Oliva
J.I. Epstein

Definition
Tumours of the urinary bladder that originate from an extravesical, non-urothelial tract neoplasm.

Localization
The most frequent locations of metastases to the urinary bladder are the bladder neck and the trigone.

Clinical features
Metastases or, in most cases, direct extension of colonic carcinomas to the bladder are most frequent at 21%, followed by carcinomas of the prostate (19%), rectum (12%), and uterine cervix (11%). Much less frequent is metastatic spread to the urinary bladder of neoplasias of the stomach, skin, breast, and lung at 2,5-4% {184}.

Macroscopy
The lesions may mimic a primary urothelial carcinoma or may manifest as multiple nodules.

Histopathology
Some metastatic or secondary tumours, such as malignant lymphomas, leukemias, malignant melanomas, or prostatic adenocarcinomas may be diagnosed by routine microscopy. However, tumours with less characteristic histological features, poorly or undifferentiated high grade tumours require immunohistochemical work-up {849,1954,2415, 2708,2777}.
Multifocality and prominent vascular involvement in tumours with unusual morphology should raise suspicion of metastatic tumours.

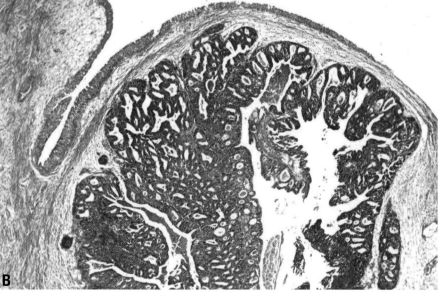

Fig. 2.85 A Metastatic prostate cancer to urinary bladder. **B** Metastatic colon cancer to urinary bladder.

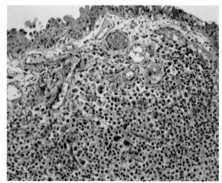

Fig. 2.86 Metastic breast cancer to urinary bladder.

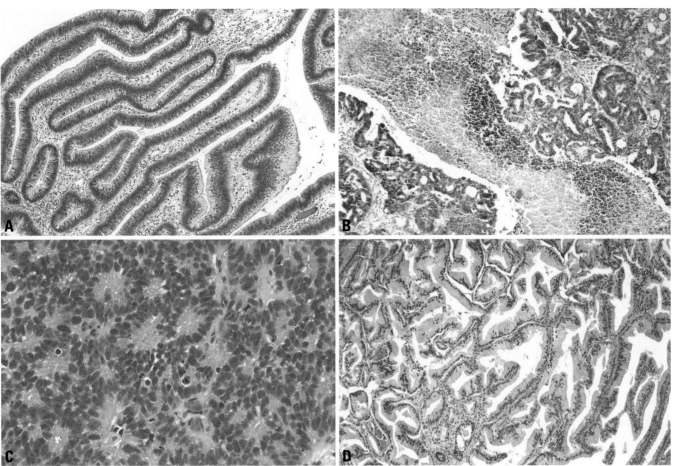

Fig. 2.87 Metastatic tumours to the urinary bladder. **A** Well differentiated adenocarcinoma of the colon infiltrating the bladder. **B** Moderately differentiated colonic adenocarcinoma infiltrating the bladder with extensive areas of necrosis. **C** Prostatic carcinoma with neuroendocrine features. **D** Well differentiated carcinoma of the prostate infiltrating the bladder.

Tumours of the renal pelvis and ureter

B. Delahunt
M.B. Amin
F. Hofstädter
A. Hartmann
J.E. Tyczynski

Definition
Benign and malignant tumours arising from epithelial and mesenchymal elements of the renal pelvis and ureter.

Epidemiology
Tumours of the ureter and renal pelvis account for 8% of all urinary tract neoplasms and of these greater than 90% are urothelial carcinomas {1582}. The incidence of these tumours is 0.7 to 1.1 per 100,000 and has increased slightly in the last 30 years. There is a male to female ratio of 1.7 to 1 with an increasing incidence in females. As with bladder cancer, tumours of the ureter and renal pelvis are more common in older patients with a mean age of incidence of 70 years {1834}.

Malignant epithelial tumours

Urothelial neoplasms

Clinical features
Malignant tumours of the pelvicalyceal system are twice as common as those of the ureter and multifocality is frequent {1655}. 80% of tumours arise following diagnosis of a bladder neoplasm {1910} and in 65% of cases, urothelial tumours develop at other sites {183}. Haematuria and flank pain are the chief presenting symptoms.

Epidemiology of urothelial renal pelvis cancer
Renal pelvis is a part of the lower urinary tract, which consists also of ureter, urinary bladder and urethra. As in the urinary bladder, a majority of renal pelvis tumours are urothelial carcinomas. {602}. Tumours of renal pelvis are rare. In males, they constitute 2.4% of tumours of lower urinary tract and 0.1% of all cancers in Europe. Corresponding figures for North America are 2.7% and 0.1%. In females, cancer of the renal pelvis

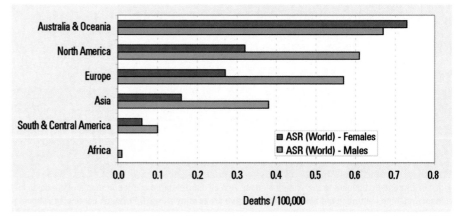

Fig. 2.88 Renal pelvis cancer. Incidence of cancer of the renal pelvis, by sex and continents. From D.M. Parkin et al. {2016}.

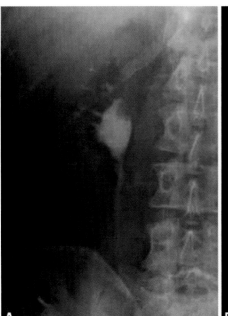
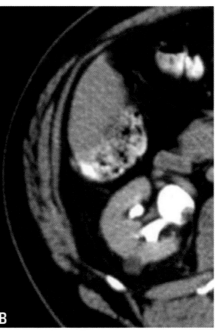

Fig. 2.89 Tumours of the ureter and renal pelvis. **A** IVP tumour renal pelvis. **B** CT tumour renal pelvis.

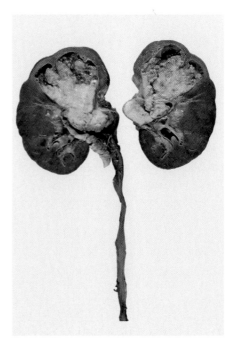

Fig. 2.90 Pelvic urothelial carcinoma.

makes 4.6% of lower urinary tract tumours and 0.07% of all cancers in Europe, and 5.2% and 0.07% respectively in North America.

The highest incidence rates of renal pelvis tumours are observed in Australia, North America and Europe, while the lowest rates are noted in South and Central America and in Africa. The highest rates in males in 1990s were observed in Denmark (1.65/105), Ferrara Province in Italy (1.45/105), Hiroshima, Japan (1.41/105), and in Mallorca, Spain (1.38/105). In females, the highest incidence rates were noted in New South Wales and Queensland in Australia (1.34 and 1.03/105 respectively), Denmark (0.95/105), Louisiana (among Blacks), USA (0.79/105), and Iceland (0.79/105) {2016}. Although limited information is available about changes of renal pelvis cancer in time, available data from US show that in 1970s and 1980s renal pelvis cancer incidence rates rose by approximately 2.2% per year in both males and females {602}.

Etiology of urothelial renal pelvis cancer
Tobacco smoking
Similar to cancers of the urinary bladder, the main risk factor for renal pelvis tumours is tobacco smoking {1680}. The relationship between tobacco smoking and renal pelvis tumours was reported already in 1970s {2324}, and confirmed by several authors {1215,1681,2245}. The risk increases with increasing lifetime consumption, as well as with

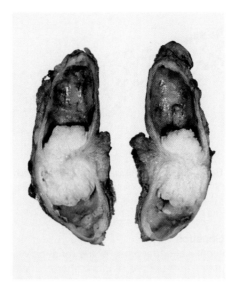
Fig. 2.91 Ureter urothelial carcinoma.

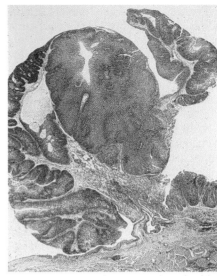
Fig. 2.92 Tumours of the ureter and renal pelvis. Inverted papillary urothelial carcinoma of the ureter with mutator phenotype.

increasing intensity of smoking, and is similar in both sexes {1215,1681}.

Analgetics
Another proven risk factor for cancer of the renal pelvis is long-term use of analgesics, particularly phenacetin. Use of analgesics increases risk of renal pelvis tumours by 4-8 times in males and 10-13 times in women, even after elimination of the confounding effect of tobacco smoking {1668,1680,2245}.

Occupational exposure
Several occupations and occupational exposures have been reported to be associated with increased risk of renal pelvis tumours {1215}. The highest risk was found for workers of chemical, petrochemical and plastic industries, and also exposed to coke and coal, as well as to asphalt and tar {1215}.

Other risk factors include papillary necrosis, Balkan nephropathy, thorium containing radiologic contrast material, urinary tract infections or stones {922, 1227,1260,1583}.

Macroscopy
Tumours may be papillary, polypoid,

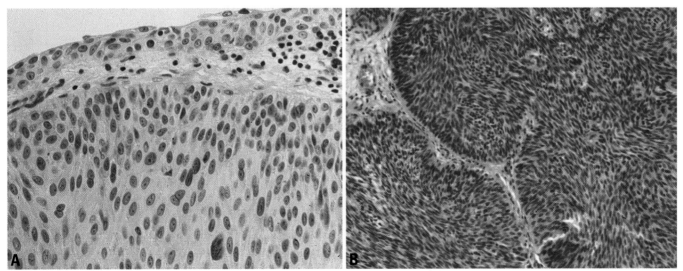
Fig. 2.93 Tumours of the ureter and renal pelvis. **A** Partly papillary predominamtly inverted growth pattern (a,c) with cytological atypia. **B** Inverted papillary urothelial carcinoma of the ureter with mutator phenotype.

nodular, ulcerative or infiltrative. Some tumours distend the entire pelvis while others ulcerate and infiltrate, causing thickening of the wall. A high grade tumour may appear as an ill defined scirrhous mass that involves the renal parenchyma, mimicking a primary renal epithelial neoplasm. Hydronephrosis and stones may be present in renal pelvic tumours while hydroureter and/or stricture may accompany ureteral neoplasms. Multifocality must be assessed in all nephroureterectomy specimens.

Tumour staging
There is a separate TNM staging system for tumours of the renal pelvis and ureter {944,2662}. Slight differences based on anatomical distinctions exist in the pT_3 designation of renal pelvis and ureteral tumours.

Histopathology
The basic histopathology of renal pelvis urothelial malignancies mirrors bladder urothelial neoplasia and may occur as papillary non-invasive tumours (papillary urothelial neoplasm of low malignant potential, low grade papillary carcinoma or high grade papillary carcinoma), carcinoma-in-situ and invasive carcinoma. The entire morphologic spectrum of vesical urothelial carcinoma is seen and tumour types include those showing aberrant differentiation (squamous and glandular), unusual morphology (nested, microcystic, micropapillary, clear cell and plasmacytoid) and poorly differentiated carcinoma (lymphoepithelioma-like, sarcomatoid and giant cell) {355,399, 656,727,2706}. Concurrence of aberrant differentiation, unusual morphology or undifferentiated carcinoma with conventional invasive poorly differentiated carcinoma is frequent.

Grading
The grading system for urothelial tumours is identical to that employed for bladder tumours.

Genetic susceptibility
Familial history of kidney cancer {2245} is generall considered a risk factor. Urothelial carcinomas of the upper urothelial tract occur in the setting of hereditary nonpolyposis colorectal cancer (HNPCC) syndrome (Lynch syndrome II) {251}.

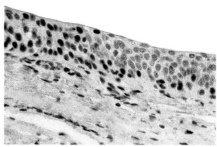

Fig. 2.94 Loss of expression of the DNA mismatch repair gene *MLH1* in an area of low grade urothelial dysplasia.

Genetics
Urothelial carcinomas of the renal pelvis, ureter and urinary bladder share similar genetic alterations {734,2197}. Deletions on chromosome 9p and 9q occur in 50-75% of all patients {734,993,2197,2554} and frequent deletions at 17p in addition to p53 mutations, are seen in advanced invasive tumours {321,993}. 20-30% of all upper urinary tract cancers demonstrate microsatellite instability and loss of the mismatch repair proteins MSH2, MLH1 or MSH6 {251,1032,1507}. Mutations in genes with repetitive sequences in the coding region (TGFβRII, bax, MSH3, MSH6) are found in 20-33% of cases with MSI, indicating a molecular pathway of carcinogenesis that is similar to some mismatch repair-deficient colorectal cancers. Tumours with microsatellite instabil-

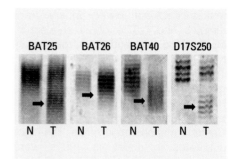

Fig. 2.95 Tumours of the ureter and renal pelvis. Microsatellite instability in 4 markers of the consensus Bethesda panel {264}.

ity have significantly different clinical and histopathological features including low tumour stage and grade, papillary and frequently inverted growth pattern and a higher prevalence in female patients {1028,1032}.

Prognosis and predictive factors
The most important prognostic factor is tumour stage and for invasive tumours the depth of invasion. A potential pitfall is that, while involvement of the renal parenchyma is categorized as a pT_3 tumour, some tumours that invade the muscularis (pT_2) may show extension into renal tubules in a pagetoid or intramucosal pattern and this should not be designated as pT_3. Survival for patients with pT_a/pT_{is} lesions is essentially 100%,

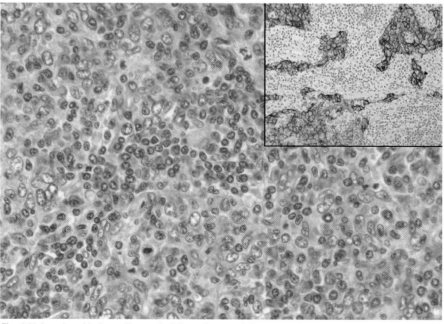

Fig. 2.96 Lymphoepithelioma-like urothelial carcinoma of the ureter. Inset shows cytokeratin AE1/AE3 immunostain.

and patients with pT_2 tumours have a survival rate of 75% {1003,1834}. Survival for patients with pT_3 and pT_4 tumours, tumours with positive nodal disease and residual tumour after surgery is poor {1995}. Other prognostic factors include patient age, type of treatment, and presence and severity of concurrent urothelial neoplasia {163,2884}.

Squamous cell carcinoma

Squamous cell carcinoma is more common in the renal pelvis than in the ureter, although it is the next most common tumour after urothelial carcinoma, it is very rare in both locations. Pure squamous cell carcinomas are usually high grade and high stage tumours and frequently invade the kidney. These tumours may occur in the background of nephrolithiasis with squamous metaplasia. Survival for 5 years is rare {248}.

Adenocarcinoma

Pure adenocarcinomas of the renal pelvis and ureters are rare and enteric, mucinous or signet-ring cell phenotypes, often occur concurrently. Glandular (intestinal) metaplasia, nephrolithiasis and repeated infections are predisposing factors. Most adenocarcinomas are high grade and are widely invasive at presentation {590}.

Benign epithelial tumours

Urothelial papilloma and inverted papilloma

Urothelial papilloma is usually a small, delicate proliferation with a fibrovascular core lined by normal urothelium. It is extraordinarily rare and often found incidentally. Inverted papilloma is also rare being twice as common in the ureter as in the renal pelvis. Most lesions are incidentally discovered.

Villous adenoma and squamous papilloma

These benign tumours are rare in the upper urinary tract. The presence of a villous adenoma histology in a limited biopsy does not entirely exclude the possibility of adenocarcinoma, and complete excision is essential.

Non-epithelial tumours of renal pelvis and ureter

Malignant tumours

The most frequent malignant stromal tumour of the ureter is leiomyosarcoma. Other malignant tumours reported are rhabdomyosarcoma, osteosarcoma, fibrosarcoma, angiosarcoma, malignant schwannoma, and Ewing sarcoma {416, 506,657,746,1745,1925,2634}.

Benign tumours

Fibroepithelial polyps are exophytic intraluminal masses of vascular connective tissue and varying amounts of inflammatory cells, covered by normal transitional epithelium. These are most frequently seen in the proximal ureter in young male adults and, in contrast to urethral polyps, children are rarely affected {2828}. Renal pelvic and ureteric leiomyoma, neurofibroma, fibrous histiocytoma, haemangioma, and periureteric lipoma, including hibernoma, have been reported {91,974, 1456,2449,2573,2712,2870}.

Miscellaneous tumours

Neuroendocrine tumours

Few cases of ureteric phaeochromocytoma have been reported {128}. Pelvic and ureteric carcinoid is similarly rare {45,1217,2260} and must be differentiated from metastatic disease {231}. Carcinoids also occur in ureteroileal conduits {1343}. Small cell carcinoma of the renal pelvis is confined to elderly patients {971,1347}. These aggressive tumours usually contain foci of urothelial carcinoma {971,1321,1326} and have a typical neuroendocrine immunohistochemical profile {971,1326,1347}.

Lymphoma

Renal pelvic and ureteric lymphomas are usually associated with systemic disease {200,331,2635}, while localized pelvic plasmacytoma has been reported {1165}.

Other

Rare cases of *sarcomatoid carcinoma* of the pelvis and ureter can show either homologous or heterologous stromal elements {621,774,2727,2882}. The tumours may be associated with urothelial carcinoma in situ {2727,2882} and have a poor prognosis {621,774,2882}. *Wilms tumour* confined to the renal pelvis or extending into the ureter {1114} and cases of *malignant melanoma* and *choriocarcinoma* of the renal pelvis have been described {669,800,2680}.

Tumours of the urethra

F. Hofstädter
M.B. Amin
B. Delahunt
A. Hartmann

Definition

Epithelial and non-epithelial neoplasms of the male and female urethra, frequently associated with chronic HPV infection.

Introduction and epidemiology

Epithelial tumours of the urethra are distinctly rare but, when encountered, are usually malignant and perhaps unique among genitourinary malignancies, as they are three to four times more common in women than in men {85,920, 1799,2318}. Urethral carcinomas occurring in men are strikingly different in clinical and pathologic features when compared to tumours in women. The dissimilarities may chiefly be attributable to the distinct differences in the anatomy and histology of the urethra in the two sexes. Benign epithelial tumours are exquisitely rare in the urethra of either sex.

Etiology

Human papilloma virus plays a crucial role in the etiology of condyloma of the urethra. Congenital diverticulum as well as acquired strictures of the female urethra, contribute to female preponderance of carcinomas. Columnar and mucinous adenocarcinoma are thought to arise

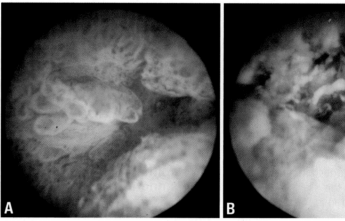

Fig. 2.97 Urethra. **A** Transurethral endoscopic view of a non-invasive warty carcinoma of the Fossa navicularis urethrae (pTa), Courtesy Dr. Peter Schneede, Dept. of Urology, LMU Munich. **B** Transurethral endoscopic view of an invasive squamous cell carcinoma of the distal urethra (pT1) (Fossa navicularis), Courtesy Dr. Peter Schneede, Dept. of Urology, LMU Munich.

from glandular metaplasia, whereas cribriform adenocarcinoma showed positive PSA staining indicating origin from prostate (male or female) {1837}. Villous adenoma has been shown to occur associated with tubulovillous adenoma and adenocarcinoma of the rectum {1782}.

Leiomyoma may show expression of estrogen receptors and is related to endocrine growth stimulation during pregnancy {72}. Leiomyoma may occur as a part of diffuse leiomyomatosis syndrome (esophageal and rectal leiomyomata).

Molecular pathology

Squamous cell carcinoma of the urethra is associated with HPV infection in female and male patients. High risk HPV 16 or 18 was detected in 60 % of urethral carcinomas in women {2822}.

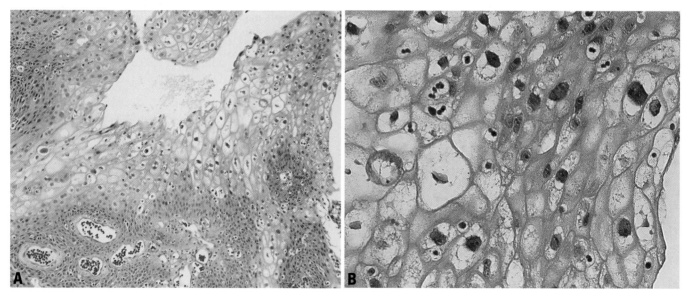

Fig. 2.98 **A, B** Non-invasive verrucous squamous cell carcinoma of the urethra with HPV infection and numerous koilocytes.

Table 2.07
Anatomic classification of epithelial tumours of the urethra.

Female
– Tumours of anterior urethra
– Tumours of posterior urethra
– Tumours of "paraurethral tissue" presenting as a urethral mass
– Skenes glands
Male
– Tumours of penile urethra
– Tumours of bulbomembranous urethra
– Tumours of prostatic urethra
– Tumours of "paraurethral tissue" presenting as a urethral mass
– Prostate
– Littres glands
– Cowpers glands

In men, approximately 30% of squamous cell carcinomas tested positive for HPV16 {529,2821}. All tumours were located in the pendulous part of the urethra whereas tumours in the bulbar urethra were negative. HPV16-positive tumours had a more favourable prognosis {2821}. There is no convincing evidence for an association of urothelial carcinoma with HPV, both in the urethra and the urinary bladder. One squamous cell carcinoma of the urethra was investigated cytogenetically and showed a complex karyotype with alterations at chromosomes 2,3,4,6,7,8,11,20 and Y, but not at chromosomes 9 and 17 {732}.

Epithelial tumours of the urethra

Female urethra

Malignant tumours
Macroscopy
Tumours may develop anywhere from urinary bladder to external vaginal orifice including accessory glands (Cowper and Littre glands as well as Skene glands in the female). Tumours involving the distal urethra and meatus are most common and appear as exophytic nodular, infiltrative or papillary lesions with frequent ulceration. Tumours involving the proximal urethra that are urothelial in differentiation exhibit the macroscopic diversity of bladder neoplasia: papillary excrescences (non-invasive tumour); erythema and ulceration (carcinoma in situ); and papillary, nodular, ulcerative or infiltrative (carcinoma with and without invasion). Adenocarcinomas are often large infiltrative or expansile neoplasms with a variable surface exophytic component and mucinous, gelatinous or cystic consistency. Carcinomas may occur within preexisting diverticuli.

Tumour staging
There is a separate TNM staging system for tumours of the urethra {944,2662}.

Histopathology
The histopathology of female urethral carcinomas corresponds to the location. Distal urethral and meatus tumours are squamous cell carcinomas (70%), and tumours of the proximal urethra are urothelial carcinomas (20%) or adenocarcinomas (10%) {85,2532}.

Squamous cell carcinomas of the urethra span the range from well differentiated (including the rare verrucous carcinoma histology) to moderately differentiated (most common) to poorly differentiated.

Urothelial neoplasms may be non-invasive, papillary (neoplasms of low malignant potential, low grade and high grade carcinomas), carcinoma in situ (CIS) or invasive. CIS may involve suburethral glands, focally or extensively mimicking invasion. Invasive carcinomas are usually high grade, with or without papillary component, and are characterized by irregular nests, sheets or cords of cells accompanied by a desmoplastic and/or inflammatory response. Tumours may exhibit variable aberrant differentiation (squamous or glandular differentiation), unusual morphology (nested, microcystic, micropapillary, clear cell or plasmacytoid), or rarely be accompanied by an undifferentiated component (small cell or sarcomatoid carcinoma).

The glandular differentiation may be broadly in the form of two patterns, clear cell adenocarcinoma (approximately 40%) and non-clear cell adenocarcinoma (approximately 60%), the latter frequently exhibiting myriad patterns that often coexist - enteric, mucinous, signet-ring cell or adenocarcinoma NOS {640, 1700,1955}. They are identical to primary bladder adenocarcinomas. Clear cell carcinomas are usually characterized by pattern heterogeneity within the same neoplasm and show solid, tubular, tubulocystic or papillary patterns. The cyto-

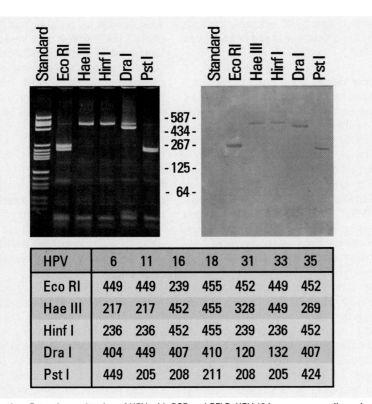

HPV	6	11	16	18	31	33	35
Eco RI	449	449	239	455	452	449	452
Hae III	217	217	452	455	328	449	269
Hinf I	236	236	452	455	239	236	452
Dra I	404	449	407	410	120	132	407
Pst I	449	205	208	211	208	205	424

Fig. 2.99 Urethra. Detection and typing of HPV with PCR and RFLP, HPV 16 in squamous cell carcinoma of the urethra, courtesy Dr. Th. Meyer, IPM, Hamburg.

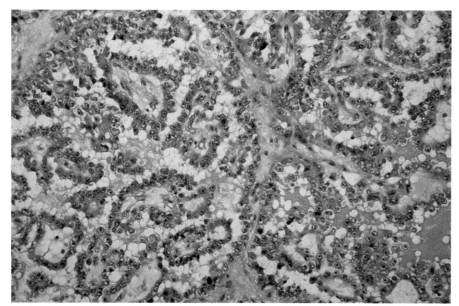

Fig. 2.100 Clear cell adenocarcinoma of urethra. This tumour demonstrates a papillary architecture in which cells have clear cytoplasm and a high nuclear grade.

logic features vary from low grade and banal (resembling nephrogenic adenoma superficially) to high grade (more frequently). Necrosis, mitotic activity and extensive infiltrative growth are commonly observed. These tumours may arise in a urethral diverticulum or, rarely, in association with mullerianosis {1954}. Relationship to nephrogenic adenoma is controversial {85}.

Benign tumours

Squamous papilloma, villous adenoma and urothelial papilloma of the urethra are the only three benign epithelial neoplasms, all being rare. The latter also includes inverted papilloma. The histologic features are identical to neoplasms described in the urinary bladder and other sites.

Male urethra

Malignant tumours

Macroscopy

Tumours may occur in the penile urethra, bulbomembranous urethra or the prostatic urethra; location often determines the gross appearance and the histopathology. Tumour appearance may be ulcerative, nodular, papillary, cauliflower-like, ill defined or reflective of histologic appearance – greyish-white or pearly with necrosis (squamous cell carcinoma) or mucoid, gelatinous, or cystic (adenocarcinoma). Abscess, sinus or fistulous

complication may be evident. In situ lesions may be erythematous erosions (urothelial CIS) or white and plaque-like (squamous CIS).

Tumour staging

There is a separate TNM staging system for tumours of the urethra. A separate subsection deals with urothelial carcinoma of the prostate and prostatic urethra {944,2662}.

Histopathology

Approximately 75% of carcinomas are squamous cell carcinoma (usually penile and bulbomembranous urethra); the remainder are urothelial carcinomas (usually prostatic urethra and less commonly bulbomembranous and penile urethra) or adenocarcinomas (usually bulbomembranous urethra) or undifferentiated {2905}. Squamous cell carcinomas are similar in histology to invasive squamous cell carcinomas at other sites.

Urothelial carcinoma may involve the prostatic urethra, exhibiting the same grade and histologic spectrum described in the female urethra. It may be synchronous or metachronous to bladder neoplasia. Features unique to prostatic urethral urothelial cancers are the frequent proclivity of high grade tumours to extend into the prostatic ducts and acini in a pagetoid fashion {2662,2905}.

Adenocarcinomas of the male urethra

usually show enteric, colloid or signet-ring cell histology, alone or in combination. Clear cell adenocarcinoma is distinctly rare {640}.

Benign tumours

Tumours occurring in males are similar to those described in the female urethra.

Grading of male and female urethral cancers

Urothelial neoplasms are graded as outlined in the chapter on the urinary bladder. Adenocarcinomas and squamous cell carcinomas are usually graded as per convention for similar carcinomas in other organs - well, moderately, and poorly differentiated carcinomas using the well established criteria of degree of differentiation.

Prognostic and predictive factors

The overall prognosis is relatively poor. Tumour stage and location are important prognostic factors. In females and males, proximal tumours have better overall survival than distal tumours (51% for proximal versus 6% for distal). In both sexes, or entire tumours in females {920,1487}, and 50% for proximal and 20% 5-year survival for distal tumours in males {1118,2154,2155}. In both sexes, high pT tumour stage and the presence of lymph node metastasis are adverse prognostic parameters {543,865,1736}. The prognosis for clear cell adenocarcinoma may not be as unfavourable as initially proposed {543,1700}.

Differential diagnosis

Nephrogenic adenoma

Nephrogenic adenoma of the urethra is similar to that found elsewhere in the urinary tract. In females it is more frequently associated with urethral diverticulum and has also been noted after urethral reconstruction of hypospadia using bladder mucosa {2801,2890}.

Fibroepithelial and prostatic polyps

Fibroepithelial polyps occur in both adults and children and are more common in the proximal urethra in males and the distal urethra in females {485,565}. Prostatic polyps may cause hematuria but do not recur following resection. These polyps are covered by urothelial and/or prostatic epithelium and have a prominent basal epithelial cell layer {2453,2549,2770}.

Condyloma acuminatum and caruncle

Urethral condylomas are flat or polypoid and are not always associated with external genital disease {583,795}. Caruncles are inflammatory polyps of the female urethra and must be distinguished from exophytic inflammatory pseudotumour, urothelial carcinoma or metastatic tumour {127,1557,2903}.

Non-epithelial tumours of the urethra

Malignant tumours

Malignant melanoma has been described in the male and female ure-thra. In male, the distal urethra is the most common site. Amelanotic melanoma may mimic urethral carcinoma {2130}.

Other reported non-epithelial tumours are *primary non-Hodgkin lymphoma* {127,1325} and *sarcomatoid carcinoma* {1352,2160}. Lymphoma or sarcomatoid carcinoma has to be differentiated from atypical stromal cells described in urethral caruncles with pseudoneoplastic histology {2897}.

Benign tumours

Leiomyoma shows immunohistochemically positive staining for vimentin, desmin and actin {72}. Periurethral leiomyoma has been described associated with esophageal and rectal leiomyomatosis {969}. Leiomyoma is more frequent in female urethra, but has been described also in the male {1740}. *Haemangioma* occurs in the bulbar {2020} or prostatic urethra {825}. *Localized plasmacytoma* has been shown to be treated by excisional biopsy {1473}.

Tumours of accessory glands

Bulbourethral gland carcinomas may show a mucinous, papillary, adenoid cystic, acinar or tubular architecture, while rare mucinous and papillary adenocarcinomas of the paraurethral glands have been reported {301,1292,2414, 2440}. Female periurethral gland adenocarcinomas are clear cell, mucinous or, rarely, prostatic. {2466}.

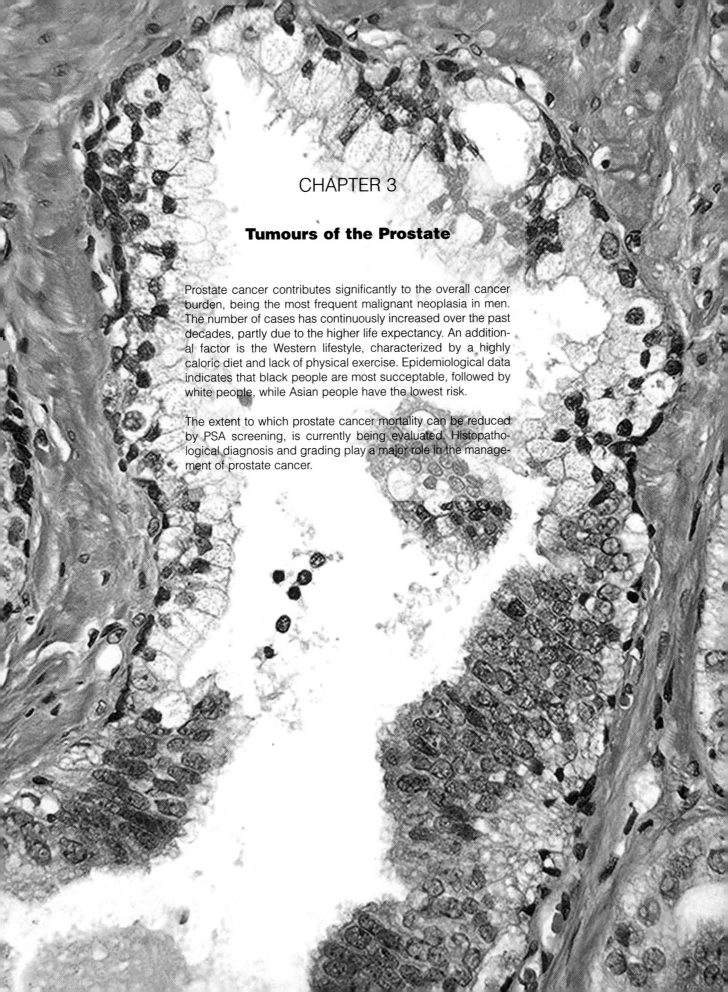

CHAPTER 3

Tumours of the Prostate

Prostate cancer contributes significantly to the overall cancer burden, being the most frequent malignant neoplasia in men. The number of cases has continuously increased over the past decades, partly due to the higher life expectancy. An additional factor is the Western lifestyle, characterized by a highly caloric diet and lack of physical exercise. Epidemiological data indicates that black people are most succeptable, followed by white people, while Asian people have the lowest risk.

The extent to which prostate cancer mortality can be reduced by PSA screening, is currently being evaluated. Histopathological diagnosis and grading play a major role in the management of prostate cancer.

WHO histological classification of tumours of the prostate

Epithelial tumours
Glandular neoplasms
Adenocarcinoma (acinar)   8140/3[1]
   Atrophic
   Pseudohyperplastic
   Foamy
   Colloid   8480/3
   Signet ring   8490/3
   Oncocytic   8290/3
   Lymphoepithelioma-like   8082/3
Carcinoma with spindle cell differentiation
(carcinosarcoma, sarcomatoid carcinoma)   8572/3

Prostatic intraepithelial neoplasia (PIN)
Prostatic intraepithelial neoplasia, grade III (PIN III)   8148/2

Ductal adenocarcinoma   8500/3
   Cribriform   8201/3
   Papillary   8260/3
   Solid   8230/3

Urothelial tumours
Urothelial carcinoma   8120/3

Squamous tumours
Adenosquamous carcinoma   8560/3
Squamous cell carcinoma   8070/3

Basal cell tumours
Basal cell adenoma   8147/0
Basal cell carcinoma   8147/3

Neuroendocrine tumours
Endocrine differentiation within adenocarcinoma   8574/3
Carcinoid tumour   8240/3
Small cell carcinoma   8041/3
Paraganglioma   8680/1
Neuroblastoma   9500/3

Prostatic stromal tumours
Stromal tumour of uncertain malignant potential   8935/1
Stromal sarcoma   8935/3

Mesenchymal tumours
Leiomyosarcoma   8890/3
Rhabdomyosarcoma   8900/3
Chondrosarcoma   9220/3
Angiosarcoma   9120/3
Malignant fibrous histiocytoma   8830/3
Malignant peripheral nerve sheath tumour   9540/3

Haemangioma   9120/0
Chondroma   9220/0
Leiomyoma   8890/0
Granular cell tumour   9580/0
Haemangiopericytoma   9150/1
Solitary fibrous tumour   8815/0

Hematolymphoid tumours
Lymphoma
Leukaemia

Miscellaneous tumours
Cystadenoma   8440/0
Nephroblastoma (Wilms tumour)   8960/3
Rhabdoid tumour   8963/3
Germ cell tumours
   Yolk sac tumour   9071/3
   Seminoma   9061/3
   Embryonal carcinoma & teratoma   9081/3
   Choriocarcinoma   9100/3
Clear cell adenocarcinoma   0/3
Melanoma   8720/3

Metastatic tumours

Tumours of the seminal vesicles

Epithelial tumours
Adenocarcinoma   8140/3
Cystadenoma   8440/0

Mixed epithelial and stromal tumours
   Malignant
   Benign

Mesenchymal tumours
Leiomyosarcoma   8890/3
Angiosarcoma   9120/3
Liposarcoma   8850/3
Malignant fibrous histiocytoma   8830/3
Solitary fibrous tumour   8815/0
Haemangiopericytoma   9150/1
Leiomyoma   8890/0

Miscellaneous tumours
   Choriocarcinoma   9100/3
Male adnexal tumour of probable Wolffian origin

Metastatic tumours

---

[1] Morphology code of the International Classification of Diseases for Oncology (ICD-O) {808} and the Systematized Nomenclature of Medicine (http://snomed.org). Behaviour is coded /0 for benign tumours, /2 for in situ carcinomas and grade III intraepithelial neoplasia, /3 for malignant tumours, and /1 for borderline or uncertain behaviour.

TNM classification of carcinomas of the prostate

T – Primary tumour

TX	Primary tumour cannot be assessed
T0	No evidence of primary tumour
T1	Clinically inapparent tumour not palpable or visible by imaging
T1a	Tumour incidental histological finding in 5% or less of tissue resected
T1b	Tumour incidental histological finding in more than 5% of tissue resected
T1c	Tumour identified by needle biopsy (e.g., because of elevated PSA)
T2	Tumour confined within prostate[1]
T2a	Tumour involves one half of one lobe or less
T2b	Tumour involves more than half of one lobe, but not both lobes
T2c	Tumour involves both lobes
T3	Tumour extends beyond the prostate[2]
T3a	Extracapsular extension (unilateral or bilateral)
T3b	Tumour invades seminal vesicle(s)
T4	Tumour is fixed or invades adjacent structures other than seminal vesicles: bladder neck, external sphincter, rectum, levator muscles, or pelvic wall[4]

Notes:
1. Tumour found in one or both lobes by needle biopsy, but not palpable or visible by imaging, is classified as T1c.
2. Invasion into the prostatic apex yet not beyond the prostate is not classified as T3, but as T2.
3. There is no pT1 category because there is insufficient tissue to assess the highest pT category.
4. Microscopic bladder neck involvement at radical prostatectomy should be classified as T3a.

N – Regional lymph nodes

NX	Regional lymph nodes cannot be assessed
N0	No regional lymph node metastasis
N1	Regional lymph node metastasis

Note: Metastasis no larger than 0.2cm can be designated pN1mi

M – Distant metastasis

MX	Distant metastasis cannot be assessed
M0	No distant metastasis
M1	Distant metastasis
M1a	Non-regional lymph node(s)
M1b	Bone(s)
M1c	Other site(s)

G Histopathological grading

GX	Grade cannot be assessed
G1	Well differentiated (Gleason 2-4)
G2	Moderately differentiated (Gleason 5-6)
G3–4	Poorly differentiated/undifferentiated (Gleason 7-10)

Stage grouping

Stage I	T1a	N0	M0	G1
Stage II	T1a	N0	M0	G2, 3–4
	T1b, c	N0	M0	Any G
	T1, T2	N0	M0	Any G
Stage III	T3	N0	M0	Any G
Stage IV	T4	N0	M0	Any G
	Any T	N1	M0	Any G
	Any T	Any N	M1	Any G

[1] {944,2662}.
[2] A help desk for specific questions about the TNM classification is available at http://www.uicc.org/tnm/

Acinar adenocarcinoma

J.I. Epstein
F. Algaba
W.C. Allsbrook Jr.
S. Bastacky
L. Boccon-Gibod
A.M. De Marzo
L. Egevad
M. Furusato
U.M. Hamper

B. Helpap
P.A. Humphrey
K.A. Iczkowski
A. Lopez-Beltran
R. Montironi
M.A. Rubin
W.A. Sakr
H. Samaratunga
D.M. Parkin

Definition
An invasive malignant epithelial tumour consisting of secretory cells.

ICD-O code   8140/3

Epidemiology
Geographical distribution
Prostate cancer is now the sixth most common cancer in the world (in terms of number of new cases), and third in importance in men {2012}. The estimated number of cases was 513,000 in the year 2000. This represents 9.7% of cancers in men (15.3 % in developed countries and 4.3% in developing countries). It is a less prominent cause of death from cancer, with 201,000 deaths (5.6% of cancer deaths in men, 3.2% of all cancer deaths). The low fatality means that many men are alive following a diagnosis of prostate cancer – an estimated 1.5 million at 5 years, in 2000, making this the most prevalent form of cancer in men. In recent years, incidence rates reflect not only differences in risk of the disease, but also the extent of diagnosis of latent cancers both by screening of asymptomatic individuals, and by detection of latent cancer in tissue removed during prostatectomy operations, or at autopsy. Thus, especially where screening is widespread, recorded 'incidence' may be very high (in the United States, for example, where it is now by far the most commonly diagnosed cancer in men). Incidence is very high also in Australia and the Scandinavian countries (probably also due to screening). Incidence rates in Europe are quite variable, but tend to be higher in the countries of northern and western Europe, and lower in the East and South. Prostate cancer remains relatively rare in Asian populations. Mortality is less affected by the effects of early diagnosis of asymptomatic cancers, but depends upon survival as well as incidence; survival is significantly greater in high-incidence countries (80% in the USA vs. 40% in developing countries). However, this more favourable prognosis could well be due to more latent cancer being detected by screening procedures {310}. Mortality rates are high in North America, North and West Europe, Australia/New Zealand, parts of South America (Brazil) and the Caribbean, and in much of sub-Saharan Africa. Mortality rates are low in Asian populations, and in North Africa. The difference in mortality between China and the U.S.A is 26 fold (while it is almost 90 fold for incidence).

These international differences are clearly reflected within the United States, where the Black population has the highest incidence (and mortality) rates, some 70% higher than in Whites, who in turn have rates considerably higher than populations of Asian origin (e.g. Chinese, Japanese and Korean males). Similarly, in São Paulo, Brazil, the risk of prostate cancer in Black males was 1.8 (95% CI 1.4–2.3) times that of White men {297}. Latent cancers are frequent in older men, and the prevalence greatly exceeds the cumulative incidence in the same population. Two international studies of latent prostate cancer {316,2874} observed that prevalence increases steeply with age, but varies much less between populations than the incidence of clinical cancer. The country/ethnic-specific ranking was much the same. The frequency of latent carcinoma of prostate in Japan is increasing (as with clinical prostate cancer) and may eventually approach the prevalence for U.S. Whites.

Migrants
Migrants from West Africa to England & Wales have mortality rates 3.5 times (95% CI 2.4–5.1) those of the local-born population, and mortality is significantly higher also among migrants from the Caribbean (RR 1.7; 95% CI 1.5–2.0); in

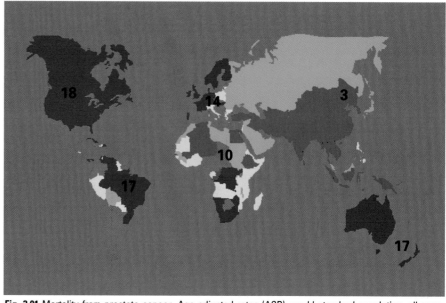

Fig. 3.01 Mortality from prostate cancer. Age adjusted rates (ASR), world standard population, all ages. From Globocan 2000 {749}.

contrast, mortality among migrants from East Africa, of predominantly Asian (Indian) ethnicity, are not high {966}. Migrants from low-risk countries to areas of higher risk show quite marked increases in incidence (for example, Japanese living in the United States). Some of this change reflects an elimination of the 'diagnostic bias" influencing the international incidence rates. Localized prostate cancer forms a small proportion of cases in Japan (24%) compared with 66-70% in the U.S.A; incidence in Japan could be 3-4 times that actually recorded if, for example, all transurethral prostatectomy (TURP) sections were carefully examined {2392}. However, rates in Japanese migrants remain well below those in the U.S. White populations, even in Japanese born in the United States, which suggests that genetic factors are responsible for at least some of the differences between ethnic groups.

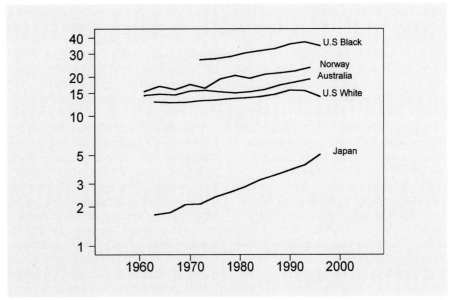

Fig. 3.02 International trends in age-standardized mortality rates of prostate cancer (world standard). Source: WHO/NCHS

Age distribution
The risk of prostate cancer rises very steeply with age. Incidence of clinical disease is low until after age 50, and then increases at approximately the 9-10th power of age, compared with the 5-6th power for other epithelial cancers {488}. Worldwide, about three-quarters of all cases occur in men aged 65 or more.

Time trends
Time trends in prostate cancer incidence and mortality have been greatly affected by the advent of screening for raised levels of serum Prostate-Specific Antigen (PSA), allowing increasing detection of preclinical (asymptomatic) disease {2100}. In the USA, prostate cancer incidence rates were increasing slowly up to the 1980's, probably due to a genuine increase in risk, coupled with increasing diagnosis of latent, asymptomatic cancers in prostatectomy specimens, due to the increasing use of TURP {2099}.

Beginning in 1986, and accelerating after 1988, there was a rapid increase in incidence. The recorded incidence of prostate cancer doubled between 1984 and 1992, with the increase being mainly in younger men (under 65) and confined to localized and regional disease. The incidence rates began to fall again in 1992 (1993 in Black males), probably because most of the prevalent latent cancers in the subset of the population reached by screening had already been detected {1467}. With the introduction of PSA screening, there was also an increase in the rate of increase in mortality, but this was very much less marked than the change in incidence. More recently, (since 1992 in White men, 1994 in Black men), mortality rates have decreased. The contribution that PSA screening and/or improved treatment has made to this decline has been the subject of considerable debate {728, 763,1015}. The increased mortality was probably partly due to mis-certification of cause of death among the large number of men who had been diagnosed with latent prostate cancer in the late 80's and early 90's. The later decline may be partly due to a reversal of this effect; it seems unlikely that screening was entirely responsible. International trends in mortality have been reviewed by Oliver et al. {1956}, and in incidence and mortality by Hsing et al. {1130}. The largest increases in incidence, especially in younger men,

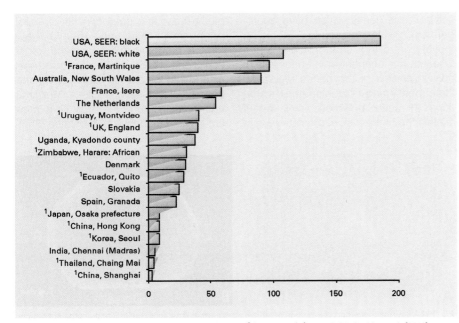

Fig. 3.03 Prostate cancer incidence: ASR (World) per 10[5] (1993-1997). [1]From D.M. Parkin et al. {2016}.

have been seen in high-risk countries, probably partly the effect of increasing detection following TURP, and, more recently, due to use of PSA. But there have been large increases also in low risk countries; 3.5 x in Shanghai, China, 3.0 x in Singapore Chinese, 2.6 x in Miyagi, Japan, 1.7 x in Hong Kong, between 1975 and 1995 {2016,2788}. Only in India (Bombay) does there seem to have been little change (+13%) in incidence. Some of this increase may be due to greater awareness of the disease, and diagnosis of small and latent cancers. But it is also probable that there is a genuine increase in risk occurring. This is confirmed by studying changes in mortality. The increases in rates in the "high risk" countries were much less than for incidence, but quite substantial nevertheless (15-25%). In low risk countries, the increase in mortality rates is large, and not much inferior to the changes observed in incidence. As in the USA, there have been declines in mortality from prostate cancer since around 1988-1991, in several high-risk populations, rather more marked in older than in younger men. In some of the countries concerned (Canada, Australia), there has been considerable screening activity, but this is not the case in others where the falls in mortality are just as marked (France, Germany, Italy, UK) {1956}. There may be a contribution from improvements in treatment which is difficult to evaluate from survival data because of lead-time bias introduced by earlier diagnosis.

Etiology

The marked differences in risk by ethnicity suggest that genetic factors are responsible for at least some of the differences between ethnic groups. Nevertheless, the changes in rates with time, and on migration, also imply that differences in environment or lifestyle are also important. Despite extensive research, the environmental risk factors for prostate cancer are not well understood.

Evidence from ecological, case–control and cohort studies implicates dietary fat in the etiology of prostate cancer, although few studies have adjusted the results for caloric intake, and no particular fat component has been consistently implicated. There is a strong positive association with intake of animal products, especially red meat. The evidence

from these studies for a protective effect of fruits and vegetables on prostate cancer, unlike many other cancer sites, is not convincing. There is little evidence for anthropometric associations with prostate cancer, or for a link with obesity {1348,2842}.

A cohort study of health professionals in the United States, found that differences in the distribution of possible dietary and lifestyle risk factors did not explain the higher risk (RR 1.81) of prostate cancer in Blacks versus Whites {2091}. Genetic factors appear therefore to play a major role in explaining the observed racial differences, and findings of elevated risk in men with a family history of the disease support this. There is a 5-11 fold increased risk among men with two or more affected first-degree relatives {2499}. A similar study involving a population-based case–control study of prostate cancer among Blacks, Whites and Asians in the United States and Canada found the prevalence of positive family histories somewhat lower among the Asian Americans than among Blacks or Whites {2815}.

It is clear that male sex hormones play an important role in the development and growth of prostate cancers. Testosterone diffuses into the gland, where it is converted by the enzyme steroid 5-alpha reductase type II (SRD5A2) to the more metabolically active form dihydrotestosterone (DHT). DHT and testosterone bind to the androgen receptor (AR), and the receptor/ligand complex translocates to the nucleus for DNA binding and transactivation of genes which have androgen-responsive elements, including those controlling cell division. Much research has concentrated on the role of polymorphisms of the genes regulating this process and how inter-ethnic variations in such polymorphisms might explain the higher risk of prostate cancer

in men of African descent {2246}. Polymorphisms in the SRD5A2 genes may provide at least part of the explanation {2389}, but more interest is focused on the AR gene, located on the long arm of chromosome X. The AR gene contains a highly polymorphic region of CAG repeats in exon 1, the normal range being 6–39 repeats. Several studies suggest that men with a lower number of AR CAG repeat lengths are at higher risk of prostate cancer {404}. Blacks in the United States have fewer CAG repeats than Whites, which has been postulated to partly explain their susceptibility to prostate cancer {2091,2246}. Other genetic mechanisms possible related to prostate cancer risk are polymorphisms in the vitamin D receptor gene {1169,1170} or in the insulin-like growth factor (IGF) signalling pathway {403}, but there is no evidence for significant inter-ethnic differences in these systems.

Other environmental factors (occupational exposures) or behavioural factors (sexual life) have been investigated, but do not seem to play a clear role.

Localization

Most clinically palpable prostate cancers diagnosed on needle biopsy are predominantly located posteriorly and posterolaterally {354,1682}. In a few cases, large transition zone tumours may extend into the peripheral zone and become palpable. Cancers detected on TURP are predominantly within the transition zone. Nonpalpable cancers detected on needle biopsy are predominantly located peripherally, although 15-25% have tumour predominantly within the transition zone {716}. Large tumours may extend into the central zone, yet cancers uncommonly arise in this zone. Multifocal adenocarcinoma of the prostate is present in more than 85% of prostates {354}.

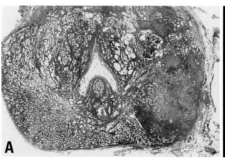 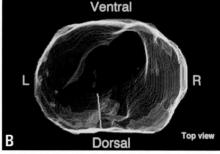

Fig. 3.04 A Low magnification of a section of radical prostatectomy showing the location of prostate cancer. **B** Computerized reconstruction of prostatectomy specimen with typical, multifocal distribution of cancer.

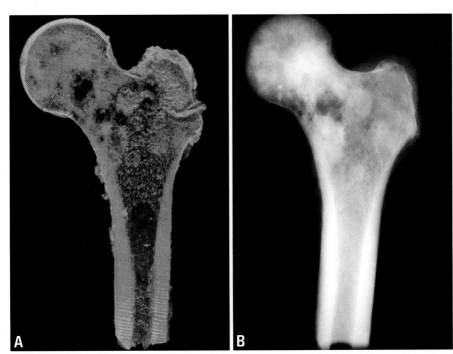

Fig. 3.05 A Gross photography of prostate carcinoma metastatic to femur (post fixation). **B** Radiography of prostate carcinoma metastatic to femur.

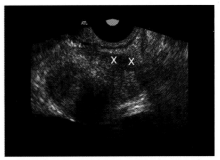

Fig. 3.06 Transrectal ultrasound of prostate shows the hypoechoic cancer is marked with 2 xs.

Clinical features

Signs and symptoms

Even before the serum prostate specific antigen test came into common usage over a decade ago, most prostate cancer was asymptomatic, detected by digital rectal examination. PSA screening has decreased the average tumour volume, and hence further lowered the percentage of cancers that present with symptoms today. Most cancers arise in the peripheral zone, so that transition zone enlargement sufficient to cause bladder outlet obstruction usually indicates hyperplasia. However, 8.0% of contemporary transurethral resection specimens disclose carcinoma {1605}, and rarely, urinary obstruction results from large-volume peri-urethral tumour. Locally extensive cancer is seen less often than in the past but may present with pelvic pain, rectal bleeding or obstruction {2348}.

Metastatic prostatic adenocarcinoma can present as bone pain, mainly in the pelvic bones and spinal cord, where it can cause cord compression {1138}. However, when bone scan discloses metastasis after diagnosis of a primary prostatic carcinoma, the metastasis is most often asymptomatic {2487}. Enlarged lymph nodes, usually pelvic, but rarely supraclavicular or axillary (typically left-sided), can sometimes be a presenting symptom. Ascites and pleural effusion are rare initial presentations of prostate cancer.

Imaging

Ultrasound imaging

Transrectal ultrasound imaging (TRUS) with high frequency transducers is a useful tool for the work-up of patients with a prostate problem. It enables the operator to evaluate gland volume, as well as delineate and measure focal lesions. Its primary application, however, remains in image guidance of transrectal prostate biopsies. It has proven to be of limited value for the detection of prostate cancer and the assessment of extraglandular spread due to lack of specificity. While the majority of early prostate cancers present as hypoechoic lesions in the peripheral zone on TRUS, this sonographic appearance is non-specific, because not all cancers are hypoechoic and not all hypoechoic lesions are malignant {1012}. Sonographic-pathologic correlation studies have shown that approximately 70-75% of cancers are hypoechoic and 25-30% of cancers are isoechoic and blend with surrounding tissues {539,2285}. These cancers cannot be detected by TRUS. A small number of cancers are echogenic or contain echogenic foci within hypoechoic lesions {1010}. The positive predictive value of a hypoechoic lesion to be cancer increases with the size of the lesion, a palpable abnormality in this region and an elevated PSA level {689}. Overall the incidence of malignancy in a sonographically suspicious lesion is approximately 20-25% {2193}. Even with high-resolution equipment many potentially clinically significant cancers are not visualized by TRUS. A large multicentre study demonstrated that up to 40% of significant cancers were missed by TRUS. In addition, the sensitivity to detect neurovascular bundle invasion has been reported to only be about 66% with a specificity of 78% {1011,2196}.

To improve lesion detection the use of colour Doppler US (CDUS) has been advocated particularly for isoechoic lesions or to initiate a TRUS guided biopsy which may not have been performed, thus tailoring the biopsy to target isoechoic yet hypervascular areas of the gland {56,1885,2195}. Results from these studies are however conflicting due to a problematic overlap in flow detected in cancers, inflammatory conditions or benign lesions. Newer colour flow techniques such as power Doppler US may be helpful as they may allow detection of slow flow in even smaller tumour vessels. Other recent developments such as intravenous contrast agents, harmonic imaging and 3-D US have shown a potential role for these US techniques to delineate subtle prostate cancers, assess extraglandular spread or monitor patients with prostate cancer undergoing hormonal treatment {364,658,1013}.

Computed tomography and magnetic resonance imaging

Cross-sectional imaging techniques such as computed tomography (CT) and magnetic resonance imaging (MRI) have

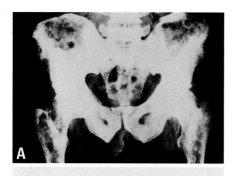

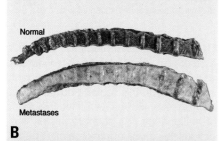

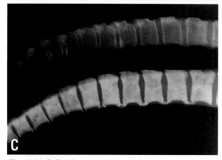

Fig. 3.07 A Pelvic metastases of prostate carcinoma. **B** Spinal osteoblastic metastases from prostate cancer. Macroscopic photograph. **C** Radiography of the same case

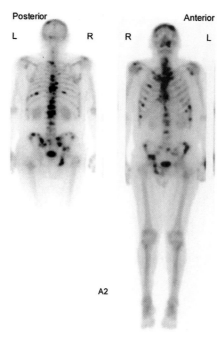

Fig. 3.08 Bone scanning showing multiple metastases of a prostate carcinoma.

not proven valuable because of low sensitivities to detect and stage prostate cancer {1011, 2149, 2594 ,2910}. MRI is sometimes reserved for staging of patients with biopsy proven prostate cancer {2605}.

The combined use of MRI and proton MRI-spectroscopy imaging (MRSI) is currently being evaluated for staging of prostate cancer. These techniques however, also appear to have limitations for imaging of microscopic disease {1412, 2911}. Knowledge obtained from MRSI may provide insight into the biological behaviour of prostate cancer, such as tumour aggressiveness and extra-prostatic extension {2911}.

Plain film radiography and nuclear medicine
Skeletal radiography (bone survey) is an insensitive method to screen for bony metastases and should be reserved to confirm skeletal abnormalities in patients with positive bone scintigraphy. Bone scintigraphy (radionuclide bone scans) provides the most sensitive method for detecting bone metastases. Upper urinary tract obstruction may also be identified on bone scintigraphy obviating the need for intravenous urography.

Monoclonal antibody radioimmuno-scintigraphy (prostate specific membrane antigen-PMSA) chelated to Indium111 (Prostacint®, Cytogen Corporation, Princeton, N.J.) has shown promise to detect microscopic metastatic deposits in regional and distant sites. However, due to limited positive predictive values reported (50-62%) its use in combination with PSA, histologic grade and clinical staging is recommended to provide increased predictive information {147,1621}. Another new development in the field of nuclear medicine is positron emission tomography (PET), which allows in vivo-characterization of tumours and may have implications for the evaluation of patients with prostate cancer in the future.

Laboratory tests
Prostate specific antigen (PSA)
PSA is produced by the epithelial cells lining the prostatic ducts and acini and is secreted directly into the prostatic ductal system. The PSA gene is located on chromosome 19 {2211,2558}. Its andro-

gen-regulated transcription results in the biosynthesis of a 261 amino acid PSA precursor. This precursor, is believed to be activated by the proteolytic liberation of a small amino-terminal fragment {2098}. Conversion from inactive proPSA to active PSA requires action of exogenous prostatic proteases, e.g. hK2, prostin (hK15), prostase (hK4) or trypsin. Different molecular forms of PSA exist in serum {392,1498,1499,2504}. These result from complex formation between free PSA and two major extracellular protease inhibitors that are synthesized in the liver. As PSA is a serine protease, its normal mode of existence in the serum is in a complex with α-1-anti-chymotrypsin (ACT), a 67 kDa single chain glycoprotein, and α-2-macroglobulin (AMG), a 720 kDa glycoprotein. Only a small percentage of the PSA found in the serum is free. Because this free form does not bind to ACT or AMG, it is thought to be either the enzymatically inactive precursor (i.e., zymogen) for PSA or an inactive nicked or damaged form of the native molecule. Subfractions of free PSA include: mature single-chain, and multi-chain, nicked free PSA forms.

Serum total PSA and age specific reference ranges
Serum PSA is determined with immunoassay techniques. No PSA epitopes that interact with anti-PSA antibodies are exposed on the PSA-AMG complex. This is thought to result from the 25-fold larger AMG molecule "engulfing" PSA and hindering recognition of PSA epitopes. Therefore, conventional assays do not measure PSA-AMG. In contrast, only one major PSA epitope is completely shielded by complex formation with ACT; PSA-ACT can therefore be readily measured in serum {1498,1667}. Monoclonal antibodies have been designed to detect the free form of PSA (29kDa), the complex of PSA and ACT (90 kDa) and the total PSA.

It has been found that total PSA correlates well with advancing age {92,483, 546,576,1937,2022,2185}. Based on the 95th percentile values in a regression model, white men under age 50 have PSA values <2.5 ng/ml, under age 60 have PSA values <3.5 ng/ml, under age 70 have PSA values <4.5 ng/ml, and under age 80 PSA levels were <6.5 ng/ml. It has been suggested that these age-related values be used as the upper limit of normal in

PSA-related diagnostic strategies.

PSA is elevated beyond the arbitrary cut-off point of 4.0 ng/ml in the majority of patients with prostate cancer. It may also be greater than 4.0 ng/ml in some benign conditions, including benign prostatic hyperplasia (BPH). Prostate cancer may also be present in men with serum PSA values lower than the above quoted cut-off points. This may be specifically true for men considered at higher risk (i.e., family history; men with faster doubling time; and in the United States African American men). Therefore, serum PSA lacks high sensitivity and specificity for prostate cancer. This problem has been partially overcome by calculating several PSA-related indices and/or evaluating other serum markers {1660,1775}. PSA tests are also useful to detect recurrence and response of cancer following therapy. The exact value used to define recurrence varies depending on the treatment modality.

Free PSA. The free form of PSA occurs to a greater proportion in men without cancer {2607} and, by contrast, the α-1-chymotrypsin complex PSA comprises a greater proportion of the total PSA in men with malignancy. The median values of total PSA and of the free-to-total PSA ratio are 7.8 ng/ml and 10.5% in prostate cancer patients, 4.3 ng/ml and 20.8% in patients with BPH, and 1.4 ng/ml and 23.6% in a control group of men without BPH {2506}. There is a significant difference in free-to-total PSA ratio between prostate cancer and BPH patients with prostate volumes smaller than 40 cm³, but not between patients in these two groups with prostate volumes exceeding 40 cm³ {2506}.

Complex PSA. Problems associated with the free-to-total PSA ratio, particularly assay variability, and the increased magnitude of error when the quotient is derived, are obviated by assays for complex PSA. Complex PSA value may offer better specificity than total and free-to-total PSA ratio {308}.

PSA density

This is the ratio of the serum PSA concentration to the volume of the gland, which can be measured by transrectal ultrasound (total PSA/prostatic volume = PSA density, PSAD). The PSAD values are divided into three categories: normal

(values equal or lower than 0.050 ng/ml/cm³), intermediate (from 0.051 to 0.099 ng/ml/cm³) and pathological (equal to or greater than 0.1 ng/ml/cm³). The production of PSA per volume of prostatic tissue is related to the presence of BPH and prostate cancer and to the proportion of epithelial cells and the histological grade of the carcinoma {1476}.

PSA density of the transition zone. Nodular hyperplasia is the main determinant of serum PSA levels in patients with BPH {139,109,1521}. Therefore, it seems logical that nodular hyperplasia volume rather than total volume should be used when trying to interpret elevated levels of serum PSA. PSA density of the transition zone (PSA TZD) is more accurate in predicting prostate cancer than PSA density for PSA levels of less than 10 ng/ml {625}.

Prostate-specific antigen epithelial density. The serum PSA level is most strongly correlated with the volume of epithelium in the transition zone. The prostate-specific antigen epithelial density (PSAED, equal to serum PSA divided by prostate epithelial volume as determined morphometrically in biopsies) should be superior to PSAD. However, the amount of PSA produced by individual epithelial cells is variable and serum levels of PSA may be related to additional factors such as hormonal milieu, vascularity, presence of inflammation, and other unrecognized phenomena {2698, 2941}.

PSA velocity and PSA doubling time

PSA velocity (or PSA slope) refers to the rate of change in total PSA levels over time. It has been demonstrated that the rate of increase over time is greater in men who have carcinoma as compared to those who do not {380,381}. This is linked to the fact that the doubling time of prostate cancer is estimated to be 100 times faster than BPH. Given the short-term variability of serum PSA values, serum PSA velocity should be calculated over an 18-month period with at least three measurements.

PSA doubling time (PSA DT) is closely related to PSA velocity {1470}. Patients with BPH have PSA doubling times of 12 ± 5 and 17 ± 5 years at years 60 and 85, respectively. In patients with prostate cancer, PSA change has both a linear and exponential phase. During the exponential phase, the doubling time for

patients with local/regional and advanced/metastatic disease ranges from 1.5-6.6 years (median, 3 years) and 0.9-8.5 years (median, 2 years), respectively {1470,1775}.

Prostate markers other than PSA

Prostatic acid phosphatase (PAP)
PAP is produced by the epithelial cells lining the prostatic ducts and acini and is secreted directly into the prostatic ductal system. PAP was the first serum marker for prostate cancer. Serum PAP may be significantly elevated in patients with BPH, prostatitis, prostatic infarction or prostate cancer. Serum PAP currently plays a limited role in the diagnosis and management of prostate cancer. The sensitivity and specificity of this tumour marker are far too low for it to be used as a screening test for prostate cancer {1660}.

Human glandular kallikrein 2 (hK2)
The gene for hK2 has a close sequence homology to the PSA gene. hK2 messenger RNA is localized predominantly to the prostate in the same manner as PSA. hK2 and PSA exhibit different proteolytic specificities, but show similar patterns of complex formation with serum protease inhibitors. In particular, hK2 is found to form a covalent complex with ACT at rates comparable to PSA. Therefore, serum hK2 is detected in its free form, as well as in a complex with ACT {2074}.
The serum level of hK2 is relatively high, especially in men with diagnosed prostate cancer and not proportional to total PSA or free PSA concentrations. This difference in serum expression between hK2 and PSA allows additional clinical information to be derived from the measurement of hK2.

Prostate specific membrane antigen (PSMA)
Although it is not a secretory protein, PSMA is a membrane-bound glycoprotein with high specificity for benign or malignant prostatic epithelial cells {142, 1125,1839,1842,2412,2846,2847}. This is a novel prognostic marker that is present in the serum of healthy men, according to studies with monoclonal antibody 7E11.C5. An elevated concentration is associated with the presence of prostate cancer. PSMA levels correlate best with advanced stage, or with a hormone-refractory state. However, studies of the

expression of PSMA in serum of both normal individuals and prostate cancer patients using western blots have provided conflicting results in some laboratories {635,1838,1841,2214}.

Reverse transcriptase-polymerase chain reaction
RT-PCR is an extremely sensitive assay, capable of detecting one prostate cell diluted in 10^8 non-prostate cells. This high degree of sensitivity mandates that extreme precaution be taken to avoid both cross-sample and environmental contamination. Because of the high sensitivity of RT-PCR, there is the possibility that extremely low-level basal transcriptions of prostate-specific genes from non-prostate cells will result in a positive RT-PCR signal. More recently, basal PSA mRNA levels were detected in a quantitative RT-PCR in individuals without prostate cancer, thus suggesting the need to quantitate the RT-PCR assay in order to control for basal transcription {2730}. These problems with RT-PCR have limited its clinical utility {1780,1927}.

Methods of tissue diagnosis
Needle biopsies
The current standard method for detection of prostate cancer is by transrectal ultrasound-guided core biopsies. Directed biopsies to either lesions detected on digital rectal examination or on ultrasound should be combined with systematic biopsies taken according to a standardized protocol {1008,1703}. The sextant protocol samples the apex, mid and base region bilaterally {1099}. Sextant biopsies aim at the centre of each half of the prostate equidistant from the midline and the lateral edge while the most common location of prostate cancer is in the dorsolateral region of the prostate.
Several modifications of the sextant protocol have been proposed. Recent studies have shown that protocols with 10 to 13 systematic biopsies have a cancer detection rate up to 35% superior to the traditional sextant protocol {105,724, 2151}. This increased yield relates to the addition of biopsies sampling the more lateral part of the peripheral zone, where a significant number of cancers are located.
Approximately 15-22% of prostate cancers arise in the transition zone, while sextant biopsies mainly sample the peripheral zone. Most studies have

found few additional cancers by adding transition zone biopsies to the sextant protocol (1.8-4.3% of all cancers detected) and transition zone biopsies are usually not taken in the initial biopsy session {778,2598}.
Handling of needle biopsies. Prostate biopsies from different regions of the gland should be identified separately. If two cores are taken from the same region, they can be placed into the same block. However, blocking more than two biopsy specimens together increases the loss of tissue at sectioning {1272}. When atypia suspicious for cancer is found, a repeat biopsy should concentrate on the initial atypical site in addition to sampling the rest of the prostate. This cannot be performed unless biopsies have been specifically designated as to their location. The normal histology of the prostate and its adjacent structures differs between base and apex and knowledge about biopsy location is helpful for the pathologist. The location and extent of cancer may be critical for the clinician when selecting treatment option {2151}. The most common fixative used for needle biopsies is formalin, although alternative fixatives, which enhance nuclear details are also in use. A potential problem with these alternative fixatives is that lesions such as high-grade prostatic intraepithelial neoplasia may be over-diagnosed.
Immunohistochemistry for high molecular weight cytokeratins provides considerable help in decreasing the number of inconclusive cases from 6-2% {1923}. It has therefore been suggested that intervening unstained sections suitable for immunohistochemistry are retained in case immunohistochemistry would be necessary. Intervening slides are critical to establish a conclusive diagnosis in 2.8% of prostate biopsies, hence, sparing a repeat biopsy {939}.

Transurethral resection of the prostate
When transurethral resection of the prostate (TURP) is done without clinical suspicion of cancer, prostate cancer is incidentally detected in approximately 8-10% of the specimens. Cancers detected at TURP are often transition zone tumours, but they may also be of peripheral zone origin, particularly when they are large {941,1685,1686}. It is recommended that the extent of tumour is reported as percentage of the total specimen area. If the tumour occupies less

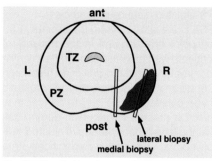

Fig. 3.09 Needle biopsies sampling the lateral part of the peripheral zone (PZ) improve detection of prostate cancer (red).

than 5% of the specimen it is stage T1a, and otherwise stage T1b. However, in the uncommon situation of less than 5% of cancer with Gleason score 7 or higher, patients are treated as if they had stage T1b disease. Most men who undergo total prostatectomy for T1a cancer have no or minimal residual disease, but in a minority there is substantial tumour located in the periphery of the prostate {711}.
Handling of TUR specimens. A TURP specimen may contain more than a hundred grams of tissue and it is often necessary to select a limited amount of tissue for histological examination. Submission should be random to ensure that the percentage of the specimen area involved with cancer is representative for the entire specimen. Several strategies for selection have been evaluated. Submission of 8 cassettes will identify almost all stage T1b cancers and approximately 90% of stage T1a tumours {1847,2223}. In young men, submission of the entire specimen may be considered to ensure detection of all T1a tumours. Guidelines have been developed for whether additional sampling is needed following the initial detection of cancer in a TURP specimen {1673}.

Fine needle aspiration cytology
Before the era of transrectal core biopsies, prostate cancer was traditionally diagnosed by fine needle aspiration (FNA). FNA is still used in some countries and has some advantages. The technique is cheap, quick, usually relatively painless and has low risk of complications. In early studies comparing FNA and limited core biopsy protocols, the sensitivity of FNA was usually found to be comparable with that of core biopsies {2765}. However, the use of FNA for diagnosing prostate cancer has disadvan-

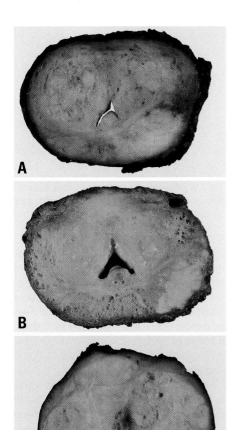

Fig. 3.10 A,B Section of prostate showing peripheral zone adenocarcinoma. **C** Section of prostate showing transition zone adenocarcinoma, difficult to distinguish from nodules of BPH.

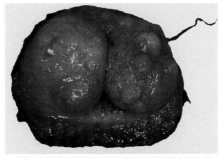

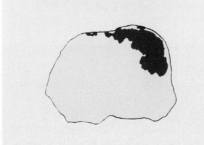

Fig. 3.11 A Transition zone cancer with yellow nodule in the anterior right area. **B** Transition zone cancer, microscopical extent of tumour.

tages. Potential sources of false positive diagnosis with FNA are inflammatory atypia, prostatic intraepithelial neoplasia and contamination of seminal vesicle epithelium. Gleason grading, which is essential for the clinician, is based on the histological architecture of glands and cannot be applied on cytology. Core biopsies, unlike FNA, provide information about tumour extent and occasionally about extra-prostatic extension and seminal vesicle invasion. Before treatment of localized prostate cancer, the diagnosis should, therefore, be confirmed by core biopsies.

Macroscopy

On section, grossly evident cancers are firm, solid, and range in colour from white-grey to yellow-orange, the latter having increased cytoplasmic lipid; the tumours contrast with the adjacent benign parenchyma, which is typically tan and spongy {289,1001,1685,2905}.

Tumours usually extend microscopically beyond their macroscopic border. Gross haemorrhage and necrosis are rare. Subtle tumours may be grossly recognized by structural asymmetry; for example, peripheral zone tumours may deform the periurethral fibromuscular concentric band demarcating the periurethral and peripheral prostate centrally, and peripherally may expand or obscure the outer boundaries of the prostate. Anterior and apical tumours are difficult to grossly identify because of admixed stromal and nodular hyperplasia {289,290,701, 1001,2905}.

In general, grossly recognizable tumours tend to be larger, of higher grade and stage, and are frequently palpable, compared with grossly inapparent tumours (usually < 5 mm), which are often non-palpable, small, low grade and low stage {2168}. Some large tumours are diffusely infiltrative, and may not be evident grossly {701,1001}. Causes of gross false positive diagnoses include confluent glandular atrophy, healed infarcts, stromal hyperplasia, granulomatous prostatitis and infection {1001}. In countries with widespread PSA testing, grossly evident prostate cancer has become relatively uncommon.

Tumour spread and staging

Local extraprostatic extension typically occurs along the anterior aspect of the gland for transition zone carcinomas, and in posterolateral sites for the more common peripheral zone carcinomas {1684}. The peripheral zone carcinomas often grow into periprostatic soft tissue by invading along nerves {2735} or by direct penetration out of the prostate. The term "capsule" has been used to denote the outer boundary of the prostate. However, as there is no well-defined capsule surrounding the entire prostate this term is no longer recommended. Extraprostatic invasion superiorly into the bladder neck can occur with larger tumours, and in advanced cases, this can lead to bladder neck and ureteral obstruction. Extension into the seminal vesicles can occur by several pathways, including direct extension from carcinoma in adjacent soft tissue, spread along the ejaculatory duct complex, and via lymphvascular space channels {1944}. Posteriorly, Denovillier's fascia constitutes an effective physical barrier {2734}, and direct prostatic carcinoma spread into the rectum is a rare event.

Metastatic spread of prostatic carcinoma begins when carcinoma invades into lymphvascular spaces. The most common sites of metastatic spread of prostatic carcinoma are the regional lymph nodes and bones of the pelvis and axial skeleton. The obturator and hypogastric nodes are usually the first ones to be involved, followed by external iliac, common iliac, presacral, and presciatic nodes. In a few patients, periprostatic/periseminal vesicle lymph nodes may be the first ones to harbour metastatic carcinoma, but these nodes are found in less than 5% of radical prostatectomy specimens {1364}. Metastasis to bone marrow, with an osteoblastic response, is a hallmark of disseminated prostate cancer {835}. The bones most frequently infiltrated by metastatic disease are, in descending order, pelvic bones, dorsal and lumbar spine, ribs, cervical spine, femur, skull, sacrum, and humerus. Visceral metastatic deposits in the lung and liver are not often clinically apparent, but are common in end-stage disease.

The TNM classification scheme {944, 2662} is the currently preferred system for clinical and pathologic staging of prostatic carcinoma.

Histopathology

Adenocarcinomas of the prostate range from well-differentiated gland forming cancers, where it is often difficult to dis-

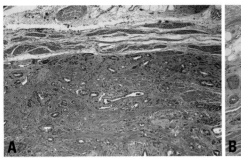
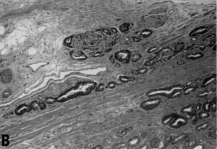
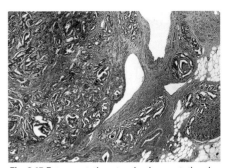

Fig. 3.12 A Organ-confined adenocarcinoma of the prostate extending to edge of gland. B Adenocarcinoma of the prostate with focal extra-prostatic extension.

Fig. 3.15 Extraprostatic extension by prostatic adenocarcinoma, with tracking along nerve, into periprostatic adipose tissue.

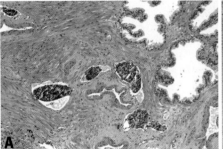
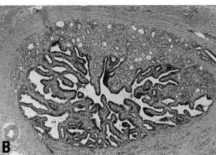

Fig. 3.13 A Intraprostatic lymphovascular space invasion by prostatic adenocarcinoma. B Ejaculatory duct invasion by prostatic adenocarcinoma, with duct wall invasion, with sparing of ejaculatory duct epithelium and lumen.

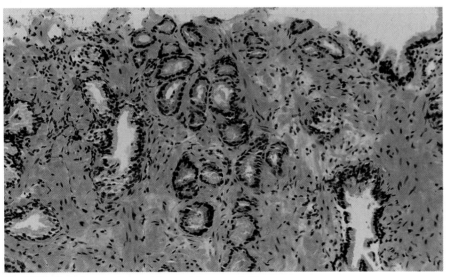

Fig. 3.14 Limited adenocarcinoma of the prostate on needle biopsy.

tinguish them from benign prostatic glands, to poorly differentiated tumours, difficult to identify as being of prostatic origin. A feature common to virtually all prostate cancers is the presence of only a single cell type without a basal cell layer. Benign prostate glands, in contrast, contain a basal cell layer beneath the secretory cells. The recognition of basal cells on hematoxylin and eosin stained sections is not straightforward. In cases of obvious carcinoma, there may be cells that closely mimic basal cells. These cells when labeled with basal cell specific antibodies are negative and represent fibroblasts closely apposed to the neoplastic glands. Conversely, basal cells may not be readily recognized in benign glands without the use of special studies. The histopathology of prostatic cancer, and its distinction from benign glands, rests on a constellation of architectural, nuclear, cytoplasmic, and intraluminal features. With the exception of three malignant specific features listed at the end of this section, all of the features listed below, while more commonly seen in cancer, can also be seen in benign mimickers of cancer.

Architectural features

Benign prostatic glands tend to grow either as circumscribed nodules within benign prostatic hyperplasia, radiate in columns out from the urethra in a linear fashion, or are evenly dispersed in the peripheral zone {1685}. In contrast, gland-forming prostate cancers typically contain glands that are more crowded than in benign prostatic tissue, although there is overlap with certain benign mimickers of prostate cancer. Glands of adenocarcinoma of the prostate typically grow in a haphazard fashion. Glands oriented perpendicular to each other and glands irregularly separated by bundles of smooth muscle are indicative of an infiltrative process. Another pattern characteristic of an infiltrative process is the presence of small atypical glands situated in between larger benign glands. With the loss of glandular differentiation and the formation of cribriform structures, fused glands, and poorly formed glands, the distinction between benign glands based on the architectural pattern becomes more apparent. Tumours composed of solid sheets, cords of cells, or isolated individual cells characterize undifferentiated prostate cancer. These architectural patterns are key components to the grading of prostate cancer (see Gleason grading system).

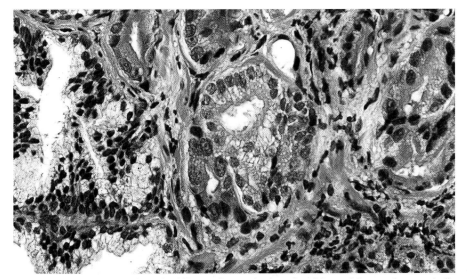

Fig. 3.16 Adenocarcinoma with amphophilic cytoplasm and enlarged nuclei containing prominent nucleoli.

Nuclear features

Nuclei in prostate cancer range from those indistinguishable from benign prostatic epithelium to those with overt malignancy. Typically, the extent of nuclear atypia correlates with the architectural degree of differentiation, although exceptions occur. In most prostate cancers, there are cytological differences in the malignant glands when compared to the surrounding benign glands. Nuclear enlargement with prominent nucleoli is a frequent finding, although not every cancer cell will display these features. Some neoplastic nuclei lack prominent nucleoli, yet are enlarged and hyperchromatic. Prostate cancer nuclei, even in cancers which lack glandular differentiation, show little variabililty in nuclear shape or size from one nucleus to another. Rarely, high-grade prostate cancer, typically seen in the terminal disseminated phase of the disease, reveals marked nuclear pleomorphism. Mitotic figures may be relatively common in high-grade cancer, yet are infrequent in lower grade tumours.

Cytoplasmic features

Glands of adenocarcinoma of the prostate tend to have a discrete crisp, sharp luminal border without undulations or ruffling of the cytoplasm. In contrast, equivalently sized benign glands have an irregular luminal surface with small papillary infoldings and a convoluted appearance. The finding of apical snouts is not helpful in distinguishing benign versus malignant glands as they can be seen in both. Cytoplasmic features of low grade prostate cancer are also often not very distinctive, since they are often pale-clear, similar to benign glands. Neoplastic glands may have amphophilic cytoplasm, which may be a useful diagnostic criterion of malignancy. Prostate cancer cytoplasm of all grades typically lacks lipofuscin, in contrast to its presence in some benign prostatic glands {314}.

Intraluminal features

A feature more commonly seen in low grade prostate cancer, as opposed to higher grade cancer is prostatic crystalloids {1111,2204}. These are dense eosinophilic crystal-like structures that appear in various geometric shapes such as rectangular, hexagonal, triangular and rod-like structures. Crystalloids, although not diagnostic of carcinoma, are more frequently found in cancer than in benign glands. The one condition that mimics cancer where crystalloids are frequently seen is adenosis (atypical adenomatous hyperplasia) {843}.

Intraluminal pink acellular dense secretions or blue-tinged mucinous secretions seen in hematoxylin and eosin stained sections are additional findings seen preferentially in cancer, especially low-grade cancer {703}. In contrast, corpora amylacea, which consists of well-circumscribed round to oval structures with concentric lamellar rings, are common in benign glands and only rarely seen in prostate cancer {2204}.

Malignant specific features

Short of seeing prostatic glands in an extra-prostatic site, there are only three features that are in and of themselves diagnostic of cancer, as they have not been described in benign prostatic

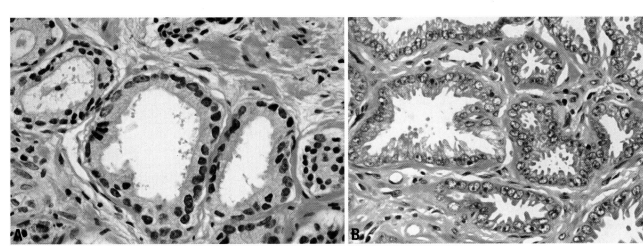

Fig. 3.17 A Well differentiated carcinoma with mild nuclear atypia. **B** Apocrine-like cytoplasmic blebing in prostatic adenocarcinoma glands.

glands. These are perineural invasion, mucinous fibroplasia (collagenous micronodules), and glomerulations {160}. Although perineural indentation by benign prostatic glands has been reported, the glands in these cases appear totally benign and are present at only one edge of the nerve rather than circumferentially involving the perineural space, as can be seen in carcinoma {379,1676}. The second specific feature for prostate cancer is known as either mucinous fibroplasia or collagenous micronodules. It is typified by very delicate loose fibrous tissue with an ingrowth of fibroblasts, sometimes reflecting organization of intraluminal mucin. The final malignant specific feature is glomerulations, consisting of glands with a cribriform proliferation that is not transluminal. Rather, these cribriform formations are attached to only one edge of the gland resulting in a structure superficially resembling a glomerulus.

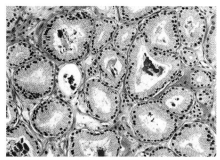

Fig. 3.18 Intraluminal crystalloids in low grade adenocarcinoma.

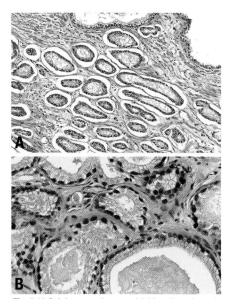

Fig. 3.19 A Adenocarcinoma with blue-tinged mucinous secretions. **B** Adenocarcinoma with straight rigid luminal borders, and dense pink secretions.

Stromal features
Ordinary acinar adenocarcinoma lacks a desmoplastic or myxoid stromal response, such that evaluation of the stroma is typically not useful in the diagnosis of prostate cancer. Typically adenocarcinoma of the prostate does not elicit a stromal inflammatory response.

Immunoprofile
Prostate specific antigen (PSA)
Following PSA's discovery in 1979, it has become a useful immunohistochemical marker of prostatic differentiation in formalin-fixed, paraffin-embedded tissue, with both polyclonal and monoclonal antibodies available {702}. PSA is localized to the cytoplasm of non-neoplastic prostatic glandular cells in all prostatic zones, but is neither expressed by basal cells, seminal vesicle/ejaculatory duct glandular cells, nor urothelial cells.
Because of its relatively high specificity for prostatic glandular cells, PSA is a useful tissue marker expressed by most prostatic adenocarcinomas {66, 702,1863,2905}. There is frequently intratumoural and intertumoural heterogeneity, with most studies indicating decreasing PSA expression with increasing tumour grade {702,906}. PSA is diagnostically helpful in distinguishing prostatic adenocarcinomas from other neoplasms secondarily involving the prostate and establishing prostatic origin in metastatic carcinomas of unknown primary {702,1863}. PSA is also helpful in excluding benign mimics of prostatic carcinoma, such as seminal vesicle/ejaculatory duct epithelium, nephrogenic adenoma, mesonephric duct remnants, Cowper's glands, granulomatous prostatitis and malakoplakia {66,309,2905}. Whereas monoclonal antibodies to PSA do not label seminal vesicle tissue, polyclonal antibodies have been shown to occasionally label seminal vesicle epithelium {2714}. PSA in conjunction with a basal cell marker is useful in distinguishing intraglandular proliferations of basal cells from acinar cells, helping to separate prostatic intraepithelial neoplasia from basal cell hyperplasia and transitional cell metaplasia in equivocal cases {66, 2374,2905}.
A minority of higher grade prostatic adenocarcinomas are PSA negative, although some of these tumours have been shown to express PSA mRNA. Some prostatic adenocarcinomas lose

PSA immunoreactivity following androgen deprivation or radiation therapy. Prostate specific membrane antigen (PSMA) (membrane bound antigen expressed in benign and malignant prostatic acinar cells) and androgen receptor may be immunoreactive in some high grade, PSA immunonegative prostatic adenocarcinomas. Extraprostatic tissues which are variably immunoreactive for PSA, include urethral and periurethral glands (male and female), urothelial glandular metaplasia (cystitis cystitica and glandularis), anal glands (male), urachal remnants and neutrophils. Extraprostatic neoplasms and tumour-like conditions occasionally immunoreactive for PSA include urethral/periurethral adenocarcinoma (female), bladder adenocarcinoma, extramammary Paget disease of the penis, salivary gland neoplasms in males (pleomorphic adenoma, mucoepidermoid carcinoma, adenoid cystic carcinoma, salivary duct carcinoma), mammary carcinoma, mature teratoma, and some nephrogenic adenomas {66,702,2905}.

Prostate specific acid phosphatase (PAP)
Immunohistochemistry for PAP is active in formalin-fixed, paraffin-embedded tissues {26,66,702,1771,1862,2905}. The polyclonal antibody is more sensitive, but less specific than the monoclonal antibody {309}. PAP and PSA have similar diagnostic utility; since a small number of prostatic adenocarcinomas are immunoreactive for only one of the two markers, PAP is primarily reserved for cases of suspected prostatic carcinoma in which the PSA stain is negative {849}. Extraprostatic tissues reported to be immunoreactive for PAP include pancreatic islet cells, hepatocytes, gastric parietal cells, some renal tubular epithelial cells and neutrophils. Reported PAP immunoreactive neoplasms include some neuroendocrine tumours (pancreatic islet cell tumours, gastrointestinal carcinoids), mammary carcinoma, urothelial adenocarcinoma, anal cloacogenic carcinoma, salivary gland neoplasms (males) and mature teratoma {66,702,2905}.

High molecular weight cytokeratins detected by 34βE12 (Cytokeratin-903)
Prostatic secretory and basal cells are immunoreactive for antibodies to broad

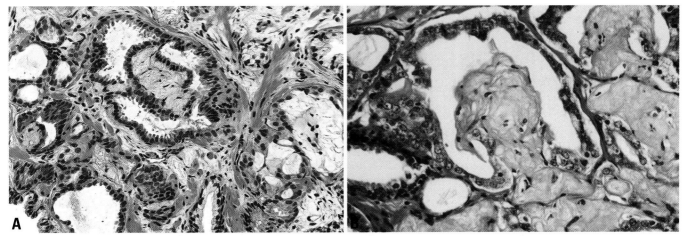

Fig. 3.20 A, B Adenocarcinoma with mucinous fibroplasia (collagenous micronodules).

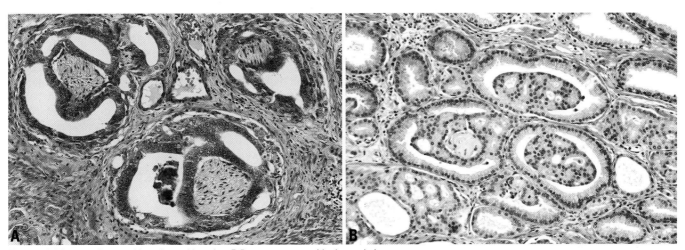

Fig. 3.21 A Adenocarcinoma with perineural invasion. **B** Prostate cancer with glomerulations.

spectrum and low molecular weight cytokeratins. However, only basal cells express high molecular weight cytokeratins {309}. One high molecular monoclonal cytokeratin antibody, clone 34βE12, recognizes 57 and 66 kilodalton cytokeratins in stratum corneum corresponding to Moll numbers 1, 5, 10 and 14, and is widely used as a basal cell specific marker active in paraffin-embedded tissue following proteolytic digestion {66,309,918,1048,1765,2374,2905}. 34βE12 is also immunoreactive against squamous, urothelial, bronchial/pneumocyte, thymic, some intestinal and ductal epithelium (breast, pancreas, bile duct, salivary gland, sweat duct, renal collecting duct), and mesothelium {918}. An immunoperoxidase cocktail containing monoclonal antibodies to cytokeratins 5 and 6 is also an effective basal cell stain {1286}. Since uniform absence of a basal cell

layer in prostatic acinar proliferations is one important diagnostic feature of invasive carcinoma and basal cells may be inapparent by H&E stain, basal cell specific immunostains may help to distinguish invasive prostatic adenocarcinoma from benign small acinar cancer - mimics which retain their basal cell layer, e.g. glandular atrophy, post-atrophic hyperplasia, adenosis (atypical adenomatous hyperplasia), sclerosing adenosis and radiation induced atypia {66,1048,2905}. Because the basal cell layer may be interrupted or not demonstrable in small numbers of benign glands, the complete absence of a basal cell layer in a small focus of acini cannot be used alone as a definitive criterion for malignancy; rather, absence of a basal cell layer is supportive of invasive carcinoma only in acinar proliferations which exhibit suspicious cytologic and / or architectural features

on H&E stain {1048}. Conversely, some early invasive prostatic carcinomas, e.g. microinvasive carcinomas arising in association with or independent of high grade prostatic intraepithelial neoplasia, may have residual basal cells {1952}. Intraductal spread of invasive carcinoma and entrapped benign glands are other proposed explanations for residual basal cells {66,2905}. Rare prostatic adenocarcinomas contain sparse neoplastic glandular cells, which are immunoreactive for 34βE12, yet these are not in a basal cell distribution {66,2374}. The use of antibodies for 34βE12 is especially helpful for the diagnosis for of deceptively benign appearing variants of prostate cancer. Immunohistochemistry for cytokeratins 7 and 20 have a limited diagnostic use in prostate pathology with the exception that negative staining for both markers, which can occur in prostate

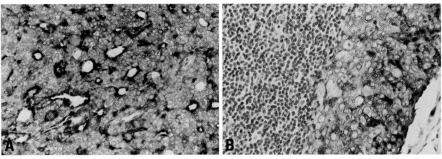

Fig. 3.22 A Prostate specific antigen (PSA) expression in prostatic adenocarcinoma with accentuation of glandular luminal spaces. **B** Metastatic adenocarcinoma to a supraclavicular lymph node labeled staining positively for prostate specific antigen.

adenocarcinoma, would be unusual for transitional cell carcinoma {849}.

p63

p63, a nuclear protein encoded by a gene on chromosome 3q27-29 with homology to p53 (a tumour suppressor gene), has been shown to regulate growth and development in epithelium of the skin, cervix, breast and urogenital tract. Specific isotypes are expressed in basal cells of pseudostratified epithelia (prostate, bronchial), reserve cells of simple columnar epithelia (endocervical, pancreatic ductal), myoepithelial cells (breast, salivary glands, cutaneous apocrine/eccrine glands), urothelium and squamous epithelium {1286}. A

monoclonal antibody is active in paraffin-embedded tissue following antigen retrieval. p63 has similar applications to those of high molecular weight cytokeratins in the diagnosis of prostatic adenocarcinoma, but with the advantages that p63: 1) stains a subset of 34βE12 negative basal cells, 2) is less susceptible to the staining variability of 34βE12 (particularly in TURP specimens with cautery artefact), and 3) is easier to interpret because of its strong nuclear staining intensity and low background. Interpretative limitations related to presence or absence of basal cells in small numbers of glands for 34βE12 apply to p63, requiring correlation with morphology {2374}. Prostatic adenocarcinomas

have occasional p63 immunoreactive cells, most representing entrapped benign glands or intraductal spread of carcinoma with residual basal cells {1286}.

α-Methyl-CoA racemase (AMACR)

AMACR mRNA was recently identified as being overexpressed in prostatic adenocarcinoma by cDNA library subtraction utilizing high throughput RNA microarray analysis {2856}. This mRNA was found to encode a racemase protein, for which polyclonal and monoclonal antibodies have been produced which are active in formalin-fixed, paraffin- embedded tissue {187,1220,2856,2935}. Immunohistochemical studies on biopsy material with an antibody directed against AMACR (P504S) demonstrate that over 80% of prostatic adenocarcinomas are labeled {1221,1593}. Certain subtypes of prostate cancer, such as foamy gland carcinoma, atrophic carcinoma, pseudohyperplastic, and treated carcinoma show lower AMACR expression {2936}. However, AMACR is not specific for prostate cancer and is present in nodular hyperplasia (12%), atrophic glands, high grade PIN (>90%) {2935}, and adenosis (atypical adenomatous hyperplasia) (17.5%) {2869}. AMACR may be used as a confirmatory stain for prostatic adenocarcinoma, in conjunction with H&E morphology and a basal cell specific marker {2935}. AMACR is expressed in other non-prostatic neoplasms including urothelial and colon cancer.

Androgen receptor (AR)

AR is a nuclear localized, androgen binding protein complex occurring in prostatic glandular, basal, stromal cells. The activated protein serves as a transcription factor, mediating androgen dependent cellular functions, e.g. PSA transcription in secretory cells and promoting cellular proliferation. AR monoclonal and polyclonal antibodies are active in formalin-fixed, paraffin-embedded tissue following antigen retrieval {1592,2559}. Positive nuclear staining indicates immunoreactive protein, but does not distinguish active from inactive forms of the protein. AR immunoreactivity was demonstrated in a minority (42.5%) cases of high grade prostatic intraepithelial neoplasia. Most invasive prostatic adenocarcinomas are immunoreactive for AR; one study demonstrated that 85% of untreated

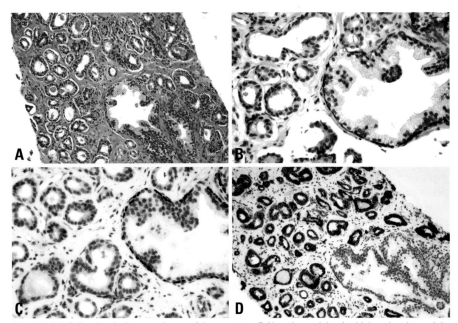

Fig. 3.23 A H & E stain of adenocarcinoma of the prostate. **B** Negative staining for high molecular weight cytokeratin in prostate cancer. Note cytoplasmic labeling of basal cells in adjacent benign glands. **C** Negative staining for p63 in prostate cancer. Note nuclear labeling of basal cells in adjacent benign glands **D** Positive staining for racemase in adenocarcinoma of the prostate.

prostate adenocarcinomas exhibit AR immunoreactivity in greater than 50% of tumour cells, with increasing heterogeneity occurring with increasing histologic grade and pathologic stage {1592}. Some studies have shown AR heterogeneity or loss in a subset of AR independent tumours, suggesting one mechanism of androgen resistance may be AR loss {1592,2559}. Because androgen insensitivity may occur without loss of AR immunoreactivity, positive AR immunophenotype may not reliably distinguish androgen dependent from independent tumours {1592}. Imumunostaining for AR is not in routine clinical use.

Histologic variants

The following histologic variants of prostate adenocarcinoma are typically seen in association with ordinary acinar adenocarcinoma. However, on limited biopsy material, the entire sampled tumour may demonstrate only the variant morphology.

Atrophic variant

As described under histopathology, most prostate cancers have abundant cytoplasm. An unusual variant of prostate cancer resembles benign atrophy owing to its scant cytoplasm. Although ordinary prostate cancers may develop atrophic cytoplasm as a result of treatment (see carcinoma affected by hormone therapy), atrophic prostate cancers are usually unassociated with such a prior history {467,664}. The diagnosis of carcinoma in these cases may be based on several features. First, atrophic prostate cancer may demonstrate a truly infiltrative process with individual small atrophic

glands situated between larger benign glands. In contrast, benign atrophy has a lobular configuration. A characteristic finding in some benign cases of atrophy is the presence of a centrally dilated atrophic gland surrounding by clustered smaller glands, which has been termed "post-atrophic hyperplasia (PAH)" {83}. Although the glands of benign atrophy may appear infiltrative on needle biopsy, they are not truly infiltrative, as individual benign atrophic glands are not seen infiltrating in between larger benign glands. Whereas some forms of atrophy, are associated with fibrosis, atrophic prostate cancer lack such a desmoplastic stromal response. Atrophic prostate cancer may also be differentiated from benign atrophy by the presence of marked cytologic atypia. Atrophy may show enlarged nuclei and prominent nucleoli, although not the huge eosinophilic nucleoli seen in some atrophic prostate cancers. Finally, the concomitant presence of ordinary less atrophic carcinoma can help in recognizing the malignant nature of the adjacent atrophic cancer glands.

Pseudohyperplastic variant

Pseudohyperplastic prostate cancer resembles benign prostate glands in that the neoplastic glands are large with branching and papillary infolding {1146, 1485}. The recognition of cancer with this pattern is based on the architectural pattern of numerous closely packed glands as well as nuclear features more typical of carcinoma. One pattern of pseudohyperplastic adenocarcinoma consists of numerous large glands that are almost

back-to-back with straight even luminal borders, and abundant cytoplasm. Comparably sized benign glands either have papillary infoldings or are atrophic. The presence of cytologic atypia in some of these glands further distinguishes them from benign glands. It is almost always helpful to verify pseudohyperplastic cancer with the use of immunohistochemistry to verify the absence of basal cells. Pseudohyperplastic cancer, despite its benign appearance, may be associated with typical intermediate grade cancer and can exhibit aggressive behaviour (ie., extraprostatic extension).

Foamy gland variant

Foamy gland cancer is a variant of acinar adenocarcinoma of the prostate that is characterized by having abundant foamy appearing cytoplasm with a very low nuclear to cytoplasmic ratio. Although the cytoplasm has a xanthomatous appearance, it does not contain lipid, but rather empty vacuoles {2637}. More typical cytological features of adenocarcinoma such as nuclear enlargement and prominent nucleoli are frequently absent, which makes this lesion difficult to recognize as carcinoma especially on biopsy material. Characteristically, the nuclei in foamy gland carcinoma are small and densely hyperchromatic. Nuclei in foamy gland cancer are round, more so than those of benign prostatic secretory cells. In addition to the unique nature of its cytoplasm, it is recognized as carcinoma by its architectural pattern of crowded and/or infiltrative glands, and frequently present dense pink acellular secretions {1880}. In most cases, foamy gland cancer is seen in association with ordinary

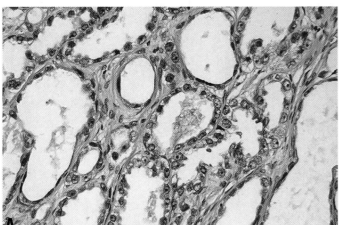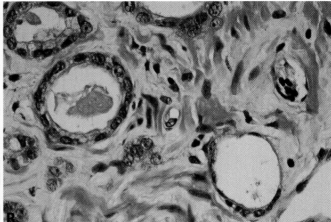

Fig. 3.24 Atrophic adenocarcinoma. **A** Note the microcystic pattern and **B** the prominent nucleoli.

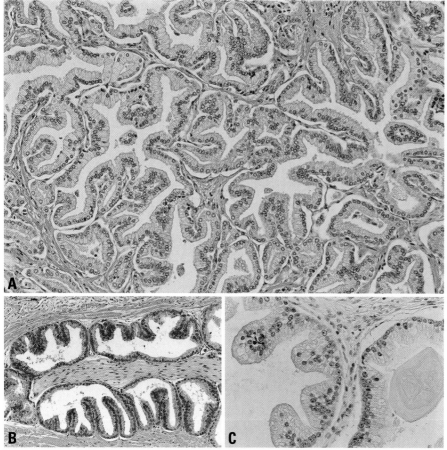

Fig. 3.25 A Pseudohyperplastic adenocarcinoma. Branding and pepillary type of and growth is typical. **B** Perineural invasion. **C** Higher magnification, showing prominent nucleoli.

adenocarcinoma of the prostate. In almost all such cases, despite foamy glands cancer's benign cytology, the ordinary adenocarcinoma component is not low grade. Consequently, foamy gland carcinoma appears best classified as intermediate grade carcinoma.

Colloid & signet ring variant
Using criteria developed for mucinous carcinomas of other organs, the diagnosis of mucinous adenocarcinoma of the prostate gland should be made when at least 25% of the tumour resected contains lakes of extracellular mucin. On biopsy material, cancers with abundant extracellular mucin should be diagnosed as *carcinomas with mucinous features*, rather than *colloid carcinoma*, as the biopsy material may not be reflective of the entire tumour. Mucinous (colloid) adenocarcinoma of the prostate gland is one of the least common morphologic variants of prostatic carcinoma {710,2207,2274}. A cribriform pattern tends to predominate in the mucinous areas. In contrast to bladder adenocarcinomas, mucinous adenocarcinoma of the prostate rarely contain mucin positive signet cells. Some carcinomas of the prostate will have a signet-ring-cell appearance, yet the vacuoles do not contain intracytoplasmic mucin {2206}. These vacuolated cells may be present as singly invasive cells, in single glands, and in sheets of cells. Only a few cases of prostate cancer have been reported with mucin positive signet cells {1057,2660}. One should exclude other mucinous tumours of non-prostatic origin based on morphology and immunohistochemistry and if necessary using clinical information. Even more rare are cases of in-situ and infiltrating mucinous adenocarcinoma arising from glandular metaplasia of the prostatic urethra with invasion into the prostate {2636}. The histologic growth pattern found in these tumours were identical to mucinous adenocarcinoma of the bladder consisting lakes of mucin lined by tall columnar epithelium with goblet cells showing varying degrees of nuclear atypia and in some of these cases, mucin-containing signet cells. These tumours have been negative immunohistochemically for PSA and PAP.

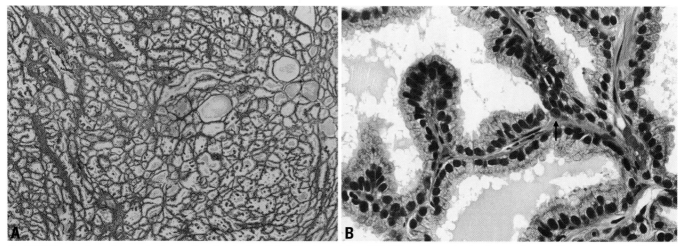

Fig. 3.26 A Cancer of pseudohyperplastic type. Crowded glands with too little stroma to be a BPH. **B** Pseudohyperplastic adenocarcinoma with prominent nucleoli (arrow).

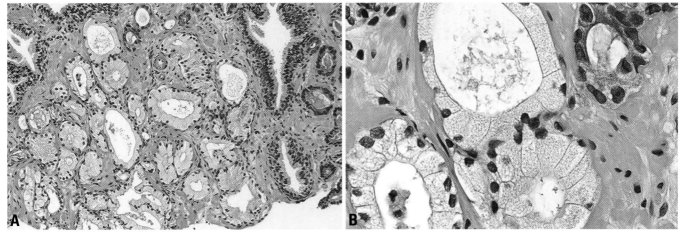

Fig. 3.27 A, B Foamy gland adenocarcinoma.

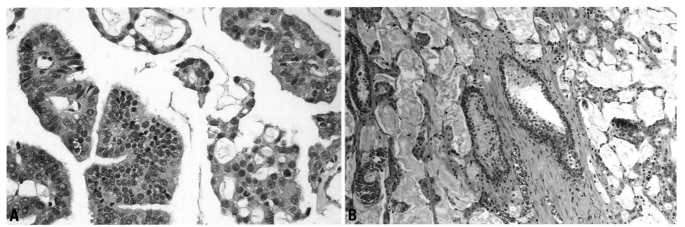

Fig. 3.28 A Colloid adenocarcinoma. **B** Acinar adenocarcinoma of the prostate, colloid variant left part.

Mucinous prostate adenocarcinomas behave aggressively {710,2207,2274}. In the largest reported series, 7 of 12 patients died of tumour (mean 5 years) and 5 were alive with disease (mean 3 years). Although these tumours are not as hormonally responsive as their non-mucinous counterparts, some respond to androgen withdrawal. Mucinous prostate adenocarcinomas have a propensity to

develop bone metastases and increased serum PSA levels with advanced disease.

Oncocytic variant
Prostatic adenocarcinoma rarely is composed of large cells with granular eosinophilic cytoplasm. Tumour cells have round to ovoid hyperchromatic nuclei, and are strongly positive for PSA. Numerous mitochondria are seen on ultra-

structural examination. A high Gleason grade {1972,2080}, elevated serum PSA {2080} and metastasis of similar morphology {1972} have been reported.

Lymphoepithelioma-like variant
This undifferentiated carcinoma is characterized by a syncytial pattern of malignant cells associated with a heavy lymphocytic infiltrate. Malignant cells are

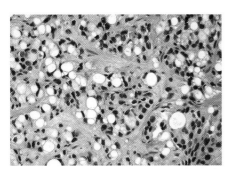

Fig. 3.29 Adenocarcinoma of the prostate with signet-ring cell-like features.

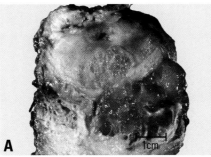 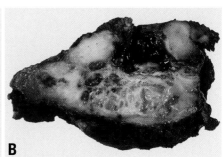

Fig. 3.30 A Mucinous adenocarcinoma. **B** Colloid carcinoma.

PSA positive. Associated acinar adenocarcinoma has been noted {34,2145}. In situ hybridization has been negative for Epstein-Barr virus {34}. Clinical significance is uncertain.

Sarcomatoid variant (carcinosarcoma)
There is considerable controversy in the literature regarding nomenclature and histogenesis of these tumours. In some series, carcinosarcoma and sarcomatoid carcinoma are considered as separate entities based on the presence of specific mesenchymal elements in the former. However, given their otherwise similar clinico-pathologic features and identically poor prognosis, these two lesions are best considered as one entity. Sarcomatoid carcinoma of the prostate is a rare neoplasm composed of both malignant epithelial and malignant spindle-cell and/or mesenchymal elements {207,588,644,1555,2175,2376}. Sarcomatoid carcinoma may be present in the initial pathologic material (synchronous presentation) or there may be a previous history of adenocarcinoma treated by radiation and/or hormonal therapy {1578}. The gross appearance often resembles sarcomas. Microscopically, sarcomatoid carcinoma is composed of a glandular component showing variable Gleason score {644,2093}. The sarcomatoid component often consists of a non-specific malignant spindle-cell proliferation. Amongst the specific mesenchymal elements are osteosarcoma, chondrosarcoma, rhabdomyosarcoma, leiomyosarcoma, liposarcoma, angiosarcoma or multiple types of heterologous differentiation {644,1578}. Sarcomatoid carcinoma should be distinguished from the rare carcinoma with metaplastic, benign-appearing bone or cartilage in the stroma. By immunohistochemistry, epithelial elements react with antibodies against PSA and/or pan-cytokeratins, whereas spindle-cell elements react with markers of soft tissue tumours and variably express cytokeratins. Serum PSA is within normal limits in most cases. Nodal and distant organ metastases at diagnosis are common {644,1578,2093}. There is less than a 40% five-year survival {644}.

Treatment effects
Radiation therapy
Radiation therapy can be given as either external beam or interstitial seed implants or as a combination of the two. After radiation therapy the prostate gland is usually small and hard. Radiation therapy affects prostate cancer variably with some glands showing marked radiation effect and others showing no evidence of radiation damage. Architecturally, carcinoma showing treatment effect typically loses their glandular pattern, resulting in clustered cells or individual cells. Cytologically, the cytoplasm of the tumour cells is pale, increased in volume and often vacuolated. There is often a greater variation of nuclear size than in non-irradiated prostate cancer and the nuclei may be pyknotic or large with clumped chromatin. Nucleoli are often lost {607,842,1060,1061,1065,1086, 1584}. Paradoxically the nuclear atypia in prostate carcinoma showing radiation effect is less than that seen in radiation atypia of benign glands. By immunohistochemistry, tumour cells with treatment effect are usually positive for PAP and PSA. These antibodies along with pan-cytokeratins are very helpful to detect isolated residual tumour cells, which can be overlooked in H&E stained sections. The stroma is often sclerosed, particularly following radioactive seed implantation. In the latter the stromal hyalinization is often sharply delineated. Following radiation therapy, prostatic biopsy should be diagnosed as no evidence of cancer, cancer showing no or minimal radiation effect, or cancer showing significant radiation effect, or a combination of the above. Although there exists various systems to grade radiation effects, these are not recommended for routine clinical practice. Biopsy findings predict prognosis with positive biopsies showing no treatment effect having a worse outcome than negative biopsies, and cancer with treatment effect having an intermediate prognosis {511}.

Hormone therapy
The histology of prostate cancer may be significantly altered following its treatment with hormonal therapy {2358}. One pattern is that neoplastic glands develop pyknotic nuclei and abundant xanthomatous cytoplasm. These cells then desquamate into the lumen of the malignant glands where they resemble histiocytes and lymphocytes, sometimes resulting in empty clefts. In some areas, there may be only scattered cells within the stroma resembling foamy histiocytes with pyknotic nuclei and xanthomatous cytoplasm. A related pattern is the presence of individual tumour cells resembling inflammatory cells. At low power, these areas may be difficult to identify, and often the only clue to areas of hormonally treated carcinoma is a fibrotic background with scattered larger cells.

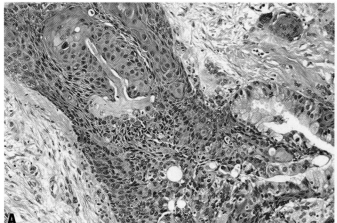
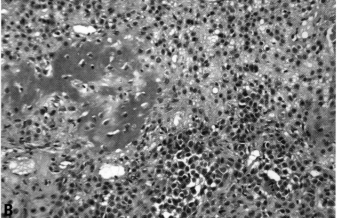

Fig. 3.31 A Sarcomatoid carcinoma with adenosquamous carcinoma. **B** Sarcomatoid carcinoma with osteoid formation.

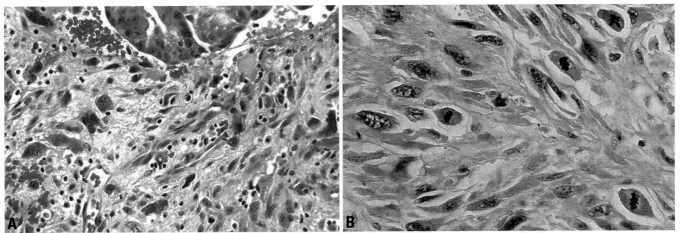

Fig. 3.32 A Sarcomatoid carcinoma. Note both epithelial (upper centre) and mesenchymal differentiation. **B** High-magnification view of spindle cell component of sarcomatoid carcinoma of prostate.

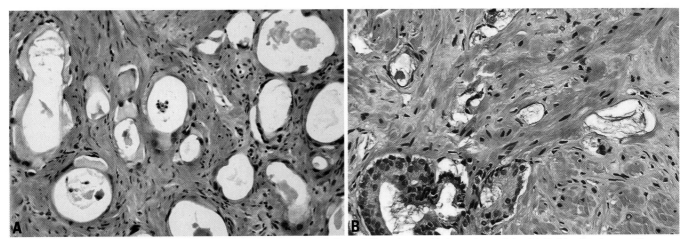

Fig. 3.33 A Cancer with radiation effect. The degenerating tumour cells are ballooned. Note pleomorphic hyperchromatic nuclei. **B** Adenocarcinoma with cancer showing radiation effect adjacent to cancer without evidence of radiation effect.

Immunohistochemistry for PSA or pancytokeratin can aid in the diagnosis of carcinoma in these cases by identifying the individual cells as epithelial cells of prostatic origin. Cancer cells following hormonal therapy demonstrate a lack of high molecular weight cytokeratin staining, identical to untreated prostate cancer. Following a response to combination endocrine therapy, the grade of the tumour appears artefactually higher, when compared to the grade of the pretreated tumour. As with radiation, the response to hormonal therapy may be variable, with areas of the cancer appearing unaffected {117,340,470, 1059,1852,2176,2447,2681}.

Gleason grading system
Numerous grading systems have been designed for histopathological grading of prostate cancer. The main controversies have been whether grading should be based on glandular differentiation alone or a combination of glandular differentiation and nuclear atypia, and also whether prostate cancer should be graded according to its least differentiated or dominant pattern. The Gleason grading system named after Donald F. Gleason is now the predominant grading system, and in 1993, it was recommended by a WHO consensus conference {1840}. The Gleason grading system is based on glandular architecture; nuclear atypia is not evaluated {894,895}. Nuclear atypia as adopted in some grading systems, correlates with prognosis of prostate cancer but there is no convincing evidence that it adds independent prognostic information to that obtained by grading glandular differentiation alone {1801}. The Gleason grading system defines five histological patterns or grades with decreasing differentiation. Normal prostate epithelial cells are arranged around a lumen. In patterns 1 to 3, there is retained epithelial polarity with luminal differentiation in virtually all glands. In pattern 4, there is partial loss of normal polarity and in pattern 5, there is an almost total loss of polarity with only occasional luminal differentiation. Prostate cancer has a pronounced morphological heterogeneity and usually more than one histological pattern is present. The primary and secondary pattern, i.e. the most prevalent and the second most prevalent pattern are added to obtain a Gleason score or sum. It is recommended that the primary and secondary pattern as well as the score be reported, e.g. Gleason score 3+4=7. If the tumour only has one pattern, Gleason score is obtained by doubling that pattern, e.g. Gleason score 3+3=6. Gleason scores 2 and 3 are only exceptionally

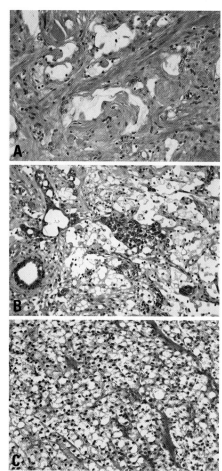

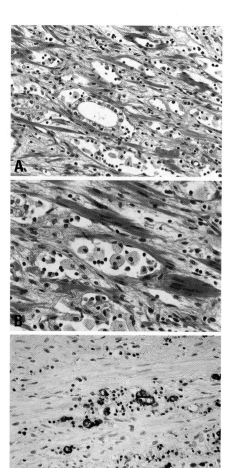

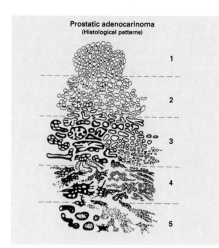

Fig. 3.36 Schematic diagram of the Gleason scoring system, created by Dr. D.F. Gleason.

Fig. 3.34 A Anti-androgen therapy induced tumour suppression leading to cystic spaces. **B** In the center a group of tumour cells with eosinophilic granular cytoplasm indicating paracrine-endocrine differentiation. Surrounding tumour cells are degenerated. **C** Tumour cells are vacuolated, clear with focal loss of cell membranes.

Fig. 3.35 A Adenocarcinoma following anti-androgen therapy with tumour undergoing pyknosis. **B** Adenocarcinoma following anti-androgen therapy with tumour undergoing pyknosis leading to tumour resembling foamy histiocytes. **C** Isolated tumour cells following anti-androgen therapy expressing pancytokeratin.

assigned, because Gleason pattern 1 is unusual. Gleason score 4 is also relatively uncommon because pattern 2 is usually mixed with some pattern 3 resulting in a Gleason score 5. Gleason score 2-4 tumour may be seen in TURP material sampling the transitional zone. In needle biopsy material, it has been proposed that a Gleason score of 2-4 should not be assigned {704,2283}. Gleason scores 6 and 7 are the most common scores and include the majority of tumours in most studies.

Gleason pattern 1
Gleason pattern 1 is composed of a very well circumscribed nodule of separate, closely packed glands, which do not infiltrate into adjacent benign prostatic tissue. The glands are of intermediate size

and approximately equal in size and shape. This pattern is usually seen in transition zone cancers. Gleason pattern 1 is exceedingly rare. When present, it is usually only a minor component of the tumour and not included in the Gleason score.

Gleason pattern 2
Gleason pattern 2 is composed of round or oval glands with smooth ends. The glands are more loosely arranged and not quite as uniform in size and shape as those of Gleason pattern 1. There may be minimal invasion by neoplastic glands into the surrounding non-neoplastic prostatic tissue. The glands are of intermediate size and larger than in Gleason pattern 3. The variation in glandular size and separation between glands is less than that seen in pattern 3. Although not eval-

uated in Gleason grading, the cytoplasm of Gleason pattern 1 and 2 cancers is abundant and pale-staining. Gleason pattern 2 is usually seen in transition zone cancers but may occasionally be found in the peripheral zone.

Gleason pattern 3
Gleason pattern 3 is the most common pattern. The glands are more infiltrative and the distance between them is more variable than in patterns 1 and 2. Malignant glands often infiltrate between adjacent non-neoplastic glands. The glands of pattern 3 vary in size and shape and are often angular. Small glands are typical for pattern 3, but there may also be large, irregular glands. Each gland has an open lumen and is circumscribed by stroma. Cribriform pattern 3 is rare and difficult to distinguish from cribriform high-grade PIN.

Gleason pattern 4
In Gleason pattern 4, the glands appear fused, cribriform or they may be poorly defined. Fused glands are composed of a group of glands that are no longer completely separated by stroma. The edge of a group of fused glands is scalloped and there are occasional thin strands of connective tissue within this group. Cribriform pattern 4 glands are large or they may be irregular with jagged edges. As opposed to fused glands, there are no strands of stroma within a cribriform gland. Most cribriform invasive cancers should be assigned a pattern 4 rather than pattern 3. Poorly defined glands do not have a lumen that is completely encircled by epithelium.

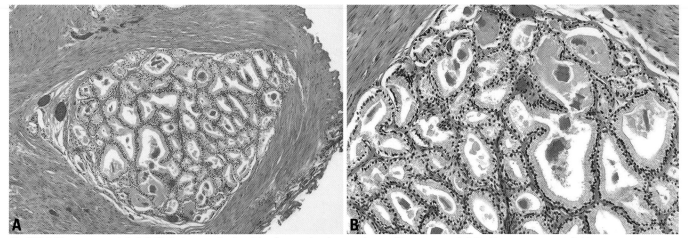

Fig. 3.37 A Gleason score 1+1=2. **B** Well-circumscribed nodule of prostatic adenocarcinoma, Gleason score 1+1=2 with numerous crystalloids.

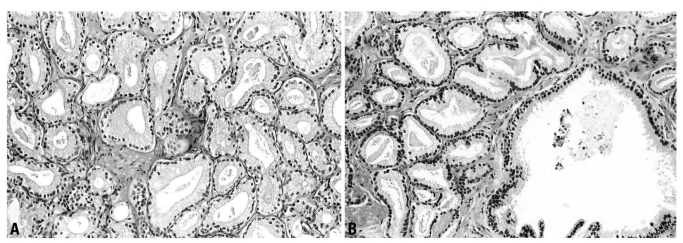

Fig. 3.38 A Prostate cancer Gleason pattern 2. **B** Prostate cancer Gleason pattern 2.

The hypernephromatoid pattern described by Gleason is a rare variant of fused glands with clear or very pale-staining cytoplasm.

Gleason pattern 5
In Gleason pattern 5, there is an almost complete loss of glandular lumina. Only occasional lumina may be seen. The epithelium forms solid sheets, solid strands or single cells invading the stroma. Care must be applied when assigning a Gleason pattern 4 or 5 to limited cancer on needle biopsy to exclude an artefact of tangential sectioning of lower grade cancer. Comedonecrosis may be present.

Grade progression
The frequency and rate of grade progression is unknown. Tumour grade is on average higher in larger tumours {1688}. However, this may be due to more rapid growth of high grade cancers. It has

been demonstated that some tumours are high grade when they are small {707}. Many studies addressing the issue of grade progression have a selection bias, because the patients have undergone a repeat transurethral resection or repeat biopsy due to symptoms of tumour progression {526}. The observed grade progression may be explained by a growth advantage of a tumour clone of higher grade that was present from the beginning but undersampled. In patients followed expectantly there is no evidence of grade progression within 1-2 years {717}.

Grading minimal cancer on biopsy. It is recommended that a Gleason score be reported even when a minimal focus of cancer is present. The correlation between biopsy and prostatectomy Gleason score is equivalent or only marginally worse with minimal cancer on

biopsy {668,2257,2498}. It is recommended that even in small cancers with one Gleason pattern that the Gleason score be reported. If only the pattern is reported, the clinician may misconstrue this as the Gleason score.

Tertiary Gleason patterns
The original Gleason grading system does not account for patterns occupying less than 5% of the tumour or for tertiary patterns. In radical prostatectomy specimens, the presence of a tertiary high grade component adversely affects prognosis. However, the prognosis is not necessarily equated to the addition of the primary Gleason pattern and the tertiary highest Gleason pattern. For example, the presence of a tertiary Gleason pattern 5 in a Gleason score 4+3=7 tumour worsens the prognosis compared to the same tumour without a tertiary high grade component. However, it is not

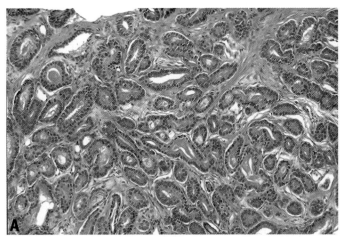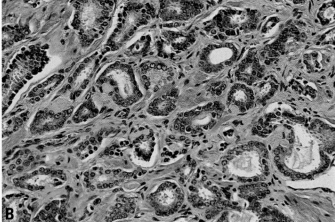

Fig. 3.39 A Gleason score 3+3=6. **B** Gleason pattern 3 with small glands.

associated with as adverse prognosis as a Gleason score 4+5=9 {2005}. When this tertiary pattern is pattern 4 or 5, it should be reported in addition to the Gleason score, even when it is less than 5% of the tumour.

Although comparable data do not currently exist for needle biopsy material, in the setting of three grades on biopsy where the highest grade is the least common, the highest grade is incorporated as the secondary pattern. An alternative option is in the situation with a tertiary high grade pattern (i.e. 3+4+5 or 4+3+5) is to diagnose the case as Gleason score

8 with patterns 3, 4 and 5 also present. The assumption is that a small focus of high grade cancer on biopsy will correlate with a significant amount of high grade cancer in the prostate such that the case overall should be considered high grade, and that sampling artefact accounts for its limited nature on biopsy.

Reporting Gleason scores in cases with multiple positive biopsies
In cases where different positive cores have divergent Gleason scores, it is controversial whether to assign an averaged (composite) Gleason score or whether the highest Gleason score should be considered as the patient's grade {1407}. In practice, most clinicians take the highest Gleason score when planning treatment options.

Grading of variants of prostate cancer
Several morphological variants of prostate adenocarcinoma have been described (e.g. mucinous and ductal cancer). They are almost always combined with conven-

tional prostate cancer and their effect on prognosis is difficult to estimate. In cases with a minor component of a prostate cancer variant, Gleason grading should be based on the conventional prostate cancer present in the specimen. In the rare case where the variant form represents the major component, it is controversial whether to assign a Gleason grade.

Grading of specimens with artefacts and treatment effect
Crush artefacts. Crush artefacts are common at the margins of prostatectomy specimens and in core biopsies. Crush artefacts cause disruption of the glandular units and consequently may lead to overgrading of prostate cancer. These artefacts are recognized by the presence of noncohesive epithelial cells with fragmented cytoplasm and dark, pyknotic nuclei adjacent to preserved cells. Crushed areas should not be Gleason graded.
Hormonal and radiation treatment. Prostate cancer showing either hormonal or radiation effects can appear artefactu-

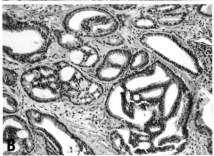

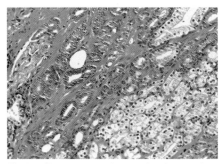

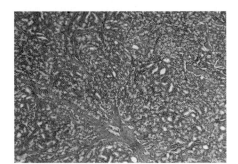

Fig. 3.40 A Cribriform Gleason score 3+3=6. **B** Prostate cancer Gleason pattern 3 of cribriform type.

Fig. 3.41 Gleason pattern 3 prostatic adenocarcinoma with amphophilic to cleared cytoplasm.

Fig. 3.42 Gleason score 4+4=8.

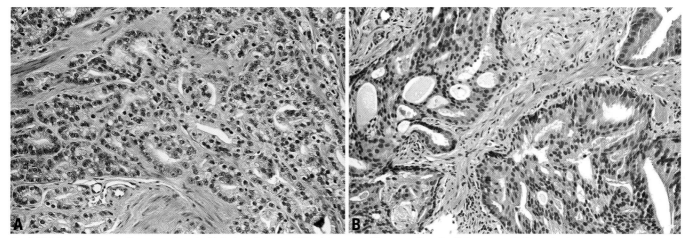

Fig. 3.43 A Prostate cancer Gleason pattern 4 with fusion of glands. **B** Prostate cancer Gleason pattern 4 with irregular cribriform glands.

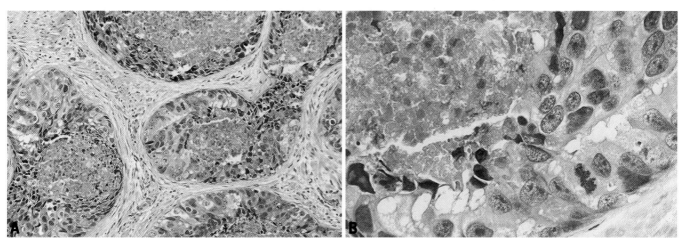

Fig. 3.44 A Gleason score 5+5=10 with comedonecrosis. **B** Gleason score 5+5=10 with comedonecrosis.

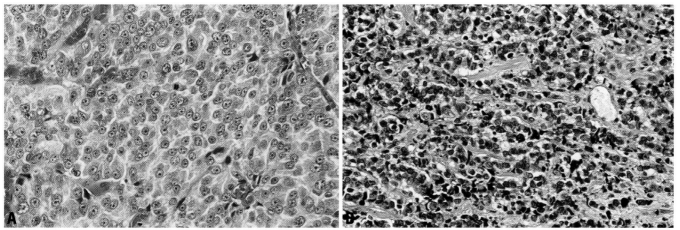

Fig. 3.45 A Gleason score 5+5=10. **B** Gleason pattern 5 with solid strands.

ally to be of higher Gleason score. Consequently, Gleason grading of these cancers should not be performed. If there is cancer that does not show treatment effect, a Gleason score can be assigned to these components.

Correlation of needle biopsy and prostatectomy grade.
Prostate cancer displays a remarkable degree of intratumoural grade heterogeneity. Over 50% of total prostatectomy specimens contain cancer of at least three different Gleason grades {41}, and cancer of a single grade is present in only 16% of the specimens {2261}. Of individual tumour foci, 58% have a single grade, but most of these foci are very small {2261}. Several studies have compared biopsy

and prostatectomy Gleason score {375,668,2498}. Exact correlation has been observed in 28.2-67.9% of the cases. The biopsies undergraded in 24.5-60.0% and overgraded in 5.2-32.2%. Causes for biopsy grading discrepencies are undersampling of higher or lower grades, tumours borderline between two grade patterns, and misinterpretation of patterns {2498}. The concordance between biopsy and prostatectomy Gleason score is within one Gleason score in more than 90% of cases {668}.

Reproducibility
Pathologists tend to undergrade {665,2498}. The vast majority of tumours graded as Gleason score 2 to 4 on core biopsy are graded as Gleason score 5 to 6 or higher when reviewed by experts in urological pathology {2498}. In a recent study of interobserver reproducibility amongst general pathologists, the overall agreement for Gleason score groups 2-4, 5-6, 7, and 8-10 was just into the moderate range {67}. Undergrading is decreased with teaching efforts and a substantial interobserver reproducibility can be obtained {665,1400}.

Prognosis
Multiple studies have confirmed that Gleason score is a very powerful prognostic factor on all prostatic samples. This includes the prediction of the natural history of prostate cancer {54,667} and the assessment of the risk of recurrence after total prostatectomy {713,1144} or radiotherapy {937}. Several schedules for grouping of Gleason scores in prognostic categories have been proposed.

Gleason scores 2 to 4 behave similarly and may be grouped. Likewise, Gleason scores 8 to 10 are usually grouped together, although they could be stratified with regard to disease progression in a large prostatectomy study {1446}. There is evidence that Gleason score 7 is a distinct entity with prognosis intermediate between that of Gleason scores 5-6 and 8 to 10, respectively {667,2590}. Although the presence and amount of high grade cancer (patterns 4 to 5) correlates with tumour prognosis, reporting the percentage pattern 4/5 is not routine clinical practice {666,2479}. Gleason score 7 cancers with a primary pattern 4 have worse prognosis than those with a primary pattern 3 {406,1447,2282}.

Genetics
In developed countries, prostate cancer is the most commonly diagnosed non-skin malignancy in males. It is estimated that 1 in 9 males will be diagnosed with prostate cancer during their lifetime. Multiple factors contribute to the high incidence and prevalence of prostate cancer. Risk factors include age, family history, and race. Environmental exposures are clearly involved as well. Although the exact exposures that increase prostate cancer risk are unclear, diet (especially those high in animal fat such as red meat, as well as, those with low levels of antioxidants such as selenium and vitamin E) job/industrial chemicals, sexually transmitted infections, and chronic prostatitis have been implicated to varying degrees. The marked increase in incidence in prostate cancer that occurred in the mid 1980s, which subsequently leveled off in the

mid to late 1990s, indicates that wide spread awareness and serum prostate specific antigen screening can produce a transient marked increase in prostate cancer incidence.

Hereditary prostate cancer
Currently the evidence for a strong genetic component is compelling. Observations made in the 1950s by Morganti and colleagues suggested a strong familial predisposition for prostate cancer {1784}. Strengthening the genetic evidence is a high frequency for prostate cancer in monozygotic as compared to dizygotic twins in a study of twins from Sweden, Denmark, and Finland {1496}. Work over the past decade using genome wide scans in prostate cancer families has identified high risk alleles, displaying either an autosomal dominant or X-linked mode of inheritance for a hereditary prostate cancer gene, from at least 7 candidate genetic loci. Of these loci, three candidate genes have been identified *HPC2/ELAC2* on 17p {2584}, RNASEL on 1q25 {377}, and MSR1 on 8p22-23 {2857}. These 3 genes do not account for the majority of hereditary prostate cancer cases. In addition, more than 10 other loci have been implicated by at least some groups. The discovery of highly penetrant prostate cancer genes has been particularly difficult for at least 2 main reasons. First, due to the advanced age of onset (median 60 years), identification of more than two generations to perform molecular studies on is difficult. Second, given the high frequency of prostate cancer, it is likely that cases considered to be hereditary during segregation studies actually repre-

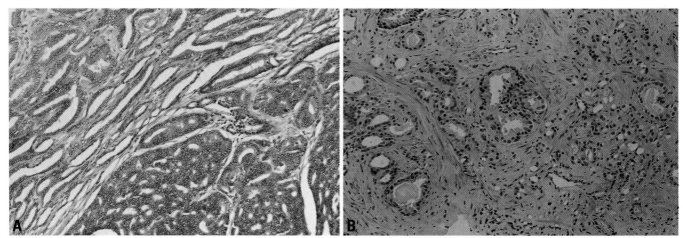

Fig. 3.46 A Gleason score 3+4=7. **B** Gleason score 3+4=7.

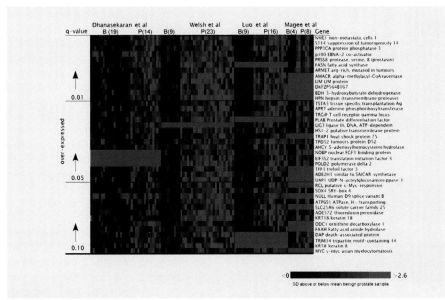

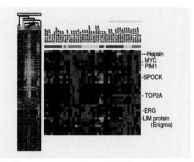

Fig. 3.48 Heat map-nature. From S.M. Dhanasekaran et al. {604}.

Fig. 3.47 Meta-analysis heat map. From D.R. Rhodes et al. {2183a}.

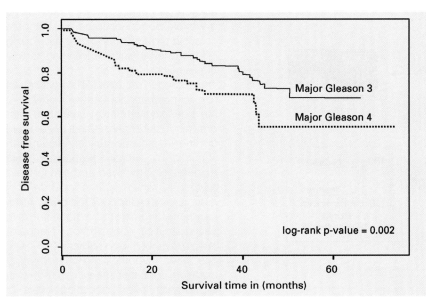

Fig. 3.49 Gleason score 7 tumours comprise a large percentage of prostate cancer in the radical prostatectomy specimens, and constitute an intermediate category in terms of prognosis between Gleason scores of ≤6 and those of ≥8. Within the score 7 tumours, the proportion of Gleason pattern 4 carcinoma is important, i.e. (4+3) are more aggressive than (3+4) tumours.

Molecular alterations in sporadic prostate cancer

While mutations in any of the classic oncogenes and tumour suppressor genes are not found in high frequency in primary prostate cancers, a large number of studies have identified non-random somatic genome alterations. Using comparative genomic hybridization (CGH) to screen the DNA of prostate cancer, the most common chromosomal alterations in prostate cancer are losses at 1p, 6q, 8p, 10q, 13q, 16q, and 18q and gains at 1q, 2p, 7, 8q, 18q, and Xq {436,1246,1924,2737}. Numerous genes have now been implicated in prostate cancer progression. Several genes have been implicated in the earliest development of prostate cancer. The pi-class of Glutathione S-transferase (GST), which plays a caretaker role by normally preventing stress related damage, demonstrates hypermethylation in high percentage of prostate cancers, thus preventing expression of this protective gene {1465, 1505,1732}. NKX3.1, a homeobox gene located at 8p21 has also been implicated in prostate cancer {304,1047,1319, 2741}. Although no mutations have been identified in this gene {2741}, recent work suggests that decreased expression is associated with prostate caner progression {304}. PTEN encodes a phosphatase, active against both proteins and lipids, is also commonly altered in prostate cancer progression {1491, 2489}. PTEN is believed to regulate the phosphatidylinositol 3'-kinase/protein kinase B (PI3/Akt) signaling pathway and therefore mutations or alterations lead to tumour progression {2850}. Mutations are less common than initially thought in prostate cancer, however, tumour suppressor activity may occur from the loss of one allele, leading to decreased expres-

sent phenocopies; currently it is not possible to distinguish sporadic (phenocopies) from hereditary cases in families with high rates of prostate cancer. In addition, hereditary prostate cancer does not occur in any of the known cancer syndromes and does not have any clinical (other than a somewhat early age of onset at times) or pathologic characteristics to allow researchers to distinguish it from sporadic cases {302}.

Perhaps even more important in terms of inherited susceptibility for prostate can-

cer are common polymorphisms in a number of low penetrance alleles of other genes - the so-called genetic modifier alleles. The list of these variants is long, but the major pathways currently under examination include those involved in androgen action, DNA repair, carcinogen metabolism, and inflammation pathways {2246,2858}. It is widely assumed that the specific combinations of these variants, in the proper environmental setting, can profoundly affect the risk of developing prostate cancer.

Table 3.01
Prostate cancer susceptibility loci identified by linkage analysis

Susceptibility loci	Locus	Mode	Putative gene	Reference
HPC1	1q24-25	AD	RNASEL	{377,2451}
PCAP	1q42.2-43	AD	?	{230}
CAPB	1p36	AD	?	{871}
HPCX	Xq27-28	X-linked/AR	?	{2855}
HPC20	20q13	AD	?	{229}
HPC2	17p	AD	HPC2/ELAC2	{2584}
	8p22-23	AD	MSR1	{2857}

Key: Mode=suggested mode of inheritance; AD=autosomal dominant; AR=autosomal recessive.

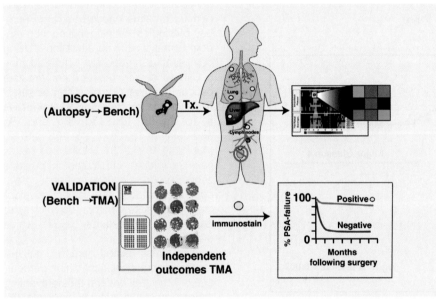

Fig. 3.50 Paradigm for gene discovery.

sion of PTEN (i.e. haploinsufficiency) {1418}. A number of other genes have also been associated with prostate cancer including p27 {496, 975,2867} and E-cadherin {1989,2674}. p53 mutations are late events in prostate cancer and tend to occur in advanced and metastatic prostate tumours {1052}.

Another very common somatic genomic alteration in prostate and other cancers is telomere shortening {1697,2461}. This molecular alteration is gaining heightened awareness as it has become clear that critically short telomere may lead to genetic instability and increased epithelial cancers in p53+/- mice {121,250}.

Recent advances in genomic and proteomic technologies suggest that molecular signatures of disease can be used for diagnosis {33,907}, to predict survival {2238,2551}, and to define novel molecular subtypes of disease {2056}. Several studies have used cDNA microarrays to characterize the gene expression profiles of prostate cancer in comparison with benign prostate disease and normal prostate tissue {604, 1574,1576,1591, 2426,2807}. Several interesting candidates include AMACR, hepsin, KLF6 and EZH2. Alpha-methylacyl-CoA racemase (AMACR), an enzyme that plays an important role in bile acid biosynthesis and β-oxidation of branched-chain fatty acids {748,1366} was determined to be upregulated in prostate cancer {604,1220, 1574,1575,2259,2807}. AMACR protein expression was also determined to be upregulated in prostate cancer {604,1220, 1575,2259}. Hepsin is overexpressed in localized and metastatic prostate cancer when compared to benign prostate or benign prostatic hyperplasia {604,1574, 1591,2481}. By immunohistochemistry, hepsin was found to be highly expressed in prostatic intraepithelial neoplasia (PIN), suggesting that dysregulation of hepsin is an early event in the development of prostate cancer {604}. Kruppel-like factor 6 (KLF6) is a zinc finger is mutated in a subset of human prostate cancer {1870}. EZH2, a member of the polycomb gene family, is a transcriptional repressor known to be active early in embryogenesis {796, 1601}, showing decreased expression as cells differentiate. It has been demonstrated that EZH2 is highly over expressed in metastatic hormone refractory prostate cancer as determined by cDNA and TMA analysis {2711}. EZH2 was also seen to be overexpressed in localized prostate cancers that have a higher risk of developing biochemical recurrence following radical prostatectomy.

The androgen receptor (AR) plays critical role in prostate development {2877}. It has been know for many years that withdrawal of androgens leads to a rapid decline in prostate cancer growth with significant clinical response. This response is short-lived and tumour cells reemerge, which are independent of androgen stimulation (androgen independent). Numerous mutations have been identified in the androgen receptor gene (reviewed by Gelmann {847}). It has been hypothesized that through mutation, prostate cancers can grow with significantly lower levels of androgens. In addition to common mutations, the amino-terminal domain encoded by exon one demonstrates a high percentage of polymorphic CAG repeats {2638}. Shorter CAG repeat lengths have been associated with a greater risk of developing prostate cancer and prostate cancer progression {884, 2337}. Shorter CAG repeat lengths have been identified in African American men {208}.

Prognosis and predictive factors
The College of American Pathologists (CAP) have classified prognostic factors into three categories:
Category I – Factors proven to be of prognostic importance and useful in clinical patient management.

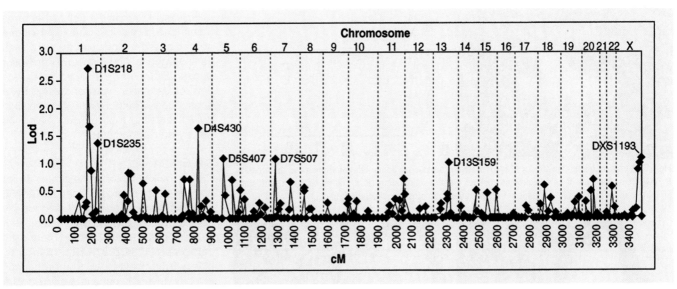

Fig. 3.51 Prostate cancer. Major susceptibility locus for prostate cancer on chromosome 1 suggested by a genome-wide search. 91 families from Sweden and NA (10cM). Reprinted with permission from J.R. Smith et al. {2451}. Copyright 1996 American Association for the Advancement of Science.

Category II – Factors that have been extensively studied biologically and clinically, but whose importance remains to be validated in statistically robust studies.

Category III – All other factors not sufficiently studied to demonstrate their prognostic value.

Factors included in category I, were pre-operative PSA, histologic grade (Gleason score), TNM stage grouping, and surgical margin status. Category II included tumour volume, histologic type and DNA ploidy. Factors in Category III included such things as perineural invasion, neuroendorcrine differentiation,

Table 3.02
Selected genes associated with prostate cancer progression.

Abbreviation	Gene Name(s)	Locus	Functional Role	Molecular Alteration
GST-pi	Glutathione S-transferase pi	11q13	Caretaker gene	Hypermethlyation
NKX3.1	NK3 transcription factor homolog A	8p21	Homeobox gene	No mutations
PTEN	Phosphatase and tensin homolog (mutated in multiple advanced cancers 1)	10q23.3	Tumour supressor gene	Mutations and haplotype insufficiency insufficiency
AMACR	Alpha-methylacyl-CoA racemase	5p13.2-q11.1	B-oxidation of branched-chain fatty acids	Overexpressed in PIN/Pca
Hepsin	Hepsin	19q11-q13.2	Transmembrane protease, serine 1	Overexpressed in PIN/Pca
KLF-6	Kruppel-like factor 6/COPEB	10p15	Zinc finger transcription factor	Mutations and haplotype insufficiency
EZH2	Enhancer of zeste homolog 2	7q35	Transcriptional memory	Overexpressed in aggressive Pca
p27	Cyclin-dependent kinase inhibitor 1B (p27, Kip1)	12p13	Cyclin dependent kinases 2 and 4 inhibitor	Down regulated with Pca progression
E-cadherin	E-cadherin	16q22.1	Cell adhesion molecule	Down regulated with Pca progression

Key: Pca=prostate cancer; PIN=prostatic intraepithelial neoplasia

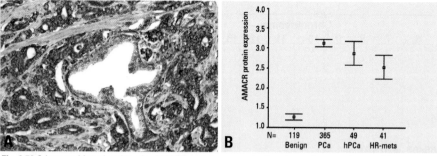

Fig. 3.52 A Immunohistochemistry for AMACR protein expression in acinar adenocarcinoma of the prostate. **B** AMACR expression in benign prostate tissue, prostate carcinoma (PCa), hormone naive metastatic prostate cancer (hPCa), and hormone refractory metastatic prostate cancer (HR-mets).

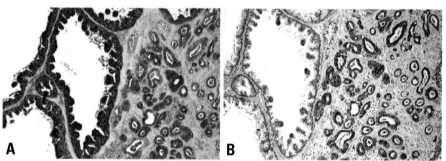

Fig. 3.53 PSA (**A**) vs AMACR (**B**) expression in an adenocarcinoma (acinar) of the prostate. PSA is expressed in all epithelial cells of prostate origin (**A**) in contrast to AMACR, which is strongly expressed in the prostate cancer but not the benign epithelial cells.

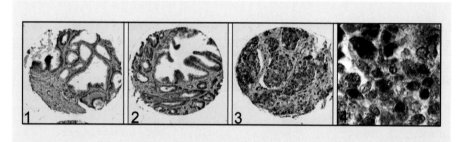

Fig. 3.54 Expression of the Polycomb Group Protien EZH2 in prostate cancer. EZH2 demonstrates negative to weak staining in benign prostate tissue (1). Moderate EZH2 expression is seen in a subset of clinically localized PCa (2). Strong nuclear EZH2 expression is seen in the majority of hormone refractory metastatic prostate cancers (3,4).

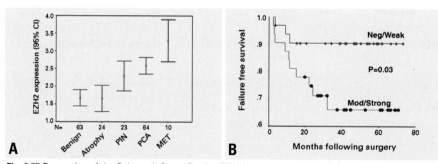

Fig. 3.55 Expression of the Polycomb Group Protien EZH2 in prostate cancer. **A** Summary of EZH2 protein expression for benign prostate tissue (benign), atrophic, high-grade prostatic intraepitheial neoplasia (PIN), localized prostate cancer (PCA), and hormone refractory prostate cancer (MET). **B** EZH2 overexpression as determined by immunohistochemistry is significantly associated with PSA-failure following radical prostatectomy for clinically localized prostate cancer.

microvessel density, nuclear features other than ploidy, proliferation markers and a variety of molecular markers such as oncogenes and tumour suppressor genes {290}.

This classification was endorsed by a subsequent World Health Organization (WHO) meeting that focused mainly on biopsy-derived factors.

Serum PSA
PSA is the key factor in the screening for and detection of prostate cancer {2448}, its serum level at the time of diagnosis is considered a prognostic marker that stratifies patients into differing prognostic categories {1284,2023}. Recent reports, however indicate that the prognostic value is driven by patients with high PSA levels, which is significantly associated with increasing tumour volume and a poorer prognosis {2478}. In recent years however, most newly diagnosed patients have only modestly elevated PSA (between 2 and 9 ng/ml), a range in which BPH and other benign conditions could be the cause of the PSA elevation. For patients within this category, it was reported that PSA has no meaningful relationship to cancer volume and grade in the radical prostatectomy specimen, and a limited relationship with PSA cure rates {2478}. Following treatment, serum PSA is the major mean of monitoring patients for tumour recurrence.

Stages T1a and T1b
Although the risk of progression at 4 years with stage T1a cancer is low (2%), between 16% and 25% of men with untreated stage T1a prostate cancer and longer (8-10 years) follow-up have had clinically evident progression {651}. Stage T1b tumours are more heterogeneous in grade, location, and volume than are stage T2 carcinomas. Stage T1b cancers tend to be lower grade and located within the transition zone as compared with palpable cancers. The relation between tumour volume and pathologic stage also differs, in that centrally located transition zone carcinomas may grow to a large volume before reaching the edge of the gland and extending out of the prostate, whereas stage T2 tumours that begin peripherally show extraprostatic extension at relatively lower volumes {461,940,1685}. This poor correlation between volume and stage is also attributable to the lower

grade in many stage T1b cancers.

Stage T2

Most of the pathological prognostic information obtained relating to clinical stage T2 disease comes from data obtained from analysis of radical prostatectomy specimens.

Pathologic examination of the radical prostatecomy specimen

The key objectives of evaluating the RP specimens are to establish tumour pathologic stage and Gleason score. It is important to paint the entire external surface of the prostate with indelible ink prior to sectioning. In most centers, the apical and bladder neck margins are removed and submitted either as shave margins *en face* [with any tumour in this section considered a positive surgical margin (+SM)], or preferably, these margins (especially the apical) are removed as specimens of varying width, sectioned parallel to the urethra, and submitted to examine the margins in the perpendicular plane to the ink. In this method, any tumour on ink is considered to be a +SM.

The extent of sampling the radical prostatectomy specimen varies, only 12% of pathologists responding to a recent survey indicated that they processed the entire prostate {705,2283, 2645}. It was reported that a mean of 26 tissue blocks was required to submit the entire prostate and the lower portion of the seminal vesicles, {1661}. Cost and time considerations result in many centers using variable partial sampling schemes that may sacrifice sensitivity for detecting positive surgical margins (+SM) or extraprostatic extension (EPE) {2354}.

Histologic grade (Gleason)

Gleason score on the radical prostatectomy specimen is one of the most powerful predictors of progression following surgery. Gleason score on the needle biopsy also strongly correlates with prognosis following radiation therapy.

Extraprostatic extension (EPE)

This is defined as invasion of prostate cancer into adjacent periprostatic tissues. The prostate gland has no true capsule although posterolaterally, there is a layer which is more fibrous than muscular that serves as a reasonable area to denote the boundary of the prostate

{143}. At the apex and everywhere anteriorly in the gland (the latter being the fibromuscular stroma), there is no clear demarcation between the prostate and the surrounding structures. These attributes make determining EPE for tumours of primarily apical or anterior distribution difficult to establish.

EPE is diagnosed based on tumour extending beyond the outer condensed smooth muscle of the prostate. When tumour extends beyond the prostate it often elicits a desmoplastic stromal reaction, such that one will not always see tumour with EPE situated in extra-prostatic adipose tissue. It has been reported that determining the extent of EPE as "focal" (only a few glands outside the prostate) and "established or non focal" (anything more than focal) is of prognostic significance {713,714}. Focal EPE is often a difficult diagnosis Modifications to this approach with emphasis on the "level" of prostate cancer distribution relevant to benign prostatic acini and within the fibrous "capsule" where it exists, has been suggested and claimed to have further value in classifying patients into prognostic categories following radical prostatectomy {2812}. More detailed analysis has not been uniformly endorsed {705}.

Seminal vesicle invasion (SVI)

Seminal vesicle invasion is defined as cancer invading into the muscular coat of the seminal vesicle {712,1944}. SVI has been shown in numerous studies to be a significant prognostic indicator {393,536,579,2589}. Three mechanisms by which prostate cancer invades the seminal vesicles were described by Ohori et al. as: (I) by extension up the ejaculatory duct complex; (II) by spread across the base of the prostate without other evidence of EPE (IIa) or by invading the seminal vesicles from the periprostatic and periseminal vesicle adipose tissue (Ib); and (III) as an isolated tumour deposit without continuity with the primary prostate cancer tumour focus. While in almost all cases, seminal vesicle invasion occurs in glands with EPE, the latter cannot be documented in a minority of these cases. Many of these patients had only minimal involvement of the seminal vesicles, or involve only the portion of the seminal vesicles that is at least partially intraprostatic. Patients in this category were reported to have a

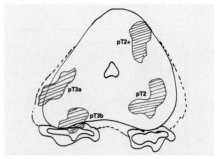

Fig. 3.56 Diagram depicting the pathologic stage categories of prostate cancer in the radical prostatectomy specimen:

pT2: Represents an organ confined tumour with no evidence of extension to inked surgical margins, extension into extraprostatic tissue or invasion of the seminal vesicles.

pT2+: Not an officially recognized category that describes an organ confined tumour with extension to inked surgical margins, but with no evidence of extension into extraprostatic tissue or invasion of the seminal vesicles. [It is important to emphasize that the status of the surgical margins while very important to document, is not a component of the TNM staging system per se as any one other pT stage categories can be associated with positive margin]

pT3a: Tumour that have extended beyond the prostate into the extraprostatic tissue. [It is preferable to specify whether the amount of tumour outside the prostate is "focal" or non focal or extensive].

pT3b: Tumour invasion of the muscularis of the seminal vesicle.

favourable prognosis, similar to otherwise similar patients without SVI and it is controversial whether SVI without EPE should be diagnosed {712}.

Lymph nodes metastases (+LN)

Pelvic lymph node metastases, when present, are associated with an almost uniformly poor prognosis in most studies. Fortunately, however, the frequency of +LN has decreased considerably over time to about 1-2% today {393,705}. Most of this decrease has resulted primarily from the widespread PSA testing and to a lesser extent from better ways to select patients for surgery preoperatively. As a consequence of this decline in patients with +LN, some have proposed that pelvic lymph node dissection is no longer necessary in appropriately selected patients {198,256}. The detection of +LN can be enhanced with special techniques such as immunohistochemistry or reverse transcriptase-polymerase chain reaction (RT-PCR) for PSA or hK2-L

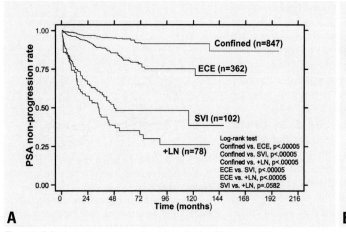 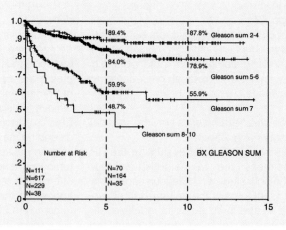

Fig. 3.57 A Pathological stage and survival. Kaplan Meir plot of the level of invasion vs progression. ECE = extracapsular extension, SVI = seminal vesicle involvement, +LN = positive for lymph node metastasis.. **B** Kaplan Meir plot of Gleason score vs recurrence.

{659}, although these tests are not used in routine clinical practice {1948}. Various prognostic parameters based on the assessment of tumour within the node have been reported. These include Gleason grade, number of positive nodes, tumour volume, tumour diameter, DNA ploidy, and perinodal tumour extension. In part because of conflicting studies, these nodal parameters are not routinely reported in clinical practice {859, 946,1477,2372,2500}. In a rare patient, a small lymph node is seen in the periprostatic soft tissue, and may be involved by metastatic prostate cancer, even in the absence of other pelvic lymph node metastases {1364}. These patients also have a poor prognosis.

Surgical margin status
Positive surgical margins (+SM) are generally considered to indicate that the cancer has not been completely excised and is an important prognostic parameter following surgery. Positive margins in a radical prostatectomy specimen may be classified as equivocal, focal, or extensive, with correspondingly worse prognosis {1661}. The site of the +SM is frequently at the same site as the area of EPE. However, a +SM may result from incision into an otherwise confined focus of prostate cancer. A +SM without EPE at the site of the +SM is not infrequently seen, having been reported in from 9-62% of cases of +SM in the literature. The most common sites of intra-prostatic incision are at the apex and at the site of the neurovascular bundle posterolaterally. Stage designations to denote a +SM in the absence of EPE anywhere in the

gland include stage pT2X and stage pT2+, because extraprostatic tumour at the site of the +SM cannot be excluded. Most studies suggest a lower risk of progression in men with positive margins as a reflection of capsular incision, as opposed to +SM with EPE {170, 1945,2790}. However, in a series of 1273 patients treated with radical prostatectomy, +SM had an impact on PSA non-progression rate over the spectrum of pathologic stages, including pT2 (confined) cancer. PSA non-progression rate at 5 years for patients with EPE (pT3a) with positive +SM was 50%, compared to 80% of patients with EPE and –SM (p<0.0005). A microscopically positive margin at the bladder neck should not be considered as pT4 disease {553}.

Perineural Invasion
Perineural invasion (PNI) by prostate cancer is seen in radical prostatectomy specimens in 75-84% of cases. Due to the near ubiquitous presence of PNI in radical prostatectomy specimens and studies have not shown radical prostatectomy PNI to be an independent prognostic parameter, this finding is not routinely reported. One study has noted that the largest diameter of PNI in the radical prostatectomy was independently related to an increased likelihood of biochemical failure after radical prostatectomy; verification of this result is needed before it can be adopted in clinical practice {1641}. Numerous studies have also evaluated the significance of PNI on cancer in needle biopsy specimens. Whereas almost all reports have noted an increased risk of EPE in the corre-

sponding radical prostatectomy specimen, there are conflicting data as to whether PNI provides independent prognostication beyond that of needle biopsy grade and serum PSA levels {180, 663,715}. It has also been demonstrated that the presence of PNI on the needle biopsy is associated with a significantly higher incidence of disease progression following radiotherapy and following radical prostatectomy {270}. As PNI is of prognostic significance and easy to assess histologically, its reporting on needle biopsy is recommended.

Tumour volume
Tumour volume can be measured most accurately with computerized planimetric methods, although a far simpler "grid" method has been described {1147}. Total tumour volume is an important predictor of prognosis and is correlated with other pathologic features. However, in several large series it was not an independent predictor of PSA progression when controlling for the other features of pathologic stage, grade and margins. These results are different from earlier series, in which many of the patients were treated in the pre-PSA era and had large tumour volumes, which resulted in a strong correlation between tumour volume and prognosis.

Multiple techniques of quantifying the amount of cancer found on needle biopsy have been developed and studied, including measurement of the: 1) number of positive cores; 2) total millimeters of cancer amongst all cores; 3) percentage of each core occupied by cancer; 4) total percent of cancer in the entire specimen

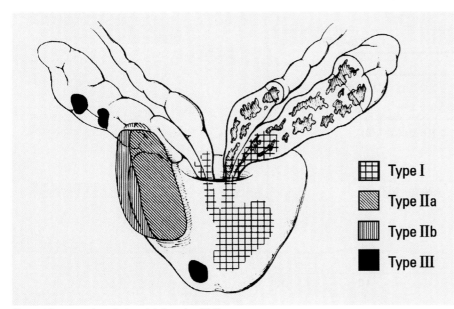

	Type I
	Type IIa
	Type IIb
	Type III

Fig. 3.58 Patterns of seminal vesicle invasion (SVI).

Lymphovascular invasion in radical prostatectomy (LVI)
The incidence rates of LVI have ranged widely from 14-53%. The differences in incidence rates amongst studies are most likely the result of the use of different criteria for the recognition of LVI. While most investigators do not recommend the use of immunohistochemistry for verification of an endothelial-lined space, retraction space artefact around tumour may cause difficulty in interpretation of LVI. Although several studies have found that LVI is important in univariate analysis, only two have reported independent significance in multivariate analysis {156,1081,2287}.

Biomarkers and nuclear morphometry (reviewed in {705,1773})
While the preponderance of studies suggest that DNA ploidy might be useful in clinical practice, a smaller number of studies analyzing large groups of patients have not found ploidy to be independently prognostically useful. A majority of studies have also demonstrated that overexpression of certain other markers (p53, BCL-2, p21^{WAF1}) and underexpression of others (Rb) is associated with more aggressive prostate cancer behaviour, but further corroboration is necessary before these tests are used

and 5) fraction of positive cores. There is no clear concensus as to superiority of one technique over the other.

Numerous studies show associations between the number of positive cores and various prognostic variables. The other widely used method of quantifying the amount of cancer on needle biopsy is measurement of the percentage of each biopsy core and/or of the total specimen involved by cancer. Extensive cancer on

needle biopsy in general predicts for adverse prognosis. However, limited carcinoma on needle biopsy is not as predictive of a favourable prognosis due to sampling limitations.

A feasible and rationale approach would be to have pathologists report the number of cores containing cancer, as well as one other system quantifying tumour extent (e.g. percentage, length).

Table 3.03
Location of positive surgical margins in radical prostatectomy specimens.

	Number of +SM	Apical	Anterior	Lateral	Posterior	Postero lateral	Bladder neck	Other
Voges et al. {2744,2745}	8	37	37	-	-	-	25	-
Rosen et al. {2231}	27	33	18	4	11	33	-	-
Epstein et al. {713}	190	22	-	-	17	14	6	-
Stamey et al. {2480}	32	69	-	-	-	6	-	
Van Poppel et al. {2699}	50	34	-	-	-	54	-	12
Watson et al. {2790}	90	38	11	-	26	17	9	-
Gomez et al. {909}	22	46	-	-	14	-	14	27

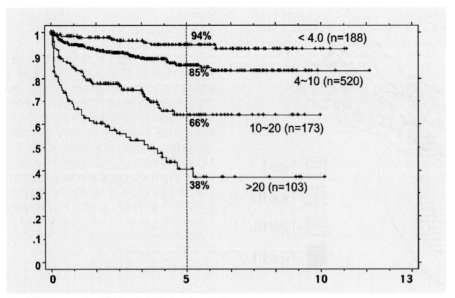

Fig. 3.59 Preoperative PSA levels (ng/ml) and prostatic cancer recurrence.

clinically. There are conflicting studies as to the prognostic significance of quantifying microvessel density counts, Ki-67 (proliferation), and chromogranin (neuroendocrine differentiation), p27[kip1], Her-2/neu, E-cadherin, and CD44. Numerous studies have correlated various nuclear measurements with progression following radical prostatectomy. These techniques have not become clinically accepted in the evaluation of prostate cancer since the majority of studies have come from only a few institutions, some of these nuclear morphometry measurements are patented and under control of private companies, and these techniques are time consuming to perform.

Preoperative and postoperative nomograms

Although there are nomograms to predict for stage prior to therapy {1284,2023}, this and other prognostic factors are best assessed, following pathologic examination of the radical prostatectomy specimen, many of which have been incorporated in a new postoperative nomogram {1284}. The prognostic factors have appreciable limitations when they are used as stand-alone. However, validation

of the several nomograms proposed in the recent times is sometimes lacking whereas comparison for superiority amongst the proposed nomograms has not always been tested. A limitation of these nomograms is that they do not provide predictive information for the individual patient.

Stages T3 and T4

In general, patients with clinical stage T3 prostate cancer are not candidates for radical prostatectomy and are usually treated with radiotherapy. Between 50% and 60% of clinical stage T3 prostate cancers have lymph node metastases at the time of diagnosis. More than 50% of patients with clinical stage T3 disease develop metastases in 5 years, and 75% of these patients die of prostate carcinoma within 10 years.

Distant metastases appear within 5 years in more than 85% of patients with lymph node metastases who receive no further treatment. In patients with distant metastases, the mortality is approximately 15% at 3 years, 80% at 5 years, and 90% at 10 years. Of the patients who relapse after hormone therapy, most die within several years.

Prostatic intraepithelial neoplasia

W.A. Sakr
R. Montironi
J.I. Epstein
M.A. Rubin

A.M. De Marzo
P.A. Humphrey
B. Helpap

Definition

Prostatic intraepithelial neoplasia (PIN) is best characterized as a neoplastic transformation of the lining epithelium of prostatic ducts and acini. By definition, this process is confined within the epithelium therefore, intraepithelial.

ICD-O code   8148/2

Epidemiology

There is limited literature characterizing the epidemiology of high grade prostatic intraepithelial neoplasia (HGPIN) as the lesion has been well defined relatively recently with respect to diagnostic criteria and terminology. Based on few recent autopsy studies that included HGPIN in their analysis, it appears that similar to prostate cancer, HGPIN can be detected microscopically in young males, its prevalence increases with age and HGPIN shows strong association with cancer in terms of coincidence in the same gland and in its spatial distribution {1683,1993}. In a contemporary autopsy series of 652 prostates with high proportion of young men, Sakr et al. identified HGPIN in 7, 26, 46, 72, 75 and 91% of African Americans between the third and eighth decades compared to: 8, 23, 29, 49, 53 and 67% for Caucasian men {2278}. In addition to higher the prevalence, this study also suggested a more extensive HGPIN in younger African American men compared to Caucasians {2279}. In an autopsy series of 180 African and White-Brazilian men older than 40, more extensive and diffuse HGPIN in African Brazilians tended to appear at a younger age compared to Whites {244}.

Prevalence of HGPIN in surgical prostate samples

Biopsy specimens

There are significant variations in the reported prevalence of HGPIN in needle biopsies of the prostate. This is likely to result from several reasons:
– Population studied (ethnicity, extent of screening/early detection activities).
– Observers variability as there is an inherent degree of subjectivity in applying diagnostic criteria and in setting the threshold for establishing diagnosis.
– The technical quality of the material evaluated (fixation, section thickness and staining quality).
– The extent of sampling (i.e., number of core biopsies obtained).

The majority of large recent series, have reported a prevalence of 4-6% {296, 1133,1435,1926,2830}. The European and the Japanese literature indicate a slightly lower prevalence of HGPIN on needle biopsies {58,572,594,1913,2046, 2434}.

TURP specimens

The incidence of HGPIN in transurethral resection of the prostate is relatively uncommon with two studies reporting a rate of 2.3% and 2.8%, respectively {845,1996}.

HGPIN in radical prostatectomy/ cystoprostatectomy specimens

The prevalence of HGPIN in radical prostatectomy specimens is remarkably high reflecting the strong association between the lesion and prostate cancer. Investigators have found HGPIN in 85-100% of radical prostatectomy specimens {568,2122,2125,2824}.

In a series of 100 cystoprostatectomy specimens, Troncoso et al. found 49% and 61% of the prostates to harbour HGPIN and carcinoma, respectively {2644}. In 48 men who underwent cystoprostatectomy for reasons other than prostate cancer, Wiley et al. {2046} found 83% and 46% of the prostates to contain HGPIN and incidental carcinoma, respectively. More extensive HGPIN predicted significantly for the presence of prostate cancer in this study {2824}.

Morphological relationship of HGPIN to prostate carcinoma

The associations of HGPIN and prostate cancer are several {1776}:
– The incidence and extent of both lesions increase with patient age {2280}.
– There is an increased frequency, severity and extent of HGPIN in prostate with cancer {1683,1993,2122,2279,2644}.
– Both HGPIN and cancer are multifocal with a predominant peripheral zone distribution {2122}.
– Histological transition from HGPIN to cancer has been described {1687}.
– High-grade PIN shares molecular

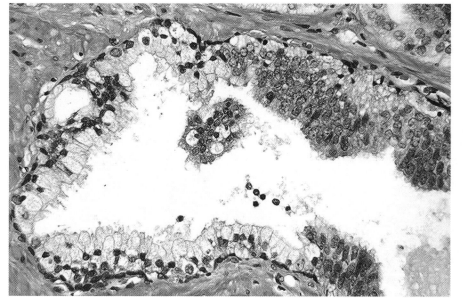

Fig. 3.60 Focal high grade PIN (upper and lower right) in otherwise normal prostatic gland.

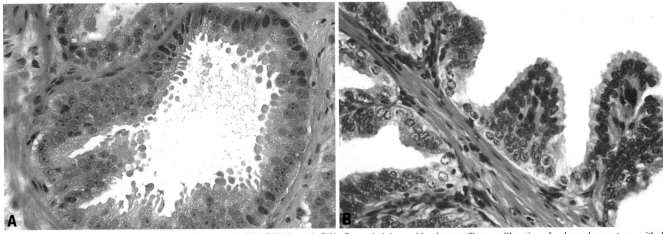

Fig. 3.61 A Flat and tufting pattern of growth of high grade PIN. **B** High grade PIN. Expanded duct with micropapillary proliferation of enlarged secretory epithelial cells with high nuclear cytoplasmic ratio and enlarged nucleoli.

genetics features with cancer {2121}. HGPIN is more strongly associated with intermediate-high grade prostatic carcinoma {708,721,995,1777,2007,2122, 2281}.

There is limited data addressing the relationship between the presence and extent of HGPIN in the prostate and the pathologic stage of prostate cancer. It has been reported that the total volume of HGPIN increases with increasing pathologic stage with a significant correlation between volume of HGPIN and the number of lymph node metastases {2122}.

Molecular genetic associations of HGPIN and prostate cancer

There is extensive literature indicating that HGPIN demonstrates a range of genetic abnormalities and biomarker

expression profile that is more closely related to prostate cancer than to benign prostatic epithelium. These studies investigated aspects ranging from cell proliferation and death, histomorphometric analysis and a host of genetic alterations, inactivation of tumour suppressor genes or overexpression of oncogenes {721,1777,2007,2121,2281}.

Clinical features

HGPIN does not result in any abnormalities on digital rectal examination. HGPIN may appear indistinguishable from cancer, manifesting as a hypoechoic lesion on transrectal ultrasound examination {1012}. HGPIN by itself does not appear to elevate serum PSA levels {57,2144, 2227}.

Histopathology

Initially, PIN was divided into three grades based on architectural and cytologic features recognizing that the changes cover a continuum. Subsequently, it has been recommended that the classification should be simplified into a two-tier system: low (previous grade I) and high (previous grades II and III) grade lesions {638}. The distinction between low and high grade PIN is based on the degree of architectural complexity and more importantly, on the extent of cytologic abnormalities. In *low grade PIN*, there is proliferation and "piling up" of secretory cells of the lining epithelium with irregular spacing. Some nuclei have small, usually inconspicuous nucleoli while a few may contain more prominent nucleoli. The basal cell layer

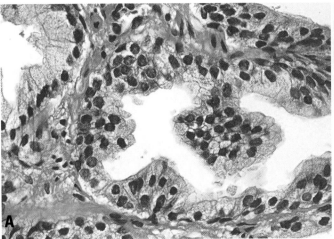
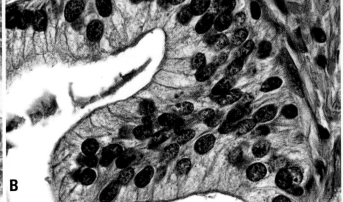

Fig. 3.62 A Low grade PIN. **B** Low grade PIN. Higher magnification.

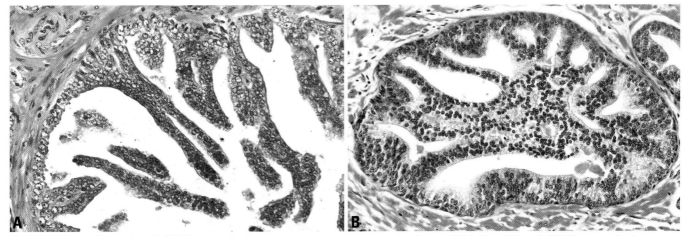

Fig. 3.63 A Micropapillary high grade PIN. Note more benign appearing cytology towards center of gland. **B** Cribriform high grade PIN. Note more benign appearing cytology towards center of gland.

normally rimming ducts and acini is intact in low grade PIN. It is difficult to reproducibly distinguish low grade PIN from normal and hyperplastic epithelium {709}. *High grade PIN* is characterized by a more uniform morphologic alteration. Cytologically, the acini and ducts are lined by malignant cells with a variety of architectural complexity and patterns. The individual cells are almost uniformly enlarged with increased nuclear/cytoplasmic ratio, therefore showing less variation in nuclear size than that seen in low grade PIN. Many cells of HGPIN contain prominent nucleoli and most show coarse clumping of the chromatin that is often present along the nuclear membrane. HGPIN can be readily appreciated at low power microscopic examination by virtue of the darker "blue" staining of the lining that reflects the expanded nuclear chromatin area {294}.

Architectural patterns of HGPIN

Four patterns of HGPIN have been described, which are flat, tufting, micropapillary, and cribrifrom: nuclear atypia without significant architectural changes (*flat pattern*); nuclei become more piled up, resulting in undulating mounds of cells (*tufting pattern*); columns of atypical epithelium that typically lack fibrovascular cores (*micropapillary pattern*); more complex architectural patterns appear such as Roman bridge and cribriform formation (*cribriform pattern*). The distinction between cribriform high grade PIN and ductal carcinoma in-situ is controversial (see duct carcinoma in-situ) {288}. In high grade PIN, nuclei towards the centre of the gland tend to have blander cytology, as compared to peripherally located nuclei. The grade of PIN is assigned based on assessment of the nuclei located up against the basement membrane.

Histologic variants

Signet-ring variant. High grade prostatic intraepithelial neoplasia (PIN) with signet-ring cells is exceedingly rare with only three reported cases {2181}. In all cases signet-ring cell PIN was admixed with adjacent, invasive signet-ring carcinoma. Histologically, cytoplasmic vacuoles displace and indent PIN cell nuclei. The vacuoles are mucin-negative by histochemical staining (mucicarmine, Alcian blue, PAS).

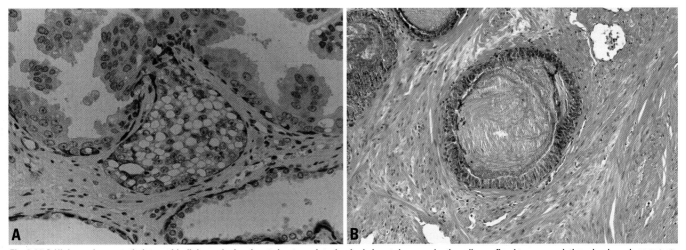

Fig. 3.64 A High-grade prostatic intraepithelial neoplasia, signet ring type. Intraluminal signet ring neoplastic cells confined to a pre-existing gland, as demonstrated by positive basal cell staining (34BE12 immunostain). **B** High-grade prostatic intraepithelial neoplasia, of mucinous type, with a flat pattern of growth. Note intraluminal filling of the gland by blue mucin.

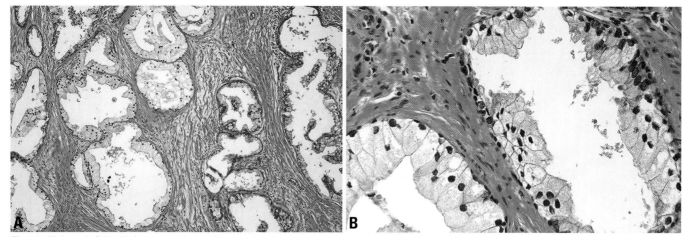

Fig. 3.65 High grade PIN with foamy cytoplasmic features. **A** Tufted growth pattern. **B** Higher magnification demonstrates foamy cytoplasmic features.

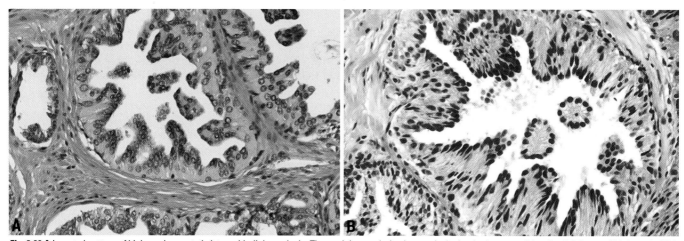

Fig. 3.66 A Inverted pattern of high grade prostatic intraepithelial neoplasia. The nuclei are polarized towards the luminal aspect of the gland. **B** Inverted high grade PIN.

Mucinous variant. Mucinous high grade PIN exhibits solid intraluminal masses of blue tinged mucin that fill and distend the PIN glands, resulting in a flat pattern of growth. This is a rare pattern, with five reported cases. It is associated with adjacent, invasive, typical acinar adenocarcinoma (of Gleason score 5-7), but not mucinous adenocarcinoma {2181}.

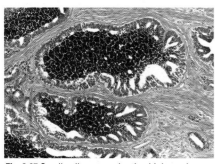

Fig. 3.67 Small cell neuroendocrine high-grade prostatic intraepithelial neoplasia.

Foamy variant. Two cases of foamy gland high-grade PIN have been published {223}. Microscopically, foamy PIN glands are large, with papillary infoldings lined by cells with bland nuclei and xanthomatous cytoplasm. In one case there was extensive associated Gleason grade 3+3=6 acinar adenocarcinoma, but no associated invasive foamy gland adenocarcinoma.

Inverted variant. The inverted, or hobnail, variant is typified by polarization of enlarged secretory cell nuclei toward the glandular lumen of high-grade PIN glands with tufted or micropapillary architectural patterns. The frequency was estimated to be less than 1% of all PIN cases. In six of 15 reported needle biopsy cases, there was associated usual, small acinar Gleason score 6-7 adenocarcinoma {111}.

Small cell neuroendocrine variant. Extremely rare examples with small cell neuroendocrine cells exist {2181,2474}. Small neoplastic cells, with rosette-like formations, are observed in the centre of glands, which display peripheral, glandular-type PIN cells. In one case there was admixed, invasive mixed small cell-adenocarcinoma. The small neoplastic cells are chromogranin and synaptophysin-positive, and harbour dense-core, membrane-bound, neurosecretory granules at the ultrastructural level.

Intraductal carcinoma is controversial as it has overlapping features with cribriform high grade PIN and can not be separated from intraductal spread of adenocarcinoma of the prostate {479,1689, 2256}. All three entities consist of neoplastic cells spanning prostatic glands, which are surrounded by basal cells. The most salient morphologic feature distin-

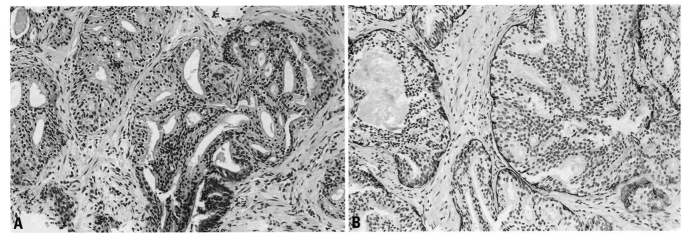

Fig. 3.68 A Ductal carcinoma in-situ with typical cribriform pattern on growth. **B** Ductal carcinoma in-situ with necrosis demonstrating retention of basal cell layer as revealed by high molecular weight cytokeratin staining.

guishing "intraductal carcinoma" from high-grade cribriform PIN is the presence of multiple cribriform glands with prominent cytological atypia containing comedo necrosis. In practice, this distinction rarely poses a problem in the evaluation of a prostatectomy specimen as invasive cancer is always concurrently present. In prostate needle biopsies and TURP, this process may rarely be present without small glands of adenocarcinoma, where some experts consider it prudent to refer to the lesion as high grade cribriform PIN {2256,2823} with a strong recommendation for repeat biopsy. Other experts will use the term "intraductal carcinoma" on biopsy with the recognition that definitive therapy may be undertaken, recognizing that infiltrating cancer will be identified upon further prostatic sampling {719}.

Somatic genetics
Germ-line heritable alterations
There is no evidence that the frequency or extent of high grade PIN is increased in patients with familial prostate cancer {181}.

Somatic genomic alterations
Genetic changes tend to be very similar to the chromosomal aberrations identified in prostatic adenocarcinoma {204,1214,1588,2120}. Frequent changes in PIN include both increases and decreases in chromosome 8 centromeric region, often with simultaneous loss of regions from 8p and gains of 8q. Other fairly common numeric changes include gains of chromosomes 10, 7, 12, and Y. Other regions of loss in both prostate cancer and PIN include chro-

mosomes 10q, 16q and 18q. The overall incidence of any aneuploidy in high grade PIN using FISH is approximately 50-70%, which is usually found to be similar to, or somewhat lower than, invasive carcinoma, and usually lower than metastatic disease. While carcinoma foci generally contain more anomalies than paired PIN foci, at times there are foci of PIN with more anomalies than nearby carcinoma {2120}. Loss of regions of chromosome 8p, have been reported to be very common in high grade PIN {694}, as is known for prostate cancer {276}.

While many of the acquired chromosome aberrations in PIN do not appear random, high grade PIN shares with invasive cancer some degree of chromosomal instability, as evidenced by telomere shortening {204,1696,1698}. Telomerase activity has been reported to occur in 16% of high grade PIN lesions {1344} and 85% of invasive prostatic carcinomas {2461} and may serve as an important biomarker in prostate carcinogenesis.

Specific genes involved in the pathogenesis of PIN
There is decreased protein expression in HGPIN of NKX3.1 and p27, paralleling that seen in carcinoma {17,237,304,569, 752,1520,2333}. *TP53* mutations and protein overexpression may be identified in at least some PIN lesions {48,2873}. *C-MYC* may be over-represented at times and PSCA is overexpressed in some lesions at the mRNA level {2165}. GSTP1 is hypermethylated in approximately 70% of HGPIN lesions {325}. GSTP1, which is known to inactivate carcino-

gens, gives rise to prostate cells with an increased burden of DNA adducts and hence mutations {1879}. Fatty acid synthetase (FAS), inhibitors of which may be selectively toxic to prostate cancer cells, has been seen to be consistently overexpressed in prostate cancer and high grade PIN {2401,2546}. The BCL-2 protein is present in at least a subset of high grade PIN lesions {271}. Many other genes have been shown to be overexpressed in PIN as compared to normal epithelium {295}. AMACR is also increased in at least a subset of high grade PIN lesions {604,1220,1574-1576,2259,2856}.

Prognosis and predictive factors
Needle biopsy
High-grade PIN in needle biopsy tissue is, in most studies, a risk factor for the subsequent detection of carcinoma, while low-grade PIN is not. The mean incidence of carcinoma detection on re-biopsy after a diagnosis of high-grade PIN in needle biopsy tissue is about 30% {559,1398,1926}. In comparison, the re-biopsy cancer detection frequency is about 20% after a diagnosis of benign prostatic tissue {715,1293}, and 16% after a diagnosis of low-grade PIN. The large majority (80-90%) of cases of carcinoma are detected on the first re-biopsy after a high-grade PIN diagnosis {1398}. Re-biopsy may also detect persistent high-grade PIN in 5-43% of cases {559, 1398,1399,1926}.

High-grade PIN with adjacent atypical glands seems to confer a higher risk for subsequent diagnosis of carcinoma compared to high-grade PIN alone, averaging 53% {70,1399,1926}. Due to the magnitude of the risk, all men with this finding should undergo re-biopsy {1399}. It is not settled whether serum PSA and digital rectal examination findings provide further information beyond PIN presence on risk for subsequent detection of carcinoma {995,1398,2010}. There are inconsistent data as to whether the extent of HGPIN and its architectural pattern predict risk of subsequent carcinoma {559,1294,1398}. Genetic abnormali-

Table 3.04
Risk of subsequent carcinoma detection after re-biopsy.

Needle biopsy diagnosis	Percentage of patients with carcinoma on re-biopsy
Benign prostatic tissue	20%
High grade PIN	30%
PINATYP[2]	53%

[1] PIN: prostatic intraepithelial neoplasia.
[2] PINATYP: high grade PIN with adjacent small atypical glands.

ties and/or immunophenotype of high-grade PIN are not currently utilized to stratify risk for subsequent detection of carcinoma.

Current standards of care recommend that patients with isolated high-grade PIN be re-biopsied in 0-6 months, irrespective of the serum PSA level and DRE findings. However, this recommendation may change with emerging data indicating a lower risk of prostate carcinoma following a needle biopsy showing HGPIN. The re-biopsy technique should entail at least systematic sextant re-biopsy of the entire gland {277,1435,2386}, since high-grade PIN is a general risk factor for carcinoma throughout the gland. For example, in one study fully 35% of carcinomas would have been missed if only the side with the high-grade PIN had been re-biopsied {2386}. Radical prostatectomy specimens removed for carcinoma detected after a diagnosis of high-grade PIN contain mostly organ-confined cancer, with a mean Gleason score of 6 (range 5-7) {1294}.

Treatment is currently not indicated after a needle biopsy diagnosis of high-grade PIN {994}. Patients with isolated high-grade PIN in needle biopsy may be considered for enrollment into clinical trials

with chemoprevention agents {1929, 2278}.

TURP

Several studies have found that high grade PIN on TURP places an individual at higher risk for the subsequent detection of cancer {845,1996}, whereas a long-term study from Norway demonstrated no association between the presence of high grade PIN on TURP and the incidence of subsequent cancer {1034}. In a younger man with high grade PIN on TURP, it may be recommended that needle biopsies be performed to rule out a peripheral zone cancer. In an older man without elevated serum PSA levels, clinical follow-up is probably sufficient. When high grade PIN is found on TURP, some pathologists recommend sectioning deeper into the corresponding block and most pathologists recommend processing the entire specimen {1996}.

Ductal adenocarcinoma

X.J. Yang
L. Cheng
B. Helpap
H. Samaratunga

Definition
Subtype of adenocarcinoma composed of large glands lined by tall pseudostratified columnar cells.

ICD-O code   8500/3

Synonyms
Several terms used in the past are no longer appropriate. *Endometrial carcinoma* was originally used to describe this entity because of its morphologic similarity to endometrium. This tumour was previously believed to be derived from a Müllerian structure named prostatic utricle {1706,1707}. However, subsequent studies on favourable response to orchiectomy, ultrastructural studies, histochemistry and immunohistochemistry have proven the prostatic origin of this tumour {1990,2205,2888,2919}. Therefore, the term *endometrial* or *endometrioid* carcinoma should not be used. *Prostatic duct carcinoma* should be used with caution, because it could also refer to urothelial carcinoma involving prostatic ducts.

Epidemiology
In pure form, ductal adenocarcinoma accounts for 0.2-0.8% of prostate cancers {292,718,938}. More commonly it is seen with an acinar component.

Etiology
No specific etiologic factors have been defined for this particular type.

Localization
Ductal adenocarcinoma may be located centrally around the prostatic urethra or more frequently located peripherally admixed with typical acinar adenocarcinoma. Both centrally and peripherally located ductal adenocarcinoma components can be present in the same prostate. A centrally located adenocarcinoma may also be associated with a peripherally located acinar adenocarcinoma.

Clinical features
Signs and symptoms
Periurethral or centrally located ductal adenocarcinoma may cause haematuria, urinary urgency and eventually urinary retention. In these cases, there may be no abnormalities on rectal examination. Tumours arising peripherally may lead to enlargement or induration of the prostate. Although ductal adenocarcinoma strongly expresses prostate specific antigen (PSA) immunohistochemically, they are associated with variable serum PSA levels {323}.

Methods of diagnosis
Serum PSA levels may be normal particularly in a patient with only centrally located tumour. In most cases, transurethral resections performed for diagnosis or relief of the urinary obstruction will provide sufficient diagnostic tis-

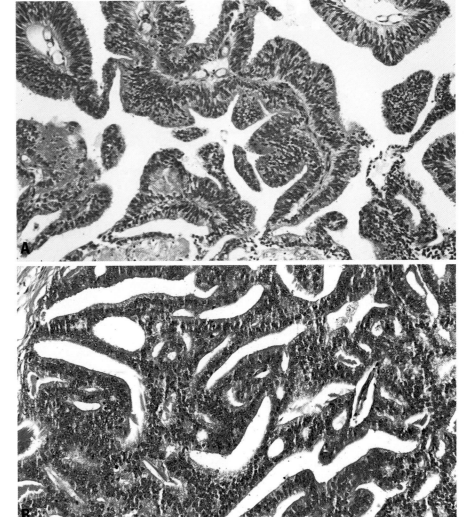

Fig. 3.69 Ductal adenocarcinoma of the prostate. **A** Papillary type of growth. **B** Cribriform pattern.

sue. Transrectal needle core biopsies may also obtain diagnostic tissue when the tumour is more peripherally located {323}. In addition, areas of ductal adenocarcinoma may be incidentally identified in prostatectomy specimens.

Macroscopy/Urethroscopy

Centrally occurring tumours appear as exophytic polypoid or papillary masses protruding into the urethra around the verumontanum. Peripherally occurring tumours typically show a white-grey firm appearance similar to acinar adenocarcinoma.

Tumour spread and staging

Ductal adenocarcinoma usually spread along the urethra or into the prostatic ducts with or without stromal invasion. Other patterns of spread are similar to that of acinar prostatic adenocarcinoma with invasion to extraprostatic tissues and metastasis to pelvic lymph nodes or distal organs. However, ductal adenocarcinomas appear to have a tendency to metastasize to lung and penis {491, 2654}. The metastasis of ductal adenocarcinoma may show pure ductal, acinar or mixed components.

Histopathology

Ductal adenocarcinoma is characterized by tall columnar cells with abundant usually amphophilic cytoplasm, which form a single or pseudostratified layer reminiscent of endometrial carcinoma. The cytoplasm of ductal adenocarcinoma is often amphophilic and may occasionally appear clear. In some cases, there are numerous mitoses and marked cytological atypia. In other cases, the cytological atypia is minimal, which makes a diagnosis difficult particularly on needle biopsy. Peripherally located tumours are often admixed with cribriform, glandular or solid patterns as seen in acinar adenocarcinoma. Although ductal adenocarcinomas are not typically graded, they are mostly equivalent to Gleason patterns 4. In some cases comedo necrosis is present whereby they could be considered equivalent to Gleason pattern 5. In contrast to ordinary acinar adenocarcinoma, some ductal adenocarcinomas are associated with a prominent fibrotic response often including haemosiderin-laden macrophages. Ductal adenocarcinoma displays a variety of architectural patterns, which are often intermingled {286,720}.

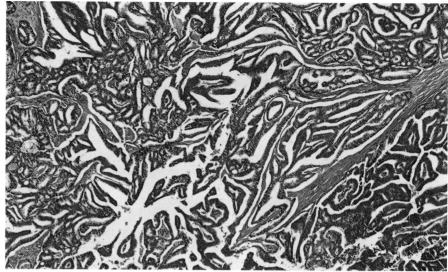

Fig. 3.70 Ductal adenocarcinoma. Infiltrating cribriform and pepillary growth pattern.

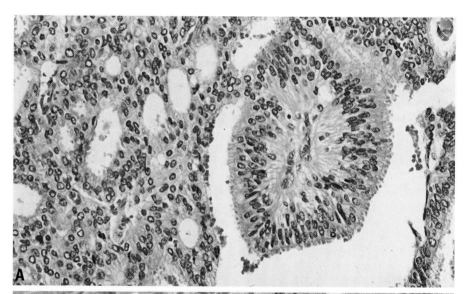

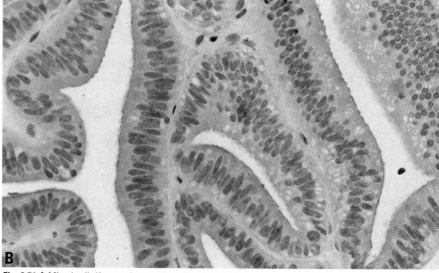

Fig. 3.71 A Mixed cribriform acinar and papillary ductal adenocarcinoma. **B** High magnification shows tall pseudostratified arrangement of nuclei diagnosed as ductal adenocarcinoma despite bland cytology.

Papillary pattern can be seen in both centrally or peripherally located tumours, yet is more common in the former.

Cribriform pattern is more commonly seen in peripherally located tumours, although they may be also present in centrally located tumours. The cribriform pattern is formed by back-to-back large glands with intraglandular bridging resulting in the formation of slit-like lumens.

Individual gland pattern is characterized by single glands.

Solid pattern can only be identified when it is associated with other patterns of ductal adenocarcinoma. The solid nests of tumour cells are separated by incomplete fibrovascular cores or thin septae.

Ductal adenocarcinoma must be distinguished from urothelial carcinoma, ectopic prostatic tissue, benign prostatic polyps, and proliferative papillary urethritis. One of the more difficult differential diagnoses is cribriform high grade prostatic intraepithelial neoplasia. Some patterns of ductal adenocarcinoma may represent *ductal carcinoma in situ*.

Immunoprofile

Immunohistochemically ductal adenocarcinoma is strongly positive for PSA and PAP. Tumour cells are typically negative for basal cell specific high molecular weight cytokeratin (detected by 34βE12), however, preexisting ducts may be positive for this marker.

Prognosis and predictive factors

Most studies have demonstrated that ductal adenocarcinoma is aggressive. Some reported that 25-40% of cases had metastases at the time of diagnosis with a poor 5-year survival rate ranging from 15-43% {462,718,2205}. It is not known whether prognosis correlates with the degree of cytological atypia or growth patterns. Even limited ductal adenocarcinoma on biopsy warrants definitive therapy. Androgen deprivation therapy may provide palliative relief, even though these cancers are less hormonally responsive than acinar adenocarcinoma.

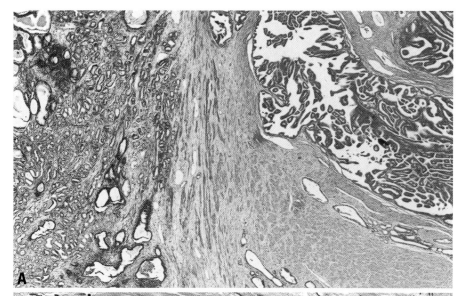

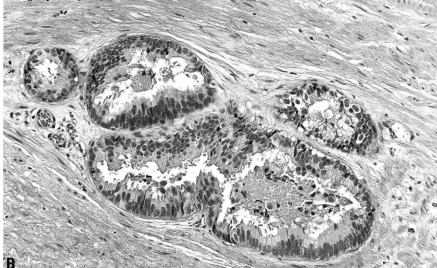

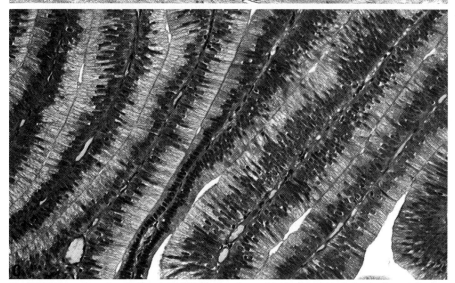

Fig. 3.72 A Separate acinar (left) and ductal adenocarcinoma (right). **B** Individual glands of prostatic duct adenocarcinoma, resembling colonic adenocarcinoma. **C** Ductal adenocarcinoma of the prostate showing close morphologic resemblance to endometrial carcinoma.

Urothelial carcinoma

D.J. Grignon

Definition
Urothelial carcinoma involving the prostate.

ICD-O code   8120/3

Epidemiology
The frequency of primary urothelial carcinoma ranges from 0.7-2.8% of prostatic tumours in adults {942,943}. Most patients are older with a similar age distribution to urothelial carcinoma of the bladder (range 45-90 years) {942,1231}. In patients with invasive bladder carcinoma, there is involvement of the prostate gland in up to 45% of cases {1596, 1907,2837}. This is highest when there is multifocality or carcinoma in situ associated with the invasive carcinoma {1907}.

Etiology
Primary urothelial carcinomas presumably arise from the urothelial lining of the prostatic urethra and the proximal portions of prostatic ducts. It has been postulated that this may arise through a hyperplasia to dysplasia sequence, possibly from reserve cells within the urothelium {696,1278,2673}. Secondary urothelial carcinoma of the prostate is usually accompanied by CIS of the prostatic urethra {2673}. Involvement of the prostate appears to be by direct extension from the overlying urethra, since in the majority of cases the more centrally located prostatic ducts are involved by urothelial neoplasia to a greater extent than the peripheral ducts and acini. Less commonly, deeply invasive urothelial carcinoma from the bladder directly invades the prostate.

Localization
Primary urothelial carcinoma is usually located within the proximal prostatic ducts. Many cases are locally advanced at diagnosis and extensively replace the prostate gland.

Clinical features
Signs and symptoms
Primary urothelial carcinoma presents in a similar fashion to other prostatic masses including urinary obstruction and haematuria {943,2159}. Digital rectal examination is abnormal in the majority but is infrequently the presenting sign {1951}. There is limited data on PSA levels in patients with urothelial carcinoma of the prostate. In one series 4 of 6 patients had elevated serum PSA (>4 ng/ml) in the absence of prostatic adenocarcinoma {1951}. In some cases patients present with signs and symptoms related to metastases {2159}.

Methods of diagnosis
Most cases are diagnosed by transurethral resection or less often needle biopsy {1951}. In all suspected cases the possibility of secondary involvement from a bladder primary must be excluded; the bladder tumour can be occult and random biopsies may be necessary to exclude this possibility {2313,2905}. Biopsies of the prostatic urethra and suburethral prostate tissue are often recommended as a staging procedure to detect secondary urothelial cancer involving the prostate of patients undergoing conservative treatment for superficial bladder tumours.

Tumour spread and staging
In situ carcinoma can spread along ducts and involve acini, or the tumour can spread along ejaculatory ducts and into seminal vesicles. Subsequent spread is by invasion of prostatic stroma. Local spread beyond the confines of the prostate may occur. Metastases are to regional lymph nodes and bone {2556}. Bone metastases are osteolytic. These tumours are staged as urethral tumours {944}. For tumours involving the prostatic ducts, there is a T1 category for invasion of subepithelial connective tissue distinct from invasion of prostatic stroma (T2). The prognostic importance of these categories has been confirmed in clinical studies {442}.

Histopathology
The full range of histologic types and grades of urothelial neoplasia can be

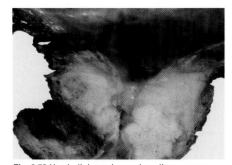
Fig. 3.73 Urothelial carcinoma invading prostate.

seen in primary and secondary urothelial neoplasms of the prostate {442}. A few examples of papillary urothelial neoplasms arising within prostatic ducts are described {1278}. The vast majority, however, are high-grade and are associated with an in situ component {442, 899,1893,1951,2445,2580}. The in situ component has the characteristic histologic features of urothelial carcinoma in situ elsewhere with marked nuclear pleomorphism, frequent mitoses and apoptotic bodies. A single cell pattern of pagetoid spread or burrowing of tumour cells between the basal cell and secretory cell layers of the prostate is characteristic. With extensive tumour involvement, urothelial carcinoma fills and expands ducts and often develops central comedonecrosis. Stromal invasion is associated with a prominent desmoplastic stromal response with tumour cells arranged in small irregular nests, cords and single cells. Inflammation in the adjacent stroma frequently accompanies in situ disease but without desmoplasia. With stromal invasive tumours, squamous or glandular differentiation can be seen. Angiolymphatic invasion is often identified. Incidental adenocarcinoma of the prostate is found in up to 40% of cystoprostatectomy specimens removed for urothelial carcinoma of the bladder and can accompany primary urothelial carcinoma {1772}.

In cases of direct invasion of the prostate from a poorly differentiated urothelial carcinoma of the bladder, a common prob-

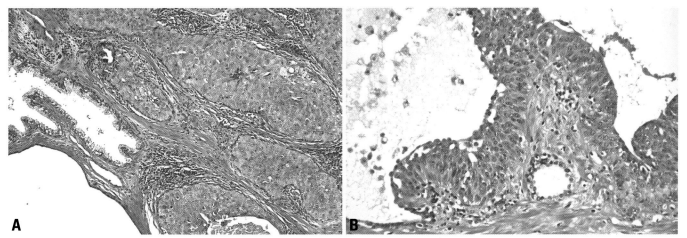

Fig. 3.74 A Inflammation without desmoplasia accompanying in situ carcinoma. **B** Pagetoid spread of tumour cells between the basal cell and secretory cell layers.

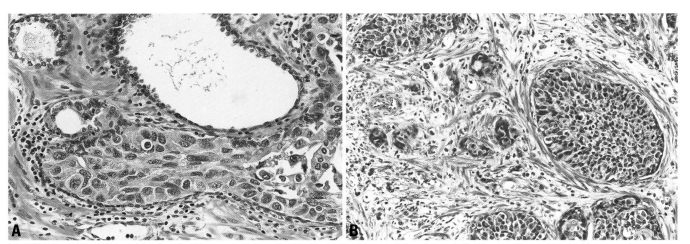

Fig. 3.75 A Urothelial carcinoma extensively involving prostatic ducts. **B** Infiltrating high grade urothelial carcinoma (left) with more pleomorphism than adenocarcinoma of the prostate.

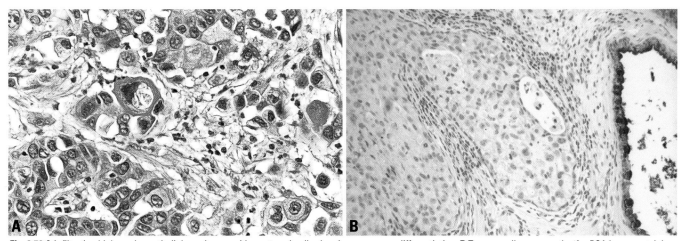

Fig. 3.76 A Infiltrating high grade urothelial carcinoma with scattered cells showing squamous differentiation. **B** Tumour cells are negative for PSA immunostaining, whereas the adjacent prostatic gland epithelium expresses PSA.

lem is its distinction from a poorly differentiated prostatic adenocarcinoma. Poorly differentiated urothelial carcinomas have greater pleomorphism and mitotic activity compared to poorly differentiated adenocarcinomas of the prostate. Urothelial carcinomas tend to have hard glassy eosinophilic cytoplasm or more prominent squamous differentiation, in contrast to the foamy, pale cytoplasm of prostate adenocarcinoma. Urothelial cancer tends to grow in nests,

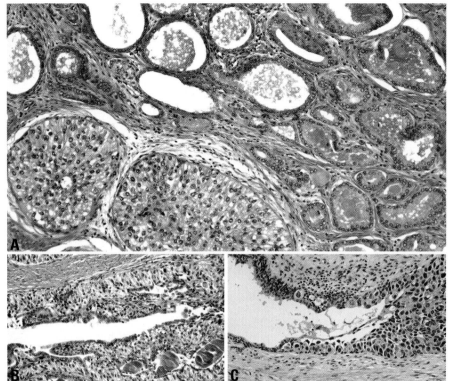

Fig. 3.77 A Urothelial carcinoma (lower left) and adenocarcinoma of the prostate (upper right). **B** Urothelial carcinoma in situ extending into large periurethral prostatic duct. **C** Urothelial carcinoma in situ with involvement of prostatic epithelium with undermining and pagetoid spread.

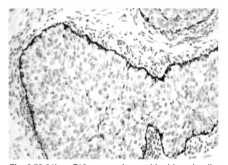

Fig. 3.78 34betaE12 expressing residual basal cells delineate in situ areas of urothelial carcinoma.

as opposed to cords of cells or focal cribriform glandular differentiation typical of prostatic adenocarcinoma.

Immunoprofile
The tumour cells are negative for PSA and PAP {440,1951}. Prostatic secretions in the ductal lumens can react positively resulting in faint staining of tumour cells at the luminal surface, a finding that should not be misinterpreted as positive staining. Tumour cells express CK7 and CK20 in the majority of cases and high molecular weight cytokeratin or P63 in about 50% of cases {1951}. Residual basal cells are frequent in the in situ areas {440}. Urothelial cancers may also express thrombomodulin and uroplakins, which are negative in prostate adenocarcinoma.

Prognosis and predictive factors
For patients with either primary or secondary urothelial carcinoma of the prostate the single most important prognostic parameter is the presence of prostatic stromal invasion. In one series, survival was 100% for patients with noninvasive disease treated by radical cystoprostatectomy {442}. With stromal invasion or extension beyond the confines of the prostate prognosis is poor {261,442,943,1437}. In one series, overall survival was 45% at 5 years in 19 patients with stromal invasion {442}. In 10 cases of primary urothelial carcinoma reported by Goebbels et al. mean survival was 28.8 months (range 1 to 93 months) {899}. However, even if only intraductal urothelial carcinoma is identified on TURP or transurethral biopsy in a patient followed for superficial bladder cancer, patients usually will be recommended for radical cystoprostatectomy as intravesical therapy is in general not thought to be effective in treating prostatic involvement.

Squamous neoplasms

T.H. Van der Kwast

Definition
Tumours with squamous cell differentiation involving the prostate.

ICD-O codes
Adenosquamous carcinoma   8560/3
Squamous cell carcinoma   8070/3

Epidemiology
The incidence of squamous cell carcinoma of the prostate is less than 0.6% of all prostate cancers {1814,1861}. There are 70 cases reported in literature. Even more rare is adenosquamous carcinoma of the prostate, with about 10 cases reported so far. For primary prostatic squamous cell carcinoma an association with Schistosomiasis infection has been described {44}. Approximately 50% of adenosquamous carcinomas may arise in prostate cancer patients subsequent to endocrine therapy or radiotherapy {179}.

Localization
Squamous cell carcinomas may originate either in the periurethral glands or in the prostatic glandular acini, probably from the lining basal cells, which show a divergent differentiation pathway {606,931}. Adenosquamous carcinomas are probably localized more commonly in the transition zone of the prostate accounting for their more frequent detection in transurethral resection specimens {179,2613}.

Clinical features
Most, if not all pure squamous cell carcinomas become clinically manifest by local symptoms such as urinary outflow obstruction, occasionally in association with bone pain and haematuria. Most patients have at the time of diagnosis metastatic disease, and bone metastases are osteolytic. PSA levels are not typically elevated. The age range of patients is between 52 and 79 years {1861}. Hormone treatment and chemotherapy are not effective, except for a single case with non-progressive disease after local irradiation and systemic chemotherapy {2657}. In cases of organ-confined disease, radical prostatectomy or cystoprostatectomy, including total urethrectomy is recommended {1513}.
Adenosquamous carcinomas may be detected by increased serum PSA, but more typically by obstruction of the urinary outflow, requiring transurethral resection {179}. Patients may also present with metastatic disease. A proportion of cases show an initial response to hormone therapy {32,1176}.

Tumour spread
Both squamous cell carcinomas and adenosquamous carcinomas tend to metastasize rapidly with a predilection for the skeletal bones {841,1861}.

Histopathology
By definition pure *squamous cell carcinoma* does not contain glandular features and it is identical to squamous cell carcinoma of other origin. With rare exception, it does not express PSA or PAP {1861,2657}. Primary prostatic squamous cell carcinoma must be distinguished on clinical grounds from secondary involvement of the gland by bladder or urethral squamous carcinoma. Histologically, squamous cell carcinoma must be distinguished from squamous metaplasia as may occur in infarction or after hormonal therapy.

Adenosquamous carcinoma is defined by the presence of both glandular (acinar) and squamous cell carcinoma components. Some authors considered the possibility that adenosquamous carcinomas consist of collision tumours with a de novo origin of adenocarcinoma and squamous cell carcinoma {841}. The glandular tumour component generally expresses PSA and PAP, whereas the squamous component displays high molecular weight cytokeratins {179}.

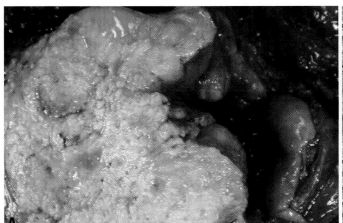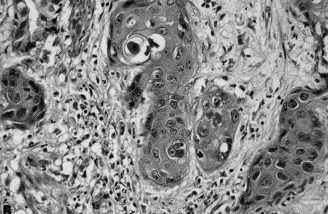

Fig. 3.79 A Cross section of squamous cell carcinoma. **B** Squamous cell carcinoma of the prostate with focal keratinization.

Basal cell carcinoma

P.H. Tan
A. Billis

Definition
This is a neoplasm composed of prostatic basal cells. It is believed that a subset of basal cells are prostatic epithelial stem cells, which can give rise to a spectrum of proliferative lesions ranging from basal cell hyperplasia to basal cell carcinoma {271,1139,2007,2410}.

ICD-O code   8147/3

Clinical features
Patients are generally elderly, presenting with urinary obstruction with TURP being the most common tissue source of diagnosis. The youngest reported case was 28 years old {597}.

Histopathology
Some tumours resemble its namesake in the skin, comprising large basaloid nests with peripheral palisading and necrosis. Other patterns have histologic similarity to florid basal cell hyperplasia or the adenoid basal cell pattern of basal cell hyperplasia (the latter pattern of cancer occasionally referred to as adenoid cystic carcinoma). Histologic criteria for malignancy that distinguish it from basal cell hyperplasia include an infiltrative pattern, extraprostatic extension, perineural invasion, necrosis and stromal desmoplasia.

Basal cell carcinoma shows immunoreactivity for keratin 34βE12, confirming its relationship with prostatic basal cells. S-100 staining is described as weak to intensely positive in about 50% of tumour cells {954,2893}, raising the possibility of myoepithelial differentiation; but there is no corroborative anti-smooth muscle actin (HHF35) reactivity {954} nor ultrastructural evidence of a myoepithelial nature {2893}. Distinction from basal cell hyperplasia with a pseudoinfiltrative pattern or prominent nucleoli can be difficult; basal cell carcinoma shows strong BCL2 positivity and high Ki-67 indices as compared to basal cell hyperplasia {2868}.

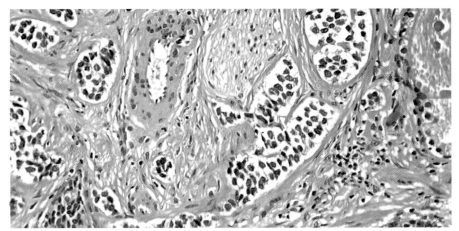

Fig. 3.80 Basal cell carcinoma resembling basal cell hyperplasia.

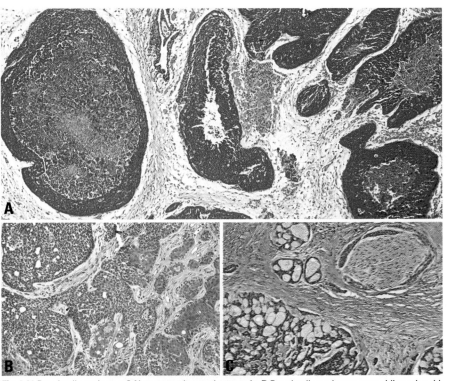

Fig. 3.81 Basal cell carcinoma **A** Note central comedonecrosis. **B** Basal cell carcinoma resembling adenoid cystic carcinoma. **C** Perineural invasion.

Prognosis
The biologic behaviour and treatment of basal cell carcinoma is not well elucidated in view of the few cases with mostly short follow-up. Local extra-prostatic extension may be seen, along with distant metastases {597,1160}. A benign morphologic counterpart to basal cell carcinoma (basal cell adenoma) has been proposed, although it should be considered as florid nodular basal cell hyperplasia.

Neuroendocrine tumours

P.A. di Sant'Agnese
L. Egevad
J.I. Epstein
B. Helpap
P.A. Humphrey

R.Montironi
M.A. Rubin
W.A. Sakr
P.H. Tan

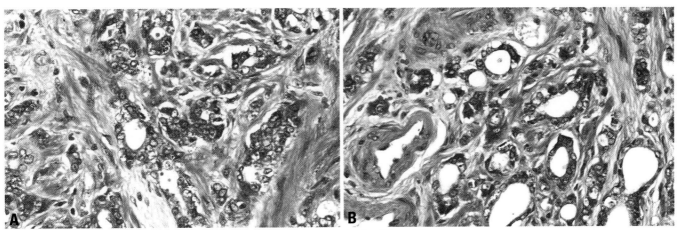

Fig. 3.82 A, B Adenocarcinoma with fine eosinophilic granules indicating neuroendocrine differentiation.

Definition

Neuroendocrine differentiation in prostatic carcinoma has three forms:
1. Focal neuroendocrine differentiation in conventional prostatic adenocarcinoma
2. Carcinoid tumour (WHO well differentiated neuroendocrine tumour) and
3. Small cell neuroendocrine carcinoma (new WHO classification poorly differentiated neuroendocrine carcinoma)

ICD-O codes

Focal neuroendocrine differentiation in prostatic adenocarcinoma 8574/3
Carcinoid 8240/3
Small cell carcinoma 8041/3

Focal neuroendocrine differentiation in prostatic adenocarcinoma

All prostate cancers show focal neuroendocrine differentiation, although the majority shows only rare or sparse single neuroendocrine cells as demonstrated by neuroendocrine markers. In 5-10% of prostatic carcinomas there are zones with a large number of single or clustered neuroendocrine cells detected by chromogranin A immunostaining {29,31,272, 609-611,1016,1064,1066}. A subset of these neuroendocrine cells may also be serotonin positive. Immunostaining for neuron-specific enolase, synaptophysin,

bombesin/gastrin-releasing peptide and a variety of other neuroendocrine peptides may also occur in individual neoplastic neuroendocrine cells, or in a more diffuse pattern {1178} and receptors for serotonin {16} and neuroendocrine peptides {1017,2537} may also be present. Vascular endothelial growth factor (VEGF) may also be expressed in foci of neuroendorine differentiation {1026}. The definitional context of these other neuroendocrine elements (other than chromogranin A and serotonin) remains to be elucidated. There are conflicting studies as to whether advanced androgen deprived and androgen independent carcinomas show increased neuroendocrine differentiation {446,1185,1222, 1395,1822,2582}.

The prognostic significance of focal neuroendocrine differentiation in primary untreated prostatic carcinoma is controversial with some showing an independent negative effect on prognosis {267,478,2802}, while others have not shown a prognostic relationship {30, 335,384,1915,2352,2465}. In advanced prostate cancer, especially androgen independent cancer, focal neuroendocrine differentiation portends a poor prognosis {446,1222,1395,2582} and may be a therapeutic target {228,2317, 2918}. Serum chromogranin A levels (and potentially other markers such as

pro-gastin-releasing peptide) {2537, 2582,2853,2802,2871} may be diagnostically and prognostically useful, particularly in PSA negative, androgen independent carcinomas {227,1183,1500, 2871,2918}.

Carcinoid tumours

True carcinoid tumours of the prostate, which meets the diagnostic criteria for carcinoid tumour elsewhere are exceedingly rare {609,2472,2583}. These tumours show classic cytologic features of carcinoid tumour and diffuse neuroendocrine differentiation (chromogranin A and synaptophysin immunoreativity). They should be essentially negative for PSA. The prognosis is uncertain due to the small number of reported cases. The

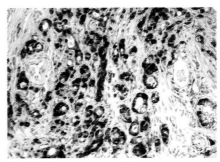

Fig. 3.83 Chromogranin positivity in adenocarcinoma with eosinophilic granules.

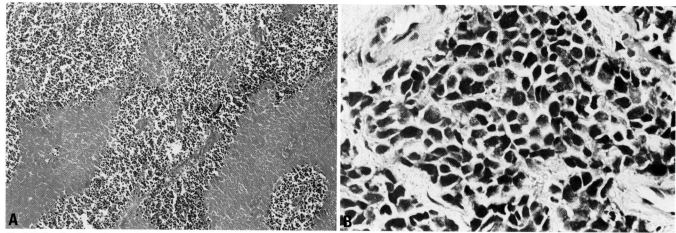

Fig. 3.84 Small cell carcinoma. **A** Note extensive necrosis. **B** Typical cytological appearance of small cell carcinoma.

term "carcinoid-like tumours" has been used to refer to a variety of miscellaneous entities, most of which refer to ordinary acinar adenocarcinoma of the prostate with an organoid appearance and focal neuroendorcrine immunoreactivity.

Small cell carcinoma

Clinical features

Many patients have a previous history of a hormonally treated acinar adenocarcinoma. As the small cell carcinoma component predominates, serum PSA level falls and may be undetectable. While most small cell carcinomas of the prostate lack clinically evident hormone production, they account for the majority of prostatic tumours with clinically evident ACTH or antidiuretic hormone production.

Histopathology

Small cell carcinomas of the prostate histologically are identical to small-cell carcinomas of the lung {2210,2600}. In approximately 50% of the cases, the tumours are mixed small cell carcinoma and adenocarcinoma of the prostate. Neurosecretory granules have been demonstrated within several prostatic small cell carcinomas. Using immunohistochemical techniques small cell components are negative for PSA and PAP. There are conflicting studies as to whether small cell carcinoma of the prostate is positive for thyroid transcription factor-1 (TTF-1), in order to distinguish them from a metastasis from the lung {37,1969}.

Prognosis

The average survival of patients with small cell carcinoma of the prostate is less than a year. There is no difference in prognosis between patients with pure small cell carcinoma and those with mixed glandular and small cell carcinoma. The appearance of a small cell component within the course of adenocarcinoma of the prostate usually indicates an aggressive terminal phase of the disease. In a review of the literature of genitourinary small cell carcinoma, whereas cisplatin chemotherapy was beneficial for bladder tumours, only surgery was prognostic for prostate small cell carcinomas {1587}. While this study concluded that hormonal manipulation and systemic chemotherapy had little effect on the natural history of disease in the prostate, the number of patients were small and others suggest to treat small cell carcinoma of the prostate with the same combination chemotherapy used to treat small cell carcinomas in other sites {75,2254}.

Mesenchymal tumours

J. Cheville   L. Cheng
F. Algaba   J.I. Epstein
L. Boccon-Gibod   M. Furusato
A. Billis   A. Lopez-Beltran

Definition

A variety of rare benign and malignant mesenchymal tumours that arise in the prostate {1063,1774}.

ICD-O codes

Stromal tumour of uncertain malignant potential	8935/1
Stromal sarcoma	8935/3
Leiomyosarcoma	8890/3
Rhabdomyosarcoma	8900/3
Malignant fibrous histiocytoma	8830/3
Osteosarcoma	9180/3
Chondrosarcoma	9220/3
Malignant peripheral nerve sheath tumour	9540/3
Synovial sarcoma	9040/3
Undifferentiated sarcoma	8805/3
Leiomyoma	8890/0
Granular cell tumour	9580/0
Fibroma	8810/0
Solitary fibrous tumour	8815/0
Haemangioma	9120/0
Chondroma	9220/0

Epidemiology

Sarcomas of the prostate account for 0.1-0.2% of all malignant prostatic tumours.

Tumours of specialized prostatic stroma

Sarcomas and related proliferative lesions of specialized prostatic stroma are rare. Lesions have been classified into *prostatic stromal proliferations of uncertain malignant potential (STUMP)* and *prostatic stromal sarcoma* based on the degree of stromal cellularity, presence of mitotic figures, necrosis, and stromal overgrowth {844}.

There are several different patterns of STUMP, including: those that resemble benign phyllodes tumour; hypercellular stroma with scattered atypical yet degenerative cells; and extensive overgrowth of hypercellular stroma with the histology of a stromal nodule. STUMPs are considered neoplastic, based on the observations that they may diffusely infiltrate the prostate gland and extend into adjacent tissues, and often recur. Although most cases of STUMP do not behave in an aggressive fashion, occasional cases have been documented to recur rapidly after resection and a minority have progressed to stromal sarcoma. STUMPs encompass a broad spectrum of lesions, a subset of which is focal as seen on simple prostatectomy, which neither recurs nor progresses, and could be termed in these situations as glandular-stromal or stromal nodule with atypia. The appropriate treatment of STUMPs is unknown. When these lesions are extensive or associated with a palpable mass definitive therapy may be considered. Stromal sarcomas may have the overall

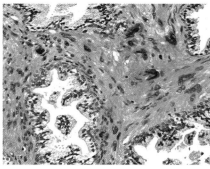

Fig. 3.85 STUMP (prostatic stromal proliferations of uncertain malignant potential) with benign glands and atypical stromal cells.

glandular growth pattern of phyllodes tumours with obviously malignant stroma with increased cellularity, mitotic figures, and pleomorphism. Other stromal sarcomas consist of sheets of hypercellular atypical stroma without the fascicular growth pattern of leiomyosarcomas. The behaviour of stromal sarcomas is not well understood due to their rarity, although some cases have gone on to metastasize to distant sites. Rare cases of adenocarcinoma of the prostate involving a phyllodes tumour have been identified. Immunohistochemical results show that STUMP and stromal sarcomas both are typically positive for CD34 and may be used to distinguish them from other prostatic mesenchymal neoplasms, such as rhabdomyosarcoma and leiomyosarco-

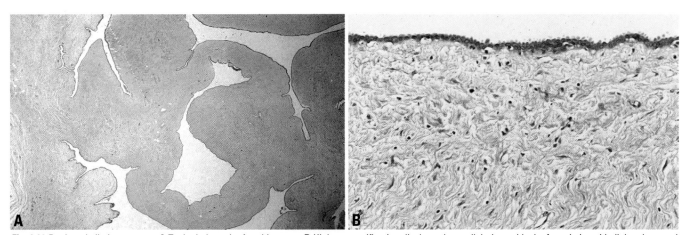

Fig. 3.86 Benign phyllodes tumour. **A** Typical clover leaf architecture. **B** Higher magnification discloses low cellularity and lack of atypia in epithelial and stromal elements.

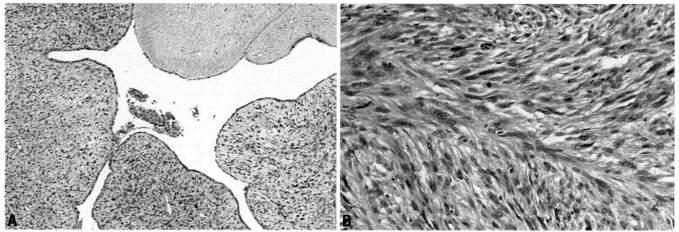

Fig. 3.87 A Malignant phyllodes tumour. High cellularity and cellular pleomorphism are obvious even at this magnification. B Leiomyosarcoma. Fascicular arrangement, high cellularity and mitotic activity are characteristic.

ma. Both STUMP and stromal sarcomas characteristically express progesterone receptors (PR) and uncommonly express estrogen receptors (ER), supporting the concept that STUMP and stromal sarcomas are lesions involving hormonally responsive prostatic mesenchymal cells, the specialized prostatic stroma. STUMPS typically react positively with actin, whereas prostatic stromal sarcomas react negatively, suggesting that the expression of muscle markers in these lesions is a function of differentiation.

Leiomyosarcoma

Leiomyosarcomas are the most common sarcomas involving the prostate in adults {443}. The majority of patients are between 40 and 70 years of age, though in some series up to 20% of leiomyosarcomas have occurred in young adults. Leiomyosarcomas range in size between 2 cm and 24 cm with a median size of 5 cm. Histologically, leiomyosarcomas range from smooth muscle tumours showing moderate atypia to highly pleomorphic sarcomas. As with leiomyosarcomas found elsewhere, these tumours immunohistochemically can express cytokeratins in addition to muscle markers. There have been several well circumscribed lesions with a variable amount of nuclear atypia and scattered mitotic activity which have been referred to as atypical leiomyoma of the prostate {2233}, giant leiomyoma of the prostate {2162}, or circumscribed leiomyosarcoma of the prostate {2505}. Following either local excision or resection of prostatic leiomyosarcomas, the clinical course tends to be characterized by multiple recurrences. Metastases, when present, are usually found in the lung. The average survival with leiomyosarcoma of the prostate is between 3 and 4 years. Because smooth muscle tumours of the prostate are rare, the criteria for distinguishing between leiomyosarcoma and leiomyoma with borderline features have not been elucidated. Although most "atypical leiomyomas" have shown no evidence of disease with short follow-up, a few have recurred.

Rhabdomyosarcoma

Rhabdomyosarcoma is the most frequent mesenchymal tumour within the prostate in childhood {1522}. Rhabdomyosarcomas of the prostate occur from infancy to early adulthood with an average age at diagnosis of 5 years. Most present with stage III disease, in which there is gross residual disease following incomplete resection or biopsy. A smaller, but significant proportion of patients present with distant metastases. Localized tumour that may be complete-

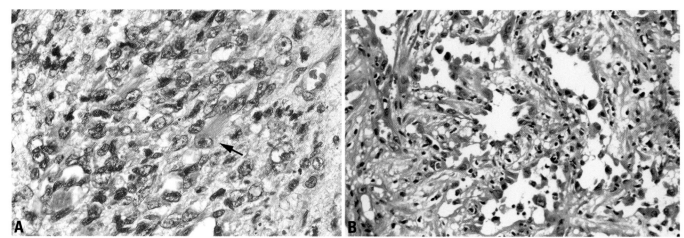

Fig. 3.88 A Rhabdomyosarcoma. Note strap cells. B Angiosarcoma with slit-like spaces lined by atypical cells.

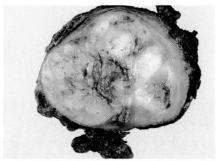

Fig. 3.89 Sarcoma of the prostate.

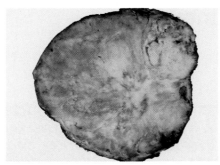

Fig. 3.90 Solitary fibrous tumour.

ly resected is only rarely present. Because of their large size at the time of diagnosis, distinction between rhabdomyosarcoma originating in the bladder and that originating in the prostate may be difficult. Histologically, most prostate rhabdomyosarcomas are of the embryonal subtype and are considered to be of favourable histology. The use of immunohistochemical, ultrastructural, and molecular techniques may be useful in the diagnosis of embryonal rhabdomyosarcoma. Following the development of effective chemotherapy for rhabdomyosarcomas, those few patients with localized disease (stage I) or microscopic regional disease (stage II) stand an excellent chance of being cured. While the majority of patients with gross residual disease (stage III) have remained without evidence of disease for a long period of time, approximately 15-20% die of their tumour. The prognosis for patients with metastatic tumour (stage IV) is more dismal, with most patients dying of their tumour. Following biopsy or partial excision of the tumour, the usual therapy for localized disease is intensive chemotherapy and radiotherapy. If tumour persists despite several courses of this therapy, then radical surgery is performed.

It is important to identify those rare cases of alveolar rhabdomyosarcoma involving the prostate since this histologic subtype is unfavourable and necessitates more aggressive chemotherapy.

Miscellaneous sarcomas

Rare cases of malignant fibrous histiocytoma {158,450,1403,1741,2369}, angiosarcoma {2446}, osteosarcoma {59, 1899}, chondrosarcoma {631}, malignant peripheral nerve sheath tumours {2143}, and synovial sarcoma {1189} have been reported.

Leiomyoma

The arbitrary definition of a leiomyoma, to distinguish it from a fibromuscular hyperplastic nodule, is a well-circumscribed proliferation of smooth muscle measuring 1 cm or more {1724}. According to this definition, less than one hundred cases are reported. Its morphology is similar to uterine leiomyoma, and even subtypes, such as the bizarre leiomyoma, are described {1277}.

Miscellaneous benign mesenchymal tumours

Various benign soft tissue tumours have been described as arising in the prostate including granular cell tumour {824}, and solitary fibrous tumour {928,1912,2079}. Other benign mesenchymal tumours such as haemangiomas {1112}, chondromas {2439}, and neural tumours {1872} have also been described.

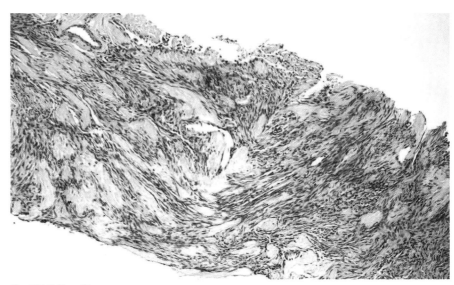

Fig. 3.91 Solitary fibrous tumour.

Haematolymphoid tumours

K.A. Iczkowski
A. Lopez-Beltran
W.A. Sakr

The prostate is a rare site of extranodal lymphoma with a total of 165 cases arising in or secondarily involving the prostate reported. Of patients with chronic lymphocytic leukaemia, 20% are reported to have prostate involvement at autopsy {2731}. The most frequent symptoms are those related to lower urinary obstruction.

In a recent large series of 62 cases, 22, 30 and 10 cases were classified as primary, secondary and indeterminate respectively. Sixty cases were non-Hodgkin lymphoma (predominately diffuse large cell followed by small lymphocytic lymphoma). Rarely Hodgkin lymphoma and mucosa-associated lymphoid tissue (MALT) lymphoma were reported {291,1216}.

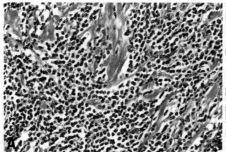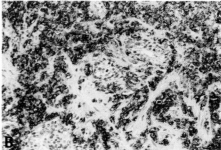

Fig. 3.92 A Lymphocytic lymphoma. Small lympocyte - like cells infiltrate the prostatic stroma. **B** Diffuse large cell lymphoma labeled with CD20.

Secondary tumours involving the prostate

M.C. Parkinson

Definition
Metastatic tumours arise outside of the prostate and spread to the gland by vascular channels. Contiguous spread from other pelvic tumours into the prostate does not constitute a metastasis. Haematolymphoid tumours of the prostate are discussed separately.

Epidemiology
True metastases from solid tumours were reported in 0.1% and 2.9% of all male postmortems {185,1699} and 1% and 6.3% of men in whom tumours caused death {1699,2930} and in 0.2% of all surgical prostatic specimens {185}. Lung was the most common primary site of metastases to the prostate {185}. In all series direct spread of bladder carcinoma is the commonest secondary prostatic tumour {185,2905}.

Histopathology and prognosis
Metastases from lung, skin (melanoma), gastrointestinal tract, kidney, testis and endocrine glands have been reported {185,2905,2930}. Clinical context, morphological features and immunocytochemical localization of PSA and PSAP clarify the differential diagnosis. Prognosis reflects the late stage of disease in which prostatic metastases are seen.

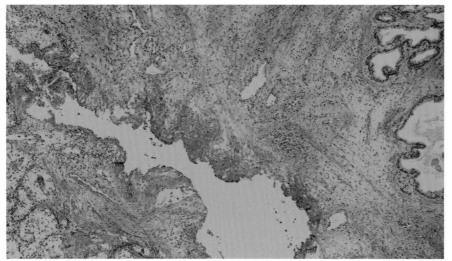

Fig. 3.93 Metastatic renal cell carcinoma to the prostate.

Miscellaneous tumours

P.H. Tan
L. Cheng
M. Furusato
C.C. Pan

ICD-O codes

Cystadenoma	8440/0
Wilms tumour (nephroblastoma)	8960/3
Malignant rhabdoid tumour	8963/3
Clear cell adenocarcinoma	8310/3
Melanoma of the prostate	8720/3
Paraganglioma	8680/1
Neuroblastoma	9500/3

Cystadenoma

Also known as multilocular cyst or giant multilocular prostatic cystadenoma, it is a rare entity characterized by benign multilocular prostatic cysts that can enlarge massively. Affected men are aged 20-80 years, presenting with obstructive urinary symptoms, with or without a palpable abdominal mass {1324}. Postulated causes include obstruction, involutional atrophy {1594}, or retrovesical ectopic prostatic tissue with cystic change {2872}.

It occurs between the bladder and the rectum {62,1501,1611,2872}, either separate from the prostate or attached to it by a pedicle. Similar lesions can be found within the prostate gland.

Cystadenomas weigh up to 6,500 grams, ranging from 7.5 cm to 20 cm in size. They are well-circumscribed, resembling nodular hyperplasia with multiple cysts macroscopically. Atrophic prostatic epithelium lines the cysts, reacting with antibodies to PSA and PSAP, with high grade prostatic intraepithelial neoplasia reported in one case {62}. When cystadenomas occur within the prostate, distinction from cystic nodular hyperplasia may be difficult. Intraprostatic cystadenoma should be diagnosed only when half the prostate appears normal, while the remaining gland is enlarged by a solitary encapsulated cystic nodule {1323,1704}.

Prostatic cystadenomas are not biologically aggressive {1611}, but can recur if incompletely excised. Extensive surgery may be necessary because of their large size and impingement on surrounding structures.

Wilms tumour (nephroblastoma)

Wilms tumour rarely occurs in the prostate {386}.

Malignant rhabdoid tumour

Malignant rhabdoid tumour may be found in the prostate {673}.

Germ cell tumours

Primary germ cell tumours of the prostate have been rarely described {1046,1725, 2586}. It is critical to exclude a metastasis from a testicular primary.

Clear cell adenocarcinoma

Clear cell adenocarcinoma resembling those seen in the Müllerian system may affect the prostate. It can develop from the prostatic urethra {636}, Müllerian derivatives such as Müllerian duct cyst {874}, or exceptionally, from the peripheral parenchyma {2004}. Histologically, it is composed of tubulocystic or papillary structures lined by cuboidal or hobnail cells with clear to eosinophilic cytoplasm. The tumour cells immunohistochemically do not express prostate specific antigen and prostate acid phosphatase, but may express CA-125. The patient may have elevated serum level of CA-125.

Melanoma of the prostate

Primary malignant melanomas of the prostate are extremely rare {2493}. Malignant melanoma of the prostate should be distinguished from melanosis and cellular blue nevus of the prostate {2208}.

Paraganglioma

Several case reports of paragangliomas originating in the prostate have been reported, including one in a child {599, 2747}. Although extra-adrenal paragan-

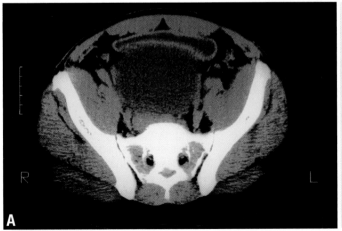 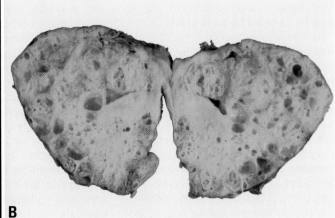

Fig. 3.94 Cystadenoma. **A** CT scan showing a large multinucleated cystic mass within the pelvis, consistent with prostatic cystadenoma. **B** Gross section discloses large multicystic tumour.

gliomas should not be designated as "phaeochromocytomas", they have been published as such. Clinical symptoms are similar to those of the adrenal (hypertension, headaches, etc.). The laboratory tests used to diagnose prostatic paragangliomas are the same as used to diagnose paragangliomas occurring elsewhere in the body. In some cases, symptoms have been exacerbated by urination (micturition attacks), identical to what is seen with paragangliomas occurring in the bladder. Malignant behaviour has not been reported.

Neuroblastoma

Neuroblastoma, a primitive tumour of neuroectodermal origin, rarely affects the prostate. {1420}. Pelvic organs may also be involved secondarily.

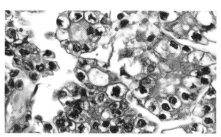
Fig. 3.95 Clear cell adenocarcinoma.

Tumours of the seminal vesicles

K.A. Iczkowski   M.C. Parkinson
H.M. Samaratunga   X.J. Yang
L. Cheng   I. Sesterhenn
B. Helpap

Epithelial tumours of the seminal vesicle

Primary adenocarcinoma

ICD-O code   8140/3

The seminal vesicle is involved by secondary tumours much more frequently than it contains primary adenocarcinoma. Strict criteria for this diagnosis of this lesion require the exclusion of a concomitant prostatic, bladder, or rectal carcinoma {1977}.

Acceptable reported cases numbered 48 {1977}. Although most were in older men, 10 men were under age 40 {212, 1322}.

Presenting symptoms usually included obstructive uropathy due to a nontender peri-rectal mass {212,1940} and less commonly haematuria or haematospermia. Serum carcinoembryonic antigen may be elevated up to 10 ng/ml.

The tumours are usually large (3-5 cm) and often invaded the bladder, ureter, or rectum {212,1940}. Tumours can show a mixture of papillary, trabecular and glandular patterns with varying degrees of differentiation. Carcinomas with colloid features have been described. Tumour cytoplasm may show clear cell or hobnail morphology. It is important to exclude a prostatic primary using PSA and PAP. Immunoreactive carcinoembryonic antigen (CEA) is detectable in normal seminal vesicle and seminal vesicle adenocarcinoma. Besides CEA, tumour should be positive for cytokeratin 7 (unlike many prostatic adenocarcinomas), negative for cytokeratin 20 (unlike bladder and colonic carcinoma), and positive for CA-125 (unlike carcinoma arising in a Müllerian duct cyst and all the above).

The prognosis of primary seminal vesicle adenocarcinoma is poor, but can be improved with adjuvant hormonal manipulation {212}. Most patients presented with metastases and survival was less than 3 years in 95% of cases; five of 48 patients survived more than 18 months {1977}.

Cystadenoma of the seminal vesicles

ICD-O code   8440/0

Cystadenomas are rare benign tumours of the seminal vesicle. Patients range in age from 37-66 years and may be asymptomatic or have symptoms of bladder outlet obstruction {177,2292}. Ultrasound reveals a complex, solid-cystic pelvic mass {1427}. Histologically, this is a well-circumscribed tumour containing variable-sized glandular spaces with branching contours and cysts with an investing spindle cell stroma. The glands are grouped in a vaguely lobular pattern, contain pale intraluminal secretions and are lined by one or two layers of cuboidal to columnar cells. No significant cytologic atypia, mitotic activity or necrosis is seen {177,1659,2292}. Incompletely removed tumours may recur.

Benign and malignant mixed epithelial stromal tumours

Epithelial-stromal tumours fulfill the following criteria: they arise from the seminal vesicle and there is no normal seminal vesicle within the tumour; they usually do not invade the prostate (one exception {1451}), have a less conspicuous, less cellular stromal component than cystadenoma, and are not immunoreactive for prostatic markers or CEA {737, 1451,1600,1656}. Benign types include *fibroadenoma* and *adenomyoma*. These tumours have occurred in men aged 39-66 who presented with pain and voiding difficulty. Tumours were grossly solid and cystic, ranging from 3 to 15 cm. The distinction from malignant epithelial-stromal tumour NOS, *low-grade* (below) is based on stromal blandness and inconspicuous mitotic activity.

Four cases of malignant or probably malignant epithelial-stromal tumours have been reported {737,1451,1600,1656}. These were categorized as *low-grade* or *high-grade* depending on mitotic activity and necrosis. The tumours occur in men in the sixth decade of life, who usually have urinary obstruction as the main presenting symptom. Grossly, the tumours were either multicystic or solid and cystic. Microscopically, the stroma was at least focally densely cellular and tended to condense around distorted glands lined by cuboidal to focally stratified epithelium. One man was cured by cystoprostatectomy {1451}; two had pelvic recurrence after 2 years, one cured by a second exci-

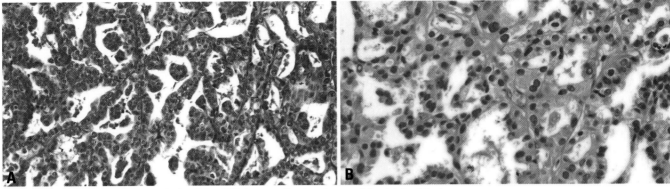

Fig. 3.96 A Adenocarcinoma of the seminal vesicles. **B** Higher magnification shows cellular details of the tumour.

sion {1656} and one surgically incurable {1600}; and one developed lung metastasis 4 years postoperatively {737}.

Mesenchymal tumours of the seminal vesicles

Mesenchymal tumours that arise in the seminal vesicles as a primary site are rare. The frequency of these tumours, in order from highest to lowest, is leiomyosarcoma, leiomyoma, angiosarcoma, malignant fibrous histiocytoma, solitary fibrous tumour, liposarcoma and haemangiopericytoma. Clinical presentations include pelvic pain and urinary or rectal obstructive symptoms. Some may be asymptomatic, and detected by digital rectal examination and sonography. Needle or open biopsy is required to establish the diagnosis. It may be difficult to ascertain the site of origin when adjacent pelvic organs are involved.

Leiomyoma

ICD-O code   8890/0

Leiomyoma of the seminal vesicles is asymptomatic and exceedingly rare. Among seven reported cases, six were detected on digital rectal examination and one, by magnetic resonance imaging {155,850}. The tumour, probably of Müllerian duct origin, measures up to 5 cm {850}. Local excision has yielded no recurrences.

Leiomyosarcoma

ICD-O code   8890/3

By digital rectal examination and pelvic computed tomography as well as magnet-ic resonance imaging, a large pelvic mass in the region of the seminal vesicles of the prostate may be detected. Six patients with reported seminal vesicle leiomyosarcoma presented with pelvic pain and obstructive symptoms but not haematuria (unlike with prostatic sarcoma) {87,1823, 2332}. When possible, resection of the tumour mass by radical prostatectomy and vesiculectomy is the therapy of choice. One patient was cured by radical cystoprostatectomy at 13-month follow-up {87}, although another developed renal metastasis after 2 years {1823}.

Angiosarcoma

ICD-O code   9120/3

Angiosarcoma of the seminal vesicles is a highly aggressive tumour, refractory to traditional surgical and adjuvant therapeutic modalities. Three cases were reported {451,1432,2006} and all presented with pelvic pain; two died of distant metastasis within two months after the diagnosis {451,1432}.

Liposarcoma

ICD-O code   8850/3

There is one case described as a "collision" tumour composed of liposarcoma of the seminal vesicles and prostatic carcinoma {1252}. The patient died of distant metastasis from prostatic carcinoma.

Malignant fibrous histiocytoma

ICD-O code   8830/3

This tumour is exceedingly rare in the seminal vesicle {538}. Sonographic studies are important to establish the site of origin. The therapy should be the complete surgical resection, in most cases by radical prostatectomy and vesiculectomy.

Solitary fibrous tumour

ICD-O code   8815/0

Three cases were reported {1785,2808}, and all were located in the right seminal vesicle. The clinical presentations were pelvic pain or haematuria. The origin of the tumour was established by transrectal ultrasonography, magnetic resonance imaging, or computed tomography. Complete local excision appears to be curative.

Haemangiopericytoma

ICD-O code   9150/1

A case of malignant haemangiopericytoma of the seminal vesicle has been reported {122}. The patient presented with hypoglycemia, and was treated by cystoprostatectomy and vesiculectomy. He died of disseminated haemangiopericytoma 10 years later.

Miscellaneous tumours of the seminal vesicle

Choriocarcinoma

ICD-O code   9100/3

One case has been reported of primary choriocarcinoma of the seminal vesicles. {738}. However, this case is not definitive as there was tumour in multiple organs, excluding the testes, with the largest deposit present in the seminal vesicle.

CHAPTER 4

Tumours of the Testis and Paratesticular Tissue

Germ cell tumours are the most frequent and important neoplasms at this site. They mainly affect young males and their incidence is steadily increasing in affluent societies. In several regions, including North America and Northern Europe, they have become the most common cancer in men aged 15 - 44. There is circumstantial epidimiological evidence that the steep increase in new cases is associated with the Western lifestyle, characterized by high caloric diet and lack of physical exercise.

Despite the increase in incidence rates, mortality from testicular cancer has sharply declined due to a very effective chemotherapy that includes cis-platinum. In most countries with an excellent clinical oncology infrastructure, 5-year survival rates approach 95%.

WHO histological classification of testis tumours

Germ cell tumours
Intratubular germ cell neoplasia, unclassified — 9064/2[1]
Other types

Tumours of one histological type (pure forms)
Seminoma — 9061/3
    Seminoma with syncytiotrophoblastic cells
Spermatocytic seminoma — 9063/3
    Spermatocytic seminoma with sarcoma
Embryonal carcinoma — 9070/3
Yolk sac tumour — 9071/3
Trophoblastic tumours
    Choriocarcinoma — 9100/3
    Trophoblastic neoplasms other than choriocarcinoma
        Monophasic choriocarcinoma
        Placental site trophoblastic tumour — 9104/1
Teratoma — 9080/3
    Dermoid cyst — 9084/0
    Monodermal teratoma
    Teratoma with somatic type malignancies — 9084/3

Tumours of more than one histological type (mixed forms)
Mixed embryonal carcinoma and teratoma — 9081/3
Mixed teratoma and seminoma — 9085/3
Choriocarcinoma and teratoma/embryonal carcinoma — 9101/3
Others

Sex cord/gonadal stromal tumours
Pure forms
Leydig cell tumour — 8650/1
Malignant Leydig cell tumour — 8650/3
Sertoli cell tumour — 8640/1
    Sertoli cell tumour lipid rich variant — 8641/0
    Sclerosing Sertoli cell tumour
    Large cell calcifying Sertoli cell tumour — 8642/1
Malignant Sertoli cell tumour — 8640/3
Granulosa cell tumour — 8620/1
    Adult type granulosa cell tumour — 8620/1
    Juvenile type granulosa cell tumour — 8622/1
Tumours of the thecoma/fibroma group
    Thecoma — 8600/0
    Fibroma — 8810/0

Sex cord/gonadal stromal tumour:
Incompletely differentiated — 8591/1
Sex cord/gonadal stromal tumours, mixed forms — 8592/1
Malignant sex cord/gonadal stromal tumours — 8590/3
Tumours containing both germ cell and sex cord/gonadal stromal elements
    Gonadoblastoma — 9073/1
    Germ cell-sex cord/gonadal stromal tumour, unclassified

Miscellaneous tumours of the testis
Carcinoid tumour — 8240/3
Tumours of ovarian epithelial types
    Serous tumour of borderline malignancy — 8442/1
    Serous carcinoma — 8441/3
    Well differentiated endometrioid carcinoma — 8380/3
    Mucinous cystadenoma — 8470/0
    Mucinous cystadenocarcinoma — 8470/3
    Brenner tumour — 9000/0
Nephroblastoma — 8960/3
Paraganglioma — 8680/1

Haematopoietic tumours

Tumours of collecting ducts and rete
Adenoma — 8140/0
Carcinoma — 8140/3

Tumours of paratesticular structures
Adenomatoid tumour — 9054/0
Malignant mesothelioma — 9050/3
Benign mesothelioma
    Well differentiated papillary mesothelioma — 9052/0
    Cystic mesothelioma — 9055/0
Adenocarcinoma of the epididymis — 8140/3
Papillary cystadenoma of the epididymis — 8450/0
Melanotic neuroectodermal tumour — 9363/0
Desmoplastic small round cell tumour — 8806/3

Mesenchymal tumours of the spermatic cord and testicular adnexae

Secondary tumours of the testis

---

[1] Morphology code of the International Classification of Diseases for Oncology (ICD-O) {808} and the Systematized Nomenclature of Medicine (http://snomed.org). Behaviour is coded /0 for benign tumours, /2 for in situ carcinomas and grade III intraepithelial neoplasia, /3 for malignant tumours, and /1 for borderline or uncertain behaviour.

TNM classification of germ cell tumours of the testis

TNM classification [1,2]

T – Primary tumour

Except for pTis and pT4, where radical orchiectomy is not always necessary for classification purposes, the extent of the primary tumour is classified after radical orchiectomy; see pT. In other circumstances, TX is
used if no radical orchiectomy has been performed

N – Regional lymph nodes
NX   Regional lymph nodes cannot be assessed
N0   No regional lymph node metastasis
N1   Metastasis with a lymph node mass 2 cm or less in greatest dime-
     nion or multiple lymph nodes, none more than 2 cm in greatest
     dimension
N2   Metastasis with a lymph node mass more than 2 cm but not more
     than 5 cm in greatest dimension, or multiple lymph nodes, any one
     mass more than 2 cm but not more than 5 cm in greatest dimension
N3   Metastasis with a lymph node mass more than 5 cm in greatest
     dimension

M – Distant metastasis
MX   Distant metastasis cannot be assessed
M0   No distant metastasis
M1   Distant metastasis
M1a Non regional lymph node(s) or lung
M1b Other sites

pTNM pathological classification

pT – Primary tumour
pTX   Primary tumour cannot be assessed (See T–primary tumour, above)
pT0   No evidence of primary tumour (e.g. histologic scar in testis)
pTis Intratubular germ cell neoplasia (carcinoma in situ)
pT1   Tumour limited to testis and epididymis without vascular/lymphatic
      invasion; tumour may invade tunica albuginea but not tunica vagi-
      nalis
pT2   Tumour limited to testis and epididymis with vascular/lymphatic
      invasion, or tumour extending through tunica albuginea with
      involvement of tunica vaginalis
pT3   Tumour invades spermatic cord with or without vascular/lymphatic
      invasion
pT4   Tumour invades scrotum with or without vascular/lymphatic
      invasion

pN – Regional lymph nodes

pNX   Regional lymph nodes cannot be assessed
pN0   No regional lymph node metastasis
pN1   Metastasis with a lymph node mass 2 cm or less in greatest dimen-
      sion and 5 or fewer positive nodes, none more than 2 cm in greatest
      dimension
pN2   Metastasis with a lymph node mass more than 2 cm but not more
      than 5 cm in greatest dimension; or more than 5 nodes positive,
      none more than 5 cm; or evidence of extranodal extension of tumour
pN3   Metastasis with a lymph node mass more than 5 cm in greatest
      dimension

S – Serum tumour markers
SX   Serum marker studies not available or not performed
S0   Serum marker study levels within normal limits

	LDH	hCG (mIU/ml)	AFP (ng/ml)
S1	$<1.5 \times N$	and $<5,000$	and $<1,000$
S2	$1.5–10 \times N$	or $5,000–50,000$	or $1,000–10,000$
S3	$>10 \times N$	or $>50,000$	or $>10,000$

N indicates the upper limit of normal for the LDH assay

Stage grouping

Stage				
Stage 0	pTis	N0	M0	S0, SX
Stage I	pT1–4	N0	M0	SX
Stage IA	pT1	N0	M0	S0
Stage IB	pT2	N0	M0	S0
	pT3	N0	M0	S0
	pT4	N0	M0	S0
Stage IS	Any pT/TX	N0	M0	S1–3
Stage II	Any pT/TX	N1–3	M0	SX
Stage IIA	Any pT/TX	N1	M0	S0
	Any pT/TX	N1	M0	S1
Stage IIB	Any pT/TX	N2	M0	S0
	Any pT/TX	N2	M0	S1
Stage IIC	Any pT/TX	N3	M0	S0
	Any pT/TX	N3	M0	S1
Stage III	Any pT/TX	Any N	M1, M1a	SX
Stage IIIA	Any pT/TX	Any N	M1, M1a	S0
	Any pT/TX	Any N	M1, M1a	S1
Stage IIIB	Any pT/TX	N1–3	M0	S2
	Any pT/TX	Any N	M1, M1a	S2
Stage IIIC	Any pT/TX	N1–3	M0	S3
	Any pT/TX	Any N	M1, M1a	S3
	Any pT/TX	Any N	M1b	Any S

[1] {944,2662}.
[2] A help desk for specific questions about the TNM classification is available at http://tnm.uicc.org.

Table 4.01
Staging of germ cell tumours by the Paediatric Oncology Group (POG) {5,282}.

Stage I: Tumour is limited to testis. No evidence of disease beyond the
testis by clinical, histologic, or radiographic examination. An appropriate
decline in serum AFP has occurred (AFP t1/2 = 5 days).
Stage II: Microscopic disease is located in the scrotum or high in the spermatic cord (<5 cm from the proximal end). Retroperitoneal lymph node
involvement is present (<2cm). Serum AFP is persistently elevated.
Stage III: Retroperitoneal lymph node involvement (>2cm) is present. No
visible evidence of visceral or extra abdominal involvement.
Stage IV: Distant metastases are present.

Introduction

F.K. Mostofi
I.A. Sesterhenn

The large majority of primary testicular tumours originate from germ cells. More than half of the tumours contain more than one tumour type: seminoma, embryonal carcinoma, yolk sac tumour, polyembryoma, choriocarcinoma, and teratoma. In over 90%, the histology of the untreated metastasis is identical to that of the primary tumour. Every cell type in the primary tumour, irrespective of its benign histological appearance or volume, is capable of invasion and metastasis. Thus, the information provided by the pathologist guides the urologic surgeon and the oncologist toward the best mode of therapy. The report of the pathologist can explain the relationship of the histology of the tumour to tumour markers and the response of the metastasis to the specific postorchiectomy treatment. If the metastases do not respond to the treatment, they may consist of some form of teratoma for which surgical intervention is the method of treatment.

In 10% of cases, the histological features of the untreated metastases may be different from those of the initial sections of the primary tumour. Further sectioning may identify an additional element in the primary tumour or a scar referred to as a regressed or burned out tumour, with or without intra- and extratubular malignant germ cells.

Therefore, it is essential that the specimen be examined adequately with extensive slicing and macroscopic description, including the major dimensions. Tissue available for microscopic examination must include the tumour (at least one block for each 1 cm maximum tumour diameter and more if the tissue is heterogeneous), the non neoplastic testis, the tunica nearest the neoplasm, the epididymis, the lower cord, and the upper cord at the level of surgical resection. The specimen should not be discarded until the clinician and the pathologist have agreed that the pathology report and diagnosis correlate with the clinical features. The presence of discordant findings (e.g. elevated AFP in a seminoma) indicates a need for further sectioning of the gross specimen.

The age of the patient provides a clue to the most likely type of tumour present. In the newborn, the most frequent testicular tumour is the juvenile granulosa cell tumour. Most germ cell tumours occur between the ages of 20 and 50 years. Before puberty, seminoma is extremely uncommon, while yolk sac tumour and the better differentiated types of teratoma are the usual germ cell tumours. Spermatocytic seminoma and malignant lymphoma usually occur in older patients, although both may also occur in younger individuals.

In addition to histological typing of the tumour, the estimated quantity of cell types, determination of vascular/lymphatic invasion and the pathological stage of the tumour should be reported. The TNM staging system is recommended.

Germm cell tumours

P.J. Woodward
A. Heidenreich
L.H.J. Looijenga
J.W. Oosterhuis
D.G. McLeod
H. Møller
J.C. Manivel

F.K. Mostofi
S. Hailemariam
M.C. Parkinson
K. Grigor
L. True
G.K. Jacobsen
T.D. Oliver

A. Talerman
G.W. Kaplan
T.M. Ulbright
I.A. Sesterhenn
H.G. Rushton
H. Michael
V.E. Reuter

Epidemiology

The incidence of testicular germ cell tumours shows a remarkable geographical variation. The highest level of incidence, around 8-10 per 100,000 world standard population (WSP) are found in Denmark, Germany, Norway, Hungary and Switzerland {749}. The only population of non European origin with a similar high level of incidence is the Maori population of New Zealand with 7 per 100,000 WSP {2016}. In populations in Africa, the Caribbean and Asia the level of incidence is typically less than 2 per 100,000 WSP.

In general, the incidence of testicular germ cell tumours has been increasing in most populations of European origin in recent decades {481}.

The age distribution of testicular germ cell tumour is unusual. The incidence increases shortly after the onset of puberty and reaches a maximum in men in the late twenties and thirties. Thereafter, the age specific incidence rate decreases to a very low level in men in their sixties or older. Consistent with the geographical variation in incidence, the area under the age incidence curve

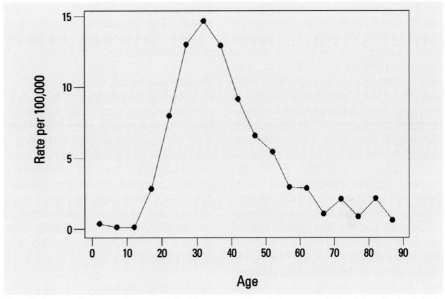

Fig. 4.01 Germ cell tumours. Age specific incidence rates of testicular cancer in South East England, 1995-1999. Source: Thames Cancer Registry.

is very different in populations with different levels of incidence, but the general shape of the curve is the same in low risk and in high risk populations {1766}. The age incidence curves of seminoma and

non-seminoma are similar, but the modal age of non-seminoma is about ten years earlier than seminoma. This probably reflects the more rapid growth and the capacity of haematogenic spread and metastasis of non-seminomas.

In Denmark, Norway and Sweden the generally increasing incidence over time was interrupted by unusual low incidence in men who were born during the Second World War {222,1766}. The reasons for this phenomenon are not known but it illustrates several important characteristics. Firstly, that the risk of developing testicular cancer in men in high risk populations is not a constant, but appears to be highly and rapidly susceptible to increasing as well as decreasing levels of exposure to casual factors. Secondly, the risk of developing testicular tumour is susceptible to changes in everyday living conditions and habits, as these occurred with respect to changes in the supply and consumption situation in the Nordic countries during the Second World War. Finally, the relatively low level of incidence throughout life of men in the

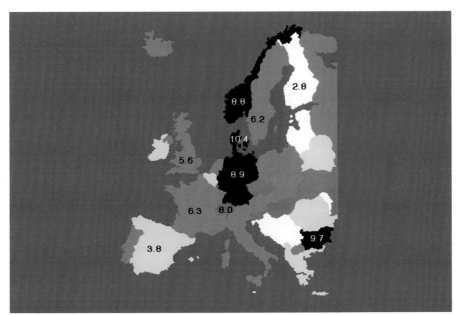

Fig. 4.02 Germ cell tumours. European annual incidence per 100,000 of testicular cancer. From Globocan 2000 {749}.

wartime birth cohorts illustrate that the propensity to develop testicular cancer is established early in life.

Testicular germ cell tumours are associated with intratubular germ cell neoplasia, unclassified (IGCNU). The association is very strong and very specific {1766}. The prevalence of carcinoma in situ in a population of men corresponds almost exactly to the lifetime risk of testicular cancer in these men, ranging from less than 1% in normal men in Denmark {891} to about 2-3% in men with a history of cryptorchidism {887} and 5% in the contralateral testicle in men who have already had one testicular germ cell tumour {614}. Intratubular germ cell neoplasia, unclassified is practically always present in the tissue surrounding a testicular germ cell tumour and the condition has never been observed to disappear spontaneously. From these observations it may be inferred that the rate limiting step in testicular germ cell tumour is the abnormal differentiation of primordial germ cells leading to the persisting unclassified intratubular germ cell neoplasia which then almost inevitably progresses to invasive cancer. The area under the age incidence curve may reflect the rate of occurrence of IGCNU. The decline in the age specific incidence rates after about forty years of age may be due to the depletion of the pool of susceptible individuals with ITCGNU as these progress to invasive cancer {1766}.

Etiology

The research for the causes of testicular germ cell tumours has been guided by the hypothesis that the disease process starts in fetal life and consists of the abnormal differentiation of the fetal population of primordial germ cells. There are several strong indications that testicular germ cell tumour is associated with abnormal conditions in fetal life.

Associations with congenital malformations of the male genitalia

Cryptorchidism (undescended testis) is consistently associated with an increased risk of testicular germ cell tumour. The incidence is about 3-5 fold increased in men with a history of cryptorchidism {3}. In those with unilateral cryptorchidism, both the undescended testicle and the normal, contralateral testicle have increased risk of testicular

cancer {1768}. The incidence of testicular cancer is possibly increased in men with hypospadias and in men with inguinal hernia, but the evidence is less strong than for cryptorchidism {2105}. Atrophy adds to the risk of germ cell tumours in maldescent {613,1020} and the normal, contralateral testicle has an increased risk of testicular cancer {1768}. The presence of atrophy in maldescended testes is a major factor in germ cell neoplasia.

Prenatal risk factors

Case control studies have shown consistent associations of testicular cancer with low birth weight and with being born small for gestational age, indicating a possible role of intrauterine growth retardation {43,1769}. A similar association is evident for cryptorchidism and hypospadias {2797}. Other, less consistent associations with testicular cancer include low birth order, high maternal age, neonatal jaundice and retained placenta {2186,2270,2775}.

Exposures in adulthood

There are no strong and consistent risk factors for testicular cancer in adulthood. Possible etiological clues, however, include a low level of physical activity and high socioeconomic class {4}. There is no consistent evidence linking testicular cancer to particular occupations or occupational exposures. Immunosuppression, both in renal transplant patients and in AIDS patients seem to be associated with an increased incidence {245,900}.

Male infertility

Subfertile and infertile men are at increased risk of developing testicular cancer {1203,1770}. It has been hypothesized that common causal factors may exist which operate prenatally and lead to both infertility and testicular neoplasia.

Specific exposures

For more than twenty years, research in testicular cancer etiology has been influenced by the work of Brian Henderson and his colleagues who hypothesized an adverse role of endogenous maternal estrogens on the development of the male embryo {1070}. More recently, the emphasis has changed away from endogenous estrogens to environmental exposures to estrogenic and anti androgenic substances {2378}. The empirical

evidence, however, for these hypotheses remains rather weak and circumstantial. Follow-up of a cohort of men who were exposed in utero to the synthetic estrogen diethylstilboestrol have shown an excess occurrence of cryptorchidism and a possible, but not statistically significant, increase in the incidence of testicular cancer (about two fold) {2520}.

From the studies, which have attempted to analyse the etiology of seminoma and non-seminoma separately, no consistent differences have emerged. It is most likely that the etiological factors in the two clinical subtypes of testicular germ cell tumour are the same {1769,2186}.

Epidemiology and etiology of other testicular germ cell tumours

Apart from testicular germ cell tumours in adult men, several other types of gonadal tumours should be mentioned briefly. A distinct peak in incidence of testicular tumours occurs in infants. These are generally yolk sac tumour or teratoma. These tumours do not seem to be associated with carcinoma in situ and their epidemiology and etiology are not well known. Spermatocytic seminoma occurs in old men. These tumours are not associated with ITCGNU and are not likely to be of prenatal origin. This may be a tumour derived from the differentiated spermatogonia. Their etiology is unknown. Finally, it may be of interest to note that there is a female counterpart to testicular germ cell tumours. Ovarian germ cell tumours such as dysgerminoma (the female equivalent of seminoma) and teratomas may share important etiological factors with their male counterparts, but their incidence level is much lower than in males {1767}.

Familial predisposition and genetic susceptibility are important factors in the development of testis tumours, which will be discussed in the genetic section.

Clinical features
Signs and symptoms

The usual presentation is a nodule or painless swelling of one testicle. Approximately one third of patients complain of a dull ache or heaviness in the scrotum or lower abdomen. Not infrequently, a diagnosis of epididymitis is made. In this situation, ultrasound may reduce the delay.

In approximately 10% of patients evidence of metastasis may be the presenting symptom: back or abdominal pain, gastrointestinal problems, cough or dyspnoea. Gynecomastia may also be seen in about 5% of cases. Occasionally, extensive work ups have resulted without an adequate examination of the genitalia.

Imaging
Ultrasound (US) is the primary imaging modality for evaluating scrotal pathology. It is easily performed and has been shown to be nearly 100% sensitive for identifying scrotal masses. Intratesticular versus extratesticular pathology can be differentiated with 98-100% sensitivity {211,378,2194}. The normal testis has a homogeneous, medium level, granular echo texture. The epididymis is isoechoic to slightly hyperechoic compared to the testis. The head of the epididymis is approximately 10-12 mm in diameter and is best seen in the longitudinal plane, appearing as a slightly rounded or triangular structure on the superior pole of the testis. Visualization of the epididymis is often easier when a hydrocele is present. When evaluating a palpable mass by ultrasound, the primary goal is localization of the mass (intratesticular versus extratesticular) and further characterization of the lesion (cystic or solid). With rare exception, solid intratesticular masses should be considered malignant. While most extratesticular masses are

benign, a thorough evaluation must be performed. If an extratesticular mass has any features suspicious of malignancy it must be removed.

The sonographic appearance of testicular tumours reflects their gross morphology and underlying histology. Most tumours are hypoechoic compared to the surrounding parenchyma. Other tumours can be heterogeneous with areas of increased echogenecity, calcifications, and cyst formation {211,378,927,1007, 2194,2347}. Although larger tumours tend to be more vascular than smaller tumours, colour Doppler is not of particular use in tumour characterization but does confirm the mass is solid {1126}.

Epididymal masses are more commonly benign. It can, however, be difficult to differentiate an epididymal mass from one originating in the spermatic cord or other paratesticular tissues. This is especially true in the region of the epididymal body and tail where normal structures can be difficult to visualize.

Since ultrasound is easily performed, inexpensive, and highly accurate, magnetic resonance (MR) imaging is seldom needed for diagnostic purposes. MR imaging can, however, be a useful problem solving tool and is particularly helpful in better characterizing extratesticular solid masses {507,2362}. Computed tomography (CT) is not generally useful for differentiating scrotal pathology but is

the primary imaging modality used for tumour staging.

Tumour markers
There are two principal serum tumour markers, alpha fetoprotein (AFP) and the beta subunit of human chorionic gonadotropin (ßhCG). The former is seen in patients with yolk sac tumours and teratomas, while the latter may be seen in any patients whose tumours include syncytiotrophoblastic cells.

AFP is normally synthesized by fetal yolk sac and also the liver and intestine. It is elevated in 50-70% of testicular germ cell tumours and has a serum half life of 4.5 days {305,1333}.

hCG is secreted by placental trophoblastic cells. There are two subunits, alpha and beta, but it is the beta subunit with a half life of 24-36 hours that is elevated in 50% of patients with germ cell tumours. Patients with seminoma may have an elevation of this tumour marker in 10-25% of cases, and all those with choriocarcinoma have elevated ßhCG {1333}.

If postorchiectomy levels do not decline as predicted by their half lives to appropriate levels residual disease should be suspected. Also a normal level of each marker does not necessarily imply the absence of disease.

Lactate dehydrogenase (LDH) may also be elevated, and there is a direct relationship between LDH and tumour burden. However, this test is nonspecific although its degree of elevation correlates with bulk of disease.

Tumour spread and staging
The lymphatic vessels from the right testis drain into lymph nodes lateral, anterior, and medial to the vena cava. The left testis drains into lymph nodes distal, lateral and anterior to the aorta, above the level of the inferior mesenteric artery. These retroperitoneal nodes drain from the thoracic duct into the left supraclavicular lymph nodes and the subclavian vein.

Somatic genetics
Epidemiology, clinical behaviour, histology, and chromosomal constitution define three entities of germ cell tumours (GCTs) in the testis {1540,1541,1965}: teratomas and yolk sac tumours of neonates and infants, seminomas and non-seminomas of adolescents and young adults, the so called TGCTs, and the spermatocytic seminomas of elderly.

Table 4.02
Overview of the three different subgroups of testicular germ cell tumours, characterized by age at clinical presentation, histology of the tumour, clinical behaviour and genetic changes.

Age of the patient at clinical presentation (years)	Histology of the tumour	Clinical behaviour	Chromosomal imbalances
0-5	Teratoma and/or yolk sac tumour	Benign Malignant	Not found Loss: 6q Gain: 1q , 20q, 22
Adolescents and young adults (i.p. 15-45)	Seminoma Non-seminoma (embryonal carcinoma, teratoma, yolk sac tumour, choriocarcinoma)	Malignant Malignant	Aneuploid, and Loss: 11, 13, 18, Y Gain: 12p*, 7, 8, X
Elderly (i.p. over 50)	Spermatocytic Seminoma	Benign, although can be associated with sarcoma	Gain: 9

* found in all invasive TGCTs, regardless of histology.

Similar tumours as those of group 1 and 2 can be found in the ovary and extragonadal sites, in particular along the midline of the body. Relatively little is known on the genomic changes of these GCTs. Supposedly the findings in the GCTs of the testis are also relevant for classification and understanding of the pathogenesis of ovarian and extragonadal GCTs.

Genetic susceptibility (familial tumours)
Familial testicular germ cell tumours of adolescents and adults (TGCTs), account for 1.5-2% of all germ cell tumours of adults. The familial risks of TGCTs increase 3.8-fold for fathers, 8.3 for brothers and 3.9 for sons indicating that genetic predisposition is a contributor to testicular cancer {532}. Earlier age of onset, a higher frequency of bilaterality and an increased severity of disease suggest that genetic anticipation is responsible for many father-son TGCTs {1014}.
Recently, environmental and heritable

causes of cancer have been analysed by structural equation modelling {532}. The estimate of proportion of cancer susceptibility due to genetic effects was 25% in adult TGCTs. The childhood shared environmental effects were also important in testicular cancer (17%).
Numerous groups have attempted to identify candidate regions for a TGCT susceptibility gene or genes {1386,1457, 2148,2435}. No differences were detected between familial/bilateral and sporadic TGCT in chromosomal changes {2435}. However, a TGCT susceptibility gene on chromosome Xq27, that also predisposes to undescended testis, has been proposed by the International Testicular Cancer Linkage Consortium {2148}.
Although the role of genetic factors in the etiology of TGCTs appears to be established, the existence of a single susceptibility gene is doubtful. Most probably genetic predisposition shared with intrauterine or childhood environmental

effects are involved in the molecular pathogenesis of TGCTs.

Inter-sex individuals
Persons with 46,XY or 45,X/46,XY gonadal dysgenesis are at very high risk of gonadal germ cell tumour. The absolute risk is reported to be as high as 10-50% {2267,2728}.

Genomic imprinting
Genomic imprinting refers to the unique phenomenon in mammals of the different functionality of a number of genes due to their parental origin. This difference is generated during passage through the germ cell lineage. The pattern of genomic imprinting has significant effects on the developmental potential of cells {2459}. TGCTs show a consistent biallelic expression of multiple imprinted genes {882,1537,1544,1742,1914,2129,2697,2 726} as do mouse embryonic germ cells {2548}. This suggests that biallelic expression of imprinted genes in TGCTs is not the result of loss of imprinting (LOI) but is intrinsic to the cell of origin. This could also explain the presence of telomerase activity in TGCTs, except in (mature) teratomas {53}. The teratomas and yolk sac tumours of infants show a slightly different pattern of genomic imprinting {2243,2334}, supporting the model that these tumours originate from an earlier stage of germ cell development than TGCTs. Although little is known about the pattern of genomic imprinting of spermatocytic seminomas {2726} the available data indicate that these tumours have already undergone paternal imprinting.

Testicular germ cell tumours of adolescents and adults:
Seminomas and non-seminomas

Chromosomal constitution
All TGCTs, including their precursor, intratubular germ cell neoplasia unclassified (IGCNU) are aneuploid [{567,676, 1962}, for review]. Seminoma and IGCNU cells are hypertriploid, while the tumour cells of non-seminoma, irrespective of their histological type are hypotriploid. This suggests that polyploidization is the initial event, leading to a tetraploid IGCNU, followed by net loss of chromosomal material {1962}. Aneuploidy of TGCTs has been related to the presence of centrosome amplification {1653}.

Table 4.03
Tumour suppressor genes involved in the pathogenesis of testicular germ cell tumours (TGCTs).

(Putative) Pathway	Gene	Chromosomal mapping	Reference(s)
Cell cycle control	CDKN2C	1p32	{175}
	CDKN1A	6p21	{175}
	CDKN2B	9p21	{1053}
	CDKN2A	9p21	{417,1041,1053}
	CDKN1B	12p12-13	{175}
	RB1	13q14	{2519}
	CDKN2D	19p13	{176}
Cell survival/ Apoptosis	BCL10	1p22	{740,2703,2829}
	FHIT	3p14	{1384}
	TP53	17p13	{1301} (for review)
Transcription	MXI1	10q24	{2436}
	WT1	11p13	{1536}
Signaling	APC	5q21-22	{2045}
	MCC	5q21-22	{2045}
	NME1,2	17q23	{161}
	DCC	18q21	{1856,2516}
	SMAD4	18q21	{299}
Methylation	DNMT2	10p15.1	{2436}
Proteolysis	Testisin	16p13	{1116}
	KALK13	19q13	{409}
	NES1/KLK10	19q13	{1577}
Protein interaction	RNF4	4p16.2	{2055}
Unknown	hH-Rev107	11q12-13	{2407}

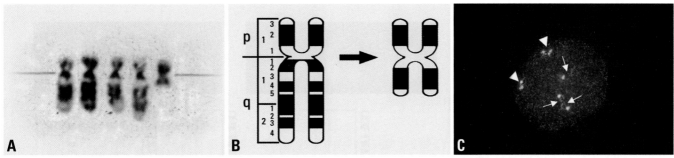

Fig. 4.03 Germ cell tumours genetics. **A** Example of G-banding of chromosomes 12 (left) and an isochromosome 12p (i(12p), right) isolated from a primary non-seminoma of the adult testis. **B** Schematic representation of a normal chromosome 12 (left) and an i(12p) (right). **C** Representative example of fluorescent in situ hybridization on an interphase nucleus of a cell line derived from a primary non-seminoma of the adult testis. The centromeric region of chromosome 12 is stained in red, while part of 12p is stained in green. Note the presence of three normal chromosomes 12 (paired single red and green signals, indicated by an arrow), and two i(12p)s (paired single red and double green signals, indicated by an arrowhead).

Karyotyping, FISH, CGH and spectral karyotyping (SKY) {388-390,1360,1794, 1854,1988,2217,2535,2692} revealed a complex but highly similar pattern of over- and underrepresentation of (parts of) chromosomes in seminomas and non-seminomas. Parts of chromosomes 4, 5, 11, 13, 18 and Y are underrepresented, while (parts of) chromosomes 7, 8, 12 and X are overrepresented. Seminomas have significantly more copies of the chromosomes 7, 15, 17, 19, and 22, explaining their higher DNA content {2235,2692}. This supports a common origin of all histological subtypes of these tumours, in accordance to findings in TGCTs, composed of both a seminoma and a non-seminoma component {388, 880,2250}.

Overrepresentation of 12p and candidate genes
The only consistent structural chromoso-

mal aberration in invasive TGCTs is gain of 12p-sequences, most often as i(12p) {2290}, for review. The i(12p) was initially reported in 1982 by Atkin and Baker {129,130}, and subsequently found to be characteristic for TGCTs [{1743}, for review]. Molecular analysis showed that the i(12p) is of uniparental origin {2428} indicating that its mechanism is doubling of the p-arm of one chromosome, and loss of the q-arm, instead of non sister

chromatin exchange {1827}. Interestingly, i(12p) is not restricted to the seminomas and non-seminomas of the testis, but is also detected in these types of tumours in the ovary, anterior mediastinum and midline of the brain. The majority of TGCTs, up to 80%, have i(12p) {2692}, while the remaining cases also show additional copies of (part of) 12p {2216,2529}. This leads to the conclusion that gain of 12p-sequences is

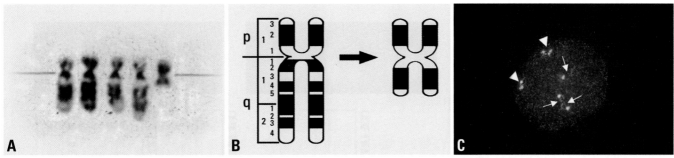

Fig. 4.04 Teratoma of the adult testis. Fluorescent immunohistochemical detection of centrosome hypertrophy on a histological section. The centrosomes are stained in red, and the nuclei are counterstained in blue (DAPI). Normal centrosomes are indicated by an arrow, and hypertrophic centrosomes by an arrowhead.

Table 4.04
Summary of the investigated proto-oncogenes studied for their involvement in the pathogenesis of TGCTs. The candidates are classified based on the supposed biological pathway. Their chromosomal localization is indicated, as well as the references.

(Putative) pathway	Gene	Chromosomal localization	Reference(s)
Cell cycle control	CCNB	5q12	{175}
	CCND2	12p13	{174,1128,2325,2436}
	CCNA	13q12.3-13	{175}
	CCNE	19q1	{175}
Cell survival/ apoptosis	c-KIT	4q12	{2135,2517,2518,2615}
	FAS	10q24	{2557}
	DAD-R	12p11.2	{2914}
	MDM2	12q14-15	{1301,2199}
	TCL1	14q32.1	{1869}
Translation	E1F3S8	16p11.2	{2251}
Transcription	MYCL1	1p34	{2436}
	MYCN	2p24	{2436}
	MYBL2	20q13	{2436}
Signalling	RHOA	3p21	{1262}
	KRAS2	12p12	{834,1829,1953,2192,2436}
	GRB7	17q11	{2436}
	JUP1	17q11	{2436}
Stem cell biology	HIWI	12q24	{2123}
Unknown	POV1	11q12	{2436}

crucial for the development of this cancer, in particular related to invasive growth {2236}.

Several candidate genes have been proposed to explain the gain of 12p in TGCTs. These included KRAS2, which is rarely mutated and sometimes overexpressed in TGCTs {1818,1829,1953, 2192,2436}, and cyclin D2 (CCND2) {1128,2325,2404,2436}. The latter might be involved via a deregulated G1-S checkpoint. A more focused approach to the identification of candidate genes was initiated by the finding of a metastatic seminoma with a high level of amplification of a restricted region of 12p, cytogenetically identified as 12p11.2-p12.1 {2530}. Subsequently, primary TGCTs have been found with such an amplification {1360,1793,1795,2147,2221,2914}. The 12p-amplicon occurs in about 8-10% of primary seminomas, particularly in those lacking an i(12p) {2914}, and it is much rarer in non-seminomas. This suggests the existence of two pathways leading to overrepresentation of certain genes on 12p, either via isochromosome formation, or an alternative mechanism, possibly followed by high level amplification. The seminomas with amplification have a reduced sensitivity to apoptosis for which DAD-R is a promising candidate {2914}. Probably more genes on 12p, in particular in the amplicon, help the tumour cells to overcome apoptosis {807}.

Molecular genetic alterations
Multiple studies on the possible role of inactivation of tumour suppressor genes and activation of proto-oncogenes in the development of TGCTs have been reported. Interpretation of the findings must be done with caution if the data derived from the tumours are compared to normal testicular parenchyma, which does not contain the normal counterpart of the cell of origin of this cancer.

A significant difference in genome methylation has been reported between seminomas (hypomethylated) and non-seminomas (hypermethylated) {882,2443}. This could reflect simply their embryonic origin, and the capacity of the non-seminomas to mimic embryonal and extra embryonal development. This is for example supported by their pattern of expression of OCT3/4, also known as POU5F1 {2003} X-inactivation {1538}, as well as their telomerase activity.

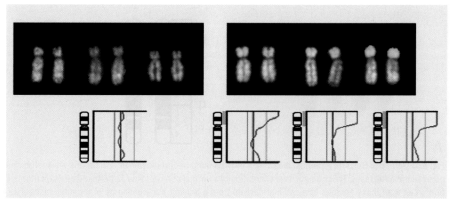

Fig. 4.05 Comparative genomic hybridization on isolated intratubular germ cell neoplasia unclassified (left) and three different histological variants of an invasive primary non-seminoma of the adult testis (left is embryonal carcinoma, middle is teratoma, and right is yolk sac tumour). Note the absence of gain of 12p in the precursor lesion, while it is present in the various types of invasive elements.

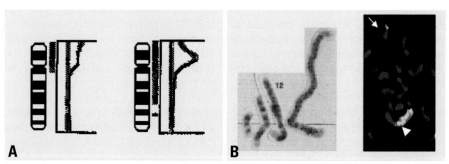

Fig. 4.06 Germ cell tumours genetics. **A** Representative comparative genomic hybridization results on chromosome 12 of a seminoma with an i(12p) (left panel), and gain of the short arm of chromosome 12, and additionally a restricted high level amplification. **B** G-banding (left) and fluorescent in situ hybridization with a 12p-specific probe stained in green on a metaphase spread of a primary testicular seminoma with a restricted 12p amplification (chromosomes are counterstained in red) (right). Note the presence of a normal chromosome 12 (indicated by an arrow) and a chromosome 12 with a high level amplification (indicated by an arrowhead).

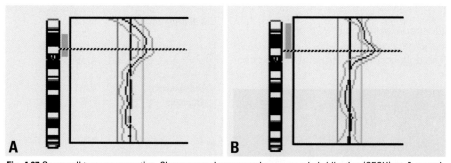

Fig. 4.07 Germ cell tumours genetics. Chromosomal expressed sequence hybridization (CESH) on **A** a seminoma with an isochromosome 12p, and **B** a seminoma with a restricted 12p amplification. Note the predominant expression of genes mapped within the 12p11.2-p12.2 region in both the seminoma with and without the restricted amplification. These data indicate that genes from this region are involved in the development of this cancer, even without the presence of a restricted amplification.

Several studies have been done to identify genomic deletions, in particular by means of detection of loss of heterozygosity (LOH), with the goal to identify candidate tumour suppressor gene-loci. However, because of the aneuploid DNA content of TGCTs, as well as their embryonic nature, these data have to be interpreted with caution {1536}. In fact, aneuploid cells are thought to predominantly loose genomic sequences, resulting in LOH, expected to affect about 200.000 regions, which might not be involved in initiation of the malignant process at all {1524}. In addition, pluripotent embryonic stem cells show a different mutation frequency and type compared to somatic cells {397}. In fact, embryonic cells show a higher tendency to chromosome loss and reduplication, leading to uniparental disomies, which are detected as LOH.

So far, the majority of LOH studies focused on parts of chromosomes 1, 3, 5, 11, 12 and 18 {162,672,1384,1536, 1560,1645,1853,1855,1856,2045}. Recurrent losses have been identified on 1p13, p22, p31.3-p32, 1q32, 3p, 5p15.1-p15.2, q11, q14, q21, and q34-qter, 12q13 and q22, and 18q. No candidate gene has yet been identified at 12q22 {162} in spite of the identification of a homozygous deletion. Some of the candidate tumour suppressor genes mapped in the deleted genomic regions in TGCTs have been investigated; for review see ref. {1541}.

TP53 and microsatellite instability and treatment response

Immunohistochemistry demonstrates a high level of wild type TP53 protein in TGCTs. However, inactivating mutations are hardly found. This led to the view that high levels of wild type TP53 might explain the exquisite chemosensitivity of TGCTs. However, it has been shown that this is an oversimplification [{1301}, for review], and that inactivation of TP53 explains only a minority of treatment resistant TGCTs {1129}. In fact, the overall sensitivity of TGCTs might be related to their embryonic origin, in contrast to the majority of solid cancers.

Chemoresistance of seminomas and non-seminomas has been related to high level genomic amplifications at 1q31-32, 2p23-24, 7q21, 7q31, 9q22, 9q32-34, 15q23-24, and 20q11.2-12 {2147}. The *XPA* gene, involved in DNA repair, maps to 9q22. Low expression of *XPA* has been related to the sensitivity of TGCT to cisplatin based chemotherapy {1342}, possibly due to a reduced nucleotide excision repair. A high expression of the DNA base excision repair has been suggested for chemoresistance in TGCTs {2212}. Another mechanism of resistance against cisplatin is interruption of the link between DNA damage and apoptosis. The mismatch repair pathway (MMR) is most likely involved in the detection of DNA damage, and initiation of apoptotic programs rather than

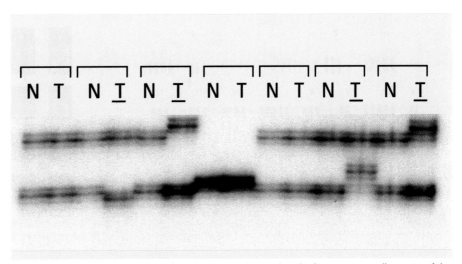

Fig. 4.08 Microsatellite instability (MSI) at locus D2S123 in a series of refractory germ cell tumours of the adult. Shown are the results in normal peripheral blood DNA (indicated by "N") and matched tumour DNA ("T"). The underlined cases show MSI.

repair. Disturbed MMR, apparent from microsatellite instability (MSI), is a frequent finding in cisplatin refractory non-seminomas {1652}, but not in TGCTs in general {603,1561,1652,1857,2044}. However, so far, immunohistochemical demonstration of MMR factors cannot predict MSI in these cancers.

Expression profiles

Three independent studies using array DNA and cDNA CGH on TGCTs have been reported. The first {2436} showed that gene expression profiling is able to distinguish the various histological types of TGCTs using hierarchical cluster analysis based on 501 differentially expressed genes. In addition, it was found that the GRB7 and JUP genes are overexpressed from the long arm of chromosome 17 and are therefore interesting candidates for further investigation. The other two studies focus on the short arm of chromosome 12, i.p. the p11.2-p12.1 region. That this region is indeed of interest is demonstrated by the finding that TGCTs without a restricted 12p amplification do show preferential overexpression of genes from this region {2219}. Two putative candidate genes (related to the ESTs Unigene cluster Hs.22595 and Hs.62275) referred to as GCT1 and 2 genes were identified to be overexpressed in TGCTs {300}. However, these candidates map outside the region of interest as found by earlier studies and are expressed ubiquitously. The second study on 12p {2219}, reports that BCAT1

is an interesting candidate for non-seminomas specifically, while a number of candidates were identified within the region of interest on 12p, including *EKI*1, and amongst others a gene related to ESTs AJ 511866. Recent findings indicating specific regions of amplification within the amplicon itself {1545,2915} will facilitate further investigation of the gene(s) involved.

Animal models

A number of animal models have been suggested to be informative for the development of TGCTs, like the mouse teratocarcinoma {1580,1581,2771}, the seminomas of the rabbit {2717}, horse {2716}, and dog {1539}, as well as the HPV-{1351}, and more recently the *GDNF* induced seminomatous tumours in mice {1712}. However, none of these include all the characteristics of human TGCTs, like their origin from IGCNU, embryonic characteristics, their postpubertal manifestation, and the possible combination of seminoma and non-seminoma. Therefore, data derived from these models must be interpreted with caution in the context of the pathogenesis of TGCTs. However, the mouse teratocarcinomas and canine seminomas, are most likely informative models for the infantile teratomas and yolk sac tumours and the spermatocytic seminomas, respectively.

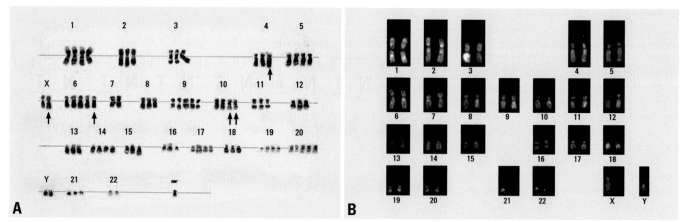

Fig. 4.09 Spermatocytic seminoma. **A** Example of G-banding on a metaphase spread. **B** Comparative genomic hybridization of DNA isolated from the same tumour. Note the almost complete absence of structural anomalies, while numerical changes are present. Gain of chromosome 9 is the only consistent anomaly identified.

Precursor lesions

Intratubular germ cell neoplasia, unclassified type (IGCNU)

Definition
Germ cells with abundant vacuolated cytoplasm, large, irregular nuclei and prominent nucleoli located within the seminiferous tubules.

ICD-O code   9064/2

Synonyms
Intratubular malignant germ cell, carcinoma in situ, intratubular preinvasive tumour, gonocytoma in situ, testicular intraepithelial neoplasia, intratubular atypical germ cells and intratubular malignant germ cells.

Epidemiology
Adults
In adults with history of cryptorchidism intratubular germ cell neoplasia, unclassified are seen in 2-4% {345,787,887, 1010,1124,2040,2131,2222} in contrast to 0.5% in young children {501}. In infertility studies, the prevalence is about 1% {233,345,1900,2346, 2430,2943} ranging from 0-5%. Patients with intersex syndrome, and a Y chromosome have intratubular germ cell neoplasia of the unclassified type (IGCNU) in 6-25% of cases {118,387,1831,2140, 2826}. Testes harbouring a germ cell tumour contain IGCNU in a mean of 82.4% of cases, ranging from 63 {889} -99% {346}. Since the risk of tumour development in the contralateral testis is increased about 25-50 fold {615,1985, 2774}, some centres in Europe have initiated biopsies of the contralateral testis, with detection rates of IGCNU of 4.9-5.7% {613,2749}. IGCNU is detected in 42% of patients who presented with retroperitoneal germ cell tumours {262,555,1100} but is rarely found in patients with mediastinal tumours {997}.

Several autopsy studies have shown that the incidence of IGCNU is the same as the incidence of germ cell tumours in the general population {616,891}.

Children
In contrast to their adult counterpart, the true incidence of prepubertal IGCNU is difficult to assess. IGCNU has only rarely been described in association with testicular maldescent, intersex states and in a very few case reports of infantile yolk sac tumour and teratoma {1134,1381, 2018,2167,2482,2483}.
IGCNU is seen in association with cryptorchidism is 2–8% of patients {1381}. Four of 4 patients with gonadal dysgenesis in one series had intratubular germ cell neoplasia of the unclassified type (IGCNU) {1833} as did 3 of 12 patients with androgen insensitivity (testicular feminization) syndrome {1831}. In review of the literature Ramani et al. found IGCNU in 2 of 87 cases of different intersex states {2140}.

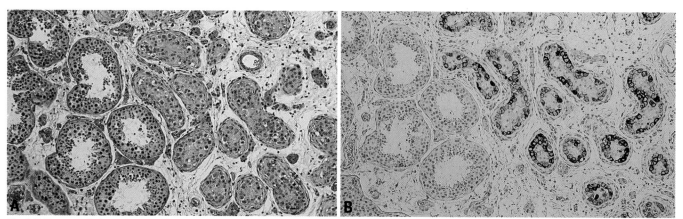

Fig. 4.10 Precursor lesions of germ cell tumours. **A** Intratubular germ cell neoplasia (IGCNU) adjacent to normal seminiferous tubules. **B** Positive PLAP staining in the intratubular germ cell neoplasia (IGCNU) adjacent to normal seminiferous tubules.

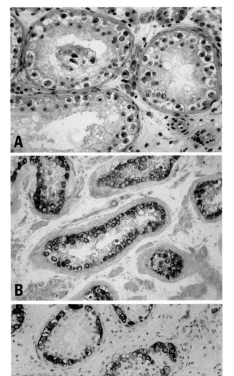

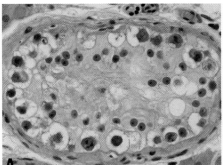

Fig. 4.11 Precursor lesions of germ cell tumours. **A** Typical pattern of intratubular germ cell tumour unclassified. **B** PAS staining for glycogen in the malignant germ cells. **C** Positive PLAP staining in the malignant germ cells.

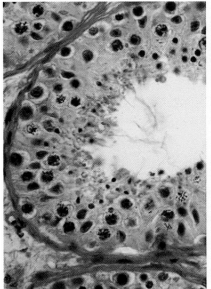

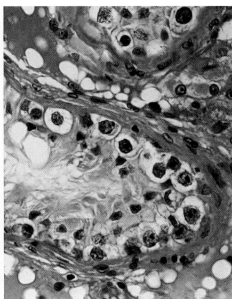

Fig. 4.12 Comparison of morphological features of normal seminiferous tubules (left part) and intratubular germ cell neoplasia (IGCNU) in seminiferous tubules (right part).

The morphologic and the immunohistochemical features of normal prepubertal germ cells resemble those of IGCNU and can persist up to 8 months to one year of age {118}. Therefore, the validity of prepubertal IGCNU needs further investigation. One study found no testicular cancer in 12 of the 22 prepubertal patients, with mean 25 years follow up, who were biopsied during orchidopexy and found to have placental alkaline phosphatase (PLAP) positive atypical appearing germ cells {996}. The absence of isochromosome 12p in testicular germ cell tumours of childhood, suggests that the pathogenesis of germ cell tumours in children may be different than in adults.

Clinical features

The symptoms and signs are those of the associated findings, including atrophic testis, infertility, maldescended testis, overt tumour and intersex features.

Macroscopy

There is no grossly visible lesion specific for IGCNU.

Histopathology

The malignant germ cells are larger than normal spermatogonia. They have abundant clear or vacuolated cytoplasm that is rich in glycogen, as demonstrated by periodic acid-Schiff (PAS) stains. The nuclei are large, irregular and hyperchromatic with one or more large, irregular nucleoli. Mitoses, including abnormal ones, are not uncommon. The cells are usually basally located between Sertoli cells. Spermatogenesis is commonly absent, but occasionally one can see a pagetoid spread in tubules with spermatogenesis. The tubular involvement is often segmental but may be diffuse. The malignant germ cells are also seen in the rete and even in the epididymal ducts. Isolated malignant germ cells in the interstitium or lymphatics represent microinvasive disease. A lymphocytic response often accompanies both intratubular and microinvasive foci.

Immunoprofile

PLAP can be demonstrated in 83-99% of intratubular germ cell neoplasia of the unclassified type (IGCNU) cases and is widely used for diagnosis {189,345,346, 888,1100,1199,1345,1615,2763}. Other markers include: CD117 (c-kit) {1191, 1302,1619,2518}, M2A {157,890}, 43-9F {889,1054,2061} and TRA-1-60 {97,151, 886}. These markers are heterogeneously expressed in IGCNU, for example: TRA-1-60 is seen in tubules adjacent to

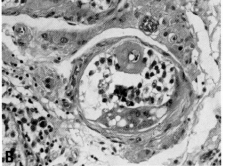

Fig. 4.13 Precursor lesions of germ cell tumours. **A** Intratubular germ cell neoplasia, unclassified. Note the large nuclei with multiple nucleoli. **B** Syncytiotrophoblasts in a tubule with intratubular germ cell neoplasia (IGCNU).

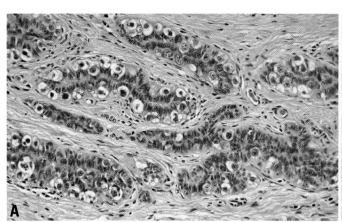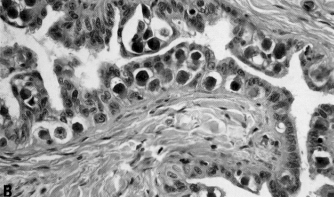

Fig. 4.14 Intratubular germ cell neoplasia (IGCNU). A Spread of malignant germ cells to rete. B Higher magnification discloses cytological features of IGCNU.

non-seminomatous germ cell tumours but not seminoma {886}. If both tumour types are present, the expression is even more heterogeneous.

Ultrastructure
By electron microscopy the IGCNU are very similar to prespermatogenic germ cells in their early stage of differentiation {911,1895,2409}.

Differential diagnosis
IGCNU has to be distinguished from spermatogenic arrest at spermatogonia stage, which lacks the nuclear features of IGCNU and PLAP reactivity. Giant spermatogonia have a round nucleus with evenly dispersed chromatin and are solitary and widely scattered. Intratubular seminoma distends and completely obliterates the lumina of the involved tubules. Intratubular spermatocytic seminoma shows the 3 characteristic cell types.

Genetics
The DNA content of IGCNU has been reported to be between hypotriploid and hypopentaploid {567,676,1830,1900}. In fact, the chromosomal constitution of IGCNU, adjacent to an invasive TGCT is highly similar to the invasive tumours, with the absence of gain of 12p being the major difference {1543,2216,2236,2536}. It can therefore be concluded that gain of 12p is not the initiating event in the development of TGCTs, in line with earlier observations {861}. This demonstrates that polyploidization precedes formation of i(12p). These findings support the model that IGCNU in its karyotypic evolution is only one step behind invasive TGCTs {1964}. CGH has shown that IGCNU adjacent to invasive TGCTs have

less frequent loss of parts of chromosome 4 and 13, and gain of 2p {2694}.

Prognosis
About 50% of cases progress to invasive germ cell tumours in 5 years and about 90% do so in 7 years. These statements are based on retrospective follow-up of infertile men with IGCNU or prospective surveillance of patients with a treated TGCT or IGCNU in the contralateral testis {233,2750}. Rare cases may not progress {345,892,2116,2431}.

Tumours of one histological type

Seminoma

Definition
A germ cell tumour of fairly uniform cells, typically with clear or dense glycogen

containing cytoplasm, a large regular nucleus, with one or more nucleoli, and well defined cell borders.

ICD-O code   9061/3

Epidemiology
The increase in the incidence of testicular germ cell tumours in white populations affects seminoma and non-seminomatous neoplasms equally, the rate doubling about every 30 years. In non white populations trends in incidence are not uniform including both an increase (Singapore Chinese, New Zealand Maoris and Japanese) and no increase (US Blacks) {2017,2132}.

Clinical features
Signs and symptoms
The most common mode of presentation is testicular enlargement, which is usually painless. Hydrocele may be present.

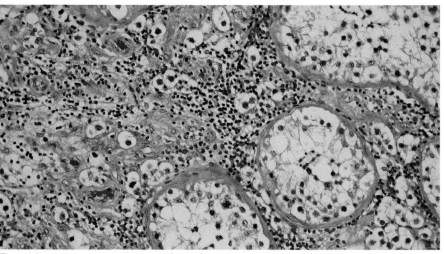

Fig. 4.15 Intratubular germ cell neoplasia (IGCNU) and microinvasion. Note the lymphocytic infiltration.

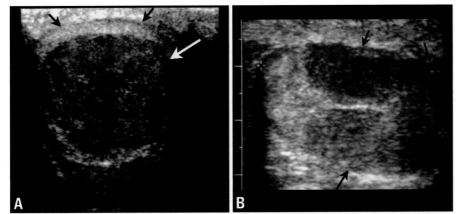

Fig. 4.16 Seminoma. **A** Transverse ultrasound image of the testis shows a large, well defined, uniformly hypoechoic mass (white arrow). A small rim of normal, more hyperechoic, parenchyma remains (black arrows). **B** Longitudinal ultrasound image of the testis shows lobular, well defined, hypoechoic mass (arrows).

Imaging

Seminoma has one of the more sonographically characteristic appearances of the testicular tumours. They are generally well defined and uniformly hypoechoic. Seminomas can be lobulated or multinodular; however, these nodules are most commonly in continuity with one another. Larger tumours can completely replace the normal parenchyma and may be more heterogeneous.

Tumour spread

Seminoma metastasizes initially via lymphatics to the paraaortic lymph nodes, and afterward to the mediastinal and supraclavicular nodes. Haematogeneous spread occurs later and involves liver, lung, bones and other organs.

Macroscopy

The affected testis is usually enlarged although a proportion of seminomas occurs in an atrophic gonad. A small hydrocoele may be present but it is unusual for seminoma to spread into the vaginal sac. Veins in the tunica are prominent. Characteristically a seminoma forms a grey, cream or pale pink soft homogeneous lobulated mass with a clear cut edge and may have irregular foci of yellow necrosis. Cyst formation and haemorrhage are uncommon. Nodules separate from the main mass may be seen and occasionally the tumour is composed of numerous macroscopically distinct nodules. Tumour spread into the epididymis and cord is rare.

Histopathology

Seminomas are typically composed of uniform cells arranged in sheets or divided into clusters or columns by fine fibrous trabeculae associated with a lymphocytic infiltrate, which may be dense with follicle formation. Plasma cells and eosinophils may also occur on occasion. Less frequently appearances include dense fibrous bands and "cystic" spaces produced by oedema within the tumour. Granulomatous reaction and fibrosis are common and occasionally so extensive that the neoplasm is obscured. Seminomas usually obliterate testicular architecture but other growth patterns include: interstitial invasion (or microinvasion) in a small tumour insufficient to produce a palpable or macroscopic mass or at the edge of a large tumour; intratubular infiltration; pagetoid spread along the rete. Seminoma cells are round or polygonal with a distinct membrane. Cytoplasm is usually clear reflecting the glycogen or lipid content. Less commonly, they have more densely staining cytoplasm. Nuclei contain prominent nucleoli, which may be bar shaped. Mitoses are variable in number.

Variants

Cribriform, pseudoglandular and tubular variants of seminoma

The seminoma cells may be arranged in a nested pseudoglandular/alveolar or "cribriform" pattern with sparse lymphocytes {549}. A tubular pattern may occur, resembling Sertoli cell tumour {2892}. Confirmation of pure seminoma may require demonstration of positive staining for placental alkaline phosphatase (PLAP) and CD117 (C-Kit) with negative staining for inhibin, alpha-fetoprotein (AFP) and CD30.

Seminoma with high mitotic rate

Seminomas with a greater degree of cellular pleomorphism, higher mitotic activity and a sparsity of stromal lymphocytes have been called atypical seminoma,

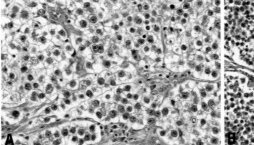
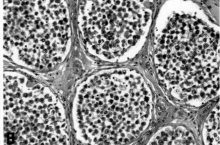
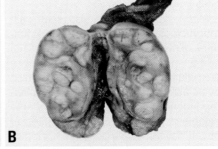
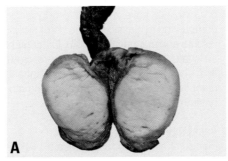

Fig. 4.17 Seminoma. **A** Typical homogenous whitish seminoma. **B** Nodular architecture.

Fig. 4.18 Seminoma. **A** Seminoma cells with finely granular eosinophilic cytoplasm. **B** Intratubular typical seminoma.

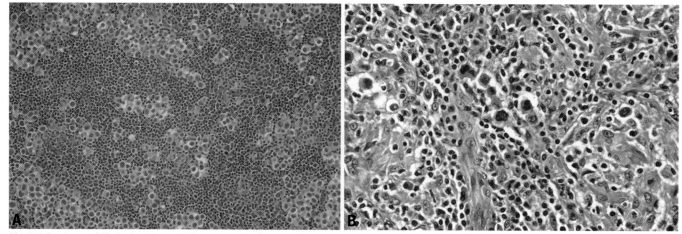

Fig. 4.19 Seminoma. **A** Typical seminoma with pronounced infiltration of lymphocytes. **B** Granulomatous stromal response.

anaplastic seminoma, or seminoma with high mitotic index {1805,1809,2603}. These are not always subdivided into a separate category of seminoma because their clinical outcome is similar to classical seminoma {2542,2946}. However, some studies indicate that seminomas with high mitotic counts, higher S-phase fraction, increased mean nuclear volume, and aneuploidy have a poorer prognosis {1778,2780}, higher incidence of metastasis {817,1122}, and are at a higher stage at clinical presentation {1873,2616}. The prognostic significance of these features, however, remains controversial {444}.

Seminoma with syncytiotrophoblastic cells

Tumour giant cells are also seen with morphological and ultrastructural features of syncytiotrophoblastic cells (STC) {2355}. The STCs are usually multinucleate with abundant slightly basophilic cytoplasm, and may have intracytoplasmic lacunae, although some have sparse cytoplasm with crowded aggregates of nuclei having a "mulberry-like" appear-ance. They may be surrounded by localized areas of haemorrhage although they are not associated with cytotrophoblastic cells, and do not have the features of choriocarcinoma. These cells stain for hCG and other pregnancy related proteins and cytokeratins {550}.

Up to 7% of classical seminomas have recognizable STCs, however, hCG positive cells may be identified in up to 25% of seminomas {1202,1803} some of which are mononuclear cells.

The presence of hCG positive cells is frequently associated with elevated serum hCG (typically in the 100s mIU/ml) {1033}. Higher levels may indicate bulky disease but possibly choriocarcinoma {1123,2806}. Seminomas with STCs or elevated serum hCG do not have a poorer prognosis in comparison to classic seminoma of similar volume and stage {1123,2806}. Other giant cells are frequently seen in seminomas and may be non neoplastic Langhans giant cells associated with the inflammatory stromal response.

Immunoprofile

Placental alkaline phosphatase (PLAP) is seen diffusely in 85-100% of classical seminomas with a membranous or perinuclear dot pattern {444,2664} and persists in necrotic areas {780}. C-Kit (CD117) has a similar established incidence and distribution {1478,2616}. VASA is extensively positive {2929}. Angiotensin 1-converting enzyme (CD 143) resembles PLAP and CD117 in distribution {2618} but is not in widespread diagnostic use. In contrast, pancytokeratins (Cam 5.2 and AE1/3) and CD30 are less frequently seen and usually have a focal distribution {444,2616}. In differential diagnostic contexts the following are helpful:

Seminoma versus embryonal carcinoma – a combination of negative CD117 and positive CD30 {1478,2664}, widespread membranous pancytokeratins, CK8, 18 or 19 {2664}, support embryonal carcinoma; classical seminoma versus spermatocytic seminoma – widespread PLAP indicates the former.

Differential diagnosis

Seminomas are occasionally misdiagnosed {1463,2353}. Rarely, the distinc-

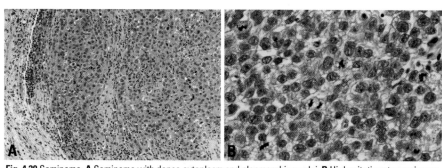

Fig. 4.20 Seminoma. **A** Seminoma with dense cytoplasm and pleomorphic nuclei. **B** High mitotic rate seminoma.

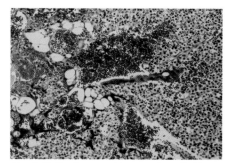

Fig. 4.21 Seminoma with syncytiotrophoblasts. Note the association with haemorrhage.

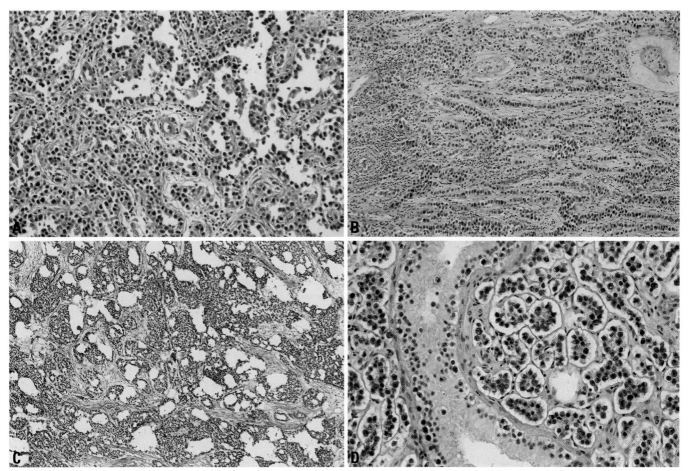

Fig. 4.22 Seminoma. **A** Pseudoglandular variant of seminoma. **B** Cords of tumour cells in seminoma. **C** Cribriform variant of seminoma. **D** Alveolar variant of seminoma.

tion between seminoma and embryonal carcinoma is difficult with respect to an area within a tumour or the entire neoplasm. Morphological discrimination features include: the discrete uniform cells of seminoma which contrast with the pleomorphic overlapping cells of embryonal carcinoma; the lymphocytic and granulomatous response typical of seminoma but rare in embryonal carcinoma. PLAP and CD117 are distributed more diffusely in seminoma than embryonal

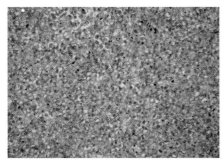

Fig. 4.23 Positive staining for PLAP in typical seminoma.

carcinoma, whereas CD30 and pancytokeratin are more pronounced in embryonal carcinoma. The florid lymphocytic or granulomatous response within seminoma occasionally prompts the misdiagnosis of an inflammatory lesion, especially on frozen section. Extensive sampling and a high power search for seminoma cells (supported by PLAP and CD117 content) help reduce such errors. Conversely, other tumours are occasionally misinterpreted as classical seminoma, possibly as a consequence of their rarity, these include: spermatocytic seminoma, Leydig cell tumours, (especially those with clear/vacuolated cytoplasm); Sertoli cell tumours, in which tubule formation may resemble the tubular variant of seminoma; metastases (e.g. melanoma). In all these neoplasms, the absence of IGCNU and the demonstration of either the typical seminoma immunophenotype or the immunocytochemical features of Leydig, Sertoli or the specific metastatic tumour should limit error.

Prognosis and predictive factors

The size of the primary seminoma, necrosis, vascular space, and tunical invasion have all been related to clinical stage at presentation {1626,2616}. With respect to patients with stage I disease managed on high surveillance protocols, retrospective studies have emphasized the size of the primary and invasion of the rete testis as independent predictors of relapse {1202,2781}. The 4 year relapse free survivals were 94, 82 and 64% for tumours <3, 3-6 and ≥6 cm, respectively {2751}. Blood and lymphatic channel invasion was seen more commonly in association with relapse but statistical significance is not consistent. Views are not uniform on the value of cytokeratins and CD30 for predicting prognosis {444,2616}.

Spermatocytic seminoma

Definition

A tumour composed of germ cells that

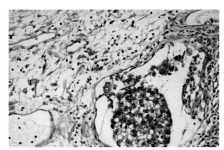

Fig. 4.24 Seminoma. Vascular invasion.

vary in size from lymphocyte-like to giant cells of about 100 μm in diameter, with the bulk of the tumour composed of cells of intermediate size.

ICD-O code   9063/3

Epidemiology

Spermatocytic seminoma is rare, its frequency varying from 1.2 to 4.5 percent {347,1195,2565}. There is no difference in race predilection from other germ cell tumours. In a series of 79 cases {347} none of the patients had a history of cryptorchidism.

Clinical features

Most tumours occur in the older male with an average age of 52 years but it can also be encountered in patients in their third decade of life. Spermatocytic seminoma occurs only in the testis, unlike other germ cell tumours, which may be seen in the ovary and elsewhere. Most tumours are unilateral. Bilateral tumours are more often metachronous {220,347,2565}. Generally symptoms

consist of painless swelling of variable duration {347}. Serum tumour markers are negative.

Macroscopy

The size ranges from 2 to 20 cm with an average of 7 cm {347}. The tumours are often soft, well circumscribed with bulging mucoid cut surfaces. They have been described as lobulated, cystic, haemorrhagic and even necrotic. Extension into paratesticular tissue has been rarely reported {2349}.

Histopathology

The tumour cells are noncohesive and are supported by a scant or oedematous stroma. The oedema may cause a "pseudoglandular" pattern. Collagen bands may enclose tumour compartments. Lymphocytic infiltration and granulomatous stromal reaction are only rarely seen. The tumour consists typically of 3 basic cell types {347,1195,1644, 1800,1805,2229,2349}. The predominant cell type is round of varying size with variable amounts of eosinophilic cytoplasm. Glycogen is not demonstrable. The round nucleus often has a lacy chromatin distribution with a filamentous or spireme pattern similar to that seen in spermatocytes. The second type is a small cell with dark staining nuclei and scant eosinophilic cytoplasm. The third cell type is a mono-, rarely multinucleated giant cell with round, oval or indented nuclei. These often have the typical spireme like chromatin distribution. Sometimes, the cells are relatively monotonous with prominent nucleoli

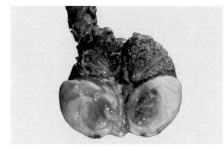

Fig. 4.25 Spermatocytic seminoma. Note the mucoid appearence.

although wider sampling reveals characteristic areas {55}. Mitoses, including abnormal forms are frequent.

There may be vascular, tunical and epididymal invasion. The adjacent seminiferous tubules often show intratubular growth. The malignant germ cells (IGCNU) in adjacent tubules typically associated with other germ cell tumours are not present.

Immunoprofile

Many of the markers useful in other types of germ cell tumour are generally negative in spermatocytic seminoma. VASA is diffusely reactive {2929} PLAP has been observed in isolated or small groups of tumour cells {346,347,582}. Cytokeratin 18 has been demonstrated in a dot-like pattern {527,784}. NY-ESO-1, a cancer specific antigen, was found in 8 of 16 spermatocytic seminomas but not in other germ cell tumours {2299}. AFP, hCG, CEA, actin, desmin, LCA, CD30 are not demonstrable. CD117 (c-kit) has been reported to be positive {2299}, but others had negative results. Germ cell

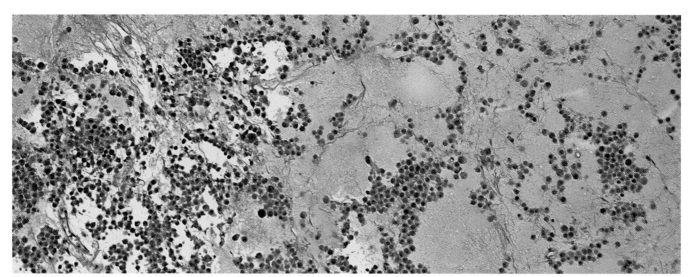

Fig. 4.26 Spermatocytic seminoma devoid of stroma and very edematous.

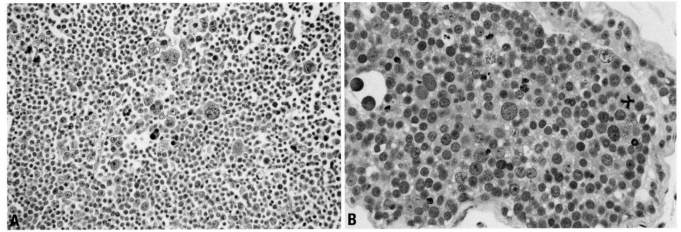

Fig. 4.27 Spermatocytic seminoma. **A** Note the three different cell types of spermatocytic seminoma. **B** Intratubular spread of spermatocytic seminoma.

maturation stage specific markers, including SCP1 (synaptonemal complex protein 1), SSX (synovial sarcoma on X chromosome) and XPA (xeroderma pigmentosum type A1), have been demonstrated {2512}.

Ultrastructure
The cell membranes lack folds and indentations. There are intercellular bridges like those between primary spermatocytes {2226}. Gap junctions and macula adherens type junctions can be observed. The chromatin is either homogeneously dispersed or has dense condensations and nucleoli have net-like nucleolonema {2299}.

Differential diagnosis
Spermatocytic seminoma, when misinterpreted, is most frequently classified as typical seminoma or lymphoma. Seminoma, however, usually has a fibrous stroma, a lymphocytic and/or granulomatous stromal reaction and cells with abundant glycogen, PLAP positivity, and IGCNU component. Lymphoma has a predominant interstitial growth pattern and lacks the spireme chromatin distribution.

Genetics
The DNA content of spermatocytic seminoma is different from that of seminoma, including diploid or near hyperdiploid values {582,1832,2234,2568}. Small cells have been reported to be diploid or near diploid by cytophotometry {2555}, the intermediate cells have intermediate values and the giant tumour cells up to 42C. Haploid cells have not been reported {1385,2568}. These data are in keeping with the finding that spermatocytic semi-

noma cells show characteristics of cells undergoing meiosis, a feature that is diagnostically helpful {2512}. CGH and karyotyping show mostly numerical chromosomal aberrations. The gain of chromosome 9 in all spermatocytic seminomas appears to be a nonrandom chromosome imbalance {2234}. The presence of common chromosomal imbalances in a bilateral spermatocytic seminoma and immunohistochemical characteristics {2512} suggests that the initiating event may occur during intra-uterine development, before the germ cells populate the gonadal ridges. This might explain the relatively frequent occurrence of bilateral spermatocytic seminoma (5% of the cases). No gene or genes involved in the pathogenesis of spermatocytic seminomas have been identified yet, although *puf-8* recently identified in C. *elegans* might be an interesting candidate {2524}.

Prognosis
Only one documented case of metastatic pure spermatocytic seminoma has been reported {1646}.

Spermatocytic seminoma with sarcoma

Definition
A spermatocytic seminoma associated with an undifferentiated or, less frequently, with a differentiated sarcoma.

Clinical features
Approximately a dozen cases of this tumour have been reported. The age range is 34-68 years. There is no familial

association, and no etiologic agents have been identified. The typical patient has a slowly growing mass that suddenly enlarges within months of diagnosis. Fifty percent of patients have metastases at diagnosis. Levels of serum alpha-fetoprotein and human chorionic gonadotropin are normal.

Macroscopy
Typically the tumour is a large (up to 25 cm), bulging mass with variegated cut surface exhibiting areas of induration, necrosis, and focal myxoid change.

Histopathology
The spermatocytic seminoma component frequently has foci of marked pleomorphism {647}, and is histologically contiguous with the sarcoma component. The sarcoma can exhibit various patterns - rhabdomyosarcoma, spindle cell sarcoma, and chondrosarcoma {347,783, 1649,1800,2646}.

Differential diagnosis
The primary differential diagnosis is sarcomatous transformation of a testicular germ cell tumour {2665}. Absence of teratoma and recognition of the spermatocytic seminoma excludes this possibility. The differential diagnosis of a tumour where only the sarcoma component is sampled includes primary testicular sarcoma {408,2786,2950}, paratesticular sarcoma, and metastatic sarcoma or sarcomatoid carcinoma {510,753,769, 2146}.

Tumour spread and prognosis
The sarcomatous component metastasizes widely. Most patients die of metastatic tumour, with a median sur-

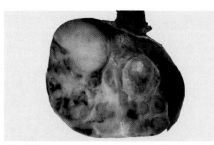

Fig. 4.28 Spermatocytic seminoma with sarcoma. Cut section: irregular, focally fibrotic, vaguely multinodular, variegated white to tan surface with foci of hemorrhage.

vival of one year. Only two have survived more than a year without disease. Systemic therapy has no effect {347,783, 1649 ,2646}.

Embryonal carcinoma

Definition
A tumour composed of undifferentiated cells of epithelial appearance with abundant clear to granular cytoplasm and a variety of growth patterns.

ICD-O code 9070/3

Synonym
Malignant teratoma, undifferentiated.

Epidemiology
Embryonal carcinoma occurs in pure form and as a tumour component in germ cell tumours of more than one histologic type (mixed germ cell tumours). In pure form embryonal carcinoma comprises only 2-10% while it occurs as a component in more than 80% of mixed germ cell tumours {1808}.

Clinical features
Signs and symptoms
It occurs first at puberty and has a peak incidence around 30 years of age, which is approximately 10 years before the peak incidence of classical seminoma. A painless swelling is the commonest clinical feature, though because of their propensity to grow faster than seminoma, they are more prone to present with testicular pain, which may mimic torsion. It may be found in a testis, which had been traumatized but did not appropriately resolve. Some patients present with symptoms referable to metastases and/or gynaecomastia.

Imaging
Embryonal carcinoma is often smaller than seminoma at the time of presentation and more heterogeneous and ill defined. The tunica albuginea may be invaded and the borders of the tumour are less distinct, often blending imperceptibly into the adjacent parenchyma. They are indistinguishable from mixed germ cell tumours.

Macroscopy
Embryonal carcinoma causes a slight or moderate enlargement of the testis often with distortion of the testicular contour. The average diameter at presentation is 4.0 cm. Local extension into the rete testis and epididymis or even beyond is not uncommon. The tumour tissue is soft and granular, grey or whitish to pink or tan often with foci of haemorrhage and necrosis. It bulges extensively from the cut surface and is often not well demarcated from the surrounding testicular tissue. It may contain occasional fibrous septae and ill defined cysts or clefts {1201,2664}.

Histopathology
The growth pattern varies from solid and syncytial to papillary with or without stromal fibrovascular cores, forming clefts or gland-like structures.
The tumour cells are undifferentiated, of epithelial appearance and not unlike the cells that form the inner cell mass of the very early embryo. They are large, polygonal or sometimes columnar with large irregular nuclei that usually are vesicular with a see through appearance, or they may be hyperchromatic. One or more large irregular nucleoli are present and the nuclear membranes are distinct. The cytoplasm is abundant, usually finely granular but may also be more or less clear. It stains from basophilic to amphophilic to eosinophilic. The cell borders are indistinct and the cells often tend to crowd with nuclei abutting or overlapping. Mitotic figures are frequent, includ-

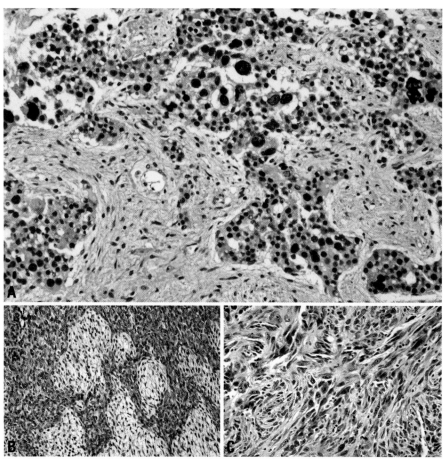

Fig. 4.29 Spermatocytic seminoma. **A** Spermatocytic seminoma associated with sarcoma. **B** Sarcomatous component of spermatocytic seminoma. **C** A sarcoma component that consists of a storiform pattern of undifferentiated, spindle shaped tumour cells.

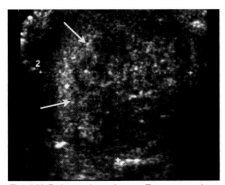

Fig. 4.30 Embryonal carcinoma. Transverse ultrasound image of the testis (cursors) shows an ill defined, irregular, heterogeneous mass (arrows).

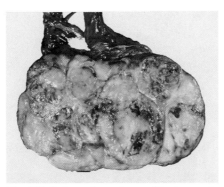

Fig. 4.31 Embryonal carcinoma. The tumour is fleshy and has foci of haemorrhage and necrosis.

ing abnormal forms. Syncytiotrophoblastic cells may occur scattered among the tumour cells as single cells or in small cell groups. Cells at the periphery of the solid tumour formations may appear degenerated, smudged or apoptotic resulting in a biphasic pattern that may mimic choriocarcinoma.

The stroma that varies from scant within the solid formations, to more abundant at the periphery of the tumour is usual fibrous, more or less cellular and with or without lymphocytic infiltration. Eosinophils are rarely present as is granulomatous reaction.

In the adjacent testicular tissue intratubular embryonal carcinoma is often present, and is often more or less necrotic, and sometimes calcified. In the surrounding tissue vascular and lymphatic invasion are also common and should be carefully distinguished from the intratubular occurrence and from artificial implantation of tumour cells into vascular spaces during handling of the specimen. Loose, "floating" tumour cells in vascular spaces, usually associated with surface implants of similar cells should be considered artefactual.

Immunoprofile
Embryonal carcinoma contains a number of immunohistochemical markers reflecting embryonic histogenesis but the majority have hitherto not been very useful diagnostically. CD30 can be demonstrated in many cases {2202}. Cytokeratins of various classes are present while epithelial membrane antigen (EMA) and carcinoembryonic antigen (CEA) and vimentin can usually not be demonstrated {1894}. Placental alkaline phosphatase (PLAP) occurs focally as a membranous and/or cytoplasmic stain-

ing {1615}. Many embryonal carcinomas are strongly positive for TP53 in up to 50% of the tumour cells {2667}. AFP may occur in scattered cells {1196,1198}. Human placental lactogen (HPL) is occasionally found focally in the tumour cells {1198,1807}. HCG occurs in the syncytiotrophoblastic cells, which may be present in the tumour, but not in the embryonal carcinoma cells and the same applies to pregnancy specific β_1 glycoprotein (SP1) {1807}.

Ultrastructure
Ultrastructural examinations have not proven to be diagnostically useful although it may differentiate embryonal carcinoma from seminoma and glandular like pattern of embryonal carcinoma from somatic type adenocarcinomas.

Differential diagnoses
Differential diagnoses include, among the germ cell tumours, seminoma, solid type of yolk sac tumour, and choriocarcinoma. Among other tumours anaplastic large cell lymphoma, malignant Sertoli cell tumour and metastases are considerations. The age of the patient, microscop-

ic examination of representative sections from the tumour including all growth patterns, and a small panel of immunohistochemical stains yields the correct diagnosis in the majority of the cases.

Prognosis
The most important prognostic factor is clinical tumour stage. In general, the tumour spread is lymphatic, first to the retroperitoneal lymph nodes and subsequently to the mediastinum. Haematogeneous spread to the lung may also be seen. Patients with pure embryonal carcinoma and with vascular invasion tend to have higher stage disease {1200}. This is emphasized by studies defining high risk patients as those with pure embryonal carcinoma, predominant embryonal carcinoma, embryonal carcinoma unassociated with teratoma, and/or tumours with vascular/lymphatic invasion and advanced local stage {1803,1817}.

Yolk sac tumour

Definition
A tumour characterized by numerous patterns that recapitulate the yolk sac, allantois and extra embryonic mesenchyme.

ICD-O code   9071/3

Synonym
Endodermal sinus tumour, orchioblastoma.

Epidemiology
In the testis yolk sac tumour (YST) is seen in two distinct age groups, infants and young children and postpubertal males. In children, it is the most common testicular neoplasm {1274} and occurs in all races. It is less common in Blacks, Native Americans, and in Indians {490,

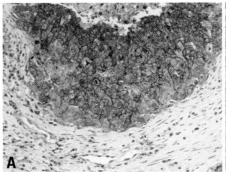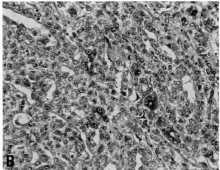

Fig. 4.32 Embryonal carcinoma. **A** Positive staining for CD30 in embryonal carcinoma. **B** Positive staining for AFP in scattered cells of embryonal carcinoma.

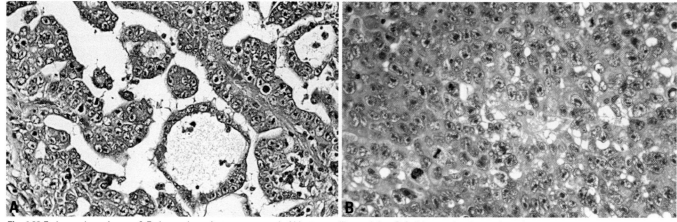

Fig. 4.33 Embryonal carcinoma. **A** Embryonal carcinoma composed of blastocyst-like vesicles. **B** Solid type of embryonal carcinoma.

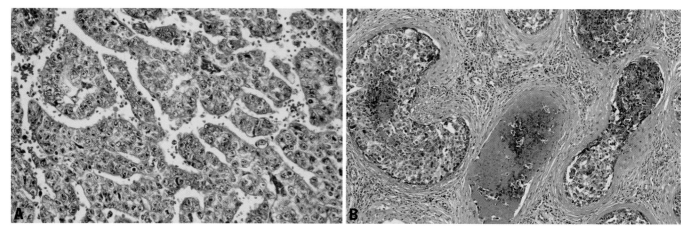

Fig. 4.34 Embryonal carcinoma. **A** Papillary type of embryonal carcinoma. **B** Intratubular embryonal carcinoma. Note the tumour necrosis.

1490} and may be more common in Orientals when compared to Caucasians {1276}. In adults, it usually occurs as a component of a mixed germ cell tumour and is seen in approximately 40% of NSGCTs. In adults, it is much more common in Caucasians than in other races. The age incidence corresponds to the age incidence of testicular malignant mixed germ cell tumours {2564}.

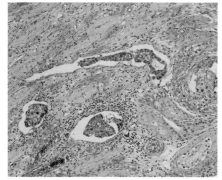

Fig. 4.35 Embryonal carcinoma. Vascular invasion of embryonal carcinoma.

Clinical features
Signs and symptoms
In children, the median age at the presentation is 16-17 months but may extend to 11 years {1274,2244}. There is a right sided preponderance {1274}. Almost ninety percent of cases present with an otherwise asymptomatic scrotal mass {1274}. Seven percent of cases present with a history of trauma or acute onset pain and 1 percent present with a hydrocele {1274}. Alpha fetoprotein levels are elevated in 90 percent of cases {1274, 2595}. Ultrasound examination reveals a solid intratesticular lesion with a different echo texture from that of the testis.

Tumour spread
Ten to twenty percent of children have metastases at presentation {1274,2078}. The nodal spread is to the retroperitoneum {1274,2244}. In children there appears to be a predilection for haematogenous spread, 40% presenting with haematogenous spread alone {326}. In 20-26 percent of cases the first site of

clinical involvement is the lungs {326, 1274}. Although it is not clear if retroperitoneal nodes are also involved in those cases, in adults, the pattern of spread is similar to that seen in other NSGCTs.

Macroscopy
Macroscopically pure yolk sac tumours are solid, soft, and the cut surface is typically pale grey or grey-white and somewhat gelatinous or mucoid {1021,1274}. Large tumours show haemorrhage and necrosis {2564}.

Histopathology
The histopathological appearance is the same, regardless of patient age {1021, 1274,2564}. Several different patterns are usually admixed, and may be present in equal amounts, although not infrequently one pattern may predominate {1201}. Tumours composed entirely of a single histologic pattern are rare {2564}.

Histologic patterns

Microcystic or reticular pattern

The microcystic pattern consists of a meshwork of vacuolated cells producing a honeycomb appearance. The tumour cells are small and may be compressed by the vacuoles, which may contain pale eosinophilic secretion. The nuclei vary in size, but generally are small. Mitotic activity is typically brisk. Hyaline globules are often present {1201,2593}. This pattern is the most common one.

Macrocystic pattern

The macrocystic pattern consists of collections of thin-walled spaces of varying sizes. They may be adjacent to each other, or separated by other histologic patterns.

Solid pattern

The solid pattern consists of nodular collections or aggregates of medium sized polygonal tumour cells with clear cytoplasm, prominent nuclei, and usually showing brisk mitotic activity. It is often associated with a peripheral microcystic pattern which helps distinguish it from typical seminoma and embryonal carcinoma. Sometimes the cells may show greater pleomorphism and giant cells may be present.

Glandular-alveolar pattern

This pattern consists of collections of irregular alveoli, gland-like spaces and tubular structures lined by cells varying from flattened to cuboidal or polygonal. The gland-like spaces or clefts form a meshwork of cavities and channels, sometimes interspersed with myxomatous tissue.

Endodermal sinus pattern

This pattern consists of structures composed of a stalk of connective tissue containing a thin walled blood vessel and lined on the surface by a layer of cuboidal cells with clear cytoplasm and prominent nuclei. Mitotic activity is usually present and may be brisk. These structures, also known as Schiller-Duval bodies, are considered a hallmark of YST {2593}. They are seen scattered within the tumour in varying numbers. Their absence does not preclude the diagnosis.

Papillary pattern

This pattern has numerous, usually fine papillae consisting of connective tissue cores lined by cells with prominent nuclei and often showing brisk mitotic activity. The connective tissue cores vary from loose and oedematous to fibrous and hyalinized. Sometimes there may be considerable deposits of hyaline material forming wider and more solid brightly eosinophilic and amorphous papillae.

Myxomatous pattern

This pattern consists of collections of myxomatous tissue containing sparse cords, strands or collections of individual cells showing prominent nuclei and mitotic activity {1201}.

Polyvesicular vitelline pattern

This pattern consists of collections of vesicles or cysts varying in shape and size surrounded by connective tissue which may vary from cellular and oedematous to dense and fibrous. The vesicles are lined by columnar to flattened cells. Sometimes the vesicles are small and adhere to each other, and some may

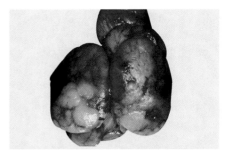

Fig. 4.36 Yolk sac tumour in the testis of a one year old.

be hourglass shaped {2593}. This pattern is uncommon.

Hepatoid pattern

Collections of hepatoid cells are present in some tumours, and is more frequently seen in tumours from postpubertal patients. Hyaline globules are frequently seen {1197,2669}. Sometimes, collections of such cells may be numerous and of considerable size, although usually they are small.

Enteric pattern

Individual or collections of immature glands are not uncommon {1201,2669}. They usually resemble allantois, enteric or endometrioid glands. They are similar to some glands in teratomas, but the association with other yolk sac tumour patterns and absence of a muscular component aid in their distinction. Hyaline globules may be present and numerous.

Immunoprofile

Positive staining for AFP is helpful in diagnosis but the reaction is variable and sometimes weak. Negative staining does not exclude a diagnosis of YST.

YST shows strong positive immunocyto-

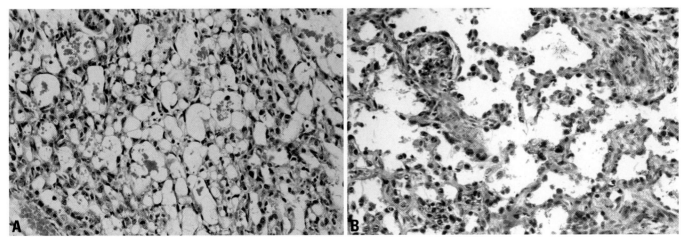

Fig. 4.37 Yolk sac tumour. **A** Microcystic pattern of yolk sac tumour. **B** Glandular-alveolar pattern of yolk sac tumour.

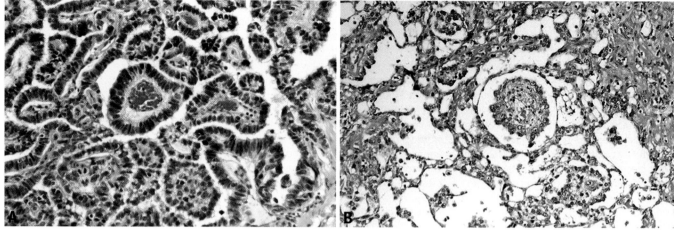
Fig. 4.38 Yolk sac tumour. **A** Endodermal sinus pattern. **B** Endodermal sinus structure (Schiller-Duval body).

chemical staining with low molecular weight cytokeratin. Other proteins present in fetal liver such as alpha-1 antitrypsin, albumin, ferritin, and others, may also be present {1201}.

Genetics

Recurrent anomalies have been detected in the infantile yolk sac tumours of the testis, including loss of the short arm of chromosome 1 (in particular the p36 region), the long arm of chromosome 6, and gain of the long arm of chromosomes 1, and 20, and the complete chromosome 22 {1792,2054,2693}. High level amplification of the 12q13-q14 region (of which *MDM2* might be the target), and to a lesser extent the 17q12-q21 region, has been demonstrated in one tumour. However, no gene or genes involved in the yolk sac tumour of neonates and infants have been identified yet. The yolk sac tumours of adults, being a pure or a part of a mixed TGCTs are also aneuploid

{1543}. Interestingly, loss of 6q also seems to be a recurrent change, which might indicate that it is related to the histology of the tumour.

Prognosis and predictive factors
Clinical criteria
Age does not appear to be prognostically important {1274,2244}. Clinical stage and degree of AFP elevation are of prognostic value {1274,2244,2595}.

Morphologic criteria
Except for lymphovascular invasion, there are no established morphologic prognostic criteria.

Trophoblastic tumours

Choriocarcinoma

Definition
Choriocarcinoma is a malignant neo-

plasm composed of syncytiotrophoblastic, cytotrophoblastic, and intermediate trophoblastic cells.

ICD-O codes
Choriocarcinoma   9100/3
Trophoblastic neoplasms
other than choriocarcinoma
    Monophasic choriocarcinoma
    Placental site trophoblastic
    tumour   9104/1

Epidemiology
Pure choriocarcinoma represents less than 1% (0.19%) of testicular germ cell tumours; choriocarcinoma is admixed with other germ cell tumour elements in 8% of testicular germ cell tumours {1382}. Its estimated incidence, occurring either as a pure tumour or as a component of a mixed germ cell tumour, is approximately 0.8 cases per year per 100,000 male population in those countries with the highest frequency of testicular cancer.

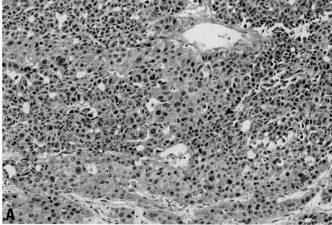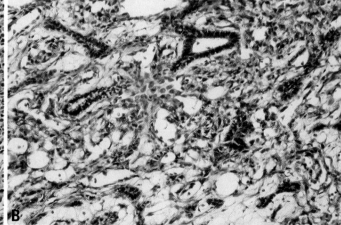
Fig. 4.39 Yolk sac tumour. **A** Hepatoid pattern. **B** Enteric pattern.

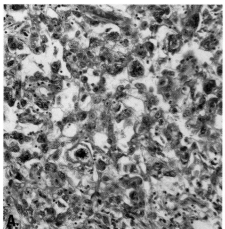
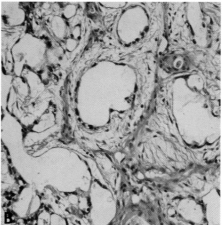
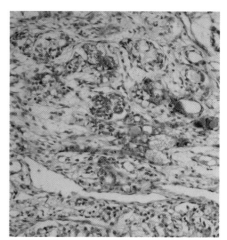

Fig. 4.40 Yolk sac tumour. **A** Pleomorphic cell type. **B** Polyvesicular vitelline pattern.

Fig. 4.41 Yolk sac tumour. AFP positive staining.

Clinical features

Signs and symptoms

Patients with choriocarcinoma are young, averaging 25-30 years of age. They most commonly present with symptoms referable to metastases. The haematogenous distribution of metastases explains the common presenting symptoms: haemoptysis, dyspnoea, central nervous system dysfunction, haematemesis, melena, hypotension, and anaemia. Haemorrhage in multiple visceral sites represents the hallmark of a "choriocarcinoma syndrome" {1529}. Patients typically have very high levels of circulating human chorionic gonadotropin (hCG) (commonly greater than 100,000 mIU/ml). Because of the cross reactivity of hCG with luteinizing hormone, the consequent Leydig cell hyperplasia causes some patients (about 10%) to present with gynecomastia. Occasional patients develop hyperthyroidism because of the cross reactivity of hCG with thyroid stimulating hormone. Clinical examination of the testes may or may not disclose a mass. This is because the primary site may be quite small, or even totally regressed, despite widespread metastatic involvement.

Imaging

Choriocarcinomas do not have distinctive imaging characteristics to differentiate them from other non-seminomatous tumours. Their appearance varies from hypoechoic to hyperechoic. They may invade the tunica albuginea.

Macroscopy

Choriocarcinoma most commonly presents as a haemorrhagic nodule that may be surrounded by a discernible rim of white to tan tumour. In some cases with marked regression, a white/grey scar is the only identifiable abnormality.

Tumour spread

Choriocarcinoma disseminates by both haematogenous and lymphatic pathways. Retroperitoneal lymph nodes are commonly involved, although some patients with visceral metastases may lack lymph node involvement. Additionally, autopsy studies have shown common involvement of the lungs (100%), liver (86%), gastrointestinal tract (71%), and spleen, brain, and adrenal glands (56%) {1800}.

Histopathology

Choriocarcinoma has an admixture, in varying proportions, of syncytiotrophoblastic, cytotrophoblastic and intermediate trophoblastic cells. These cellular components are arranged in varying patterns, usually in an extensively haemorrhagic and necrotic background. In some examples, the syncytiotrophoblasts "cap" nests of cytotrophoblasts in a pattern that is reminiscent of the architecture seen in immature placental villi. Most commonly, they are admixed in a more or less random fashion, usually at the periphery of a nodule that has a central zone of haemorrhage and necrosis. In occasional cases, which have been descriptively termed "monophasic" {2672}, the syncytiotrophoblastic cell component is inconspicuous, leaving a marked preponderance of cytotrophoblastic and intermediate trophoblastic cells. Blood vessel invasion is commonly identified in all of the patterns.

The syncytiotrophoblastic cells are usually multinucleated with deeply staining, eosinophilic to amphophilic cytoplasm; they typically have several, large, irregularly shaped, hyperchromatic and often smudged appearing nuclei. They often

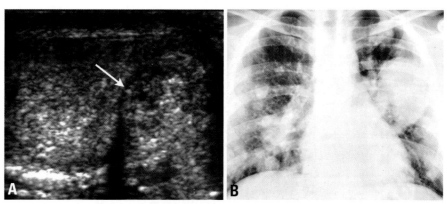

Fig. 4.42 Choriocarcinoma. **A** Longitudinal ultrasound image of the testis shows a small, slightly heterogeneous mass, which is almost isoechoic compared to the normal parenchyma (arrow). **B** Chest radiograph shows multiple lung metastases. The patient presented with hemoptysis.

have cytoplasmic lacunae that contain pink secretion or erythrocytes. The cytotrophoblastic cells have pale to clear cytoplasm with a single, irregularly shaped nucleus with one or two prominent nucleoli. Intermediate trophoblastic cells have eosinophilic to clear cytoplasm and single nuclei; they are larger than cytotrophoblastic cells but may not be readily discernible from them without the use of immunohistochemical stains.

Immunoprofile

The syncytiotrophoblasts are positive for hCG, alpha subunit of inhibin {1664,2042} and epithelial membrane antigen {1894}. Stains for hCG may also highlight large cells that possibly represent transitional forms between mononucleated trophoblastic cells and syncytiotrophoblasts. The intermediate trophoblastic cells are positive for human placental lactogen {1615, 1616} and, if comparable to the gestational examples, would be expected to stain for Mel-CAM and HLA-G {2425}. All of the cell types express cytokeratin, and placental alkaline phosphatase shows patchy reactivity in about one half of the cases.

Prognosis

Choriocarcinoma often disseminates prior to its discovery, probably because of its propensity to invade blood vessels. As a consequence, the majority of patients present with advanced stage disease. It is this aspect of choriocarcinoma that causes it to be associated with a worse prognosis than most other forms of testicular germ cell tumour. Additionally, high levels of hCG correlate with a worse prognosis, likely reflecting a greater tumour burden {7,281,575,1897}.

Trophoblastic neoplasms other than choriocarcinoma

Two cases have been described of trophoblastic testicular tumours that lacked the biphasic pattern of choriocarcinoma and were composed predominantly of cytotrophoblastic cells (monophasic choriocarcinoma) or intermediate trophoblastic cells (similar to placental site trophoblastic tumour). The latter consisted of eosinophilic mononucleated angioinvasive cells that were diffusely immunoreactive for placental lactogen and focally for chorionic gonadotrophin. Follow-up was uneventful after orchiectomy in both cases {2672}.

A favourable lesion described as cystic trophoblastic tumour has been observed in retroperitoneal metastases after chemotherapy in eighteen patients; small foci having a similar appearance may rarely be seen in the testis of patients with germ cell tumours who have not received chemotherapy. The lesions consist of small cysts lined predominantly by

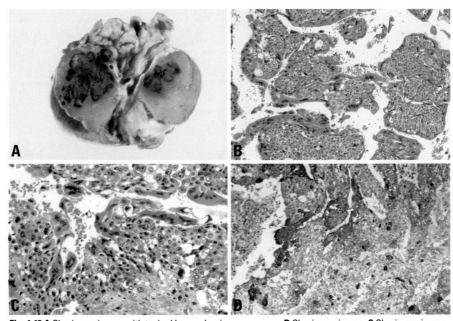

Fig. 4.43 A Choriocarcinoma with typical hemorrhagic appearance. **B** Choriocarcinoma. **C** Choriocarcinoma. Syncytiotrophoblastic cells with deeply eosinophilic cytoplasm and multiple, smudged appearing nuclei; they "cap" aggregates of mononucleated trophoblastic cells with pale to clear cytoplasm. Note the fibrin aggregates. **D** Choriocarcinoma. Positive HCG staining.

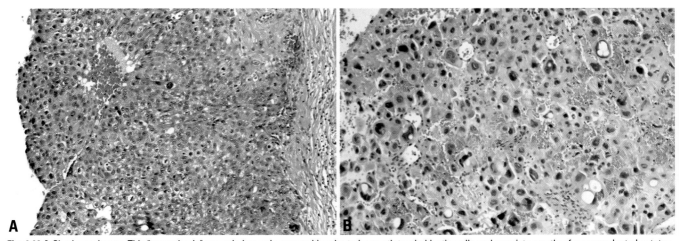

Fig. 4.44 A Choriocarcinoma. This "monophasic" example has only rare multinucleated syncytiotrophoblastic cells and consists mostly of mononucleated cytotrophoblastic and intermediate trophoblastic cells. **B** Placental site trophoblastic tumour. Mononucleated intermediate trophoblasts with eosinophilic cytoplasm.

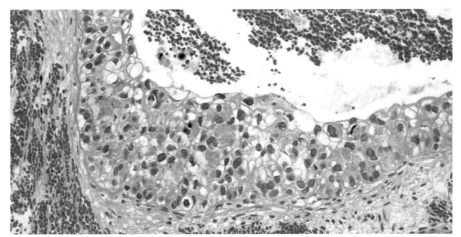

Fig. 4.45 Cystic trophoblastic tumour. The cyst is lined by relatively inactive appearing mononucleated trophoblastic cells.

mononucleated trophoblastic cells with abundant eosinophilic cytoplasm. The nuclei often have smudged chromatin; mitotic figures are infrequent. Focal reactivity for hCG is found {427}.

Teratomas

Definition
A tumour composed of several types of tissue representing different germinal layers (endoderm, mesoderm and ectoderm). They may be composed exclusively of well differentiated, mature tissues or have immature, fetal-like tissues. It has been recommended to consider these morphologies as a single entity based on genetics.
Teratomas in children and the dermoid cyst are benign. Tumours consisting of ectoderm, mesoderm, or endoderm only are classified as monodermal teratomas e.g. struma testis. A single type of differentiated tissue associated with seminoma, embryonal carcinoma, yolk sac tumour or choriocarcinoma is classified as teratomatous component. Teratoma may contain syncytiotrophoblastic giant cells.

ICD-O codes
Teratoma	9080/3
Dermoid cyst	9084/0
Monodermal teratoma	
Teratoma with somatic type	
malignancies	9084/3

Synonyms
Mature teratoma, immature teratoma, teratoma differentiated (mature), teratoma differentiated (immature).

Epidemiology
Teratoma occurs in two age groups. In adults, the frequency of pure teratoma ranges from 2.7-7% {804,1807} and 47-50% in mixed TGCTs {172,2753}. In children, the incidence is between 24-36% {326,2366}. A number of congenital abnormalities, predominantly of the GU tract have been observed {883,2664}. In the prepubertal testis, the presence of IGCNU is not proven, because the markers used are not specific at this period of life for IGCNU {1617,2264,2482}.

Clinical features
Signs and symptoms
In children, 65% of teratomas occur in the 1st and 2nd year of life with a mean age of 20 months. In postpubertal patients, most are seen in young adults. Symptoms consist of swelling or are due to metastases. Occasionally, serum levels of AFP and hCG may be elevated in adult patients {1211}.
Most patients present with a mass that is usually firm, irregular or nodular, nontender and does not transilluminate. Approximately 2-3% of prepubertal testis tumours may be associated with or misdiagnosed as a hydrocele, particularly if the tumour contains a cystic component. Since neither of these tumours is hormonally active, precocious puberty is not seen. Serum alpha-fetoprotein (AFP) levels are helpful in the differentiation of teratomas from yolk sac tumours {924,2264}.

Imaging

Teratoma
Teratomas are generally well circum-

scribed complex masses. Cartilage, calcification, fibrosis, and scar formation result in echogenic foci, which result in variable degrees of shadowing. Cyst formation is commonly seen in teratomas and the demonstration of a predominately cystic mass suggests that it is either a teratoma or a mixed germ cell tumour with a large component of teratoma within it.

Epidermoid cyst
The distinctive laminated morphology is reflected in ultrasound images. They are sharply marginated, round to slightly oval masses. The capsule of the lesion is well defined and is sometimes calcified. The mass may be hypoechoic but the laminations often give rise to an "onion-skin" or "target" appearance {813,2377}. Teratomas and other malignant tumours may have a similar appearance and great care should be taken in evaluating the mass for any irregular borders, which would suggest a malignant lesion {671,813}.

Macroscopy
The tumours are nodular and firm. The cut surfaces are heterogeneous with solid and cystic areas corresponding to the tissue types present histologically. Cartilage, bone and pigmented areas may be recognizable.

Tumour spread
Metastatic spread from teratomas in prepubertal children is not reported {326, 330,2805}. Conversely, similar tumours found after puberty are known to metastasize.

Histopathology
The well differentiated, mature tissue types consist of keratinizing and nonkeratinizing squamous epithelium, neural and glandular tissues. Organoid structures are not uncommon, particularly in children such as skin, respiratory, gastrointestinal and genitourinary tract. Thyroid tissue has rarely been observed {2792}. Of the mesodermal components, muscular tissue is the most common {548}. Virtually any other tissue type can be seen. Fetal type tissue may also consist of ectodermal, endodermal and/or mesenchymal tissues. They can have an organoid arrangement resembling primitive renal or pulmonary tissues. It can be difficult to differentiate fetal-type tissues from teratoma with somatic type malig-

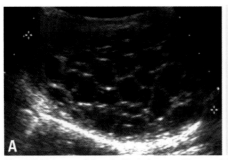

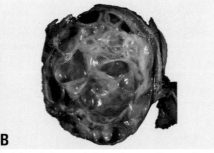

Fig. 4.46 Teratoma. A Longitudinal ultrasound image of the left testis (cursors) shows the normal parenchyma being replaced by complex, multiseptated, cystic mass. B Gross specimen confirms the cystic nature of the mass.

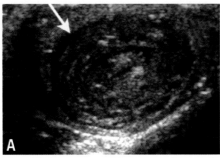

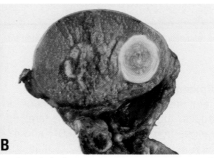

Fig. 4.47 Epidermoid cyst. A Transverse ultrasound image through the lower pole of the testis shows a well marginated, hypoechoic, oval mass (arrow). Multiple concentric rings are visualized giving an "onion-skin" appearance. B Epidermoid cyst within the stroma of the testis. Note the laminated structure.

nancies. Some have classified foci indistinguishable from primitive neuroectodermal tumours as malignant irrespective of size {1797} whereas others recognize a nodule equal to or greater than a (4x objective) microscopic field as PNET {1722}. Monodermal teratomas have been described as struma testis {2427}, pure cartilagenous teratoma {2427}, and possibly epidermal (epidermoid) cyst. Teratoma can show invasion of paratesticular tissue and intra and extratesticular vascular invasion.

Immunoprofile
The differentiated elements express the immunophenotype expected for that specific cell type. Alpha-fetoprotein pro-

duction occurs in about 19-36% of teratomas in intestinal and hepatoid areas {1196,1198,1807}. Other markers include alpha-1 antitrypsin, CEA and ferritin {1198}. hCG can be seen in syncytiotrophoblastic cells. PLAP is also demonstrable in glandular structures {346,1615, 1807,2658}.

Genetics
Teratomas of the infantile testis are diploid {1350,2413}. Karyotyping, as well as CGH, even after microdissection of the tumour cells, has failed to demonstrate chromosomal changes in these tumours [{1792,2054} for review]. It remains to be shown whether the recently identified constitutional translocation

between chromosome 12 and 15 as found in a family with a predisposition to sacral teratoma at young age {2724} is involved in the genesis of this type of tumour. In contrast to the diploidy of teratomas of neonates and infants, teratoma is hypotriploid in adult patients {1763,1963,2209}. In fact, teratomas as part of TGCTs have similar genetic changes compared to other components. In addition, the fully differentiated tumour cells found in residual teratomas as a remainder after chemotherapy of a non-seminoma of adults, are hypotriploid {1542}.

Prognosis
The behaviour of teratoma in the two different age groups is strikingly different. In the prepubertal testis, teratoma is benign {2264}. In the postpubertal testis, despite appearance, teratoma shows metastases in 22-37% of cases. Teratoma shows mostly synchronous metastases; in 13% of cases, it is metachronous {1806}. If it is associated with a scar (burned out component), the metastatic frequency is 66%. In a series from Indiana, 37% of 41 adult patients with pure teratoma showed synchronous metastases {1471}. Teratoma may metastasize as such {793,1204,1966, 2128,2509}, or in some instances precursor cells may invade vascular spaces and differentiate at the metastatic site {1800}. The cellular composition of metastases may differ from that of the respective primary tumour {548}.

Dermoid cyst

Definition
A mature teratoma with a predominance of one or more cysts lined by keratinizing squamous epithelium with skin appendages, with or without small areas of other teratomatous elements. Epidermoid cysts lack skin appendages.

ICD-O code   9084/0

Testicular dermoid cyst is a specialized, benign form of cystic teratoma that is analogous to the common ovarian tumour {2670}. It is rare, with less than 20 cases reported {126,324,349,629,976, 1392,1609,2670}. Most have been in young men who presented with testicular masses, but an occasional example has

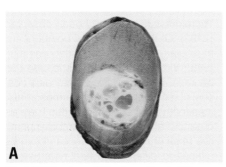

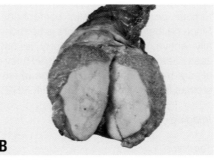

Fig. 4.48 A Teratoma. B Teratoma. Carcinoid tumour within the testis.

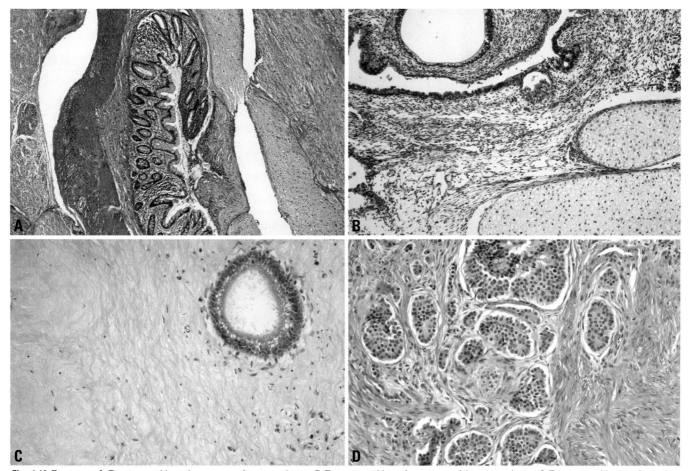

Fig. 4.49 Teratoma. **A** Teratoma with various types of mature tissue. **B** Teratoma with various types of immature tissue. **C** Teratoma with scar formation. **D** Carcinoid tumour within teratoma.

occurred in a child. On gross examination a single cyst is usually seen, and it may contain hair and "cheesy", keratinous material. On microscopic examination a keratin filled cyst is lined by stratified squamous epithelium with associated pilosebaceous units as normally seen in the skin. A surrounding fibrous wall may also contain sweat glands, glands having ciliated or goblet cell containing epithelium, bundles of smooth muscle, bone, cartilage, thyroid, fat, intestinal tis-

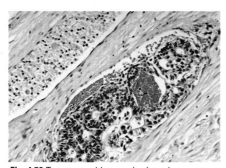

Fig. 4.50 Teratoma with vascular invasion.

sue, gastric epithelium, salivary gland and pancreatic tissue, all having bland cytological features. The seminiferous tubules usually have normal spermatogenesis and always lack intratubular germ cell neoplasia. Many examples also have an associated lipogranulomatous reaction in the parenchyma. Patients are well on follow-up.

Monodermal teratomas

Definition
A tumour that consists of only one of the three germ layers (endo-, ecto- or mesoderm.)
Primitive neuroectodermal tumour has been described {38,1903,1909,2904} either in pure form or as a component of a mixed germ cell tumour. The histology is similar to that in other sites. Only PNET occurring in the metastasis is associated with a poor prognosis {1722}. Pure cartilaginous teratoma has been described {2427}. Epidermoid cysts have been considered as a tumour like lesion.

However, recently we have encountered an epidermal cyst with diffuse intratubular malignant germ cells indicating that some may be teratomatous.

Teratoma with somatic-type malignancies

Definition
A teratoma containing a malignant component of a type typically encountered in other organs and tissues, e.g. sarcomas and carcinomas.

ICD-O code   9084/3

Clinical features
Nongerm cell malignant tumours may arise in primary or metastatic germ cell tumours (GCTs) and are most likely derived from teratomas {1720}. They are seen in 3-6% of patients with metastatic GCTs {484}.

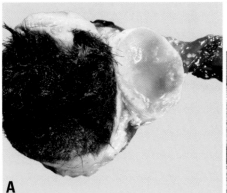
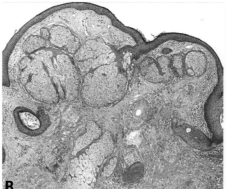
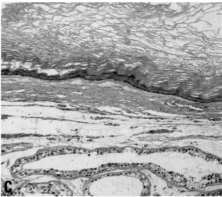

Fig. 4.51 A Cut surface of dermoid cyst, spermatic cord on the right. **B** Dermoid cyst with a stratified squamous epithelial lining and pilosebaceous units and smooth muscle bundles in its wall. **C** Epidermoid cyst with laminated keratin in the lumen and at the periphery atrophic seminiferus tubule without intratubuler germ cell neoplasia.

Histopathology

Nongerm cell malignant tumours are characterized by an invasive or solid (expansile) proliferation of highly atypical somatic cells that overgrow the surrounding GCT. How much expansile growth is required has not been clearly defined, but some authors have suggested that the tumour should fill a 4X field of view {2668}. Care must be taken not to confuse chemotherapy induced atypia with the development of a secondary malignancy. The most common type of somatic type malignancy seen in patients with testicular GCTs is sarcoma {39,40,484,998,1334,1720,1815,2200, 2597,2665,2666}. About half are undifferentiated sarcomas and most of the remainder display striated or smooth muscle differentiation. Any type of sarcoma may occur in germ cell tumours, including chondrosarcoma, osteosarcoma, malignant fibrous histiocytoma and malignant nerve sheath tumours.

Primitive neuroectodermal tumours (PNETs) have been increasingly recognized {38,1282,1722,1763,1815,1909, 2363}; they may resemble neuroblastoma, medulloepithelioma, peripheral neuroepithelioma or ependymoblastoma. Most are cytokeratin-positive and stain with synaptophysin and Leu 7. One third is chromogranin-positive. Tumours may also stain with antibodies to S-100 protein, GFAP and HBA.71. Nephroblastoma like teratomas are rare in the testis {881}, but are more common in metastases {1721}. Carcinomas are less often associated with GCTs. Adenocarcinomas, squamous carcinomas and neuroendocrine carcinomas have all been reported {40, 484,1723,1815,2665}. These tumours stain for cytokeratins, EMA and some-

times CEA. Stains for PLAP, AFP and HCG are negative.

Somatic genetics

In several cases, the nongerm cell tumour has demonstrated the i(12p) chromosomal abnormality associated with GCTs; some have demonstrated chromosomal rearrangements characteristic of the somatic tumour in conventional locations {1815}.

Prognosis

If the malignant tumour is limited to the testis, the prognosis is not affected {40,1815}. In metastatic sites, the somatic type malignancies have a poor prognosis {1525,1815}. They do not respond to germ cell tumour chemotherapy; surgical resection is the treatment of choice. Therapy designed for the specific type of somatic neoplasm may also be helpful.

Tumours of more than one histological type (mixed forms)

Definition

This category includes germ cell tumours composed of two or more types.

ICD-O codes

Tumours of more than one histological
type (mixed forms)   9085/3
Others
Polyembryoma   9072/3

Synonyms

Malignant teratoma intermediate includes only teratoma and embryonal carcinoma, combined tumour is synonymous for seminoma and any other cell type and malignant teratoma trophoblas-

tic for choriocarcinoma and non-seminomatous germ cell tumour types.

Incidence

Excluding seminoma with syncytiotrophoblastic cells and spermatocytic seminoma with sarcoma, the frequency of mixed germ cell tumours has been reported between 32-54% of all germ cell tumours {1195,1807}.

Clinical features

Signs and symptoms

The age range of these tumours depends on whether or not they contain seminoma. With seminoma, the age is intermediate between that of seminoma and pure non-seminoma; without seminoma, the age is the same as pure non-seminoma. Mixed germ cell tumours are rarely seen in prepubertal children. Patients present with painless or painful testicular swelling. Signs of metastatic disease include abdominal mass, gastrointestinal tract disturbances or pulmonary discomfort. Serum elevations of AFP and hCG are common {2265}.

Macroscopy

The enlarged testis shows a heterogeneous cut surface with solid areas, haemorrhage and necrosis. Cystic spaces indicate teratomatous elements.

Tumour spread

The tumours follow the usual route through retroperitoneal lymph nodes to visceral organs. Those with foci of choriocarcinoma or numerous syncytiotrophoblastic cells tend to involve liver and/or brain.

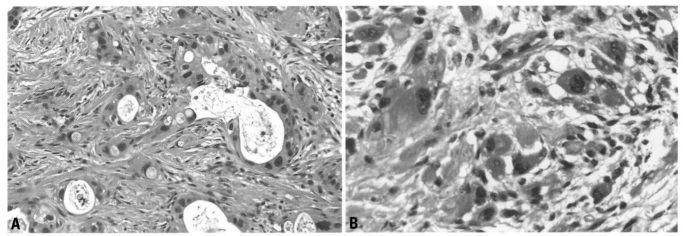

Fig. 4.52 Teratoma with somatic type malignancies. **A** Adenocarcinoma in patient with testicular GCT. Goblet cells and glands are present in desmoplastic stroma. **B** Rhabdomyosarcoma in a GCT patient. Cells with abundant eosinophilic cytoplasm are rhabdomyoblasts.

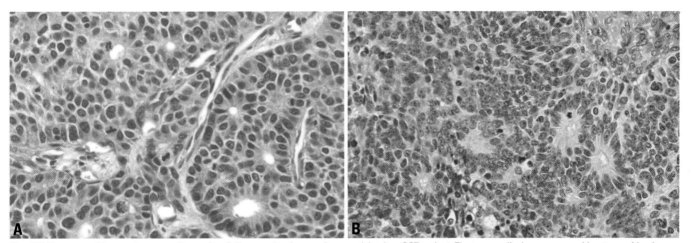

Fig. 4.53 Teratoma with somatic type malignancies. **A** Neuroendocrine carcinoma arising in a GCT patient. The tumour displays an organoid pattern with mitoses. **B** PNET in a GCT patient. The tumour is composed of small round blue cells with rosettes.

Histopathology

The various types of germ cell tumour can occur in any combination and their appearances are identical to those occurring in pure form. The diagnosis should include all components that are present and the quantity of each should be estimated. While the basic germ cell tumour types are infrequent in pure forms they are very frequent in the mixed forms. Embryonal carcinoma and teratoma are each present in 47% of cases and yolk sac tumours in 41%. The latter is frequently overlooked {2367}. 40% of mixed germ cell tumours contain varying numbers of syncytiotrophoblastic cells {1796}. The most common combination, in one series, was teratoma and embryonal carcinoma {1195} and in another, the combination of embryonal carcinoma, yolk sac tumour, teratoma and syncytiotrophoblastic cells {1796}. Polyembryoma, {730,

1868} a rare germ cell tumour composed predominantly of embryoid bodies, is considered by some as a unique germ cell tumour and is listed under one histologic type {1805}. However, the individual components consisting of embryonal carcinoma, yolk sac tumour, syncytiotrophoblastic cells and teratoma, suggest that these should be regarded as mixed germ cell tumours with a unique growth pattern. The histology of the metastases reflects that of the primary tumour in about 88% of cases. In embryonal carcinoma, teratoma and yolk sac tumour the metastases are identical to the primaries in 95, 90 and 83% of these tumours, respectively {2367}.

Treatment effect

Radiation and chemotherapy may produce the following histologic changes. 1) Necrosis is often associated with ghost-like necrotic tumour cells surrounded by a xanthogranulomatous response. 2) Fibrosis may show cellular pleomorphism. 3) Residual teratoma is often cystic and may show reactive cellular pleomorphism or frank malignant change with or without selective overgrowth. 4) Viable tumour may show loss of marker production e.g. AFP or hCG {1797,2663}.

Burned out germ cell tumour

Occasionally, germ cell tumours of the testis, particularly choriocarcinoma {1556,2252} can completely or partially undergo necrosis and regress {20,144, 145,350,556} leaving a homogeneous scar. The scar is frequently associated with haematoxylin staining bodies that contain not only calcium but also DNA {144}. The scar can be associated with intratubular malignant germ cells or residual viable tumour such as teratoma

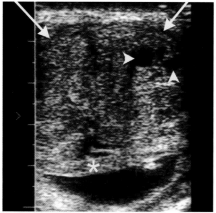

Fig. 4.54 Mixed germ cell tumour. Longitudinal ultrasound image of the testis shows a large, heterogeneous mass (arrows) with cystic areas (arrowheads). There is a small amount of normal parenchyma remaining posteriorly (asterisk).

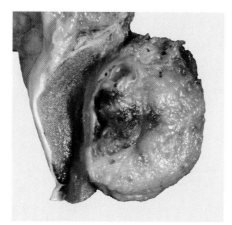

Fig. 4.55 Mixed germ cell tumour. Gross specimen showing a tumour with cystic areas.

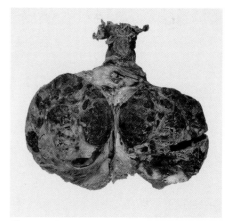

Fig. 4.56 Teratoma and choriocarcinoma (trophoblastic teratoma).

{262,556,2664}. The metastases often differ from the residual viable tumour in the testis {167}.

Immunoprofile

Most tumours show immunoreactivity for AFP in the yolk sac elements, teratomatous glands and hepatoid cells. There is a strong correlation between elevated serum levels of AFP and the presence of YST {1807,1917}. Syncytiotrophoblastic cells either singly or in association with foci of choriocarcinoma are positive for hCG and other placental glycoproteins (pregnancy specific β_1 glycoprotein, human placental lactogen and placental alkaline phosphatase).

Genetics

A vast amount of knowledge has been accumulated concerning the genetic features of mixed germ cell tumours; it is discussed in the genetic overview to germ cell tumours, earlier in this chapter.

Prognosis

Clinical criteria

Mixed germ cell tumours containing large areas of seminoma appear to respond better to treatment than those with no or only microscopic foci of seminoma.

Morphologic criteria

Vascular/lymphatic invasion in the primary tumour is predictive of nodal metastasis and relapse {802,823,1087, 2367}. The presence and percent of embryonal carcinoma in the primary tumour is also predictive of stage II disease {278,802,823,1817,2249}. In contrast, the presence of teratoma and yolk sac tumour is associated with a lower incidence of metastases following orchiectomy in clinical stage I disease {311,802,823,848,1817,2834}.

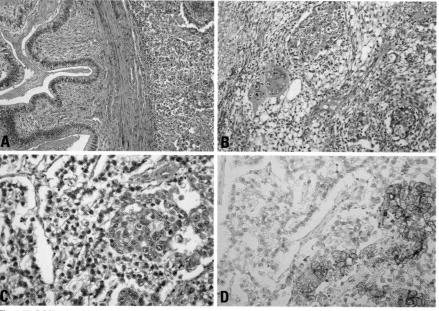

Fig. 4.57 A Mixed teratoma and embryonal carcinoma. Note seperation of two components: teratoma (left) and embryonal carcinoma (right). **B** Embryonal carcinoma, yolk sac tumour, syncytiotrophoblasts. **C** Mixed seminoma and embryonal carcinoma. **D** Mixed seminoma and embryonal carcinoma. CD30 immunoreactivity on the right.

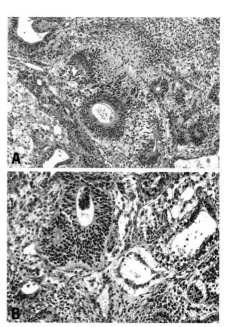

Fig. 4.58 A,B Mixed germ cell tumour: teratoma and yolk sac tumour.

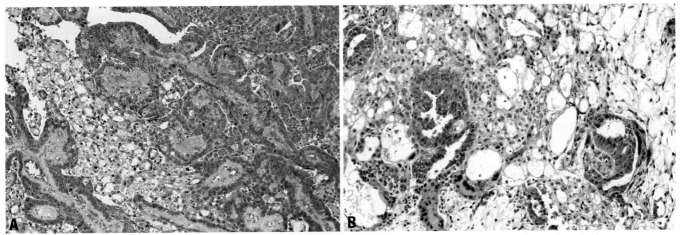

Fig. 4.59 Mixed germ cell tumours. **A** Embryonal carcinoma and yolk sac tumour. **B** Embryonal carcinoma, yolk sac tumour and syncytiotrophoblasts.

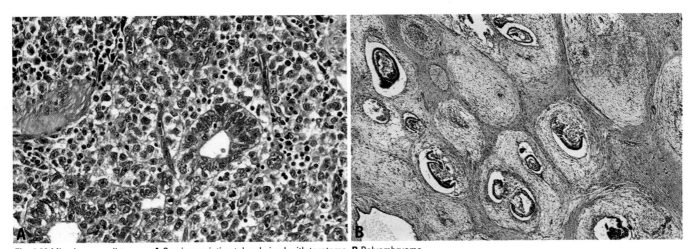

Fig. 4.60 Mixed germ cell tumour. **A** Seminoma intimately admixed with teratoma. **B** Polyembryoma.

Sex cord / gonadal stromal tumours

I.A. Sesterhenn
J. Cheville
P.J. Woodward
I. Damjanov

G.K. Jacobsen
M. Nistal
R. Paniagua
A.A. Renshaw

Sex cord / gonadal stromal tumours, pure forms

Included in this category are Leydig cell tumours, Sertoli cell tumours, granulosa cell tumours and tumours of the theco-ma/fibroma group.

These tumours constitute about 4-6% of adult testicular tumours and over 30% of testicular tumours in infants and children. The name given to this group does not indicate a preference for any particular concept of testicular embryogenesis. As with the germ cell tumours, the aim throughout this section is to closely parallel the WHO terminology and classification of ovarian tumours.

About 10% of these tumours, almost always in adults, metastasize. However, it may not be possible on histological grounds to forecast their behaviour. Some of these tumours occur in androgen insensitivity syndrome (AIS) and adrenogenital syndrome (AGS) and should be classified under tumour-like lesions.

Leydig cell tumour

Definition
A tumour composed of elements recapitulating normal development and evolution of Leydig cells.

ICD-O codes
Leydig cell tumour   8650/1
Malignant Leydig cell tumour   8650/3

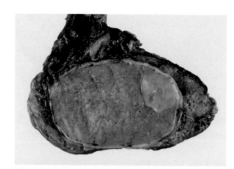

Fig. 4.61 Leydig cell tumour.

Synonym
Interstitial cell tumour.

Epidemiology
Leydig cell tumours account for 1-3% of testicular tumours {1318,1800,2664}. In infants and children, they constitute about 3% of testis tumours and 14% of stromal tumours {2366}. Unlike germ cell tumours, there is no race predilection {1800}. Occasionally, Leydig cell tumours are seen in patients with Klinefelter syndrome {1800,2664}. About 5-10% of patients have a history of cryptorchidism {1318}.

Clinical features
Signs and symptoms
The tumour is most common in the 3rd to 6th decade and in children between 3 and 9 years {1318,2366}. Painless testicular enlargement is the most common presentation. Gynecomastia is seen in about 30% of patients either as a presenting feature or at clinical evaluation for a testicular mass {979,2664}. Libido

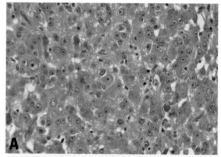

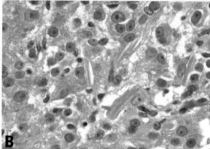

Fig. 4.62 Leydig cell tumour. **A** Typical morphological appearance. **B** Leydig cell tumour. Note the Reinke crystals.

and potency may be compromized. In children, precocious puberty is not uncommon {2831}. Leydig cell tumours produce steroids, particularly testosterone, androstenedione and dehydroepi-androsterone {298,2831}. Serum estrogen and estradiol levels may be elevated {828}. The latter may be associated with low testosterone and follicle stimulating hormone levels {213,1738}. Progesterone, urinary pregnanediol and urinary 17-ketosteroid levels may be elevated {535,2052}. Bilaterality is rare {1318,1800}.

Imaging
Leydig cell tumours are generally well defined, hypoechoic, small solid masses but may show cystic areas, haemorrhage or necrosis. The sonographic appearance is quite variable and is indistinguishable from germ cell tumours. There are no sonographic criteria, which can differentiate benign from malignant Leydig cell tumours and orchiectomy is required.

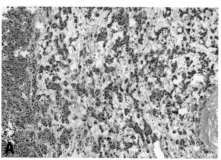

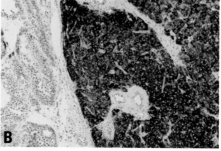

Fig. 4.63 Leydig cell tumour. **A** Leydig cell tumour with cords of tumour cells. **B** Tumour cells stain intensely for inhibin, which is also present to a lesser extend in adjacent tubules.

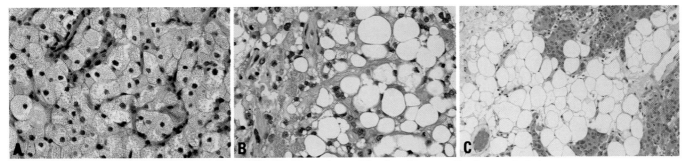

Fig. 4.64 Leydig cell tumour. **A** Note lipid rich cytoplasm. **B** Note lipomatous change. **C** Leydig cell tumour with adipose metaplasia.

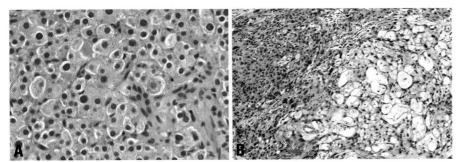

Fig. 4.65 Leydig cell tumour. **A** Leydig cell tumour with lipochrome pigment. **B** Unusual microcystic change in Leydig cell tumour.

Macroscopy

The tumours are well circumscribed, often encapsulated and 3-5 cm in size. The cut surface is usually homogeneously yellow to mahogany brown. There may be hyalinization and calcification. Expansion into paratesticular tissue can be detected in about 10-15% of cases {1318}.

Histopathology

The tumour shows variable histologic features recapitulating the evolution of Leydig cells. The most common type consists of medium to large polygonal cells with abundant eosinophilic cytoplasm and distinct cell borders. The cytoplasm may be vacuolated or foamy depending on the lipid content. Even fatty metaplasia can occur. Reinke crystals can be seen in about 30-40% of cases. The crystals are usually intracytoplasmic, but may be seen in the nucleus and interstitial tissue. Lipofuscin pigment is present in up to 15% of cases. Occasionally, the tumour cells are spindled or have scant cytoplasm. The nuclei are round or oval with a prominent nucleolus. There may be variation in nuclear size. Binucleated or multinucleated cells may be present. Some nuclear atypia can be observed. Mitoses are generally rare. The tumour has a rich vascular network as in endocrine tumours. The stro-

ma is usually scant, but may be hyalinized and prominent. Occasionally it is oedematous. Psammoma bodies can occur {165,1739}. The growth pattern is usually diffuse, but may be trabecular, insular, pseudotubular and ribbon-like.

Immunoprofile

In addition to the steroid hormones, the tumours are positive for vimentin and inhibin {218,1159,1666,1727}. S100 protein has also been described {1663}. A positive reaction for cytokeratin does not exclude the diagnosis.

Ultrastructure

The polygonal Reinke crystals can have a variable appearance depending on the plane of sectioning e.g. various dot patterns, parallel lines, prismatic or hexagonal lattice {1290,2455,2456}.

Differential diagnosis

Most importantly, Leydig cell tumours have to be distinguished from the multi-nodular tumours of the adrenogenital syndrome. These are usually bilateral, dark brown and show cellular pleomorphism and pigmentation and are associated with a hyalinized fibrous stroma {1733,2230,2269}. Similar lesions are seen in Nelson syndrome {1234,1393}. Leydig cell hyperplasia has an interstitial

and not expansile growth pattern. Stromal tumours with prominent luteinization can mimic a Leydig cell tumour. The eosinophilic histiocytes of malakoplakia can be identified by the typical cytoplasmic inclusions (Michaelis Gutman bodies) and prominent intratubular involvement.

Malignant Leydig cell tumour

ICD-O code   8650/3

Approximately 10% of Leydig cell tumours are malignant. Malignant features include large size (greater than 5 cm), cytologic atypia, increased mitotic activity, necrosis and vascular invasion {445,1318,1665}. The majority of malignant Leydig cell tumours have most or all of these features {445}. Most malignant Leydig cell tumours are DNA aneuploid and show increased MIB-1 proliferative activity, in contrast to benign Leydig cell tumours that are DNA diploid with low MIB-1 proliferation {445,1665}. On occasion, a benign Leydig cell tumour can be aneuploid. Currently, malignant Leydig cell tumours are managed by radical orchiectomy, and retroperitoneal lymphadenectomy. Malignant tumours do not respond to radiation or chemotherapy, and survival is poor with the majority of patients developing metastases that result in death.

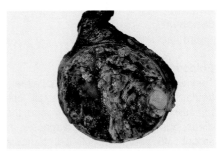

Fig. 4.66 Malignant Leydig cell tumour.

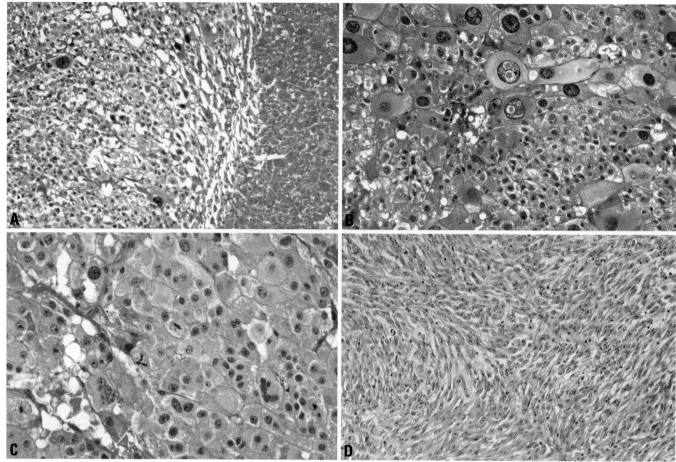

Fig. 4.67 Malignant Leydig cell tumour. **A** Necrosis. **B** Pronounced nuclear and cellular pleomorphism. **C** Note abnormal mitosis in center. **D** Leydig cell tumour with spindle change.

Sertoli cell tumour

Definition
Sertoli cell tumour is a sex cord-stromal tumour of the testis composed of cells expressing to a varying degree features of fetal, prepubertal or adult Sertoli cells.

ICD-O codes
Sertoli cell tumour	8640/1
Sertoli cell tumour lipid rich variant	8641/0
Sclerosing Sertoli cell tumour	
Large cell calcifying Sertoli cell tumour	8642/1

Synonym
Androblastoma.

Epidemiology
They account for less than 1% of all testicular tumours. Typically Sertoli cell tumours NOS occur in adults, and the mean age at the time of diagnosis, is around 45 years. Sertoli cell tumours NOS are only exceptionally found in men under the age of 20 years {2894}. Variant forms, and especially those that occur as parts of various syndromes, are more common in infants and children.

The vast majority of Sertoli cell tumours are sporadic, but some tumours have been associated with genetic syndromes such as androgen insensitivity syndrome {2268}, Carney syndrome {2785}, and Peutz-Jeghers syndrome {2894}.

Clinical features
Signs and symptoms
Patients harbouring Sertoli tumours of any type typically present with a slowly enlarging testicular mass {827}. Hormone related symptoms are not typical of Sertoli cell tumours {2894}. Sertoli cell tumours in boys with Peutz-Jeghers syndrome have signs of hyperestrinism {61,2907}.

Imaging
Sertoli cell tumours are generally hypoechoic. They can be variable echogenecity and cystic areas. The imaging characteristics are nonspecific and indistinguishable from germ cell tumours. An interesting subtype, which can often be distinguished, is the large cell calcifying Sertoli cell tumour. These

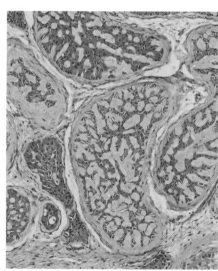

Fig. 4.68 Sertoli cell tumour. Intratubular Sertoli cell tumour in a patient with Peutz-Jeghers syndrome.

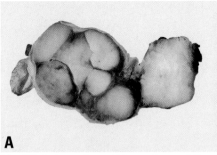

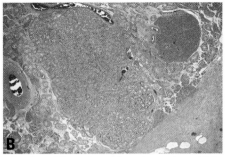

Fig. 4.69 Androgen insensitivity syndrome. **A** Sertoli - Leydig cell hamartomas in androgen insensitivity syndrome (AIS). **B** Sertoli cell hamartoma in center and nodular Leydig cell proliferation.

masses can be multiple and bilateral and, as the name implies, are characterized by large areas of calcification which are readily seen by ultrasound {410,873}. Calcifications will app`ear as brightly echogenic foci, which block the transmission of sound (posterior acoustic shadowing). This diagnosis is strongly suggested when calcified testicular masses are identified in the pediatric age group.

Macroscopy

Most tumours present as spherical or

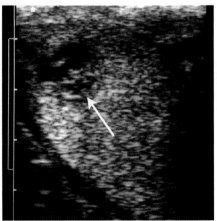

Fig. 4.70 Sertoli cell tumour. Longitudinal ultrasound image of the testis shows a small well defined mass (arrow). It is slightly heterogeneous with small cysts (anechoic areas) within it.

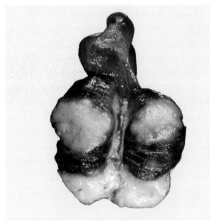

Fig. 4.71 Sertoli cell tumour of the testis.

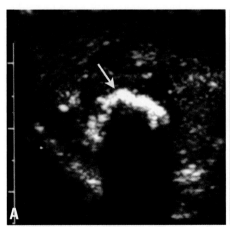

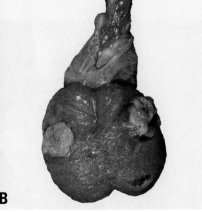

Fig. 4.72 A Large cell calcified Sertoli cell tumour shows bilateral, brightly echogenic masses with posterior acoustic shadowing (arrow). **B** Sertoli cell tumour. Large cell calcified Sertoli cell tumour. This case was malignant; note focus of yellow necrosis.

lobulated, well circumscribed masses, varying in size from 1 cm to more than 20 cm in diameter. The average size of tumours recorded in the largest series of 60 cases is 3.5 cm {2894}. On cross section the tumours appear tan-yellow or greyish white. Foci of haemorrhage may be seen. Necrosis is typically not evident. Sertoli cell tumours NOS are always unilateral. Tumours in patients with Peutz-Jeghers syndrome may be bilateral, and some large cell calcifying Sertoli cell tumours on record were also bilateral {1391}.

Histopathology

Tumour cells have oval, round, or elongated nuclei, and the nucleoli are not overtly prominent. Nuclear grooves and inclusions are usually not seen. The cytoplasm may be pale eosinophilic or clear and vacuolated due to lipids. In some instances the cytoplasm of tumour cells is prominently eosinophilic. Overall the cells appear bland and uniform. Mild nuclear pleomorphism and atypia is found in a minority of cases. Mitoses are uncommon and most cases contain fewer than 5 mitoses per ten high power fields. An increased number of mitotic figures (>5 per HPF) may be found in about 15% of cases, but in itself this finding should not be considered to be a sign of malignancy.

The tumour cells are typically arranged into tubules surrounded by a basement membrane. These tubules may be solid or hollow with a central lumen. Furthermore, tumour cells may form retiform and tubular-glandular structures. Some tumours consist predominantly of solid sheets and nodules, but even in such neoplasms, well developed or abortive tubules are usually also present. The stroma between the tubules, cords and cell nests is fibrotic and moderately cellular to acellular and hyalinized. The hyalinized stroma contains often dilated blood vessels and may be markedly oedematous. Inflammatory cells are typically absent. Minor calcifications can be found in about 10% of cases, but occasional tumours may show more prominent deposits.

Immunoprofile

Sertoli cell tumours NOS stain with antibodies to vimentin (90%) and cytokeratins (80%) and to a variable extent with antibodies to inhibin (40%), and S100

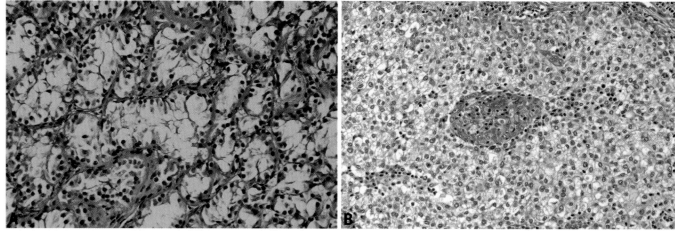

Fig. 4.73 A Sertoli cell tumour. **B** Sertoli cell tumour mimicking seminoma.

(30%) {2575,2894}. Tumour cells are invariably negative for placental alkaline phosphatase, alpha-fetoprotein, human chorionic gonadotropin.

Ultrastructure

Charcot-Böttcher crystals, composed of filaments, are rarely seen but are considered to be typical of Sertoli cells.

Variants

In addition to Sertoli cell tumours NOS two variants are recognized: large cell calcifying Sertoli cell tumour, and sclerosing Sertoli cell tumour. There are not enough data to determine whether the proposed variants such as "lipid rich variant" and "Sertoli cell tumour with heterologous sarcomatous component" {875} warrant separation from the Sertoli cell tumour NOS.

Large cell calcifying Sertoli cell tumour (LCCST)

Large cell calcifying Sertoli cell tumour

(LCCST) can be sporadic, but occur also as parts of the Carney and Peutz-Jeghers syndromes {1391}. Only about 50 cases of this neoplasm have been reported so far.

Sporadic tumours account for 60% of cases, whereas the remaining 40% are associated with genetic syndromes or have endocrine disorders {1391}. Endocrine symptoms, including precocious puberty and gynecomastia are found in a significant number of cases. In contrast to Sertoli cell tumours NOS, most patients harbouring LCCST are young and the average age is 16 years. The youngest patient on record was 2 years old. In most cases the tumours are benign, but 20% are malignant. In 40% of cases the tumours are bilateral.

Microscopic features of LCCST include nests and cords of relatively large polygonal cells with eosinophilic cytoplasm embedded in myxohyaline stroma. Tumour cells have vesicular and relatively large nuclei and prominent nucleoli,

but mitoses are rare. The stroma may be hyalinized, often with abundant neutrophils, and typically shows broad areas of calcification, though a substantial proportion lack calcification. Intratubular spread of the tumour cells is typically found in most cases {366}.

Sclerosing Sertoli cell tumour (SSCT)

Sclerosing Sertoli cell tumour (SSCT) is rare and less than 20 cases of this variant are recorded {929,2951}. They occur in adults and the average age at the time of diagnosis is 35 years.

Most tumours on record are relatively small (0.4-1.5 cm). Microscopically, features of SSCT include small neoplastic tubules surrounded by dense sclerotic stroma. The tubules may be solid or hollow, and may be discrete or anastomosing. Typically the tumours contain entrapped non neoplastic tubules.

Differential diagnosis

Sertoli cell tumours NOS need to be dis-

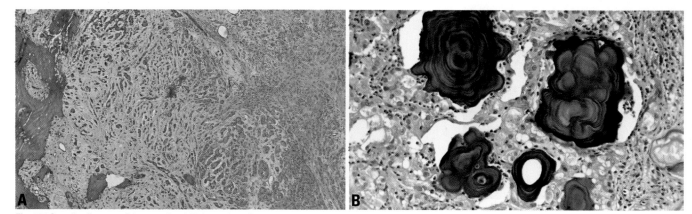

Fig. 4.74 Sertoli cell tumour **A** Large cell calcifiying variant. Cords and nests of cells in a fibrous stroma with focal ossification. **B** Large cell calcifiying Sertoli cell tumour.

tinguished from Sertoli cell nodules, and Leydig cell tumours, and rete adenomas. Sertoli cell nodules, however, are small, incidentally discovered, non neoplastic lesions composed of aggregates of small tubules lined by immature Sertoli cells and contain prominent basement membrane deposits. The rete adenomas occur within the dilated lumens of the rete testis.

Prognosis
Most Sertoli cell tumours are benign.

Malignant Sertoli cell tumour

ICD-O code   8640/3

Epidemiology
Malignant Sertoli cell tumour not otherwise specified is rare {1194}. Less than 50 cases have been reported. Age distribution does not differ from that of the benign form, occurring from childhood to old age.

Clinical features
Some patients present with metastases; most commonly to inguinal, retroperitoneal and/or supraclavicular lymph nodes. Approximately one third has gynecomastia at presentation, but apart from that no specific lesions or syndrome are known to be associated with malignant Sertoli cell tumour.

Macroscopy
They tend to be larger than the benign counterparts {2894}, usually more than 5 cm but range 2 to 18 cm. The macroscopic appearance may differ from that of the benign tumour by necrosis and haemorrhage.

Histopathology
Microscopically, the cellular features and

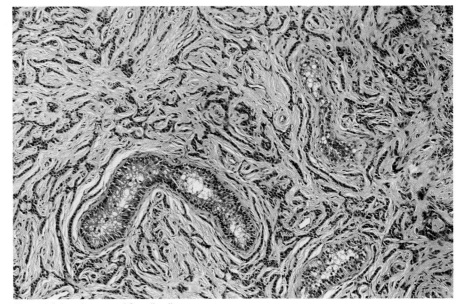

Fig. 4.75 Sclerosing type of Sertoli cell tumour.

growth patterns are similar to those of the benign counterpart but tend to be more variable within the same tumour and between tumours. The solid, sheet-like growth pattern is often prominent. The nuclei may be pleomorphic with one or more nucleoli, which are usually not very prominent. Mitotic figures may be numerous, and necrosis may occur. A fibrous, hyalinized or myxoid stroma occurs in varying amounts, but is usually sparse. Lymphovascular invasion may be seen. Lymphoplasmacytic infiltration is reported in some cases varying from sparse to pronounced and even with secondary germinal centres.

The most important differential diagnoses are classical and spermatocytic seminoma and variants of yolk sac tumour, however granulomatous reactions and intratubular germ cell neoplasia are not present in the surrounding testicular parenchyma. Endometrioid adenocarci-

noma and metastases, and among the latter especially adenocarcinomas with pale or clear cytoplasm, as well as melanoma should also be considered.

Immunohistochemical staining is helpful in defining the Sertoli cell nature of the tumour but not its malignant potential {1074,1194}. The tumour cells are cytokeratin and vimentin positive and they may also be positive for epithelial membrane antigen. They stain for inhibin A, but usually not very intensely, and they may be S100 positive. They are PLAP and CEA negative.

Granulosa cell tumour group

Definition
Granulosa cell tumours of the testis are morphologically similar to their ovarian counterparts. Two variants are distinguished: adult and juvenile types.

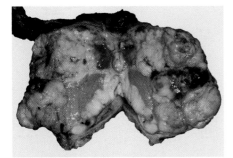

Fig. 4.76 Malignant Sertoli cell tumour.

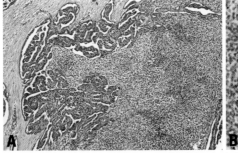
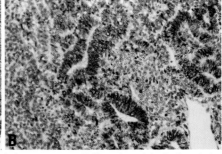

Fig. 4.77 Malignant Sertoli cell tumour. **A** Solid and tubular components. **B** Vimentin staining in the tubular component.

ICD-O codes

Granulosa cell tumour	8620/1
Adult type granulosa cell tumour	8620/1
Juvenile type granulosa cell tumour	8622/1

Adult type granulosa cell tumour

Incidence and clinical features

This tumour is rare {1,477,1443,1705,1 812,2567}, grows slowly and only two dozen cases have been reported {1901}. Some are incidental. About 25% of patients have gynecomastia. The average age at presentation is 44 years (range, 16-76 years). Patients have elevated serum levels of both inhibin, as occurs in other sex cord-stromal tumours {1781}, and Müllerian-inhibiting hormone, as occurs in similar ovarian tumours {1433}.

Macroscopy

These tumours are circumscribed, sometimes encapsulated, have a firm consistency and vary from yellow to beige. They vary from microscopic to 13 cm in diameter. The tumour surface may show cysts from 1-3 mm in diameter. Necrosis or haemorrhage are unusual.

Histopathology

Several patterns occur: macrofollicular, microfollicular, insular, trabecular, gyriform, solid and pseudosarcomatous. The microfollicular pattern is the most frequent. Microfollicles consist of palisading cells, which surround an eosinophilic material (Call-Exner bodies). Tumour cells are round to ovoid with grooved nuclei (coffee-bean nuclei) with one to two large peripheral nucleoli. Cellular pleomorphism and mitotic figures are infrequent, except for those areas showing fusiform cell pattern. The tumour may intermingle with seminiferous tubules and infiltrate the tunica albuginea. Some show focal theca cell differentiation, or have smooth muscle or osteoid {46}.
Tumour cells are immunoreactive for vimentin, smooth muscle actin, inhibin, MIC2 (013-Ewing sarcoma marker), and focally cytokeratins.

Prognosis

The tumour metastasizes in 20% or more of patients, even several years after the presentation {1223,1647}.

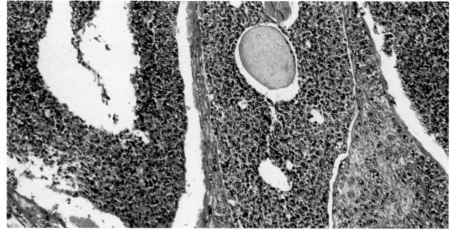
Fig. 4.78 Granulosa cell tumour, adult type.

Juvenile type granulosa cell tumour

This tumour is multicystic and its structure resembles that of Graafian follicles. Although it is rare, it is the most frequent congenital testicular neoplasm {1022, 2528}, comprising 6.6% of all prepubertal testicular tumours {1275}.

Clinical features

The tumour presents as a scrotal or abdominal asymptomatic mass, preferentially located in the left testis {1896}. It involves an abdominal testis in about 30% of cases. The contralateral testis is often undescended too. Most of the tumours are observed in the perinatal period, and presentation after the first year of life is exceptional. External genitalia are ambiguous in 20% and the most frequent associated anomaly is mixed gonadal dysgenesis, followed by hypospadias. In all cases with ambiguous genitalia the karyotype is abnormal: 45X / 46XY mosaicism or structural anomalies of Y chromosome. Neither recurrences nor metastases have been observed {400,2092,2136,2576,2895}. Neither gynecomastia nor endocrine disorders appeared associated.

Macroscopy

These tumours are usually cystic, with solid areas and partially encapsulated. The tumour size varies from 0.8 to 5 cm in size {1453}. Haemorrhage secondary to a torsion or trauma may make diagnosis difficult {407}.

Histopathology

Cysts are lined by several cell layers, depending on the degree of cystic dilation. The inner cells are similar to granulosa cells, while the outer cells resemble theca cells. Granulosa-like cells are

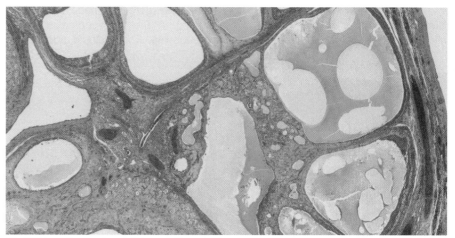
Fig. 4.79 Juvenile granulosa cell tumour. Note prominent cysts.

round and have spherical, regularly outlined, euchromatic nuclei with inconspicuous nucleoli, and scanty, vacuolated cytoplasm. Occasionally, Call-Exner bodies are seen. Theca-like cells are elongated and show scanty cytoplasm and few mitoses. In some cases, the cystic fluid is mucinous. Occasionally, the tumour is seen within adjacent tubules {1905}. Ultrastructural examination reveals a dual epithelial smooth muscle cell differentiation {2048} and a similarity between the tumoural cells and both primitive Sertoli cells and preovulatory ovarian granulosa cells {2082}.

Granulosa-like cells show diffuse immunostaining to vimentin, cytokeratins {956} and S-100 protein {2576}, and focal immunostaining to anti-Müllerian hormone {2180}. Theca-like cells immunoreact diffusely to vimentin, smooth muscle actin, and focally to desmin.

The differential diagnosis is yolk sac tumour, and this can be addressed by immunostains {65,837,1651,2661}.

Tumours of the thecoma / fibroma group

Definition
Tumours of the thecoma/fibroma group resemble their ovarian counterparts.

Most intratesticular "thecomas" that have been reported are actually fibromas of gonadal stromal origin. Fibroma of gonadal stromal origin is a benign tumour, which displays fusiform cells and variable degrees of collagenization.

ICD-O codes
Thecoma   8600/0
Fibroma   8810/0

Synonyms
Diffuse stromal form of gonadal stromal tumour {2592}, thecoma-like Sertoli cell tumour {482}, stromal tumour resembling fibroma {2547}, incompletely differentiated gonadal stromal tumour {1809}, testicular fibroma {1902}, testicular stromal tumour with myofilaments {932}, benign gonadal stromal tumour spindle fibroblastic type {64}, unclassified sex cord-stromal tumour with a predominance of spindle cells {2170}, myoid gonadal stromal tumour with epithelial differentiation {1904,2798}, theca cell tumour {2320}, and fibroma of gonadal stromal origin {1241}.

Clinical features
These tumours are rare, with only about 25 cases reported. The tumour presents as a slow growing, sometimes painful mass usually in the third and forth decades. It is not associated with hormonal alterations. Neither recurrences nor metastases have been observed.

Macroscopy
The tumour is a firm, well circumscribed, rarely encapsulated nodule, measuring 0.8 to 7 cm in diameter, and is yellow-white to white, without haemorrhage or necrosis.

Histopathology
Fusiform cells are arranged into fascicles or a storiform pattern, in slightly collagenized connective tissue with numerous small blood vessels. Cell density and amounts of collagen vary. Mitoses are usually scant, although up to four mitoses per high power field have been reported. Neither Sertoli cells nor granulosa cells are observed. Seminiferous tubules {571} with germ cells {2671} may be entrapped.

Positive immunoreaction, to both vimentin, smooth muscle actin, and occasionally, to desmin, S-100 protein and cytokeratin have been observed. Inhibin and CD99 are non reactive.

Tumour cells have ultrastructural features of both fibroblasts and myofibroblasts, although they are joined by desmosomes like Sertoli cells and granulosa cells {1726}.

The differential diagnosis includes leiomyoma, neurofibroma, and solitary fibrous tumour {601}. Some malignant tumours such as primary testicular fibrosarcoma {2683} and stromal tumours should also be considered.

Sex cord / gonadal stromal tumours: incompletely differentiated

Definition
Tumours composed largely of undifferentiated tissue in which abortive tubule formation, islands of Leydig cells, or evidence of other specific sex cord/gonadal stromal cell types are identified. These include tumours also recognizable as sex cord/gonadal stromal tumours but without specifically differentiated cell types.

ICD-O code   8591/1

Histopathology
Incompletely differentiated sex cord/gonadal stromal tumours are a heterogeneous group of testicular tumours that have been described under a variety of names but are not classifiable into more specific sex cord tumour types, including Leydig cell tumours, granulosa cell tumours and Sertoli cell tumours. Although heterogeneous, many of these tumours are similar {2170}, and are most often comprised of either short, wavy to round, spindle cells with nuclear grooves and a minor epithelioid component, or less commonly, long straight spindle cells with abundant cytoplasm, perinuclear vacuoles and blunt ended nuclei. Reticulin envelops aggregates of cells but not individual cells. Immunohistochemically, these tumours are most often reactive for both smooth muscle actin, and S-100 protein, a pattern also seen in both adult and juvenile granulosa cell tumours. Although most ovarian granulosa cell tumours are keratin positive, these tumours and most testicular granulosa cell tumours are keratin negative. Ultrastructural studies show desmosomes, numerous thin filaments, and focal dense bodies. Taken together these findings suggest granulosa cell differentiation in many of these incompletely differentiated tumours. With the exception of one large and poorly characterized tumour {1811}, the limited clinical follow-up available to date has been benign {932,2170,2860}.

Sex cord / gonadal stromal tumours, mixed forms

Definition
The mixed form may contain any combination of cell types e.g. Sertoli, Leydig, and granulosa.

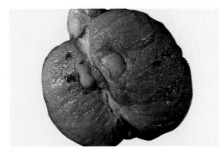

Fig. 4.80 Sex cord stromal tumour of the testis.

ICD-O code   8592/1

Clinical features
The tumours occur at all ages {1800, 1812,2664} Testicular swelling of several months or years is the most common symptom. Gynecomastia may be present {827,2906}. The tumours vary in size but may be large and replace the testis. The cut surface shows generally well circumscribed white or yellow masses. Some tumours are lobulated. The mixed forms show the histologic features of the individual well differentiated components. The Sertoli-Leydig cell tumour, common in the ovary, is rare in the testis {741,814,2053,2591,2592}. The differentiated areas react with appropriate antibodies for substances found in Sertoli, Leydig and granulosa cell tumours. The undifferentiated component may be positive for S-100 protein, smooth muscle actin, desmin, and cytokeratins {932, 1726}.

Malignant sex cord / gonadal stromal tumours

ICD-O code   8590/3

About 18-20% of gonadal stromal tumours are malignant {1454}. These tumours are usually very large. Macroscopically they often show necrosis and haemorrhage. They are poorly delineated. Histologically, they show cellular pleomorphism, nuclear anaplasia, numerous mitoses including abnormal forms and vascular invasion {652,875, 1800,1812,2664}.

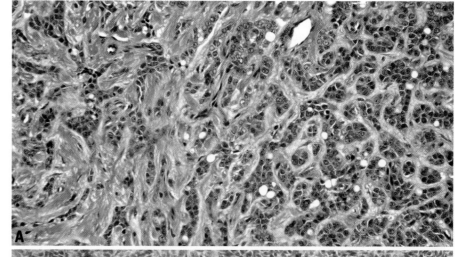
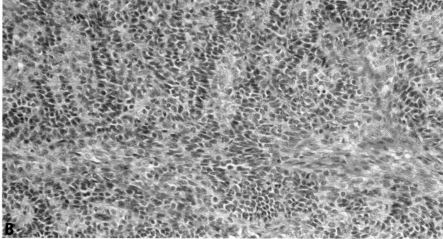

Fig. 4.81 A, B Stromal tumour, NOS

Tumours containing both germ cell and sex cord / gonadal stromal elements

T.M. Ulbright

Gonadoblastoma

Definition
A tumour composed of two principal cell types: large germ cells similar to those of seminoma and small cells resembling immature Sertoli and granulosa cells; elements resembling Leydig or lutein-like cells may also be present.

ICD-O code   9073/1

Incidence and clinical features
Gonadoblastoma is most commonly seen in mixed gonadal dysgenesis associated with ambiguous genitalia and 45,X karyotype and Y chromosome material {1389,1390,2266,2350}. The estimated risk of developing gonadoblastoma in this setting is 15-25% {2026}. In one series about 24% of patients with Turner syndrome had Y chromosome material {2026} and in another series 12.2% {930}. In the latter only 7-10% of patients had gonadoblastoma. Rarely, gonadoblastoma is found in genotypical and phenotypical males {413,2350}.

Macroscopy
The gonads contain yellowish to tan nodules with a gritty cut surface. The tumours may consist of microscopic foci or can measure up to 8 cm {2350}.

Histopathology
The lesion consists of immature Sertoli cells and germ cells which form rounded or irregularly outlined discrete aggregates. Most commonly, the Sertoli cells encircle rounded hyaline nodules and are intimately associated with basement membranes surrounding the nests. In the second growth pattern the Sertoli cells surround large germ cells or in the third pattern the germ cells occupy the center of the nests and the Sertoli cells form a peripheral ring. Mostly in the post pubertal patient, the stroma may contain large polygonal cells indistinguishable from Leydig cells. Calcifications may be focal, involving the hyaline bodies or extensive. About 50% of all patients with gonado-

blastoma irrespective of the underlying abnormality develop germ cell tumours mainly seminomas, but in 8%, other germ cell tumour types. By the age of 40, 25% of patients with mixed gonadal dysgenesis and Y component have gonadoblastoma and germ cell tumour {1620}.

Immunoprofile
The germ cells in gonadoblastoma express the VASA protein {2929}, testis specific protein Y-encoded (TSPY) {1448}, and overexpress p53 protein {1149}. They also have features of intratubular malignant germ cells expressing PLAP and c-kit {1248}. The stromal cells express inhibin and the Wilms tumour gene (WT-1) {1149}.

Differential diagnosis
Sertoli cell nodules containing germ cells may be mistaken for gonadoblastoma. Germ cell-sex cord/stromal tumours occur rarely in otherwise normal males {266,2566}. In these tumours the germ cells are seen within tubules or form cohesive nests.

Genetics
Germs cells in gonadoblastoma have been reported to be aneuploid {1248}. Gonadoblastomas contain evidence of Y-chromosome material by fluorescence in situ hybridization {1163}. The Y-chromosome contains the candidate gene of the gonadoblastoma locus {2286,2650}. Interestingly, the seminomas and non-seminomas originating in dysgenetic

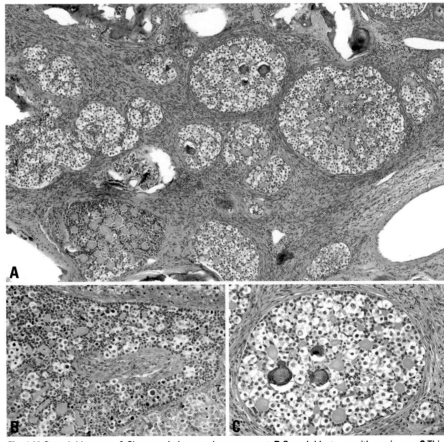

Fig. 4.82 Gonadoblastoma. **A** Characteristic nested arrangement. **B** Gonadoblastoma with seminoma. **C** This nest has cylinders of basement membrane, some of which are calcified.

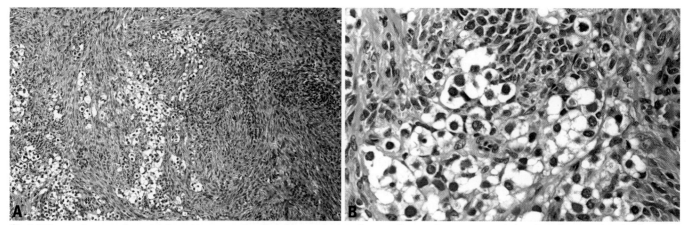

Fig. 4.83 Germ cell-sex cord/gonadal stromal tumour, unclassified. **A** Loose clusters of germ cells occur in a tumour consisting of small nests and cords of sex cord cells and spindled stromal cells. **B** The germ cells have round nuclei with fine chromatin and inconspicuous nucleoli.

gonads are most often diploid unlike those from non dysgenetic testis {351,1004,2198}.

Germ cell-sex cord/gonadal stromal tumour, unclassified

Germ cell-sex cord/gonadal stromal tumour, unclassified type is defined as a neoplasm having a combination of neoplastic germ cells and neoplastic sex cord-stromal elements arranged in a diffuse pattern, as opposed to the nested pattern of gonadoblastoma {266,1648, 2142,2563}. Recent evidence {2671}, however, casts doubt on the neoplastic nature of the germ cells, thereby providing support that most, and perhaps all, of the purported examples represent sex cord-stromal tumours with entrapped, non neoplastic germ cells. This viewpoint, however, is controversial. These tumours have occurred mostly in young men who presented with masses, although an occasional case has been in a child. The tumours are usually white, grey or tan circumscribed masses. On microscopic examination, the predominant element is the sex cord-stromal component, which is often arranged in tubules or cords with transition to spin-dled stromal cells. The germ cells are most common at the periphery but may be more diffuse or central. They are commonly loosely clustered with clear cytoplasm and round, uniform nuclei having fine chromatin. Immunostains for placental alkaline phosphatase and c-kit have been negative {2671}, while the sex-cord-stromal elements have often been positive for alpha subunit of inhibin. Malignant behaviour has not been reported, but the sex cord-stromal component should be analysed for features that are associated with metastases in sex cord-stromal tumours.

Miscellaneous tumours of the testis

F.K. Mostofi
I.A. Sesterhenn
J.R. Srigley
H.S. Levin

Carcinoid tumour

Definition
An epithelial tumour of usually monomorphous endocrine cells showing mild or no atypia and growing in the form of solid nests, trabeculae, or pseudoglandulae.

ICD-O code   8240/3

Epidemiology
The incidence is less than 1% of testicular neoplasms. In the series by Berdjis & Mostofi it accounts for 0.23% {214}.

Clinical features
The ages range from 10-83 years, with a mean age of 46. Primary carcinoid of the testis usually presents as a mass, and only rarely with carcinoid syndrome {1045}. Symptoms of testicular swelling range from a few months to 20 years {214,766,1938,2569,2923}.

Macroscopy
The tumours measure between 1.0 cm to 9.5 cm with a mean of 4.6 cm. They are solid, and yellow to dark tan. Calcifications may be present.

Histopathology
The microscopic appearance is identical to that described in other sites but the trabecular and insular pattern predominate. The larger tumours may show necrosis. Neuroendocrine granules can be identified by electron microscopy {2569,2923}. The cells are positive for endocrine markers (e.g. chromogranin) {1970,2923,2932}. Rarely, primary carcinoids of the testis are malignant metastasizing to lymph nodes, liver, skin and skeletal system {1127,1285,2393,2533}. Carcinoids in teratomas have been included in the category of teratoma with somatic type malignancy {1805}. Carcinoids from other sites (e.g. ileum) can metastasize to the testis {1823}.

Tumours of ovarian epithelial types

Definition
Tumours of testis and adjacent tissues that resemble surface epithelial tumours of the ovary.

Incidence
These are very rare tumours.

Clinical features
The patients ages range from 14-68 years. The patients present with scrotal enlargement {2664}.

Macroscopy
The macroscopic appearance varies with the tumour type. Cystic lesions are usually serous tumours of borderline malignancy or, if mucin is present, mucinous cystadenoma. The more solid tend to be carcinomas {2664,2902}. They may be located in the tunica and paratesticular tissue as well as the testis.

Histopathology
The histologic appearance is identical to their ovarian counterparts. The reader is referred to the volume dealing with ovarian tumours. Most of the lesions reported in the literature are serous tumours of borderline malignancy {570,2166,2767, 2902}. They also include serous carcinomas {1242}, well differentiated endometrioid adenocarcinoma with squamous differentiation {2902}, mucinous cystadenoma {1295}, and mucinous borderline tumours and cystadenocarcinoma {685,1906}.

Differential diagnosis
The differential diagnosis includes carcinoma of the rete and mesothelioma. The rete carcinoma should be centered around or in the rete. Immunohistochemistry will be helpful to distinguish mesothelioma from papillary serous tumours. The differential diagnosis of mucinous carcinoma and endometrioid carcinoma should include metastatic adenocarcinoma.

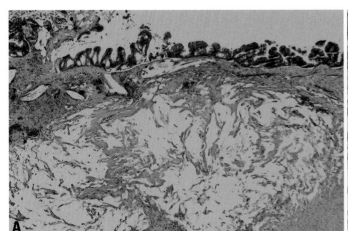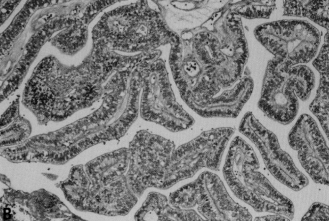

Fig. 4.84 A Mucinous borderline tumour of the paratesticular tissue. **B** Endometrioid carcinoma.

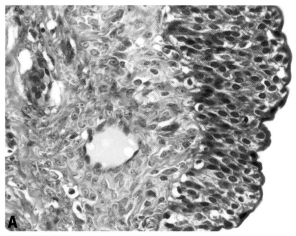
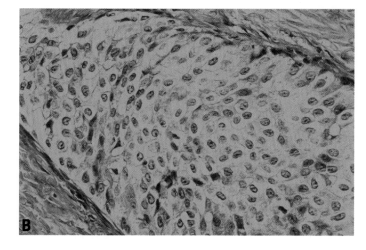

Fig. 4.85 A, B Brenner tumour of the testis.

Brenner tumour

ICD-O code   9000/0

Tumours histologically identical to Brenner tumour of ovary may be encountered in the testis and paratesticular region {312} The age range is 37-70 (mean 57.7) years. Macroscopically, the solid and cystic masses vary from less than1 to 5 cm in diameter. The histology is similar to that of ovarian Brenner tumour with cysts lined by bland transitional

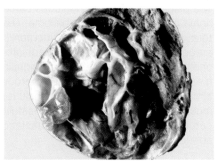

Fig. 4.86 Brenner tumour of the testis.

epithelium, solid nests of transitional type epithelium and a cellular spindle cell stroma. One mixed Brenner and adenomatoid tumour has been reported {1911}.
Most examples of Brenner tumour are benign, although one malignant example showing local invasion, lymphatic space involvement and metastatic deposits in para-aortic lymph nodes has been described {357}.

Nephroblastoma

ICD-O code   8960/3

Nephroblastoma of testicular adnexa is identical to renal nephroblastoma and is a triphasic tumour comprised of metanephric blastema, epithelial structures consisting of tubular and/or glomerular structures, and mesenchymal structures.
Nephroblastomas may occur as a paratesticular tumour {1976} or as a metastasis from a renal nephroblastoma {2303}.

Inguinal and scrotal nephroblastomas have occurred in males 3.5 years of age and younger {116}. Paratesticular tumours have been associated with heterotopic renal anlage and one paratesticular nephroblastoma metastasized to the lung {1976}. Primary nephroblastoma has been staged and treated according to NWTS protocol.

Paraganglioma

ICD-O code   8680/1

In the spermatic cord, these are rare. Five cases have been reported in the literature {605,698,729,2452} and 2 unreported cases are in the Genitourinary Tumour Registry of the Armed Forces Institute of Pathology. They vary in size from 1.5 to 10 cm and are functionally inactive. Histologically, they are indistinguishable from those in other sites.

Lymphoma and plasmacytoma of the testis and paratesticular tissues

A. Marx
P.J. Woodward

Definition

Primary lymphomas or plasmacytomas of testes or paratesticular tissues arise in the testicles, epididymis or spermatic cord and are neither associated with lymphoma elsewhere nor leukemia. Involvement of these anatomic structures by systemic lymphomas/leukemias or plasma cell myeloma defines secondary testicular or paratesticular lymphomas or plasma cell neoplasias.

Incidence and clinical features

Testicular lymphoma (TL) and plasmacytoma

The majority of primary lymphomas of the male genital tract arise in the testes {756, 1429,2944,2945}. Testicular lymphomas (TL) constitute 2% of all testicular neoplasms, 2% of all high grade lymphomas and 5% of all extranodal lymphomas in men. Primary (stage IE) TL constitute 40-60% of all TL {1429,2944,2945}. Most patients with TL are 60-80 years of age (19-91), and in this age group TL is the single most frequent testicular tumour {2001,2938,2945}.

Only single cases of primary plasmacytoma of the testis, all in older men, have been reported {1166,1968,2541}. One case was associated with HIV infection {2138}.

In children primary testicular lymphomas are rare and typically occur prior to puberty (3–10 years of age) {767,1761, 1999,2076}. Secondary involvement of the testis occurs in about 5% of childhood systemic lymphomas {547,1296}.

Paratesticular lymphoma and plasmacytoma

The majority of paratesticular lymphomas is seen in connection with TL, and 25-60% of TL show extension to paratesticular sites {509,756,767,1670,2944}. Secondary involvement of paratesticular structures in the absence of testicular lymphoma is exceedingly rare {1073}.

Primary paratesticular lymphomas {1073, 1288,1670,2718} and plasmacytomas {758} are rare as well. Primary paratesticular lymphoma appears to peak in a young (20–30 years of age) {1073} and an older (34–73 years of age) {1073, 2718} age group with a favourable clinical course only in the former {1073}.

Clinical features and macroscopy

Primary lymphoma and plasmacytoma of testis and paratesticular tissues typically present with unilateral enlargement of the scrotum or swelling in the inguinal region. "B-symptoms" are rare in primary lesions. Bilateral simultaneous involvement of the testis is typical for lymphoblastic lymphoma, but rare in other entities {756}. Bilateral paratesticular lymphoma is rare as well {1670}. By contrast, involvement of the contralateral testis during lymphoma recurrence is common (10-40%) {1429,2944,2945}.

Macroscopically, the cut surface usually reveals poorly demarcated tan, grey and necrotic or haemorrhagic single or multiple nodules or diffuse enlargement of testis or paratesticular tissues {767,1073, 1296,2076,2718}.

Imaging

Testicular lymphoma

The sonographic appearance of testicular lymphoma is variable and often indistinguishable from that of germ cell tumours. They are generally discrete hypoechoic lesions, which may completely infiltrate the testis {913,1657}. In contrast to most germ cell tumours, lymphoma is often bilateral and multifocal. It may also involve the extratesticular tissues.

Paratesticular lymphoma

Paratesticular lymphoma may appear radiologically as multiple nodules or as diffuse infiltration of the epididymis or spermatic cord {2070}. Sonographically lymphomatous masses will generally be hypoechoic. The testes are usually also involved. When multiple masses are identified involving both the testicular and extratesticular tissues lymphoma is the first consideration. Although less common, metastases can give a similar appearance.

Histopathology

Testicular lymphoma (TL) and plasmacytoma

In adult testis, primary diffuse large B-cell lymphoma (DLCL) is the single most frequent lymphoma (70-80%) {1429, 2944,2945}. DLCL cells infiltrate around seminiferous tubules, cause arrest of spermatogenesis, interstitial fibrosis, tubular hyalinization and loss of tubules {756,2825}. Primary MALT lymphomas {1174}, follicular lymphomas {756}, T-cell lymphomas {1131,2825}, and CD56+, EBV-associated T/NK-cell lymphomas of nasal type {402} are exceptional.

Primary testicular plasmacytoma is less frequent than DLCL {98,643,756,1486, 2497}. It forms nodules composed of

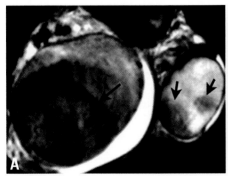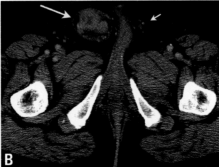

Fig. 4.87 Lymphoma. **A** Coronal T2-weighted MRI shows these lesions as hypointense masses (arrows) within the normal higher signal parenchyma. **B** Lymphoma involving the spermatic cord. Axial CT image through the level of the spermatic cord shows diffuse enlargement on the right side by a soft tissue mass (large arrow). The left spermatic cord is normal (small arrow).

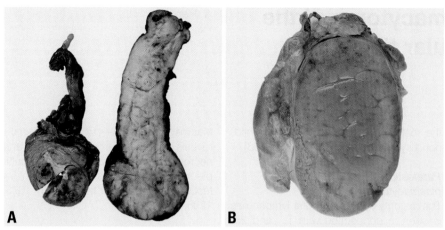

Fig. 4.88 A Lymphoma, bilateral. **B** Myeloid leukaemia (chloroma).

closely packed atypical plasma cells, that exhibit intertubular growth, while invasion of seminiferous tubules is rare {758}.

In children, the majority of testicular lymphomas represent secondary involvement by Burkitt, DLCL or lymphoblastic lymphoma {547,1296}. Primary follicular lymphoma of the testis in prepubertal children appears to be a distinct entity due to typical morphological features of grade III follicular lymphoma (+/- diffuse large cell areas) but peculiar immunohistochemical and genetic properties {767, 1761,2076} and a good prognosis.

Paratesticular lymphomas and plasmacytoma

Among lymphomas confined to the epididymis, follicular lymphomas (grade II and III) and a low grade MALT lymphoma have been described in patients 20-30 years of age {1073,1288,1670,1922, 2718}. In older patients, diffuse large B-cell lymphomas {1073,2718} and a single EBV-associated intravascular large cell lymphoma of T-lineage {137} were seen. Plasmacytoma in the paratesticular tissue is almost always associated with testicular plasmacytoma and plasma cell myeloma {1073} though exceptions occur {758}.

Immunohistochemistry

There are no immunohistochemical peculiarities in testicular and paratesticular lymphomas or plasmacytomas. However, in testicular pediatric primary follicular lymphoma absence of bcl-2 expression, variable expression of CD10 and usually strong bcl-6 positivity are characteristic {767,1568,1761,1999, 2076}.

Somatic genetics and genetic susceptibility

Specific genetic aberrations have not been published. Pediatric primary follicular lymphoma of the testis combines a typical grade III follicular morphology with combined absence of t(14;18) translocation, BCL-2 rearrangement and p53 abnormalities {1999,2076}.

Prognosis and predictive factors

In aduts the prognosis of testicular lymphoma is generally poor: taking all stages and histological lymphoma subtypes into account, the median survival was 32-53 months {1429,2370,2944}. The 5- and 10-year overall survival rates were 37-48% and 19-27%, respectively {1429,2945}.

The primary (stage IE) lymphomas of the testis and spermatic cord have the worst prognosis among all extranodal lymphomas, with 5 year overall survival rates of 70-79% {1429,2945}.

By contrast, the prognosis of primary lymphomas of the epididymis, particularly in patients <30 years, is much better {2718}. Relapses in TL occur in >50% of cases, of which 71-91% involve extranodal sites, including the contralateral testis (10-40%) and central nervous system (CNS) parenchyma (20-27%) {1429,2944,2945}. Surprisingly, CNS involvement occurs in 15-20% of stage IE TL and spermatic cord lymphomas {1429,2718}.

Prognostically favourable factors in TL and spermatic cord lymphomas are lymphoma sclerosis {756}, young age, early stage, combined modality treatment {1429,2718,2944,2945} and, in some studies, anthracyclin use {2370,2738}.

Primary testicular and paratesticular plasmacytoma has a favourable prognosis {758,1166}, while prognosis is poor in the context of plasma cell myeloma {758, 1701}.

In children, secondary testicular involvement in systemic B-cell lymphomas does not confer a poor prognosis, and these children can usually be cured by chemotherapy alone, allowing for gonadal function to be preserved {547}. Primary pediatric follicular lymphomas of testis have an excellent prognosis in spite of grade III morphology: after a follow-up of 18 – 44 months there was no death after orchiectomy and chemotherapy {767,1761,1999,2076}.

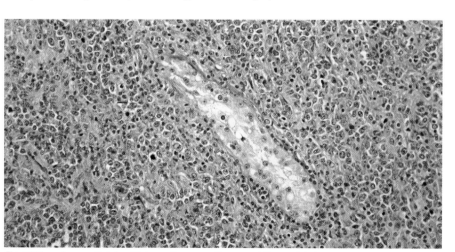

Fig. 4.89 Lymphoma with interstitial growth surrounding a seminiferous tubule.

Tumours of collecting ducts and rete

L. Nochomovitz

Adenoma

Definition
A benign tumour of rete epithelial origin that occurs within the dilated rete and typically has a tubular pattern resembling Sertoli cell tumour.

ICD-O code   8140/0

Clinical features and histopathology
This is a rare tumour that mostly occurs in adults. It typically forms polypoid nodules composed of tubules that project into the dilated lumen of the rete testis. The tubules resemble those seen in benign Sertoli cell tumours.

Adenocarcinoma

Definition
Recommended criteria for the diagnosis of adenocarcinoma of the rete testis are: no histologically similar extrascrotal primary, tumour centred on testicular hilum, absence of conventional germinal or non germinal testicular cancer, histologic transition from unaffected rete testis, solid growth pattern {1908}.

ICD-O code   8140/3

Epidemiology and clinical features
Rete testis carcinoma is rare, its etiology unknown. The tumour, predominating in the fourth through eighth decades, is usually associated with a scrotal mass, tenderness, or lumbar pain. It may be masked by an inguinal hernia, hydrocele, fistula, sinus or epididymitis. Symptoms are brief or extend over years. Locally recurrent tumour nodules and abscesses may involve the scrotal and perineal skin. A statistical analysis, based on published data, was reported {2288}.

Macroscopy
The carcinoma usually forms a non encapsulated firm, pale rubbery hilar mass. A cystic component, if any, is usually minor. Reported lesional size ranges from 1.0-10.0cm. The boundary between

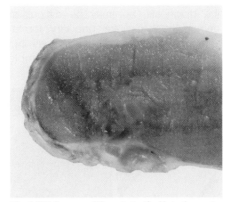

Fig. 4.90 Adenoma of the rete testis. Note the cysts.

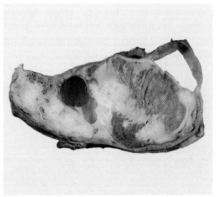

Fig. 4.91 Rete testis carcinoma.

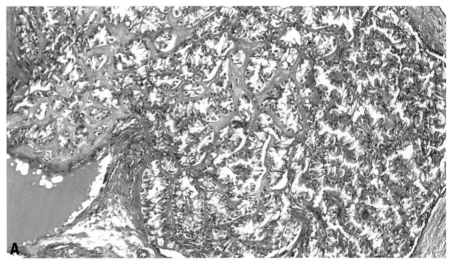

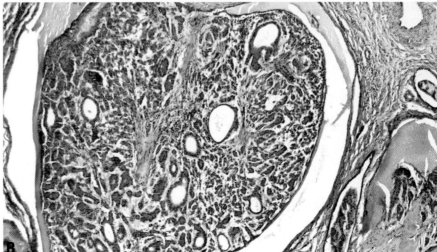

Fig. 4.92 A Sertoliform cystadenoma of the rete testis. **B** Adenoma of the rete testis. Note the cystic dilatations.

testicular parenchyma and tumour tends to be blurred where the tumour infiltrates the testicular interstitium. Nodular excrescences may stud the tunics and the spermatic cord.

Histopathology

The low power image of rete testis adenocarcinoma comprises large cellular tumour nodules with interspersed, smaller cellular clumps. Slit-like ramifications, reminiscent of Kaposi sarcoma, may permeate these cellular aggregates. The solid cellular zones may show sharply defined necrotic foci. Typically, neoplastic protuberances bulge into the residual dilated rete testis, the channels of which appear dilated. Actual and convincing transition from tumour to normal rete epithelium is the strongest evidence for the diagnosis, but may be difficult to demonstrate. Cellular papillary formations may project into open spaces, but frankly cystic lesions that resemble serous tumours analogous to those of the ovary and peritoneum should not be classified as rete testis carcinoma. Of the tumour types in the differential diagnosis, mesothelioma in particular must be carefully excluded {164,2429}.

The tumour may extend to the epididymis, spreading to the para-aortic, iliac and other lymph nodes, to various viscera, and to bone. In one analysis, 56% of 22 patients succumbed within the follow-up period.

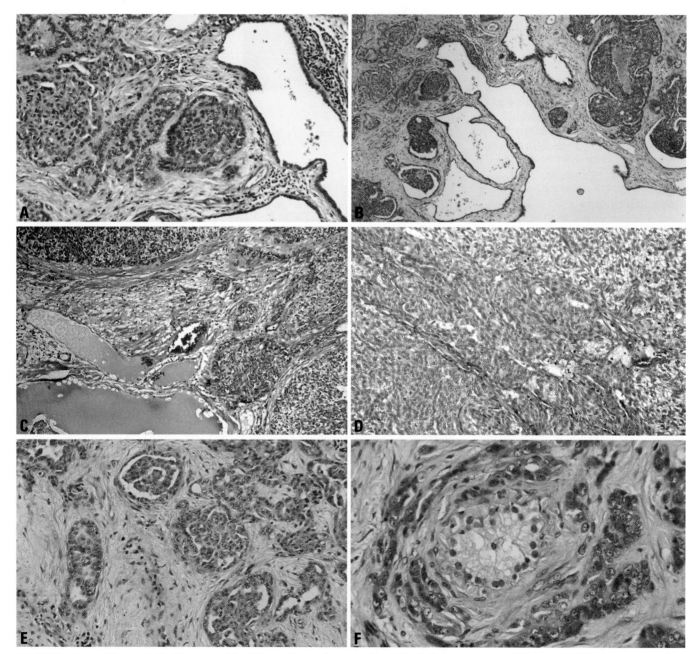

Fig. 4.93 Carcinoma of the rete testis. **A** Tumour nodules between distended spaces of rete testis. **B** Tumour aggregates elicit desmoplastic response among dilated rete testis spaces. **C** Tumour cell nodules next to dilated vessels. **D** Solid tumour area with brisk mitotic activity. **E** Tumour infiltrates between atrophic, hyalinised seminiferous tubules. **F** Tumour cells encircling an atrophic seminiferous tubule.

Tumours of paratesticular structures

C.J. Davis
P.J. Woodward
L.P. Dehner
M.A. Jones
J.R. Srigley

I.A. Sesterhenn
W.L. Gerald
M. Miettinen
J.F. Fetsch

Adenomatoid tumour

Definition
A benign tumour of mesothelial cells characterized by numerous gland-like spaces, tubules or cords.

Synonym
Benign mesothelioma.

ICD-O code   9054/0

Incidence
Adenomatoid tumours are the most common tumours of the testicular adnexa, representing 32% of all tumours in this location {287,1800} and 60% of all benign neoplasms in this area {2664}.

Clinical features
Signs and symptoms
These begin to appear in the late teens and up to 79 years and most are seen in the third through the fifth decades (mean age 36 years) {1800}. They present as small, solid intrascrotal tumours, and are usually asymptomatic. They have typically been present for several years without appreciable growth and are uniformly benign {1800,2664}.

Imaging
Adenomatoid tumours are smooth, round, and well circumscribed masses of variable size generally arising in the epididymis. They are typically described as hyperechoic and homogeneous. This should not, however, be considered characteristic as great variability has been reported {801,1475}. The most important point is to clearly identify the mass as extratesticular and if it can be shown to be arising from the epididymis, adenomatoid tumour is the most likely diagnosis. They may also arise from the spermatic cord and tunica albuginea, where they can grow intratesticularly. The latter presentation is indistinguishable from testicular germ cell neoplasms.

Localization
Most of these occur in or near the lower pole or upper pole of the epididymis but other sites include the body of the epididymis, the tunica vaginalis, tunica albuginea and rete testis. Rarely the parietal tunica or spermatic cord may be involved {1800}.

Macroscopy and histopathology
These are usually small tumours, 2.0 cm or less, but they have ranged from 0.4 to 5.0 cm {2051}. They are round or oval and well circumscribed although they can also be flattened and plaque-like. Microscopically these consist of eosinophilic mesothelial cells forming solid cords as well as dilated tubules with flattened lining cells which may initially suggest an endothelial appearance {166}. Vacuolated cytoplasm is a prominent feature of the cells. The stroma is usually fibrous but may consist largely of smooth muscle.

Ultrastructural and immunohistochemical features of these tumours support their mesothelial cell origin. There is an absence of epithelial/carcinoma markers MOC-31, Ber-Ep4, CEA, B72.3, LEA 135 and Leu M1 and also factor VIII and CD34. They invariably express cytokeratin AE1/AE3 and EMA {586,589}.

Malignant mesothelioma

Definition
Malignant tumours originating from the tunica vaginalis or tunica albuginea.

ICD-O code   9050/3

Incidence
Intrascrotal mesotheliomas are invariably described as rare although they are the most common paratesticular malignancies after the soft tissue sarcomas {287,1239,2051}. As of the year 2002

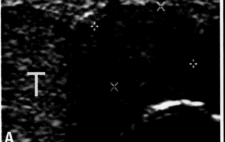
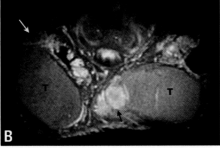

Fig. 4.94 Adenomatoid tumour. **A** Longitudinal ultrasound image shows a well defined, slightly hypoechoic, extratesticular mass in the region of the epididymal tail (cursors). (T - testis). **B** Coronal, gadolinium enhanced, T1-weighted MR image of scrotum shows an enhancing mass in the left epididymal head (black arrow). The epididymis on the right is normal (white arrow). (T - testes).

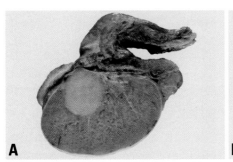
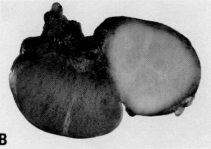

Fig. 4.95 Adenomatoid tumour. **A** Adenomatoid tumour protruding into the testis. **B** Paratesticular adenomatoid tumour.

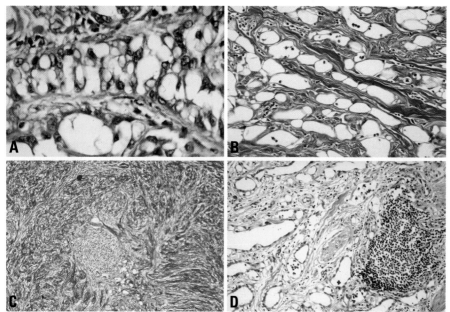

Fig. 4.96 A Adenomatoid tumour. This is the classic tubular morphology with vacuolated cells. B Vacuolated cells mimicking endothelial cells. Masson trichrome stain. C In this example the stroma is entirely smooth muscle. Masson trichrome stain. D Peripheral lymphocytic aggregates are commonly seen.

only 80 cases had been reported {353}. In one study of all mesotheliomas, including pleural, peritoneal and pericardial, only 6 of 1785 were of tunica vaginalis origin {1836}.

Clinical features

The age at presentation ranges from 6 to 91 years with most occurring between ages 55 and 75 {2051}. 10% of reported cases have been in patients younger than 25 years {2051,2664}. In descending order of frequency paratesticular mesotheliomas have been discovered incidental to hernia repair, a palpable tumour associated with a hydrocele and a palpable tumour only. There have also been sporadic cases presenting with localized soreness or swelling, acute hydrocele, recurrent hydrocele, haematocele and diffuse thickening of the spermatic cord. It is now possible to anticipate the correct diagnosis with imaging studies, particularly when combined with cytology {2051}. Demonstration of multiple nodular masses within a hydrocele, particularly if irregular contours are seen, will generally prove to be a mesothelioma {819}. The incidence of asbestos exposure in patients with tunica vaginalis mesotheliomas has been cited as 23% {2051}, 41% {1239} and even 50% in a small series {135}. To date, asbestos exposure is the only

known risk factor and the incidence of exposure correlates with that reported for pleural tumours {1239}.

Macroscopy

The common appearance of the gross specimen is thickening of the tunica vaginalis with multiple friable nodules or excrescences. The tunica albuginea may also be involved. The fluid of the hydrocele sac is described as clear or haemorrhagic {1239,1800,2051}. White or tan masses of firm tissue may be found where the tumour infiltrates into the hilus or periphery of the testis or into the epididymis or spermatic cord.

Tumour spread

Most recurrences occur in the first 2 years of follow-up {2090} and are seen in

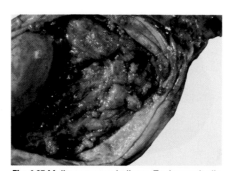

Fig. 4.97 Malignant mesothelioma. Tunica vaginalis with multiple friable excrescences.

the surgical scar and adjacent tissue of the skin, scrotum, epididymis or cord and metastasis have been found in inguinal and retroperitoneal nodes, abdominal peritoneum, lungs, mediastinum, bone and brain {1239,2051}. There have been reports of peritoneal mesotheliomas presenting initially in the tunica vaginalis {36} and of simultaneous mesotheliomas of pleura, peritoneum and tunica vaginalis {124}. We have seen other cases in which the intrascrotal lesions preceded peritoneal and/or pleural disease by up to four years.

Histopathology

Microscopically about 75% of these will be purely epithelial in type while the others are biphasic, with varying amounts of the sarcomatoid morphology {287,1239, 2051}. The epithelial type usually shows a papillary and tubulopapillary morphology, often with solid sheets of cells. The cell structure is variable; the cells covering the papillations are usually rounded or cuboidal, often with a bland appearance but may be flattened or low columnar. Where the cells are arranged in solid sheets, variation in size and shape is the rule. The cytoplasm is eosinophilic and varies in amount {1800}. Nucleoli are often prominent. The sarcomatoid element shows fascicles of spindle cells which may include a storiform pattern similar to malignant fibrous histiocytoma {1239}. Mesotheliomas of the tunica will usually show cellular atypia of the mesothelial surface indicative of in situ neoplasia {2051}.

Immunohistochemistry

By immunohistochemistry the cells are uniformly reactive with cytokeratin (AE1/AE3) in both epithelial and spindle cell elements. EMA and vimentin are also usually positive and calretinin has been

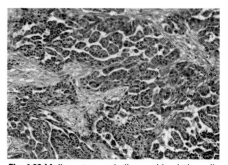

Fig. 4.98 Malignant mesothelioma with tubulopapillary morphology.

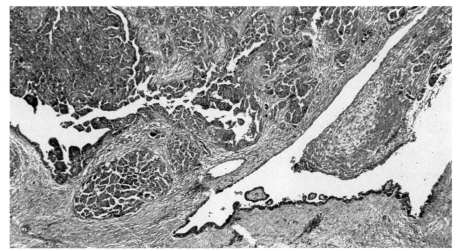

Fig. 4.99 Malignant mesothelioma. Exophytic tumour growth into the scrotal sac. Note in situ malignant change of mesothelial surface.

invariably positive {1239,2051}. CEA, B72.3, Leu M1 and Ber-Ep4 have been negative {2664}.

Ultrastructure
Ultrastructural features are characteristic of mesothelial cells.

Benign mesothelioma

This designation has been given to the rare examples of cystic mesothelioma and to the well differentiated papillary mesothelioma (WDPM) both of which are similar to those occurring in the peritoneum. The cystic mesotheliomas present as scrotal swellings suggestive of hydrocele and consist of multiple cystic structures with no cellular atypia. Lymphangioma is almost invariably the lesion to be excluded and this should be readily accomplished with the epithelial and endothelial markers {1434,2051}.

The WDPMs present as one or more superficial nodules or granular deposits over the surface of the hydrocele sac {353,2051}. Microscopically there is a single row of flattened or cuboidal mesothelial cells lining fibrovascular papillae {348,353,2051,2852}. Cellular features are bland. Most of these occur in young men in the second and third decades and have behaved in a benign fashion although it is widely regarded as a borderline mesothelioma since some have proved to be aggressive {348,353, 1239}.

Nodular mesothelial hyperplasia

Definition
A proliferative process typically discovered in a hernia sac as an incidental finding consisting of cohesive collections of polygonal cells forming one or more attached or unattached nodules.

Epidemiology
Nodular mesothelial hyperplasia (NMH) was first described in 1975 {2228}. Approximately one case of NMH occurs in 800 to 1000 hernia sacs that are examined microscopically. Approximately 70% of cases are diagnosed in patients 10 years of age or less, (median 1.5 years, range 6 weeks-84 years). There is a 3-10:1 male predilection, reflecting the predominance of inguinal hernias in male children {1519}.

Etiology
The presumptive etiology is a reaction of the hernia sac to a variety of injuries including incarceration and inflammation.

Clinical features
Clinical manifestations are those of a hernia.

Histopathology
One or more nodules, either attached or unattached to the mesothelial surface of the hernia sac are identified. Adjacent to the nodule, the surface mesothelium is hyperplastic with individual cuboidal cells and a population of submesothelial cells resembling those of the nodule. The unattached nodule is often accompanied by individual cells floating within the lumen of the hernia sac and pseudoglandular and papillary profiles of cells are present in some cases. The polygonal cells vary from innocuous to moderately pleomorphic. Mitotic activity is low. Fibrin and inflammatory cells are also present. The lesion lacks the overtly malignant features of a malignant mesothelioma, carcinoma or sarcoma. Multinucleated cells and especially strap-like cells in NMH have been confused with embryonal rhabdomyosarcoma in the past.

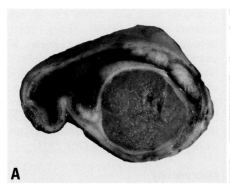
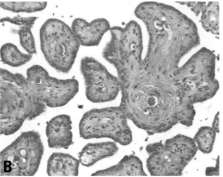

Fig. 4.100 Benign mesothelioma. **A** Well differentiated papillary mesothelioma. Note superficial nature of the tumours.g. **B** Well differentiated papillary mesothelioma. Note papillations with bland cuboidal cell lining.

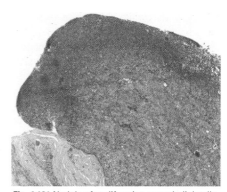

Fig. 4.101 Nodule of proliferating mesothelial cells.

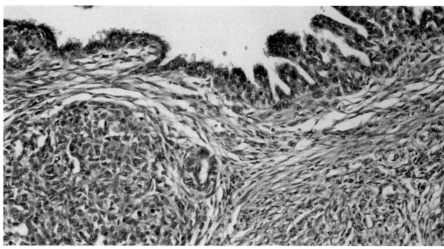

Immunoprofile

Ordóñez and associates {1973} examined one case by immunohistochemistry and concluded that the so-called mesothelial cells are histiocytes, although the originally described lesions may not represent the same process {2769}. An analogous proliferation of the pleura has been encountered and reported as nodular histiocytic hyperplasia {401,455}.

Prognosis

The lesion is benign.

Adenocarcinoma of the epididymis

Definition

Adenocarcinoma of the epididymis is a rare gland forming, malignant neoplasm derived from epididymal epithelial cells.

ICD-O code   8140/3

Incidence and clinical features

It occurs in men from 27-82 years, mean age, 67 years. Only 10 well documented cases have been reported {418,770,833, 1095,1240,1438,2814}. The clinical presentation is a palpable scrotal mass and/or testicular pain and frequently a hydrocele.

Macroscopy and histopathology

The tumours are centred in the epididymis and range from 1.0-7.0 cm. in greatest dimension with a tan or grey-white colouration. Foci of haemorrhage and necrosis may be present.
Epididymal adenocarcinoma may have tubular, tubulopapillary, papillary or cystic growth patterns often in combination {1240}. Tumour cells are columnar or cuboidal and often contain clear cytoplasm due to glycogen. The immunohistochemical profile of these tumours includes strong reactivity for cytokeratins (AE1/3) and epithelial membrane antigen. Staining for CEA, Leu M1, prostate specific antigen, Leucocyte common antigen and S100 protein have been reported as negative {418,833,1240}. Electron microscopic features include desmosomal junctions, cilia, glycogen particles and multivesicular bodies {1240}.

Prognosis

Meaningful follow-up data exists in only 5 patients, three of whom developed

Fig. 4.102 Carcinoma of the epididymis.

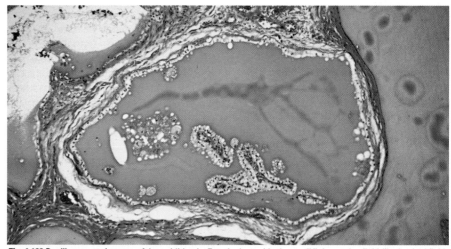

Fig. 4.103 Papillary cystadenoma of the epididymis. Ectatic duct with clear cell lining and colloid-like luminal fluid.

metastases {418,770,833,1240}. The tumour invades locally and metastatic spread is to the retroperitoneal lymph nodes and lungs.

Papillary cystadenoma of epididymis

Definition

A benign papillary epithelial tumour in the epididymal ducts.

ICD-O code   8450/0

Incidence

These benign tumours are seen in about 17% of patients with von Hippel-Lindau disease {1431,2664} but, overall, they are generally regarded as rare or uncommon {206,877}.

Clinical feature

These present as asymptomatic nodules in the region of the head of the epididymis. They have usually been present for a number of years and enlarged very little {1800}. Some have been discovered during evaluation for infertility, and this diagnosis should be considered when azoospermia is associated with an epididymal mass {2104}. They occur between 16 and 81 years (mean 36 years) although a few have been seen in females in the broad ligament and pelvic cavity {2384}. A few have also occurred in the spermatic cord {206}. The lesions have been bilateral in 30-40% of cases. In von Hippel-Lindau disease they are more frequently bilateral {287,2111}.

Macroscopy

Grossly, the tumours range from 1.6 to 6.0 cm and are solid or cystic and tan,

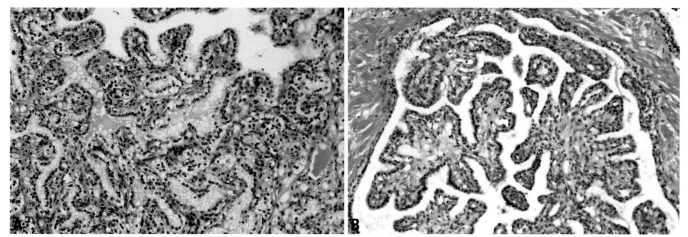

Fig. 4.104 Papillary cystadenoma of the epididymis. **A** Papillary tumour with clear cell morphology. **B** Papillary tumour fills the lumen of an ectatic epididymal duct.

brown or yellow in colour. The cut surface may be multicystic.

Histopathology
Microscopically, two findings are common to all lesions: ectasia of the efferent ducts and papillary formations. The tumours seem to arise from the efferent ducts, which show all degrees of ectasia from slight dilatation to microcyst formation {1236}. The ducts are lined by cuboidal or columnar cells with clear or vacuolated cytoplasm and often are filled with a colloid-like secretion. Papillary processes, simple or complex, arise from the walls of the ducts and may completely fill the cysts. Rarely, there have been foci of a histological pattern similar to that of the cerebellar haemangioblastoma {1800}. By immunohistochemistry they react with epithelial markers (Cam 5.2, AE1/AE3 and EMA) {877,2630}.

Genetics
The VHL gene has been identified and mapped to chromosome 3p25-26. Mutations in the VHL gene, leading to allele loss, have been detected in sporadic epididymal papillary cystadenoma {877} and also in those of patients with von Hippel-Lindau disease {206}.

Melanotic neuroectodermal tumour

Definition
Melanin containing tumour with varying proportions of two cells types in a cellular fibrous stroma.

ICD-O code   9363/0

Synonyms
Retinal anlage tumour, melanotic hamartoma, melanotic progonoma.

Epidemiology
Melanotic neuroectodermal tumour is a rare neoplasm which typically involves facial and skull bones. It may arise in the epididymis where at least two dozen examples have been reported {1073}. Most cases affect infants under the age of one and the oldest report is in an 8 year old.

Clinical features
Patients present with a firm mass, sometimes associated with hydrocele. One patient had a mild elevation of alpha-fetoprotein and there is elevation in urinary vanillylmandelic acid/homovanillic acid levels in some cases {1073}.

Macroscopy
Macroscopically, melanotic neuroectodermal tumours are circumscribed, round to oval, firm epididymal masses that measure less than 4 cm in diameter. They

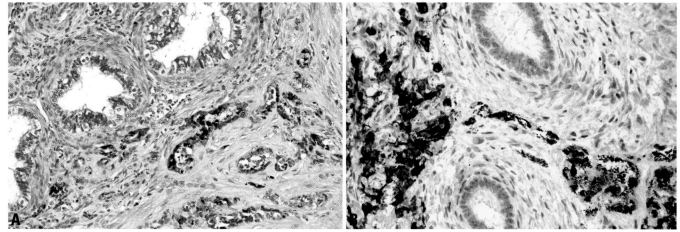

Fig. 4.105 A Melanotic neuroectodermal tumour of infancy. Bland-like structures formed by melanin containing epithelioid cells. **B** Melanotic neuroectodermal tumour of infancy. SYN expression.

often have a grey-white cut surface and may show areas of dark pigmentation.

Histopathology
There is usually a dual population of cells. Larger melanin containing epithelioid cells form nests, cords and gland-like structures. Smaller neuroblast-like cells with high nuclear to cytoplasmic ratios are closely apposed to the larger cells. Mitoses may be identified, especially in the small cell component.

Immunoprofile
Melanotic neuroectodermal tumour expresses a variety of epithelial, melanocytic and neural markers {1273, 2062}. The large cells typically stain for cytokeratins and HMB45. S100, neuron specific enolase, synaptophysin, glial fibrillary acidic protein and desmin may also be seen.

Ultrastructure
Electron microscopy shows that the small neuroblastic cells have cytoplasmic processes with microtubules and occasional dense core granules. The larger cells show evidence of both epithelial and melanocytic differentiation with desmosomal attachments and premelanosomes and mature melanosomes, respectively {2062}.

Histogenesis
The histogenesis of melanotic neuroectodermal tumour is unknown although it is thought to be a dysembryogenetic neoplasm which is nearly always congenital.

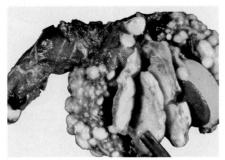

Fig. 4.106 Desmoplastic small round cell tumour.

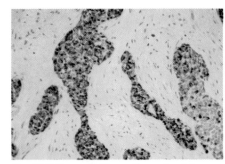

Fig. 4.107 Desmoplastic small round cell tumour. Anti desmin staining.

Prognosis
Melanotic neuroectodermal tumour of epididymis generally behaves in a benign fashion but may recur locally. Two examples have demonstrated lymph node metastasis, either inguinal or retroperitoneal {566,1235} No distant metastasis has been documented.

Desmoplastic small round cell tumour

Definition
A malignant serosa related small round cell tumour with an epithelial growth pattern in a desmoplastic stroma.

ICD-O code   8806/3

Sites of involvement
The pelvic and abdominal cavities are mostly involved followed by the paratesticular region {528,857,1971,2365}.

Clinical features
The patients range in age from 5-37 years. They present with hydroceles or scrotal masses without hydroceles.

Macroscopy
The tumours are firm and present as multiple varying sized nodules ranging from a few millimeters to 9.5 cm. The nodules are intimately associated with the tunica.

Histopathology
These consist of well delineated nests and anastomosing cords of rather uniform small cells supported by a prominent desmoplastic stroma. The nuclei are round, oval or elongated, or grooved with finely dispersed chromatin and one or two small nucleoli. The scant cytoplasm is light or eosinophilic and may contain glycogen. Cell borders are prominent. Normal and abnormal mitoses are common. Single cell necrosis and comedo like necrosis are commonly present. Occasionally, squamous metaplasia and glandular or tubular formations can be seen. One case showed sparse intra- and extra-cellular mucin production.

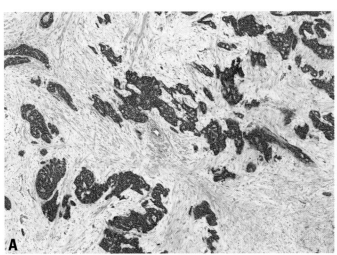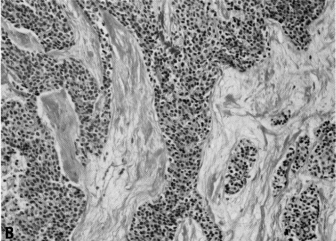

Fig. 4.108 Desmoplastic small round cell tumour. **A** Note the small nests in dense stroma. **B** Higher magnification shows nests of small cells surrounded by desmoplastic stroma.

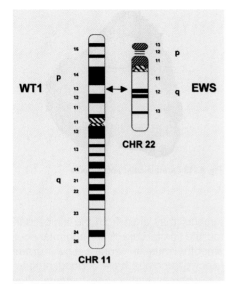

Fig. 4.109 Desmoplastic small round cell tumour DSRCT. Diagrammatic representation of chromosomal breakpoints in DSRCT with t(11;22)(p13;q12).

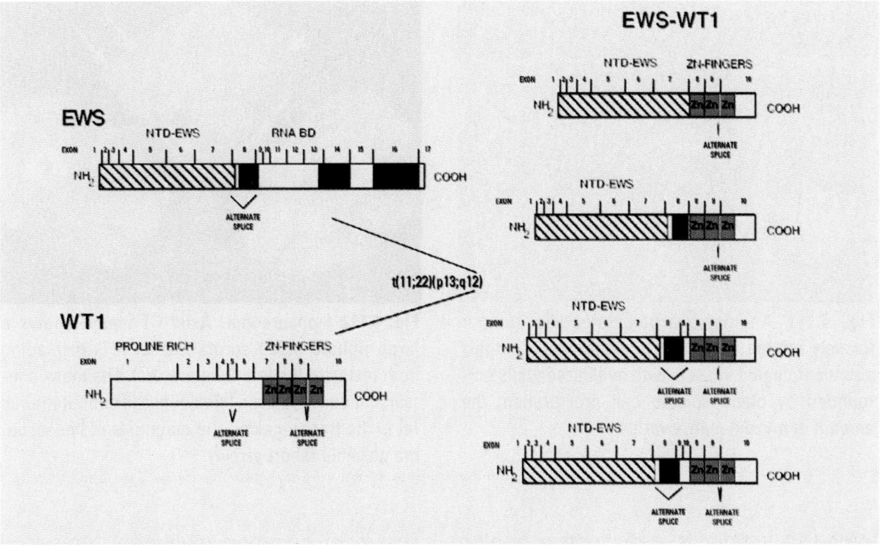

Fig. 4.110 Desmoplastic small round cell tumour DSRCT. Diagrammatic representation of chromosomal breakpoints in DSRCT with EWS-WT1 fusion transcript types. All chromosome 11 translocation breakpoints involve intron 7 of WT1, suggesting that the preservation of the last three zinc finger motifs of WT1 is crucial to the sarcomagenesis. The majority of chromosome 22 breakpoints involve the intron 7 of EWS, and very infrequently introns 8 and 9.

Immunoprofile

The tumour shows dual differentiation with keratin and desmin expression. The desmin reactivity shows a dot pattern. NSE, EMA and vimentin are also positive. About 91% of tumours express EWS-WT1 gene fusion transcript {2334}.

Differential diagnosis

Macroscopically, the tumour is similar to mesothelioma, but by microscopy it has to be separated from other small round cell tumours involving the paratesticular region. These include embryonal rhabdomyosarcoma and lymphoma. They do not show the desmoplastic stroma and nested growth pattern. Immunohistochemistry will be helpful.

Genetics

DSRCT is characterized by a specific chromosomal abnormality, t(11;22) (p13;q12), {240,2218,2314} unique to this tumour, involving two chromosomal regions previously implicated in other malignant developmental tumours. The translocation results in the fusion of the Ewing sarcoma gene, EWS, on 22q12 and the Wilms' tumour gene, WT1, on 11p13 {564,858,1423}. Interestingly, the most common primary site of DSRCT, the serosal lining of body cavities, has a high transient fetal expression of WT1 gene. WT1 is expressed in tissues derived from

the intermediate mesoderm, primarily those undergoing transition from mesenchyme to epithelium, in a specific period of development {2113,2139}. This stage of differentiation is reminiscent of DRCT with early features of epithelial differentiation. The most commonly identified EWS-WT1 chimeric transcript is composed of an in-frame fusion of the first seven exons of EWS, encoding the potential transcription modulating domain, and exons 8 through 10 of WT1, encoding the last three zinc-finger of the DNA binding domain. Rare variants including additional exons of EWS occur {102}. Intranuclear chimeric protein can be detected and shown to contain the carboxy terminus of WT1 {856}. Detection of the EWS-WT1 gene fusion and chimeric transcript serves as a sensitive and specific marker for DSRCT and has proven useful in the differential diagnosis of undifferentiated small round cell tumours of childhood {856}.

Prognosis

Most patients develop peritoneal and retroperitoneal disease within 2 years and die within 3-4 years. Metastases involve liver and lungs. One patient with a solitary tumour involving the epididymis developed retroperitoneal disease 18 years post orchiectomy.

Mesenchymal tumours of the scrotum, spermatic cord, and testicular adnexa

ICD-O codes

Lipoma	8850/0
Leiomyoma	8890/0
Neurofibroma	9540/0
Granular cell tumour	9580/0
Male angiomyofibroblastoma-like tumour (cellular angiofibroma)	8826/0
Calcifying fibrous (pseudo) tumour	
Fibrous hamartoma of infancy	
Liposarcoma	8850/3
Leiomyosarcoma	8890/3
Malignant fibrous histiocytoma	8830/3
Rhabdomyosarcoma	8900/3

Incidence

Scrotal mesenchymal tumours are rare and their etiology is poorly understood. The four most frequently reported benign tumours are haemangiomas, lymphangiomas, leiomyomas and lipomas. In our experience, many lesions designated as lipoma of the spermatic cord are reactive accumulations of fat related to hernial sac. Other benign lesions include a variety of nerve sheath tumours (neurofibroma {1182}, schwannoma and granular cell tumour). Male angiomyofibroblas-

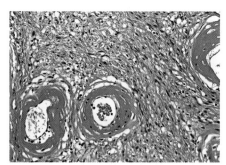

Fig. 4.111 Angiomyofibroblastoma-like tumour (closely related to cellular angiofibroma) contains abundant dilated vessels with hyalinized walls surrounded by bland spindle cell proliferation; the amount of myxoid matrix varies.

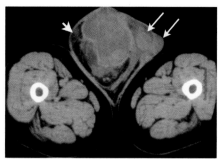

Fig. 4.112 Liposarcoma. Axial CT image shows a large righted sided scrotal mass. It is displacing both testes to the left (long arrows). The mass contains fat density tissue (similar to the subcutaneous fat in the thigh) making the diagnosis of liposarcoma possible (short arrow).

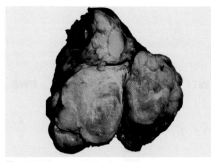

Fig. 4.113 Paratesticular liposarcoma

toma-like tumour is a distinctive benign tumour occurring in the scrotum or inguinal region of older men. Rare benign lesions of scrotum reported in infants and children include fibrous hamartoma of infancy, calcifying fibrous pseudotumour and lipoblastoma.

The most common sarcomas of the scrotum in adults are liposarcoma and leiomyosarcoma {252,769,782,1886}. According to the AFIP files, liposarcomas and malignant fibrous histiocytomas (MFH) have similar age distribution; in our experience some tumours historically diagnosed as the latter actually represent dedifferentiated liposarcomas. Liposarcoma and MFH occur predominantly in older men, and 75% of these tumours are diagnosed between the ages of 50-80 years; occurrence below the age of 30 years is very rare. Kaposi sarcoma is rare in the scrotum, and in our experience, is typically AIDS associated.

The most common malignant tumour of the scrotum in children is paratesticular embryonal rhabdomyosarcoma. These tumours occur in children of all ages, but they are most common in young adults. Nearly a third of them are diagnosed between the ages of 15-19 years and 86% are diagnosed before the age of 30.

Clinical features
Signs and symptoms
A small proportion of scrotal soft tissue tumours occur as cutaneous or subcutaneous masses, but most scrotal tumours are deep seated. Benign lesions may present as slowly enlarging, asymptomatic or mildly uncomfortable masses. Some superficial haemangiomas, often designated as angiokeratomas, can bleed {2578}. In general, malignant tumours are more likely to be symptomatic, large, and have a history of rapid growth. Superficial smooth muscle

tumours may arise from the tunica dartos, the scrotal superficial, subcutaneous smooth muscle zone. Low grade leiomyosarcomas have a good prognosis, whereas high grade tumours often develop metastases and have a significant tumour related mortality. There are no large series on paratesticular liposarcomas. In our experience, these tumours tend to have a protracted course with common recurrences and dedifferentiation in a minority of cases; dedifferentiated liposarcomas also tend to have a protracted clinical course with local recurrences, although distant metastases may also occur. Most paratesticular rhabdomyosarcomas are localized (stage, 1-2) and have an excellent prognosis with 5-year survival in the latest series at 95% {753}. However, tumours that have disseminated (group/stage 4) have a 60-70% 5-year survival. Spindle cells rhabdomyosarcomas are prognostically very favourable, whereas alveolar RMSs are unfavourable.

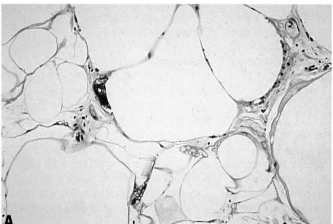

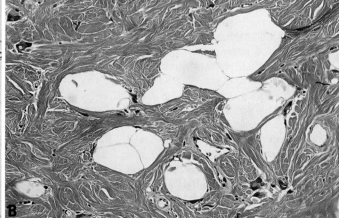

Fig. 4.114 Well differentiated liposarcoma. A Well differentiated liposarcoma is recognized by significant nuclear atypia in the adipocytes B The sclerosing variant of well differentiated liposarcoma has a dense collagenous background.

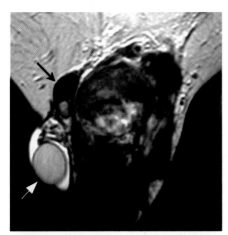

Fig. 4.115 Leiomyosarcoma. Coronal, T2-weighted, MR image shows a large heterogeneous mass filling the left hemiscrotum and extending into the inguinal canal. It is displacing the base of the penis to the right (black arrow). A normal testis is seen within the right hemiscrotum (arrow).

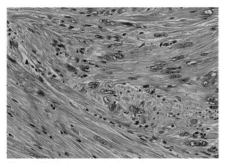

Fig. 4.116 Leiomyosarcoma of spermatic cord shows intersecting fascicles composed of atypical smooth muscle cells with blunt ended nuclei.

Imaging

Liposarcomas generally present as large extratesticular masses, which are often hyperechoic by ultrasound. However, the sonographic appearance of these tumours is variable and nonspecific. CT and MR imaging are much more specific with fat being easily recognized with both modalities {372,801}. By CT, fat will appear very low density similar to subcutaneous fat. On MR imaging the fat in a liposarcoma will follow the signal intensity of surrounding fat on all imaging sequences. Additionally a fat suppressed imaging sequence should be performed for confirmation. Fat will lose signal intensity (i.e. turn dark) on this sequence. Benign lipomas and hernias containing omentum are potential mimics, but lipomas are generally smaller and more homogeneous, and hernias are elongated masses, which can often be traced back to the inguinal canal.

With the exception of liposarcoma, none of the other sarcomas can be differentiated from one another radiologically. They all tend to be large, complex, solid masses {372}. Because of their large size, their extent is better demonstrated by CT and MR imaging rather than ultrasound.

Histopathology

Haemangiomas are classified according to the vessel type. Capillary and cavernous haemangiomas are most common within the scrotum, whereas angiokeratoma is the most common cutaneous vascular lesion {2578}. The latter features a superficial, dilated blood filled spaces initially associated with the epidermis, showing varying degrees of hyperkeratosis.

Fibrous hamartoma of infancy is a subcutaneous lesion composed of streaks of fibroblasts, mature fat, and spherical clusters of primitive mesenchymal cells {2096}. Calcifying fibrous (pseudo)tumour is a densely collagenous, paucicellullar fibroblastic tumefaction that typically contains scattered psammomatous calcifications and a patchy lymphoplasmacytic infiltration.

Granular cell tumours of the scrotum may be multifocal and are similar to those elsewhere in the skin.

Leiomyomas are composed of mature smooth muscle cells. Larger tumours often have hyalinization, myxoid change and calcification. Some of these tumours arise from the tunica dartos {1886,2406}. Focal nuclear atypia may occur, but the presence of prominent atypia should lead to a careful search for mitotic activity or coagulation necrosis which are features of leiomyosarcoma.

Leiomyosarcomas are typically composed of spindled cells with often elongated, blunt ended nuclei and variably eosinophilic, sometimes clumpy cytoplasm. Areas with round cell or pleomorphic morphology may

occur. The level of mitotic activity varies widely, but is often low.

Male angiomyofibroblastoma-like tumour is grossly circumscribed, lobulated soft to rubbery mass. Distinctive at low magnification are prominent, large vessels with perivascular fibrinoid deposition or hyalinization. The tumour cells between the vessels are tapered spindled cells with limited atypia, separated by fine collagen fibers. Focal epithelioid change is present in some cases. Nuclear palisading may occur, and a fatty component may be present; the latter has raised a question whether these tumours are fatty related neoplasms. Mitotic activity is very low. The tumour cells are immunohistochemically variably positive for desmin, muscle actins, CD34 and estrogen and progesterone receptors. This tumour is probably analogous to cellular angiofibroma as reported in females. Although some similarities with angiomyofibroblastoma of female genitalia have also been noted, these two processes are not considered synonymous {1442}.

Aggressive angiomyxoma, a tumour that typically occurs in women, has been reported in men {1162,2649}. Our review of potential male cases in the AFIP files did not reveal any diagnostic examples of this entity. It seems likely that many tumours originally reported as male aggressive angiomyxomas, in fact, represent other entities, such as the male angiomyofibroblastoma-like tumour.

Great majority of liposarcomas are well differentiated with various combinations of lipoma-like and sclerosing patterns. Presence of significant nuclear atypia in adipocytes is decisive. Multivacuolated lipoblasts may be present, but are not required for diagnosis. Dedifferentiation to spindle cell "fibrosarcoma-like" or pleomorphic "MFH-like" phenotype occurs in a proportion of paratesticular liposarco-

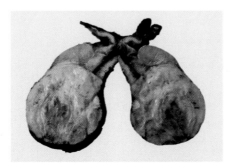

Fig. 4.117 Paratesticular rhabdomyosarcoma.

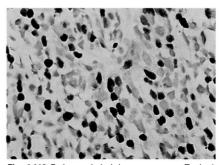

Fig. 4.118 Embryonal rhabdomyosarcoma. Typical nuclear positivity for MyoD1.

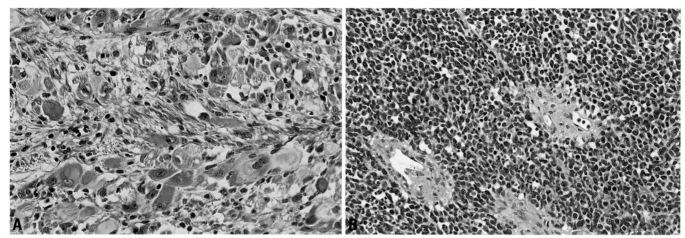

Fig. 4.119 Embryonal rhabdomyosarcoma. **A** Embryonal rhabdomyosarcoma can have a well differentiated pattern with abundant rhabdomyoblasts. **B** Embryonal rhabdomyosarcoma may be composed of primitive, hyperchromatic oval cells.

mas {1076}. The dedifferentiation may occur at the inception or in a recurrent tumour. This component can give rise to metastases. Some liposarcomas of the scrotum can have smooth muscle elements; these have been designated as combined lipoleiomyosarcomas {2539}.

Malignant fibrous histiocytoma and fibrosarcoma are diagnoses by exclusion. The former is a pleomorphic fibroblastic-myofibroblastic sarcoma, and the latter has a more uniform spindle cell pattern.

The majority of paratesticular rhabdomyosarcomas are of the embryonal type, but a small percentage (10-15%) have been classified as the alveolar type

in the largest clinicopathological series {753,1283,1563,2146}. A typical example of embryonal rhabdomyosarcoma contains large number of primitive round to oval cells and smaller numbers of differentiating rhabdomyoblasts with eosinophilic cytoplasm and possible cytoplasmic cross striations. However, the number of differentiating rhabdomyoblasts varies widely. Myxoid matrix is often present. A rare variant of embryonal rhabdomyosarcoma is composed of predominantly spindled cells, with some resemblance to smooth muscle cells. This type has been referred to as spindle cell or leiomyosarcoma-like rhabdomyosarcoma {1483}.

Although cytoplasmic cross striations may be noted, especially in the spindle cell rhabdomyosarcoma, they are not required for the diagnosis. Diagnostic confirmation should be obtained by immunohistochemistry. Virtually all RMS are positive for desmin and muscle actins (HHF35), and most have nuclear positivity for myogenic regulatory proteins, MyoD1 and myogenin (the latter demonstrated with Myf4 antibody). Cytoplasmic positivity for MyoD1 occurs in various tumours and has no diagnostic significance. Post chemotherapy specimens can show extensive rhabdomyoblastic differentiation.

Secondary tumours

C.J. Davis

Definition
Tumours of the testis which do not origi-nate in the testis or result from direct extension of tumours arising in adjacent intrascrotal sites.

Incidence
This is one of the most uncommon caus-es of testicular tumour, accounting for 2.4-3.6% {1800,2664}.

Clinical features
Most patients are over age 50, with a mean of 55-57, but one third have been under age 40 {1042,2663,2664}. It is most often found at autopsy in patients with known disseminated disease or after orchiectomy for prostatic carcino-ma {1691}, but in 6-7% of cases it has presented as the initial evidence of dis-ease as a palpable mass {548,1691, 2664}. Bilaterality has occurred in 15-20% {548, 2664}.

Origin of metastasis
A multitude of tumour types have metas-tasized to the testes, including some sar-comas but most studies have found prostate, lung, melanoma, colon and kid-ney in descending order of frequency, to be the more common ones {548,2664}. The excess of prostate cases is doubt-less related to the routine examination of orchiectomy specimens from patients with prostate carcinoma {2663}.

Macroscopy
The cut surface shows one or more nod-ules of tumour or a solitary diffuse mass.

Histopathology
The tumour exhibits an interstitial growth pattern with preservation of tubules and only uncommonly does tumour involve tubular lumina. Vascular invasion is usu-ally a prominent feature.

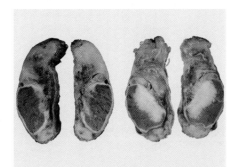

Fig. 4.120 Atrophy and metastatic carcinoma from prostate (bilateral orchiectomy).

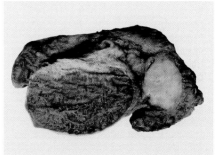

Fig. 4.121 Metastatic carcinoma from prostate in epididymis.

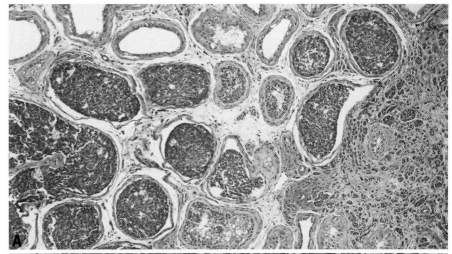

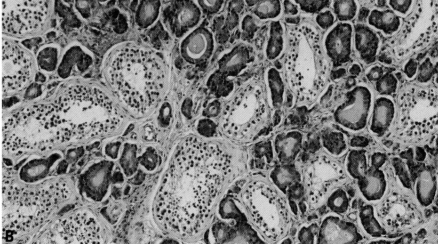

Fig. 4.122 Secondary tumours of the testis. **A** Metastatic lung carcinoma. This example, unlike most metastatic tumours, shows luminal involvement. **B** Metastatic prostatic carcinoma with PSA reactivity.

Table 4.05
Secondary tumours of the testis (surgical cases)

Primary	Total	%
Prostate	67	50%
Renal cell carcinoma	24	18%
Melanoma	14	10%
Lung*	8	6%
Bladder	5	4%
Carcinoid	3	2%
Pancreas	2	1%
Gastrointestinal	2	1%
Neuroblastoma	2	1%
Others**	8	6%
Total cases	**135**	**100%**

* Includes 4 small cell type
** One each: Thyroid, urethra, sphenoid sinus, larynx, PNET, Merkel cell tumour, nephroblastoma, adrenal.

Table 4.06
Secondary tumours of the testis (autopsy cases)

Primary	Total	%
Lung*	13	43%
Melanoma	6	20%
Prostate	3	10%
Pancreas	3	10%
Others**	5	17%
Total cases	**30**	**100%**

* Includes 5 small cell type
** One each: thyroid, ethmoid sinus, colon, renal pelvis, neuroblastoma

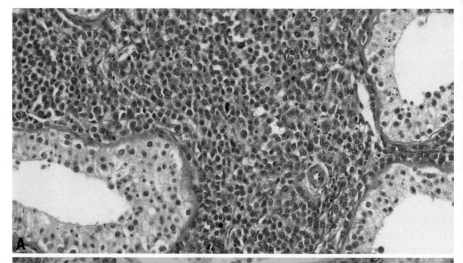
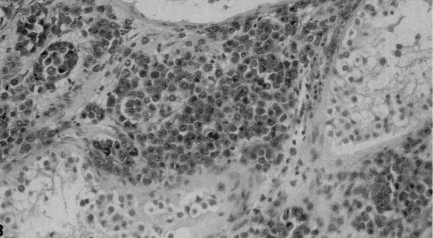

Fig. 4.123 Secondary tumours of the testis. **A** Metastatic malignant melanoma. **B** Metastatic malignant melanoma with HMB45 reactivity.

CHAPTER 5

Tumours of the Penis

The incidence of penile cancer varies worldwide, with the highest burden in some developing countries, particularly in Africa and South America. This indicates that environmental factors play an important role. Chronic papillomavirus infections have been identified with increasing frequency. Non-viral infections due to poor hygienic conditions are also established risk factors and this is underlined by the rare occurrence of penile cancer in circumcised men.

Well differentiated squamous cell carcinomas prevail. Metastasis is uncommon. However, many patients are treated in late stages of the disease, leading to the necessity of extensive surgical intervention.

WHO histological classification of tumours of the penis

Malignant epithelial tumours of the penis		Precursor lesions	
Squamous cell carcinoma	8070/3[1]	Intraepithelial neoplasia grade III	8077/2
Basaloid carcinoma	8083/3	Bowen disease	8081/2
Warty (condylomatous) carcinoma	8051/3	Erythroplasia of Queyrat	8080/2
Verrucous carcinoma	8051/3	Paget disease	8542/3
Papillary carcinoma, NOS	8050/3		
Sarcomatous carcinoma	8074/3	**Melanocytic tumours**	
Mixed carcinomas		Melanocytic nevi	8720/0
Adenosquamous carcinoma	8560/3	Melanoma	8720/3
Merkel cell carcinoma	8247/3		
Small cell carcinoma of neuroendocrine type	8041/3	**Mesenchymal tumours**	
Sebaceous carcinoma	8410/3		
Clear cell carcinoma	8310/3	**Haematopoietic tumours**	
Basal cell carcinoma	8090/3		
		Secondary tumours	

[1] Morphology code of the International Classification of Diseases for Oncology (ICD-O) {808} and the Systematized Nomenclature of Medicine (http://snomed.org). Behaviour is coded /0 for benign tumours, /2 for in situ carcinomas and grade III intraepithelial neoplasia, /3 for malignant tumours, and /1 for borderline or uncertain behaviour.

TNM classification of carcinomas of the penis

TNM classification [1,2]

T – Primary tumour

TX	Primary tumour cannot be assessed
T0	No evidence of primary tumour
Tis	Carcinoma in situ
Ta	Non-invasive verrucous carcinoma
T1	Tumour invades subepithelial connective tissue
T2	Tumour invades corpus spongiosum or cavernosum
T3	Tumour invades urethra or prostate
T4	Tumour invades other adjacent structures

N – Regional lymph nodes

NX	Regional lymph nodes cannot be assessed
N0	No regional lymph node metastasis
N1	Metastasis in a single superficial inguinal lymph node
N2	Metastasis in multiple or bilateral superficial inguinal lymph nodes
N3	Metastasis in deep inguinal or pelvic lymph node(s), unilateral or bilateral

M – Distant metastasis

MX	Distant metastasis cannot be assessed
M0	No distant metastasis
M1	Distant metastasis

Stage grouping

Stage 0	Tis	N0	M0
	Ta	N0	M0
Stage I	T1	N0	M0
Stage II	T1	N1	M0
	T2	N0,N1	M0
Stage III	T1, T2	N2	M0
	T3	N0, N1, N2	M0
Stage IV	T4	Any N	M0
	Any T	N3	M0
	Any T	Any N	M1

[1] {344,2662}.
[2] A help desk for specific questions about the TNM classification is available at http://www.uicc.org/tnm/

Malignant epithelial tumours

A.L. Cubilla
J. Dillner
P.F. Schellhammer
S. Horenblas

A.G. Ayala
V.E. Reuter
G. Von Krogh

Introduction

The vast majority of malignant tumours are squamous cell carcinomas (SCC) and they occur chiefly in the squamous epithelium of the glans, coronal sulcus and foreskin {2905}. SCC of the skin of the shaft are less frequent {695} than melanomas or Paget disease. Benign and malignant soft tissue tumours are unusual, but a large variety occurs in the penis. Whereas carcinomas affect mainly the distal penis or glans, sarcomas (excluding Kaposi sarcoma) prefer the corpora. Tumours of pendulous urethra are discussed under urothelial neoplasms.

Topographic definition of penile mucosa and anatomical levels

Penile mucosa includes the inner surface of the foreskin, coronal sulcus and glans, from the preputial orifice to the fossa navicularis. The lamina propria (LP) is similar for all sites but deeper anatomical levels are different: in the glans there are the corpus spongiosum (CS), tunica albuginea (TA) and corpus cavernosum (CC) and in the foreskin the dartos, dermis and epidermis. The penile fascia covers the shaft and inserts into the lamina propria of the coronal sulcus {171}. The fossa navicularis represents the 5-6 mm of the distal penile urethra but its squamous lining is continuous with that of the perimeatal glans.

Incidence

The incidence rates of penile cancer vary among different populations, with the highest cumulative rates (1% by age 75) seen in parts of Uganda and the lowest, 300-fold less, found among Israeli Jews. Age standardized incidence rates in the Western world are in the range of 0.3-1.0/100.000 {2016}. The incidence of penile cancer is highly correlated to the incidence of cervical cancer {280}. There is a continuous increase with advancing age. An earlier age at onset and a higher proportion of younger patients are seen in high incidence areas. The incidence rates have been slowly declining in some countries since the fifties {1607},

a decline commonly speculated to be due to improved personal hygiene.

Etiology

Etiological factors associated with penile cancer are phimosis, chronic inflammatory conditions, especially lichen sclerosus, smoking, ultraviolet irradiation, history of warts, or condylomas and lack of circumcision {620,1058,1069,1187,1590, 1871,2507}.

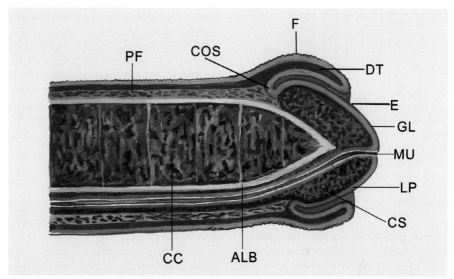

Fig. 5.01 Anatomy of the penile structures. Anatomical features: cut surface view of a partial penectomy showing anatomical sites, F= foreskin, GL= glans and COS= coronal sulcus. The anatomical levels in the glans are E= epithelium, LP= lamina propria, CS= Corpus Spongiosum and CC= corpus cavernosum. The tunica albuginea (ALB) separates CS from CC. In the foreskin additional levels are DT= dartos and F= skin. Penile fascia (PF) encases CC. The urethra is ventral and distally shows the meatus urethralis (MU).

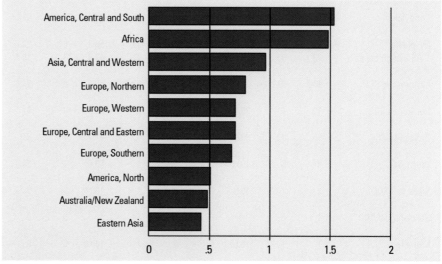

Fig. 5.02 Penis: ASR world, per 100,000, all ages. Incidence of penile cancer in some regions worldwide. From D. M. Parkin et al. {2016}.

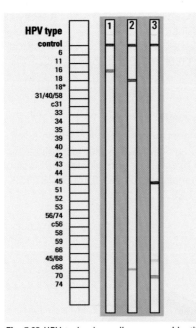

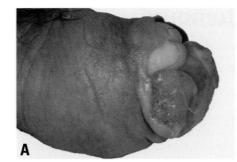
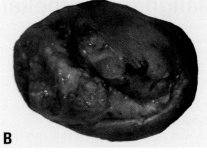

Fig. 5.04 A, B Squamous cell carcinoma of the usual type. Exophytic growth pattern.

Fig. 5.03 HPV-typing in penile cancers. Identification of HPV genotypes using a linear probe assay. LiPA strips with hybridization bands indicating a single HPV type infection: lane 1: HPV 16; lane 2: HPV 18; and a multiple HPV type infection: lane 3: HPV 45 and 70. Note: HPV 18 is reactive with two probes, 18 and c68, and HPV 45 with probes 45 and 45/68. Reprinted with permission from M.A. Rubin et al. {2258}.

Human papillomavirus (HPV) infection

HPV is present in a subset of penile SCC, with HPV 16 as the most frequent type {945,1153}. HPV DNA is preferentially found in cancers with either basaloid and/or warty features, and only weakly correlated with typically keratinizing SCC {945,2258}. Penile intraepithelial neoplasia (IN), a recognized precursor, is consistently HPV DNA positive in 70-100% of investigated cases {1153}. A possible explanation is that the HPV-negative invasive cancers do not arise from the HPV-positive IN, but from unrecognized HPV-negative precursor lesions.

Clinical features
Signs and symptoms

Mean age of presentation is 60 years {517,2905} and patients may present with an exophytic or flat ulcerative mass in the glans, a recurrent tumour in the surgical stump or a large primary tumour with inguinal nodal and skin metastases. Occasionally the lesions may be subtle, such as a blemish or an area of erythema. In patients with long foreskin and phimosis the tumour may be concealed and an inguinal metastasis be the presenting sign.

Imaging

Imaging, until very recently, has played a minimal role in the staging and direction of treatment options. A recent study compared the accuracy of physical examination, ultrasound investigation and magnetic resonance imaging (MRI) {1535} and found physical examination as the most accurate method to determine tumour site and extent of corpus spongiosum infiltration. Because of the possibility of imaging in various planes and because of the ability to visualize other structures of the penis, MRI can be useful to determine the true proximal extent of the tumour.

Recently the concept of sentinel node {356} has been explored again in penile cancer {2579}. Imaging by lymphoscintigraphy with a radioactive tracer is considered as one of the prerequisites to determine the individual drainage pattern in order to find the sentinel node. Lymphoscintigraphy visualized at least 1 sentinel node in 98% of the patients.

Tumour spread

Penile carcinoma has a fairly predictable dissemination pattern, initially to superficial lymph nodes, then to deep groin and pelvic nodes and lastly to retroperitoneal nodes. The first metastatic site is usually a superficial inguinal lymph node located in the groin upper inner quadrant (sentinel node). This pattern presents in about 70 % of the cases. Some tumours metastasize directly to deep inguinal nodes. Skip inguinal nodal metastases

Table 5.01
HPV DNA detection in penile condyloma, dysplasia and carcinoma. From Rubin et al. {2258}.

Diagnosis	n	HPV-positive		Low risk HPV		High risk HPV		Multiple HPV	
		n	%	n	%*	n	%*	n	%*
Condyloma	12	12	100.0	11	91.7	1	8.3	0	0
Dysplasia	30	27	90.0	5	18.5	16	59.3	6	22.2
All benign cases	42	39	92.8	16	41.0	17	43.6	6	15.4
Keratinizing SCC	106	37	34.9	0	0	23	62.1	8	21.6
Verrucous SCC	12	4	33.3	1	25.0	2	50.0	0	0
Basaloid SCC	15	12	80.0	0	0	11	91.7	1	8.3
Warty SCC	5	5	100.0	0	0	4	80.0	1	20.0
Clear cell SCC	2	1	50.0	0	0	1	100.0	0	0
Sarcomatoid SCC	1	0	0.0	0	0	0	0	0	0
Metastatic SCC	1	1	100.0	0	0	1	100.0	0	0
All cancer cases	142	60	42.2	1	1.6	42	70.0	10	16.6

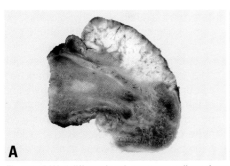 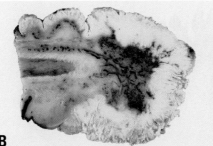 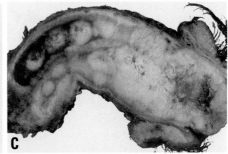

Fig. 5.05 A Well differentiated squamous cell carcinoma with invasion of corpus spongiosum. **B** Squamous cell carcinoma. Large neoplasm replacing glans surface. **C** Squamous cell carcinoma. Massive replacement of penile corpus spongiosum and cavernosum by a white neoplasm.

(primary tumour to pelvic inguinal nodes) are extremely unusual. Systemic blood borne dissemination occurs late. Common general sites of metastatic involvement are liver, heart, lungs and bone {2905}.

Prognosis

Pathologic factors related to prognosis of penile carcinomas are site of primary tumour, pattern of growth, tumour size, histological type, grade, depth and vascular invasion. Tumours exclusively in the foreskin, carry a better prognosis {1933} because of low grade and frequent superficially invasive growth {514}. The incidence of metastasis in verruciform tumours is minimal. Mortality in patients with superficially spreading carcinomas is 10% compared with 67% for patients with vertical growth pattern {521}. The 3 most important pathological factors to predict final outcome are histological grade, depth of invasion and vascular

invasion especially the combination of grade and depth. There is no consensus regarding method of grading {1121, 1608,2438}. The depths of invasion should be evaluated on penectomy specimens {2719}. Measurement of depth of invasion in mm should be performed from the basement membrane of adjacent squamous epithelium to deepest point of invasion {693}. The large destructive lesions or bulky exophytic tumours especially those of the verruciform group should be measured from the nonkeratinizing surface of the tumour to the deepest point of invasion. Evaluation of the anatomical levels of tumour invasion is limited by the variation in thickness of the corpus spongiosum. The threshold for penile metastasis is about 4-6 mm invasion into the corpus spongiosum {520}. When possible, more than one method should be utilized. A combination of histologic grade and depth is thought to better predict metastasis and

mortality, including micrometastasis {1672,2458}. One system utilizes a prognostic index from 1 to 6, combining numerical values for histologic grade (1-3) and anatomical level of invasion (1-3, LP, CS and CC in glans and LP, dartos and skin in the foreskin). Low indices (1-3) are associated with no mortality. Metastatic and mortality rates are high in patients with indexes 5 and 6 {519}. Molecular markers have been studied as prognostic predictors. Ploidy was not found to be useful as a predictor of prognosis {1002}. P53, however, appeared to be an independent risk factor for nodal metastasis, progression of disease and survival in 2 studies {1546,1640}. HPV was not found to be prognostically important {236}. Tissue associated eosinophilia has been linked with improved survival in patients with penile cancer {1961}.

Squamous cell carcinoma

Definition

A malignant epithelial neoplasm with squamous differentiation.

ICD-O codes

Squamous cell carcinoma	8070/3
Basaloid carcinoma	8083/3
Warty (condylomatous) carcinoma	8051/3
Verrucous carcinoma	8051/3
Papillary carcinoma (NOS)	8050/3
Sarcomatoid (spindle cell) carcinoma	8074/3
Adenosquamous carcinoma	8560/3

Macroscopy

Average tumour size varies from 3 to 4 cm. Three main growth patterns are noted: *superficially spreading* with horizontal growth and superficial invasion,

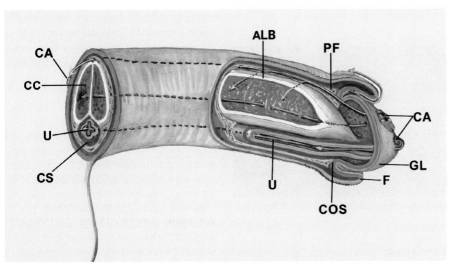

Fig. 5.06 Routes of local spread: Lines and arrows depict pathways of local tumour (CA) progression, from distal glans (GL), foreskin (F) and coronal sulcus (COS) to proximal corpus spongiosum (CS), corpora cavernosa (CC), penile fascia (PF), skin and urethra (U). (ALB) tunica albuginea.

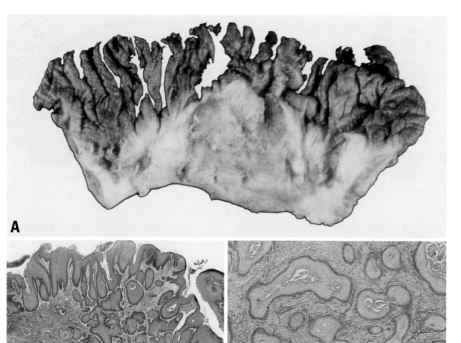

Fig. 5.07 Squamous cell carcinoma. A An irregular granular flat neoplasm involving the mucosal aspect of the foreskin. B Well differentiated SCC with irregular infiltrating borders. C Well differentiated keratinizing SCC.

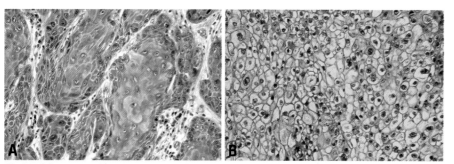

Fig. 5.08 A Squamous cell carcinoma, grade 1. B Clear cell carcinoma, a poorly differentiated squamous cell carcinoma with cytoplasmic clearing.

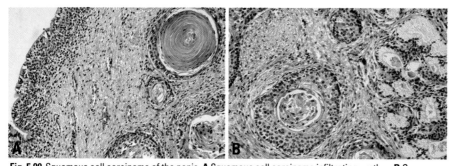

Fig. 5.09 Squamous cell carcinoma of the penis. A Squamous cell carcinoma infiltrating urethra. B Squamous cell carcinoma infiltrating periurethral glands.

vertical growth deeply invasive and *multicentric*. Any combination may occur {517}. Multicentric carcinomas are more frequent in the foreskin {1933}. The

tumours are usually white, grey, granular irregular masses partially or totally replacing the glans or foreskin. The glans surface may be flat, ulcerated or

deformed by an exophytic mass. In some patients the foreskin is abutted by underlying tumour and may show skin ulcerations. The contrast between the pale invasive tumour and the dark red colour of CS or CC permits determination of the deepest point of invasion, which is prognostically important {520}. Adjacent hyperplastic or precancerous lesions often can be visualized as a marble white 1-2 mm thickening. Mixed tumours should be suspected when different growth patterns are present.

Local spread
Penile tumours may spread from one mucosal compartment to the other. Typically, foreskin carcinomas spread to coronal sulcus or glans and carcinomas originating in the glans may spread to the foreskin. Penile SCC may spread horizontally and externally to skin of the shaft and internally to proximal urethral margin of resection. This is the characteristic spread of superficially spreading carcinomas. The vertical spread may progress from surface to deep areas {517}. An important, under recognized route of spread is the penile fascia, a common site of positive surgical margin of resection. The fascial involvement in tumours of the glans is usually through the coronal sulcus. Tumour in the fascia may secondarily penetrate into corpus cavernosum via nutritional vessels and adipose tissue traversing the tunica albugina. It is not unusual to find "satellite nodules", frequently associated with regional metastasis. Multiple urethral sites may be involved at the resection margins {2720}. Pagetoid intraepithelial spread may simulate carcinoma in situ or Paget disease. In more advanced cases penile carcinomas may spread directly to inguinal, pubic or scrotal skin.

Histopathology
There is a variable spectrum of differentiation from well to poorly differentiated. Most frequently there is keratinization and a moderate degree of differentiation. Very well differentiated and solid nonkeratinizing poorly differentiated carcinomas are unusual. Invasion can be as individual cells, small irregular nests of atypical cells, cords or large cohesive sheets present in the lamina propria or corpus spongiosum. Infrequently (about a fourth of cases) the corpus cavernosum is affected. The boundaries

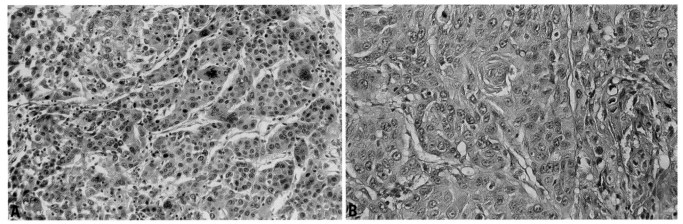

Fig. 5.10 Squamous cell carcinoma. **A** Poorly differentiated keratinizing SCC. **B** Squamous cell carcinoma of the penis, grade 3.

between stroma and tumour are irregular or finger like. Broadly based margins are unusual. Superficially invasive tumours tend to be well differentiated and deeper tumours poorly differentiated. Deeply invasive carcinomas may focally show spindle, pleomorphic, acantholytic, giant, basaloid or clear cells. In poorly differentiated tumours individual cell necrosis or comedo-like necrosis may be found as well as numerous mitotic figures {521,2905}.

Differential diagnosis
Superficial and differentiated invasive lesions should be distinguished from pseudoepitheliomatous hyperplasia. In SCC the nests detached from overlying epithelium are disorderly, show keratinization, are more eosinophilic and nucleoli are prominent. Stromal or desmoplastic reaction may be present in both conditions but is more frequent in

carcinomas. Hyperplastic nests do not involve the dartos or corpus spongiosum.

Variants of squamous cell carcinoma

Basaloid carcinoma

Basaloid carcinoma is an HPV related aggressive variant, which accounts for 5-10% of penile cancers {518,522,945}. Median age at presentation is in the sixth decade. Most commonly it arises in the glans. Grossly, it presents as a flat, ulcerated and irregular mass, which is firm, tan and infiltrative. Microscopically, it is composed of packed nests of tumour cells, often associated with comedo-type necrosis. The cells are small with scant cytoplasm and oval to round, hyperchromatic nuclei and inconspicuous nucleoli.

Mitotic rate is usually brisk. Palisading at the periphery of the nest and abrupt central keratinization is occasionally seen. They tend to infiltrate deeply into adjacent tissues, including corpora cavernosa. Spread to inguinal lymph nodes is common and the mortality rate is high.

Warty (condylomatous) carcinoma

This variant corresponds to 20% of "verruciform" neoplasms {235,521,523,945}. Median age is in the fifth decade. Grossly, it is a white to tan, cauliflower-like lesion that may involve glans, coronal sulcus or foreskin. Tumours as large as 5.0 cm have been described. Microscopically, it has a hyper-parakeratotic arborizing papillomatous growth. The papillae have thin fibrovascular cores and the tips are variably round or tapered. The tumour cells have low to intermediate grade cytology. Koilocytotic atypia is con-

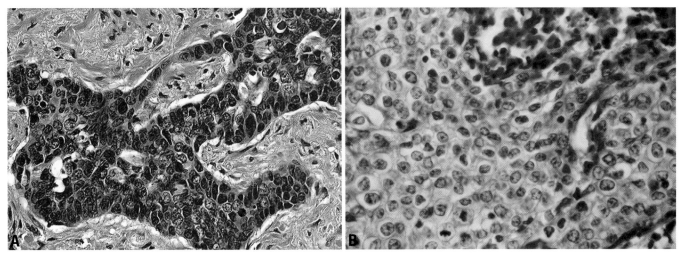

Fig. 5.11 A Basaloid carcinoma of the penis. **B** Basaloid carcinoma of the penis with comedo necrosis, upper right.

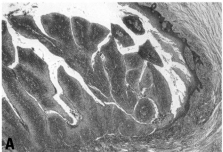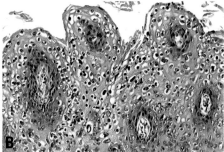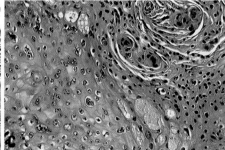

Fig. 5.12 A Warty (condylomatous) carcinoma of the penis. Note papillary growth. **B,C** Warty squamous cell carcinoma.

spicous. Nuclei may be large, hyperchromatic and wrinkled and binucleation is common. Tumours may infiltrate deeply and the interface of tumour with stroma is usually irregular. HPV DNA testing has demonstrated HPV 16 and 6 in some cases. Some have metastasized to regional lymph nodes, usually associated with deeply invasive lesions.

Verrucous carcinoma

This variant usually involves the glans or foreskin {1232,1643}. Grossly, it meas-

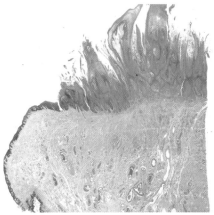

Fig. 5.13 Verrucous carcinoma. Hyperkeratosis and papillomatosis.

ures about 3.5 cm and appears as an exophytic, grey-white mass. Microscopically, it is a very well differentiated papillary neoplasm with acanthosis and hyperkeratosis. The papillations are of variable length and fibrovascular cores are inconspicuous. The nuclei are bland, round or vesicular, although slightly more atypical nuclei may be seen at the basal cell layer. Koilocytotic changes are not evident. Tumours may extend into the underlying stroma with a broad based, pushing border, making determination of invasion difficult. Verrucous carcinoma is considered not to be HPV-related. This is a slow growing tumour that may recur locally but metastasis does not occur in typical cases.

Papillary carcinoma, not otherwise specified (NOS)

This variant occurs mainly in the fifth and sixth decades {521}. Grossly, it is exophytic, grey-white and firm. The median size in one series was reported as 3.0 cm although cases as large as 14.0 cm have been reported. Microscopically, these are well differentiated, hyperkeratotic lesions with irregular, complex papillae, with or without fibrovascular cores. The interface

with the underlying stroma is infiltrative and irregular. These tumours are not HPV-related. Despite the fact that invasion into the corpus cavernosum and spongiosum has been documented, regional lymph node involvement has not been seen in the relatively few cases reported.

Sarcomatoid (spindle cell) carcinoma

Squamous cell carcinoma with a spindle cell component arises de novo, after a recurrence, or following radiation therapy {821}. The glans is a frequent site {2838} but they may occur in the foreskin as well. Grossly, they are 5-7 cm irregular white grey mixed exophytic and endophytic masses. On cut surface, corpus spongiosum and cavernosum are invariably involved. Histologically, there are atypical spindle cells with features similar to fibrosarcoma, malignant fibrous histiocytoma or leiomyosarcoma. These cells have the potential to differentiate into muscle, bone and cartilage, benign or malignant {103}. Differentiated carcinoma in situ or invasive carcinoma is usually found. Electron microscopy and immunohistochemistry are useful to rule out sarcomas and spindle cell

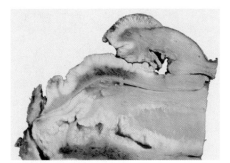

Fig. 5.14 Verrucous carcinoma. The tumour pushes into corpus spongiosum with focal involvement of tunica albuginea.

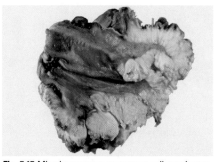

Fig. 5.15 Mixed verrucous-squamous cell carcinoma. Predominantly papillomatous appearence except in the lower central area where the neoplasm is solid.

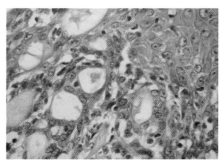

Fig. 5.16 Adenosquamous carcinoma.

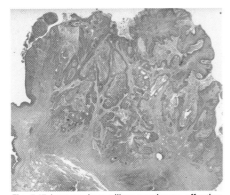

Fig. 5.17 Low grade papillary carcinoma affecting the foreskin.

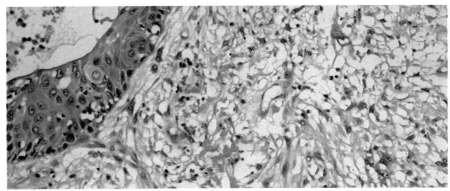

Fig. 5.18 Sarcomatoid (spindle cell) carcinoma of the penis.

melanomas {1613}. Sarcomatoid carcinomas are associated with a high rate of regional nodal metastases {521}.

Mixed carcinomas

About a fourth of penile carcinomas consist of a mixture of various types. A moderate to high grade squamous cell carcinoma in an otherwise typical verrucous carcinoma (so called 'hybridverrucous') shows metastatic potential {473,1232}. The warty-basaloid carcinoma has a high incidence of groin metastasis {2574}. Other recognized combinations include adenocarcinoma and basaloid {515} (adenobasaloid) and squamous and neuroendocrine carcinoma.

Adenosquamous carcinoma

Squamous cell carcinoma with mucinous glandular differentiation arises from surface epithelium. The origin may be related to misplaced or metaplastic mucinous glands {516,1208,1642}. Grossly, it is a firm white grey irregular mass involving the glans. Microscopically, the squamous predominates over the glandular component. The glands stain positive for CEA. Adenocarcinomas and mucoepidermoid carcinomas of the penis have also been reported {810,1455,2702}.

Other rare pure primary carcinomas

ICD-O codes

Merkel cell carcinoma	8247/3
Small cell carcinoma of neuroendocrine type	8041/3
Sebaceous carcinoma	8410/3
Clear cell carcinoma	8310/3

A small number of unusual primary penile neoplasms include the Merkel cell carcinoma {2625}, small cell carcinoma of neuroendocrine type {830}, sebaceous carcinoma {1967}, clear cell carci-

noma {2905}, and well differentiated squamous cell carcinoma with pseudo-hyperplastic features (pseudohyperplastic carcinoma) {524}. Another rare lesion is the papillary basaloid carcinoma consisting of an exophytic growth, with papillae composed of small poorly differentiated cells similar to the cells seen in invasive basaloid carcinomas {515}.

Basal cell carcinoma

ICD-O code   8090/3

Basal cell carcinoma (BCC) is a rare indolent neoplasm of the penis identical to BCC of other sites {794,1425,2041}. They may be uni- or multicentric {2041}. The localization is on the shaft and rarely on the glans {872,1674}. Of 51 BCC of regions not exposed to sun, 2 were in the penis {1244}. BCCs are differentiated and usually superficial with minimal metastatic potential {1317}. It is impor-

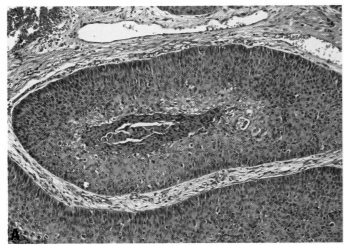
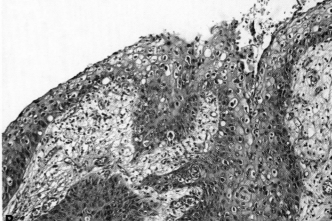

Fig. 5.19 Warty-basaloid carcinoma. **A** Invasive nests. **B** Surface appearance.

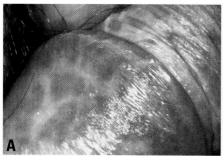
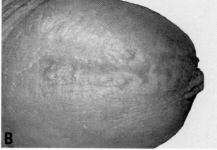

Fig. 5.20 Bowenoid papulosis. **A, B** Clinically, two types exist; macular and papular (right). The lesions may be multiple or solitary and the diameter varies from 2-10 mm.

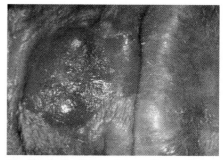

Fig. 5.21 Penile Bowen disease. Bowen disease appearing as a well demarcated reddish plaque on the inner aspect of the foreskin.

tant to distinguish them from the aggressive basaloid squamous cell carcinoma, which invades deeply, has abrupt keratinization, comedo necrosis and high mitotic rates.

Precursor lesions

HPV and penile intraepithelial neoplasia

ICD-O code

Intraepithelial neoplasia
Grade III   8077/2

Human papillomaviruses (HPV) are the most heterogeneous of human viruses {574}. About 30 sexually transmittable genotypes exist that are further classified into "low" and "high risk" types according to oncogenic potential {574,619}.

Generally, overt genital warts ("condylomas") are associated with "low risk" HPVs - including types 6 and 11. The "high risk" HPVs - most commonly types 16 and 18 - are predominantly associated with subclinical lesions {2756}. Mucosal infections mainly are transient in young people {670}. Longitudinal studies demonstrate that patients who cannot clear high risk HPV infections within about a year are at risk for malignant transformation. SCC is thought to develop via HPV-associated precursor lesions (intraepithelial neoplasia; IN) that are graded I-III in proportion to the epithelial thickness occupied by transformed basaloid cells. These vary in size and shape, with the nuclei being pleomorphic and hyperchromatic. They are accompanied by loss of polarity. In grade I, the IN occupies the lower one third, in grade II the lower two thirds, and in grade III the full

epithelial thickness ("Bowen atypia"; in situ SCC). Concurrent infection with low and high risk types is common. Condylomas and IN sometimes coexist as part of a morphological continuum.

Studies of HPV and penile cancer are limited because of the scarce occurrence and the peculiar geographical distribution of this malignancy, being rare in the USA and Europe but fairly common in many developing countries {619,2756}. The predominant HPV that is found in penile SCC is type 16, followed by type 18. HPV types 6/11 have been detected in anecdotal cases.

Most patients with IN lack physical symptoms, but itching, tenderness, pain, bleeding, crusting, scaling and difficulty in retracting the foreskin may develop {2756}. Chronic inflammation, phimosis and poor hygiene may be important contributing factors {670,2754-2756}. A pathogenic role of chronic lichen sclerosus and verrucous carcinoma has been discussed, while oncogenic HPVs have been linked more strongly to warty/basaloid carcinomas {945}.

The following comments summarize clinical features of three penile conditions presumed to be precancerous: *Giant condyloma, Bowenoid papulosis* and *Bowen disease*. Due to clinical overlap and differential diagnostic problems, a vigilant approach to diagnostic biopsy sampling cannot be overly stressed.

Giant condyloma

"Giant condyloma" (Buschke-Löwenstein) is a rare (about 100 cases published) and peculiar condyloma variant {968,2756} generally arising due to poor hygiene of uncircumcized men (range 18-86 years of age). It is characterized by a semi-malignant slowly growing condylomatous growth often larger than

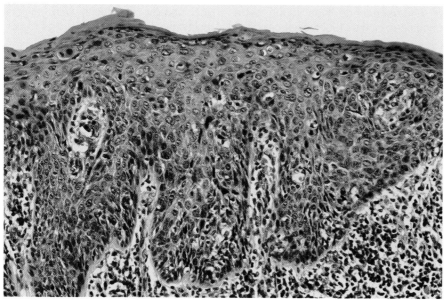

Fig. 5.22 High grade squamous intraepithelial lesion (SIL), squamous.

5 cm in diameter. The term has been used for various lesions namely: true giant condylomas, verrucous carcinoma and warty carcinoma. In some cases a complex histological pattern exists, with areas of benign condyloma intermixed with foci of atypical epithelial cells or even well differentiated in situ carcinoma. Moreover, mixed tumours have been observed in which unequivocal features of benign condyloma, warty carcinoma and either basaloid or typical squamous cell carcinoma occur adjacent to one another {2756}. It is currently believed that the giant condyloma and verrucous SCC are separate pathological lesions. The accurate diagnosis may require multiple biopsies.

Bowenoid papulosis and Bowen disease

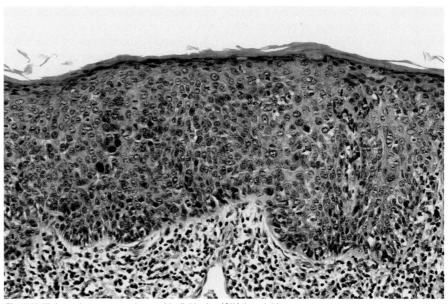
Fig. 5.23 High grade squamous intraepithelial lesion (SIL), basaloid.

ICD-O codes
Bowen disease	8081/2
Erythroplasia of Queyrat	8080/2

Genital Bowenoid papulosis (BP) is the term used for lesions in young sexually active people16-35 (mean 28) years of age that display histological features of IN III. The sharp border between the epidermis and the dermis is preserved. The histopathological presentation cannot be distinguished from that of Bowen disease (BD) although focal accumulations of uniformly round nuclei and perinuclear vacuoles in the horny layer is more common in BP {968}. Oncogenic HPV DNA, most commonly is type 16, but types 18 and/or 33-35 have repeatedly been discovered.

Reddish-brown and pigmented colour tones are more common than in benign condylomas. Typical IN III lesions tend to be small (2-10 mm), multicentric smooth velvety maculopapular reddish-brown, salmon-red, greyish-white lesions in the preputial cavity, most commonly the glans. Thicker epithelial lesions may be ashen-grey or brownish-black. BP may also be solitary or coalesce into plaques, when the clinical presentation overlaps with that of BD. Both conditions sometimes resemble lichen sclerosus, psoriasis and eczema {2756}.

BP is predominantly transient, self limiting and clinically benign in young people; spontaneous regression within a year has been reported in immunocompetent individuals below the age of 30 years. However, these lesions often show recalcitrance after surgical intervention. Possibly, some cases of persistent BP may progress to BD and invasive cancer. Bowen disease (BD) has long been considered a premalignant lesion. If left untreated, documented transformation to SCC has been reported in the range of 5-33% in uncircumcized men {2756}. Usually, the clinical appearance is that of a single, well demarcated reddish plane and/or bright red scaly papule or plaques, ranging in diameter from a 2-35 mm. When located on the glans penis it is by tradition named erythroplasia of Queyrat (EQ). Lesions on dry penile skin are brownish-red or pigmented. Occasionally they are ulcerative or may be covered by a pronounced hyperkeratosis that may appear as a "cutaneous horn" {2756}. The most important clinical hallmark in the differential diagnosis versus BP is the age. The average age on diagnosis of BD/QE is 61 years. Review of 100 cases of QE revealed that 90% of cases were white men with a median age of 51 years. From the records of 87 men with BD, 84 were uncircumcized and

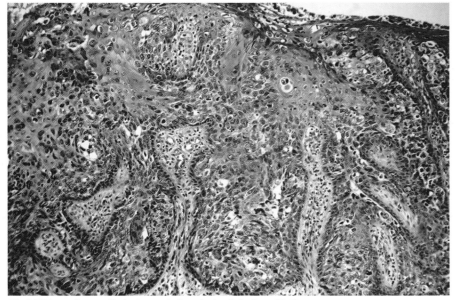
Fig. 5.24 Paget disease. Typical spread of atypical cells in the epithelium.

three had been circumcized by 9 years of age, the median age of patients with BD is 51 years {2756}.

Prognosis and follow-up of IN

It is clinically impossible to determine which individual will develop pernicious HPV infection and progress from IN III to invasive cancer. Therefore we advocate that in persons older than 40 years, as well as in immunosuppressed individuals at earlier ages (including HIV infected people and allograft recipients), lesions should always be considered as premalignant and treated surgically. In younger men, a year or so of watchful waiting may be justified.

Treatment failure may be related to indistinct margins (marginal recurrences), extension of IN down hair follicles and unrecognized foci of invasive tumour. A variety of treatments have been used.

Following treatment, the duration of follow-up is uncertain, but a clinical follow-up at 3 and 12 months seems reasonable to confirm clearance and healing. Patients remain at risk after penis sparing therapy and should be instructed to come back as soon as possible in case of suspected recurrence including the experience of a "lump", or the occurrence of local symptoms.

Paget disease

ICD-O code   8542/3

This is a form of intraepidermal adenocarcinoma, primary in the epidermis or spread from an adenocarcinoma {1067, 1401,1417}. The skin of the shaft is usually involved as part of a scrotal, inguinal, perineal or perianal tumour, but exclusive penile lesions occur {1586}. Patients are in the six or seventh decades and present with thickened red to pale plaques with scaling or oozing. Microscopically, there is an intraepithelial proliferation of atypical cells with a pale granular or vacuolated cytoplasm. Nuclei are vesicular and nucleoli prominent. Invasion into the dermis may result in metastasis to groin or widespread dissemination {1744}. Paget disease (PD) should be distinguished from pagetoid spread of penile or urothelial carcinomas {2624}, Bowen disease and melanomas. Clear cell papulosis {422} pagetoid dyskeratosis {2685} or mucinous metaplasia {2684} should also be ruled out. Frequently positive stains in PD are mucins, CEA, low molecular weight cytokeratins, EMA, gross cystic disease fluid protein and MUC 5 AC {1401}.

Melanocytic lesions

A.G. Ayala
P. Tamboli

Definition
Melanocytic lesions of the penis identical to those in other sites.

Incidence
Malignant melanocytic lesions of the penis are rare, with just over 100 cases of malignant melanoma reported since their first description by Muchison in 1859 {1229,1439,1614,1950}. Other melanocytic lesions include penile melanosis, genital lentiginosis, atypical lentiginous hyperplasia, melanocytic nevi, and atypical melanocytic nevi of the acral/genital type.

ICD-O codes
Melanocytic nevi   8720/0
Melanoma   8720/3

Epidemiology and etiology
Penile melanoma affects white men, between the ages of 50 and 70 years. Risk factors include pre-existing nevi, exposure to ultraviolet radiation, and a history of melanoma.

Localization
Sixty to eighty percent of melanomas arise on the glans penis, less than 10% affect the prepuce, and the remainder arises from the skin of the shaft.

Macroscopy
Grossly, the lesion has been described as an ulcer, papule, or nodule that is blue, brown, or red.

Histopathology
Reported histologic subtypes include nodular, superficial spreading, and mucosal lentiginous. The Breslow level (depth of invasion) is an important determinant of overall survival.

Prognosis and predictive factors
Management is similar to melanomas of other regions.

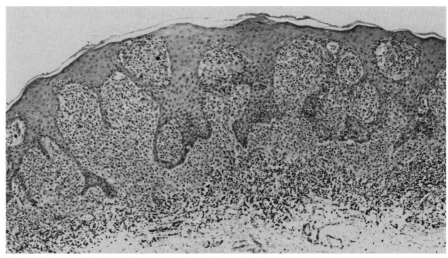

Fig. 5.25 Invasive melanoma. Perspective view of the atypical junctional component.

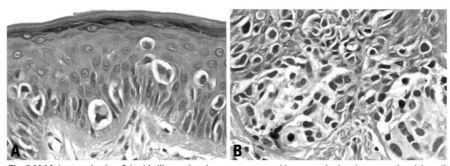

Fig. 5.26 Melanoma in situ. **A** In this illustration there are scattered large atypical melanocytes involving all layers of the epithelium. **B** This lesion shows an atypical junctional melanocytic proliferation associated with melanocytic cells that are present in the upper layers of the epithelium. Although the low power suggests a dysplastic nevus, the presence of atypical melanocytes migrating to different levels of the epithelium makes it a melanoma in situ.

Mesenchymal tumours

J.F. Fetsch
M. Miettinen

Definition
Tumours derived from the mesenchymal cells that are similar to those occuring at other sites.

Incidence
Mesenchymal tumours are very uncommon in the penis. The most frequently encountered benign mesenchymal tumours of the penis are vascular related. The most common malignant mesenchymal tumours are Kaposi sarcoma and leiomyosarcoma. With the exception of myointimoma, all of the listed tumours conform to definitions provided in other WHO fascicles (i.e., soft tissue, dermatopathology, and neuropathology fascicles). Myointimoma is a benign vascular related tumefaction with a myoid phenotype; this process is intimately associated with, and appears to be derived from, the vascular intima.

ICD-O codes
Benign

Haemangioma variants	9120/0
Lymphangioma variants	9170/0
Neurofibroma	9540/0
Schwannoma (neurilemoma)	9560/0
Granular cell tumour	9580/0
Myointimoma	
Leiomyoma	8890/0
Glomus tumour	8711/0
Fibrous histiocytoma	8830/0
Juvenile xanthogranuloma	

Intermediate Biologic Potential

Giant cell fibroblastoma	8834/1
Dermatofibrosarcoma protuberans	8832/3

Malignant

Kaposi sarcoma	9140/3
Epithelioid haemangioendothelioma	9133/3
Angiosarcoma	9120/3
Leiomyosarcoma	8890/3
Malignant fibrous histiocytoma (including myxofibrosarcoma)	8830/3
Rhabdomyosarcoma	8900/3
Epithelioid sarcoma	8804/3
Synovial sarcoma	9040/3
Clear cell sarcoma	9044/3
Malignant peripheral nerve sheath tumour	9540/3
Peripheral primitive neuroectodermal tumour	9364/3
Ewing sarcoma	9260/3
Extraskeletal osteosarcoma	9180/3

Epidemiology
Factors predisposing individuals to the development of soft tissue tumours are, for the most part, poorly understood. Genetic factors, immunodeficiency states, and human herpesvirus 8 {101,412} have been implicated in the development of Kaposi sarcoma. Irradiation has been implicated in the pathogenesis of several sarcoma types, especially malignant fibrous histiocytoma, but also, angio-

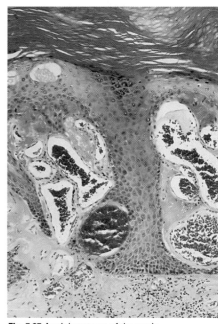

Fig. 5.27 Angiokeratoma of the penis.

sarcoma, malignant peripheral nerve sheath tumour, and others.

Most soft tissue tumours of the penis occur over a wide age range. Juvenile xanthogranuloma, giant cell fibroblastoma, and rhabdomyosarcoma are primarily paediatric tumours. Among nerve sheath tumours of the penis, neurofibromas have a peak incidence in the first and second decades, granular cell tumours primarily affect individuals in the

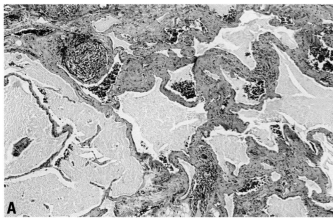
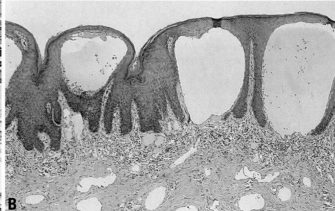

Fig. 5.28 A Lymphangioma of the penis. The presence of scattered lymphoid follicles is a helpful clue to the diagnosis. **B** Lymphangioma circumscriptum of the penis.

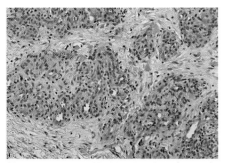

Fig. 5.29 Lobular capillary haemangioma (pyogenic granuloma) of the penis.

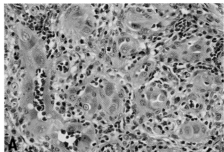
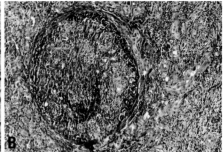

Fig. 5.30 Epithelioid haemangioma of the penis. **A** The process has immature but well formed vascular channels lined by plump epithelioid endothelial cells. A lymphocytic and eosinophilic inflammatory infiltrate is present. **B** This vascular was well demarcated and centered on a small muscular artery (note elastic lamina).

third and fourth decades, and schwannomas affect a higher percentage of patients in the fifth decade and above. Leiomyomas generally occur in mid adult life. Leiomyosarcoma, malignant fibrous histiocytoma, and angiosarcoma are usually tumours of mid and late adult life. Kaposi sarcoma of the penis diagnosed by a definitive method before the age of 60, and in the absence of other disqualifying causes for immunodeficiency (e.g. immunosuppressive/cytotoxic therapy,

certain lymphoproliferative disorders, and genetic immunodeficiency syndromes), is considered an indicator of AIDS {2}.

Localization
Most benign soft tissue tumours of the penis do not exhibit a clear predilection for a specific site except myointimomas, which affect the corpus spongiosum of the glans and coronal regions, and neurofibromas and schwannomas, which

more commonly affect the shaft and base. Among malignant tumours, Kaposi sarcoma has a strong predilection for the glans and prepuce, and leiomyosarcoma is somewhat more common on the shaft and base of the penis. Rhabdomyosarcomas of the penis are almost always located at the penopubic junction.

Clinical features
Most benign mesenchymal tumours of the penis present as a small, slowly enlarging, and often, painless mass. Malignant tumours generally occur at a later age, are more often tender or painful, and frequently grow more rapidly.
Superficial vascular tumours may exhibit erythematous or bluish colouration. Lymphangioma circumscriptum often presents as patches of translucent vesicles. Kaposi sarcoma presents as a patch, plaque, or nodule, often with a bluish or erythematous appearance.

Macroscopy
Haemangiomas and lymphangiomas have grossly apparent blood or lymph filled spaces, respectively. Neurofibromas have a well marginated, poorly marginated, or plexiform ("bag of worms") appearance and a solid off-white or myxoid cut surface. Schwannomas are typically well demarcated masses with white, pink or yellow colouration; they usually form a solitary nodule, but infrequently, they may have a multinodular appearance. Granular cell tumours tend to be poorly circumscribed and often have yellowish colouration and a scirrhous consistency. Malignant tumours tend to be poorly demarcated, infiltrative, and destructive masses, and often, are otherwise nonspecific from a gross standpoint.

Table 5.02
Soft tissue tumours of the penis: AFIP data for 116 cases (1970-1999).

Tumour type	Number of cases	Age range (mean)
Glomus tumour	1	49
Leiomyoma	1	68
Fibrous histiocytoma	1	51
Giant cell fibroblastoma	1	1
Epithelioid haemangioendothelioma	1	51
Angiokeratoma	2	23 – 47
Lymphangioma circumscriptum (LC)	2	1 – 55
Epithelioid sarcoma	2	27
Fibromyxoma, NOS	2	25 – 41
Haemangioma variants (excluding EH)	3	28 – 60
Lymphangioma (other than LC)	3	26 – 47 (35)
Angiosarcoma	3	38 – 81 (63)
Malignant fibrous histiocytoma	3	51 – 86 (74)
Epithelioid vascular tumours of UMP	4	35 – 51 (44)
Unclassified sarcoma	5	39 – 81 (59)
Neurofibroma	6	9 – 58 (26)
Schwannoma	6	20 – 73 (47)
Granular cell tumour	7	20 – 60 (41)
Epithelioid haemangioma (EH)	9	39 – 75 (50)
Myointimoma	10	2 – 61 (29)
Leiomyosarcoma	14	43 – 70 (53)
Kaposi sarcoma	30	42 – 91 (65)

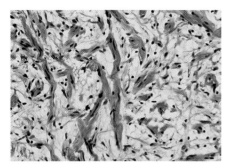

Fig. 5.31 Neurofibroma of the penis.

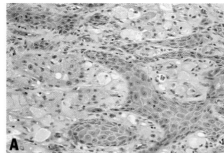
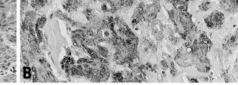

Fig. 5.32 Granular cell tumour of the penis. **A** This example was associated with prominent pseudoepitheliomatous hyperplasia of the epidermis. **B** The neoplastic cells are strongly immunoreactive for S100 protein.

Histopathology

Benign vascular lesions are classified on the basis of vessel type, growth pattern, and location. *Angiokeratoma* and *lymphangioma circumscriptum* feature superficial, dilated, blood or lymph-filled vessels, respectively. *Epithelioid haemangioma (angiolymphoid hyperplasia with eosinophilia)* contains immature, but well formed, capillary-sized vessels lined by plump epithelioid (histiocytoid) endothelial cells. This process is usually intimately associated with a small muscular artery, and it is commonly associated with a lymphocytic and eosinophilic inflammatory infiltrate.

A variety of *neurofibroma* subtypes are recognized, include solitary cutaneous, localized intraneural, plexiform, diffuse, pigmented, and epithelioid variants. All of these tumours feature S100 protein-positive Schwann cells admixed with varying numbers of EMA-positive perineurial cells, CD34-positive fibroblasts, and residual neurofilament protein-positive axons. Wagner-Meissner-like bodies are often present in diffuse neurofibroma, and melanotic stellate-shaped and spindled cells are present in pigmented neurofibroma. Atypia should not be pronounced and mitotic figures should be rare or absent.

Schwannomas (neurilemomas) are well demarcated peripheral nerve sheath tumours that classically exhibit Antoni A (cellular) and Antoni B (loose myxoid) growth patterns. Well developed Antoni A areas may exhibit nuclear palisading and contain Verocay bodies. Additional features commonly encountered in schwannomas include thick-walled vessels and perivascular xanthoma cells. In contrast with neurofibromas, atypia (often considered degenerative) is a common finding, and occasional mitoses are acceptable.

Granular cell tumours are S100 protein-positive neural neoplasms of Schwann cell derivation. These tumours feature epithelioid or spindled cells with abundant granular eosinophilic cytoplasm. Nuclear features vary, but mitotic activity is generally minimal. A fibrous connective tissue reaction may be present, and superficial examples may be associated with prominent pseudoepitheliomatous hyperplasia (sometimes mistaken for squamous carcinoma).

Myointimoma is a highly distinctive intravascular myointimal proliferation, often with multinodular or plexiform architecture, that tends to involve the corpus spongiosum. This process commonly has extensive immunoreactivity for α-smooth muscle actin, muscle-specific actin (HHF-35), and calponin, and it tends to have minimal reactivity for D33 and DE-R-11 desmin clones.

Leiomyomas consist of a proliferation of well developed smooth muscle cells with-

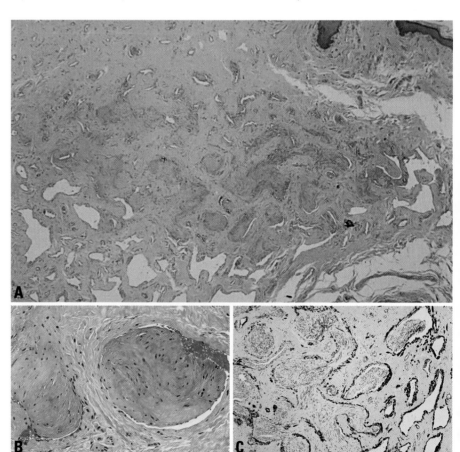

Fig. 5.33 Myointimoma of the penis. **A** Note the plexiform/multinodular appearance at low magnification. **B** This unusual process appears to originate from the vascular intima. **C** The lesional cells have immunoreactivity for calponin.

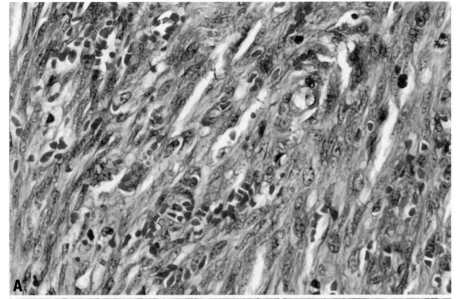

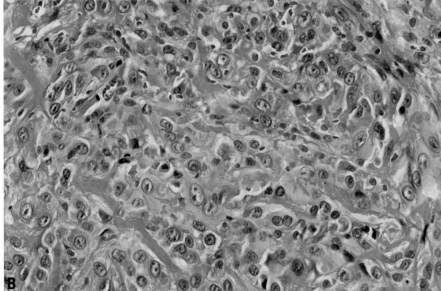

Fig. 5.34 A Kaposi sarcoma of the penis (nodular stage). Note the slit-like vascular spaces and presence of grape-like clusters of hyaline globules. **B** Epithelioid sarcoma of the penis. Note the presence of plump epithelioid tumour cells with eosinophilic cytoplasm. These cells often have an "open" chromatin pattern with a small but distinct central nucleolus. A garland growth pattern is often evident at low magnification.

out significant atypia, and generally, no mitotic activity. This diagnosis should be made only after careful examination, as leiomyomas appear to be much less common then leiomyosarcomas in this location. Early stage (patch/plaque) lesions of *Kaposi sarcoma* consist of a proliferation of small capillary-sized vessels around pre-existing dermal vessels and adnexae. The vessels may contain apoptotic nuclei. Haemosiderin deposition, a lymphoplasmacytic inflammatory infiltrate, and grapelike clusters of intracytoplas-

mic hyaline globules, when present, are helpful clues. The protrusion of small proliferating vessels into the lumen of a larger pre-existing vessel (the so-called promontory sign) is also a helpful finding. Later stage (nodular) lesions of Kaposi sarcoma are dominated by spindled cells with fascicular growth and slit-like vascular spaces. Hyaline globules are typically abundant by this stage. The lesional cells of Kaposi sarcoma are usually immunoreactive for CD34, and they may also express CD31. PCR analysis

for human herpesvirus 8 can be helpful in early stage or variant lesions.

Angiosarcoma has a broad morphologic spectrum. At one extreme, the process may closely resemble a benign haemangioma, and at the other, it may have a spindled appearance reminiscent of fibrosarcoma or an epithelioid appearance resembling carcinoma or melanoma. Infiltrative and interanastomosing growth; endothelial atypia with hyperchromasia; cell crowding and piling; and immunoreactivity for CD31, Factor VIIIr Ag and CD34 help establish the correct diagnosis.

Leiomyosarcomas contain spindled cells with nuclear atypia, mitotic activity, and a fascicular growth pattern. Longitudinal cytoplasmic striations and juxtanuclear vacuoles may be present. Immunoreactivity is usually detected for α-smooth muscle actin and desmin.

Malignant fibrous histiocytoma is a diagnosis of exclusion. This diagnosis is restricted to pleomorphic tumours (often with myxoid or collagenous matrix and a storiform growth pattern) that lack morphologic and immunohistochemical evidence for another specific line of differentiation (e.g. epithelial, melanocytic, myogenic or neural differentiation).

Grading

The grading of malignant soft tissue tumours is controversial. Some sarcomas are generally considered low-grade (e.g. Kaposi sarcoma) or high-grade (e.g. rhabdomyosarcoma and peripheral primitive neuroectodermal tumour). Others may be graded in one system but not in another (e.g. clear cell sarcoma, epithelioid sarcoma, and synovial sarcoma). For the majority of soft tissue sarcomas, we assign a numeric grade, based primarily on the modified French Federation of Cancer Centers Sarcoma Group system {970}.

Genetics

Specific cytogenetic or molecular genetic abnormalities have been identified for neurofibroma (allelic losses in 17q and/or mutations in the *NF1* gene), neurilemoma (allelic losses in 22q and/or mutations in the *NF2* gene), dermatofibrosarcoma protuberans [t(17;22)(q22;q13) or supernumerary ring chromosome derived from t(17;22)], clear cell sarcoma [t12;22)(q13;q12)], synovial sarcoma [t(X;18)((p11;q11)], peripheral primitive neuroectodermal tumour/Ewing sarcoma [primarily t(11;22)(q24;q12), t(21;22)(q22;q12), and t(7;22)(p22;q12)], and alveolar rhabdomyosarcoma [t(2;13)(q35;q14) and t(1;13)(p36;q14)] {1444}. RT-PCR tests are available for the four fully malignant tumours listed here. These tests can often be performed on fresh or formalin-fixed, paraffin-embedded tissue.

Prognosis
Superficial, benign mesenchymal lesions generally can be expected to have a low recurrence rate. Deep-seated benign lesions have a greater propensity for local recurrence. Tumours listed in the intermediate biologic potential category have a high rate of local recurrence, but only rarely give rise to metastases. The outcome for patients with Kaposi sarcoma is dependent on a variety of factors, including immune status and the extent of disease. However, the majority of patients with Kaposi sarcoma die of an unrelated event. There is insufficient data to provide site-specific prognostic information for the remainder of the sarcomas listed above.

Table 5.03
Mesenchymal tumours of the penis in the literature.

Category		Reference
Benign	Haemangioma variants	{383,761,789,811,1305,1889,1959,2361}
	Lymphangioma variants	{1356,1983}
	Neurofibroma	{1367,1599}
	Schwannoma (neurilemoma)	{1005,2300}
	Granular cell tumour	{333,2523}
	Myointimoma	{760}
	Glomus tumour	{1331,2275}
	Juvenile xanthogranuloma	{1043}
Intermediate Biological Potential	Giant cell fibroblastoma	{2398}
	Dermatofibrosarcoma protuberans	{581}
Malignant	Kaposi sarcoma	{382,1566,2232,2248}
	Epithelioid haemangioendothelioma	{1713}
	Angiosarcoma	{864,2106,2794}
	Leiomyosarcoma	{627,1173,1671,2103}
	Malignant fibrous histiocytoma (including myxofibrosarcoma)	{1714,1779}
	Rhabdomyosarcoma	{545,1998}
	Epithelioid sarcoma	{972,1136,1978,1987,2247}
	Synovial sarcoma	{49}
	Clear cell sarcoma	{2312}
	Malignant peripheral nerve sheath tumour	{581}
	Peripheral primitive neuroectodermal tumour/Ewing sarcoma	{2622}
	Extraskeletal osteosarcoma	{2271}

Lymphomas

A. Marx

Definition
Primary penile lymphomas (PL) are those that are confined to the penile skin, subcutis, and corpora cavernosa and spongiosum. Lymphomas of the urethra are counted among urinary tract lymphomas.

Synonym
Penile lymphoma.

Incidence
PL are very rare and most are considered to be primary {452}. Only 22 primary PL have been reported to date {107,123, 188,342,452,684,739,1036,1625,2508, 2787,2908}.

Clinical features and macroscopy
Painless or rarely tender swelling or ulcer of penile shaft, glans or prepuce {107}, scrotal masses {739,1503,2787}, priapism {123}, or associated Peyrone disease {2908} have been reported in PL. Systemic B symptoms appear to be an exception among primary PL {739}.

Histopathology
Several cases of diffuse large B-cell lymphomas (DLBCL) {107,1036,1625} and single cases of anaplastic large cell lymphoma (ALCL) of T-type (CD30+) {1503} and Hodgkin lymphoma have been reported as primary PL {2075}. Both nodal and cutaneous Non-Hodgkin-Lymphomas may involve the penis (secondary PL) {1416,1458}.

Precursor lesions and histogenesis (postulated cell of origin)
Precursor lesions and the histogenesis of PL are unknown. Some PL are cutaneous lymphomas {452,1458,1503}. Whether other primary PL occur due to an occult nodal lymphoma (implying systemic chemotherapy) {452} or a penile inflammatory process is unclear {107}.

Somatic genetics and genetic susceptibility
Genetic findings specific to PL have not been reported.

Prognosis and predictive factors
In the few, documented primary PL no death occurred after primary chemo- or radiochemotherapy with 42-72 months of follow-up {107,739,1514,2908}. Recurrences and dissemination were seen in a few penile lymphomas after radiotherapy {1036} or surgery as single modality treatments {684,2787}, while other cases {2508} including a probable cutaneous penile lymphoma, were apparently cured by surgery {1458,1503} or radiation {2508} alone.

Secondary tumours of the penis

C.J. Davis
F.K. Mostofi
I.A. Sesterhenn

Definition
Tumours of the penis that originate from an extra penile neoplasm.

Incidence
Metastatic carcinoma to penis is rare. By 1989 only 225 cases had been reported {2049}.

Clinical features
The presenting symptoms are frequently priapism or severe penile pain {1826}. Any patient with known cancer who develops priapism should be suspected of having metastatic disease. Other features include increased penile size, ulceration or palpable tumour nodules {2202}.

Localization
The corpus cavernosum is the most common site of metastases, but the penile skin, corpus spongiosum and mucosa of glans may be affected {2905}. A multinodular growth pattern in the CC is characteristic.

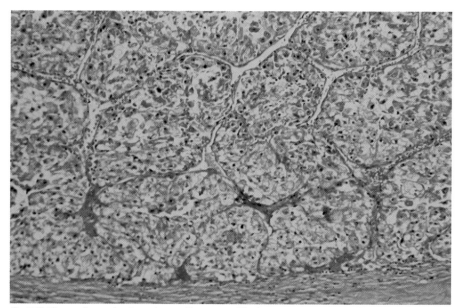

Fig. 5.35 Metastatic renal cell carcinoma. The tumour fills the corpus cavernosum. Tunica albuginea is at the top.

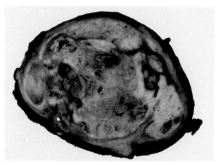

Fig. 5.36 Metastatic renal cell carcinoma. Cross section of the penis filled with RCC.

Origin of metastases
Reports invariably find prostate and bladder to be the most common primary sites with kidney and colon much less frequent {2905}. In a series of 60 cases, 21 were prostatic, 18 bladder, 14 undetermined primary sites, 3 colon, 2 kidney, 1 stomach and 1 pulmonary. Many other primary sites are occasionally reported.

Histopathology
Tumour deposits may be seen in any part of the penis but the common finding is filling of the vascular spaces of the erectile tissue and the tumour morphology will be typical of that seen in the primary tumour {2202}.

Prognosis
The prognosis is very poor since this usually occurs in the late stages in patients with known metastatic carcinoma. In one study 95% of patients died within weeks or months of diagnosis. In another, 71% died within 6 months {1826}.

Contributors

Dr Lauri A. AALTONEN
Research Professor of the Finnish
Academy of Sciences / Dept. of Med. Genetics
Biomedicum Helsinki / University of Helsinki
PO Box 63 (Haartmaninkatu 8)
FIN-00014 Helsinki / FINLAND
Tel: +358-9-1911 (direct: +358-9-19125595)
Fax: +358-9-19125105
lauri.aaltonen@helsinki.fi

Dr Ferran ALGABA*
Department of Pathology
Fundacion Puigvert (IUNA)
C. Cartagena 340-350
08025 Barcelona
SPAIN
Tel. + 349 3416 9700
Fax. + 349 3416 9730
falgaba@fundacio-puigvert.es

Dr William C. ALLSBROOK Jr.
Department of Pathology
Medical College of Georgia
Murphey Building, Room 210
Augusta, GA 30912
USA
Tel. +1 706 8631915
Fax. +1 706 721 8245
wallsbro@mail.mcg.edu

Dr Isabel ALVARADO-CABRERO
Servicio de Anatomia Patologica
National Hospital de Oncologia
Sanchez Azcona 1622 503
Col del Valle, del Benito, Juarez
C.P.03100 Mexico D.f. MEXICO
Tel. +52 56 27 69 00 / 69 57
Fax. +52 55 74 23 22 / +52 55 64 24 13
isa98@prodigy.net.mx

Dr Mahul B. AMIN*
Department of Pathology and Laboratory
Medicine, Room G 167
Emory University Hospital
1364, Clifton Road, N.E.
Atlanta, GA 30322 USA
Tel. +1 404 712 0190
Fax. +1 404 712 0148
mahul_amin@emory.org

Dr Pedram ARGANI*
Department of Pathology
The Harry & Jeannette Weinberg Building
The John Hopkins Hospital
401 N. Broadway / Room 2242
Baltimore, MD 21231-2410 USA
Tel. +1 410 614 2428
Fax. +1 410 614 9663
pargani@jhmi.edu

---

* The asterisk indicates participation
in the Working Group Meeting on the
WHO Classification of Tumours of the
Urinary System and Male Genital
Organs that was held in Lyon, France,
December 14-18, 2002.

Dr Hans ARNHOLDT
Department of Pathology
Klinikum Augsburg Tumorzentrum
Postfach 10 19 20
86009 Augsburg
GERMANY
Tel. +49 8 21 400 21 50
Fax. +49 8 21 400 21 62
hans.arnholdt@pathologie.zk.augsburg-med.de

Dr Alberto G. AYALA
Department of Pathology Box 85
M.D. Anderson Cancer Center
1515, Holcombe Boulevard
Houston, TX 77030
USA
Tel. +1 713 792 3151
Fax. +1 713 792 4049
aayala@mdanderson.org

Dr Sheldon BASTACKY
Department of Pathology
University of Pittsburgh Medical Center C622
200, Lothrop Street
Pittsburgh, PA 15213-2582
USA
Tel. +1 412 647 9612 / +1 412 648 6677
Fax. +1 412 647 3399 / 0287
bastackysi@msx.upmc.edu

Dr Louis R. BÉGIN
Division of Anatomic Pathology
Hôpital du Sacré-Coeur de Montréal
5400 Gouin Boulevard West
Montréal, QUEBEC H4J1C5
CANADA
Tel. +1 514 338 2222 (ext. 2965)
Fax. +1 514 338 2833
mdlrb@yahoo.ca

Dr Athanase BILLIS
Departmento de Anatomia Patológica
Faculdade de Ciências Médicas - UNICAMP
Caixa Postal 6111
CEP 13084-971 Campinas, SP
BRAZIL
Tel. +55 19 3788 7541
Fax. +5519 3289 3897
athanase@fcm.unicamp.br

Dr Liliane BOCCON-GIBOD
Department of Pathology
Hôpital d'enfants Armand Trousseau
26, rue du docteur Arnold Netter
75012 Paris
FRANCE
Tel. +33 1 44 73 61 82
Fax. +33 1 44 73 62 82
liliane.boccon-gibod@trs.ap-hop-paris.fr

Dr Stephen M. BONSIB*
Department of Surgical Pathology
Indiana University Medical Center
550, North University Boulevard, UH 3465
Indianapolis, IN 46202-5280
USA
Tel. +1 317 274 7005
Fax. +1 317 274 5346
sbonsib@iupui.edu

Dr Christer BUSCH*
Department of Patholog
University Hospital
SE 751 85 Uppsala
SWEDEN
Tel. +46 18611 3820
Fax. +46 706 108 750
christer.busch@genpat.uu.se

Dr Paul CAIRNS
Departments of Surgical Oncology & Pathology
Fox Chase Cancer Center
7701 Burholme Avenue
Philadelphia, PA 19111
USA
Tel. +1 215 728 5635
Fax. +1215 728 2487
P_Cairns@fccc.edu

Dr Liang CHENG
Pathology & Laboratory Medicine UM 3465
Indiana University Hospital
550, N. University Boulevard
Indianapolis, IN 46202
USA
Tel. +1 317 274 1756
Fax. +1 317 274 5346
lcheng@iupui.edu

Dr John CHEVILLE*
Department of Pathology
The Mayo Clinic
200 First Street, SW
Rochester, MN 55905-0001
USA
Tel. +1 507 284 3867
Fax. +1 507 284 1599
cheville.john@mayo.edu

Dr Carlos CORDON-CARDO
Division of Molecular Pathology
Memorial Sloan-Kettering Cancer Center
1275 York Avenue
New York, NY 10021
USA
Tel. +1 212 639 7746
Fax. +1 212 794 3186
cordon-c@mskcc.org

Dr Antonio L. CUBILLA*
Instituto de Patologia e
Investigacion
Martin Brizuela 325 y Ayala Velazquez
Asuncion
PARAGUAY
Tel. +595 21 208 963
Fax. +595 21 214 055
acubilla@institutodepatologia.com.py

Dr Ivan DAMJANOV
Department of Pathology
University of Kansas (Medicine)
3901 Rainbow Boulevard
Kansas City KS 66160-7410
USA
Tel. +1 913 588 7090
Fax. +1 913 588 7073
idamjano@kumc.edu

Dr Charles J. DAVIS*
Department of Genitourinary Pathology
Armed Forces Institute of Pathology
6825, 16th Street, NW Room 2090
Washington, DC 20306-6000
USA
Tel. +1 202 782 2755
Fax. +1 202 782 3056
DAVISC@afip.osd.mil

Dr Angelo M. DE MARZO
Department of Pathology
Bunting-Blaustein Cancer Res. Bldg, Room 153
The John Hopkins University
1650 Orleans Street
Baltimore, MD 21231-1000 USA
Tel. +1 410 614 5686
Fax. +1 410 502 9817
ademarz@jhmi.edu

Dr Louis P. DEHNER
Division of Anatomic Pathology
Washington University Medical Center
660, S. Euclid Avenue Campus Box 8118
St Louis, MO 63110-2696
USA
Tel. +1 314 362 0150 / 0101
Fax. +1 314 747 2040 / +1 314 362 0327
dehner@path.wustl.edu

Dr Brett DELAHUNT*
Dept. of Pathology & Molecular Medicine
Wellington School of Medicine & Health
Mein Street, Newtown, P.O. Box 7343
6002 Wellington South
NEW ZEALAND
Tel. +64 4 385 5569
Fax. +64 4 389 5725
bd@wnmeds.ac.nz

Dr Gonzague DE PINIEUX
Service d'Anatomie Pathologique
Hôpital Cochin, AP-HP
27, rue du Faubourg Saint Jacques
75679 PARIS Cedex 14
FRANCE
Tel. +33 1 58 41 41 41
Fax. +33 1 58 41 14 80
gonzague.de-pinieux@cch.ap-hop-paris.fr

Dr P. Anthony DI SANT'AGNESE
Department of Pathology RM 2-2115
University of Rochester Medical Center
601, Elmwood Avenue, Box 626
Rochester, NY 14642
USA
Tel. +1 585 275 0839
Fax. +1585 273 3637
anthony_disantagnese@urmc.rochester.edu

Dr Joakim DILLNER
Department of Medical Microbiology
Lund University
Malmö University Hospital Entrance 78
SE-205 02 Malmö
SWEDEN
Tel. +46 40 338126
Fax. +46 40 337312
joakim.dillner@mikrobiol.mas.lu.se

Dr John N. EBLE*
Dept. of Pathology & Laboratory Medicine
Indiana University School of Medicine
635, Barnhill Drive, MS Science Bldg. A 128
Indianapolis, IN 46202-5120
USA
Tel. +1 317 274 1738 / 7603
Fax. +1 317 278 2018
jeble@iupui.edu

Dr Diana M. ECCLES
Wessex Clinical
Genetics Service
Princess Anne Hospital
Southampton SO16 5YA
UNITED KINGDOM
Tel. +44 23 8079 8537
Fax +44 23 8079 4346
de1@soton.ac.uk

Dr Lars EGEVAD*
Department of Pathology
and Cytology
Karolinska Hospital
SE 171 16 Stockholm
SWEDEN
Tel. +46 8 5177 5492
Fax. +46 8 33 1909
lars.egevad@onkpat.ki.se

Dr M.N. EL-BOLKAINY
Lewa Building
2, Sherif street, Apt. 18
11796 Cairo
EGYPT
Tel. +20 2 3374886 /
+20 12 3470693
Fax. +20 2 3927964 /
+20 2 3644720

Dr Jonathan I. EPSTEIN*
Dept. of Pathology Weinberg Bldg, Room 2242
The John Hopkins Hospital
401, North Broadway
Baltimore, MD 21231-2410
USA
Tel. +1 410 955 5043
Fax. +1 410 955 0115
jepstein@jhmi.edu

Dr John F. FETSCH
Department of Soft Tissue Pathology
Armed Forces Institute of Pathology
14th Street & Alaska Avenue, NW
Washington, DC 20306-6000
USA
Tel. +1 202 782 2799 / 2790
Fax. +1 202 782 9182
fetsch@afip.osd.mil

Dr Masakuni FURUSATO
Department of Pathology
Kyorin University
6-20-2 Skinkawa, Mitakashi
181-8611 Tokyo
JAPAN
Tel. +81 422-47-5511 (ext. 3422)
Fax. +81 3-3437-0388
blueandwhite@earthlink.net

Dr Thomas GASSER*
Urologic Clinics
University of Basel
Rheinstrasse, 26
CH 4410 Liestal
SWITZERLAND
Tel. +41 61 925 21 70
Fax. +41 61 925 28 06
thomas.gasser@ksli.ch

Dr William L. GERALD
Department of Pathology
Memorial Sloan-Kettering Cancer Center
1275 York Avenue
New York, NY 10021
USA
Tel. +1 212 639 5858
Fax. +1 212 639 4559
geraldw@mskcc.org

Dr A. GEURTS VAN KESSEL
Department of Human Genetics 417
University Medical Center Nijmegen
P.O. Box 9101
6500 HB Nijmegen
THE NETHERLANDS
Tel. +31-24-3614107
Fax. +31-24-3540488
A.GeurtsVanKessel@antrg.umcn.nl

Dr David J. GRIGNON*
Department of Pathology
Harper University Hospital
Wayne State University
3990, John R Street
Detroit, MI 48201 USA
Tel. +1 313 745 2520
Fax. +1 313 745 8673
dgrignon@med.wayne.edu

Dr Kenneth GRIGOR
Department of Pathology
Western General Hospital
Crewe Road
Edinburgh, EH4 2XU
UNITED KINGDOM
Tel. +44 131 537 1954
Fax. +44 131 5371013
Ken.Grigor@ed.ac.uk

Dr Jay L. GROSFELD
Pediatric Surgery
J.W. Riley Children's Hospital, Suite 2500
702, Barnhill Drive
Indianapolis, IN 46202-5200
USA
Tel. +1 317 274 4966
Fax. +1 317 274 8769
jgrosfel@iupui.edu

Dr Louis GUILLOU
Institut Universitaire de Pathologie
Université de Lausanne
25, rue du Bugnon
CH-1011 Lausanne
SWITZERLAND
Tel. +41 21 314 7216 / 7202
Fax. +41 21 314 7207
louis.guillou@chuv.hospvd.ch

Dr Seife HAILEMARIAM*
Cantonal Institute of
Pathology
Rheinstrasse 37
CH-4410 Liestal
SWITZERLAND
Tel. +41 61 925 26 25
Fax. +41 61 925 20 94
seife.hailemariam@ksli.ch

Professor Ulrike Maria HAMPER
Department of Radiology
The John Hopkins University School of Medicine
600, North Wolfe Street
Baltimore, MD 21287
USA
Tel. +1 410 955 8450 / 7410
Fax. +1 410 614 9865 / +1 410 955 0231
umhamper@jhu.edu

Dr Arndt HARTMANN
Institute of Pathology
University of Regensburg
Franz-Josef-Strauss Allee 11
D-93053 Regensburg
GERMANY
Tel. +49 941 944 6605
Fax. +49 941 944 6602
arndt.hartmann@klinik.uni-regensburg.de

Dr Tadashi HASEGAWA
Pathology Division
National Cancer Center Research Institute
1-1, Tsukiji 5-chome, Chuo-ku
104-0045 Tokyo
JAPAN
Tel. +81 3 3547 5201 (ext. 7129)
Fax. +81 3 3248 2463
tdhasega@ncc.go.jp

Dr Axel HEIDENREICH
Department of Urology
University of Cologne
Joseph-Stelzmann-Str 9
50931 Köln
GERMANY
Tel. +49 221 478 3632
Fax. +49 221 478 5198
a.heidenreich@uni-koeln.de

Dr Philipp U. HEITZ
Department of Pathology
UniversitätsSpital Zurich
Schmelzbergstrasse 12
CH - 8091 Zürich
SWITZERLAND
Tel. +41 1 255 25 00
Fax. +41 1 255 44 40
philipp.heitz@pty.usz.ch

Dr Burkhard HELPAP*
Chefarzt Institut fur Pathologie
Hegau Klinikum
Virchowstrasse 10
78207 Singen
GERMANY
Tel. +49 7731 892100
Fax. +49 7731 892105
pathologie@hegau-klinikum.de

Dr Riitta HERVA
Oulu Uviversity Hospital
Department of Pathology
P.O. BOX 50
FIN-90029 OYS
FINLAND
Tel. +358-8-3155362
Fax. +358-8-3152177
riitta.herva@ppshp.fi

Professor Ferdinand HOFSTÄDTER*
Institute of Pathology
University of Regensburg, Klinikum
F.J. Strauss Allee 11
D 93053 Regensburg
GERMANY
Tel. +49 941 944 6600
Fax. +49 941 944 6602
ferdinand.hofstaedter@klinik.uni-regensburg.de

Professor Simon HORENBLAS
Department of Urology
Antoni Van Leeuwenhoek Hospital
Netherlands Cancer Institute
Plesmanlaan 121
1066 CX Amsterdam THE NETHERLANDS
Tel. +31 20 512 2553
Fax. +31 20 512 2554
shor@nki.nl

Dr Peter A. HUMPHREY*
Division of Surgical Pathology, Box 8118
Dept. of Pathology & Immunology
Washington University School of Medicine
660, S. Euclid Avenue
St Louis, MO 63110 USA
Tel. +1 314 362 0112
Fax. +1 314 747 2040
humphrey@path.wustl.edu

Dr Kenneth A. ICZKOWSKI
Dept. of Pathology, Immunology & Lab. Med.
University of Florida and Veterans
Administration Medical Center Room E126 F
1601 SW Archer Road
Gainesville, FL 32608-1197 USA
Tel. +1 352 376 1611 ext. 4522
Fax. +1 352 379 4023
iczkoka@pathology.ufl.edu

Dr Grete Krag JACOBSEN*
Department of Pathology
Gentofte Hospital University of Copenhagen
Niels Andersens Vej 65
DK-2900 Hellerup
DENMARK
Tel. +45 39 77 36 18
Fax. +45 39 77 76 24
grja@gentoftehosp.kbhamt.dk

Dr Sonny L. JOHANSSON
Deptartments of Surgical Pathology,
Cytopathology, and Urologic Pathology
University of Nebraska Med. Center at Omaha
6001 Dodge Street
Omaha, NE 68198-3135 USA
Tel. +1 402 559 7681
Fax. +1 402 559 6018
sjohanss@unmc.edu

Dr Michael A. JONES
Dept. of Pathology and Laboratory Medicine
Maine Medical Center
22, Bramhall Street
Portland, ME 04102
USA
Tel. +1 207 871 2959
Fax. +1 207 871 6268
jonesm@mmc.org

Dr Peter A. JONES
USC/Norris Comprehensive Cancer Center
& Hospital NOR 8302 L
University of Southern California
1441, East Lake Avenue
Los Angeles, CA 90089-9181 USA
Tel. +1 323 865 0816
Fax. +1 323 865 0102
jones_p@ccnt.hsc.usc.edu

Dr George W. KAPLAN
Division of Urology
Children's Specialists of San Diego
7930 Frost Street Suite 407
San Diego, CA 92123-4286
USA
Tel. +1 858 279 8527 / +1 619 279 8527
Fax. +1 858 279 8876
gkaplan@chsd.org

Dr Charles E. KEEN
Dept.of Histopathology and Cytopathology
Royal Devon and Exeter Hospital
Barrack Road
Exeter, EX2 5DW
UNITED KINGDOM
Tel. +44 1 392 402 963 / 914
Fax. +44 1 392 402 915
charlie.keen@rdehc-tr.swest.nhs.uk

Dr Kyu Rae KIM
Department of Pathology
University of Ulsan College of Medicine
Asan Medical Center
388-1 Pungnap-dong, Songpa-gu
138-736 Seoul KOREA
Tel. +82 2 3010 4514
Fax. +82 2 472 7898
krkim@amc.seoul.kr

Dr Maija KIURU
Department of Medical Genetics
Biomedicum Helsinki / University of Helsinki
P.O. Box 63 (Haartmaninkatu 8)
FIN-00014 Helsinki
FINLAND
Tel. +358-9-19125379
Fax. +358-9-19125105
E-mail maija.kiuru@helsinki.fi

Dr Paul KLEIHUES
Department of Pathology
University Hospital
CH-8091 Zurich
SWITZERLAND
Tel. +41 1 255 3516
Fax. +41 1 255 4551
paul.kleihues@usz.ch

Dr Margaret A. KNOWLES
Cancer Research UK Clinical Centre
St James' University Hospital
Beckett Street
Leeds, LS9 7TF
UNITED KINGDOM
Tel. +44 113 206 4913
Fax. +44 113 242 9886
margaret.knowles@cancer.org.uk

Dr Gyula KOVACS*
Laboratory of Molecular Oncology
Department of Urology
University of Heidelberg
Im Neuenheimer feld 325
D 69120 Heidelberg GERMANY
Tel. +49 6221 566519
Fax. +49 6221 564634
gyula.kovacs@urz.uni-heidelberg.de

Dr Marc LADANYI
Department of Pathology Room S-801
Memorial Sloan-Kettering Cancer Center
1275, York Avenue
New York, NY 10021
USA
Tel. +1 212 639 6369
Fax. +1 212 717 3515
ladanyim@mskcc.org

Dr Virpi LAUNONEN
Department of Medical Genetics
Biomedicum Helsinki / University of Helsinki
P.O. Box 63 (Haartmaninkatu 8)
FIN-00014 Helsinki
FINLAND
Tel. +358-9-1911
Fax. +358-9-19125105
virpi.launonen@helsinki.fi

Dr Ivo LEUSCHNER
Department of Pathology
University of Kiel
Michaelsstrasse 11
D-24105 Kiel
GERMANY
Tel. +49 431 597 3444
Fax. +49 431 597 3486
ileuschner@path.uni-kiel.de

Dr Howard S. LEVIN
Department of Pathology
Cleveland Clinic Foundation
9500 Euclid Avenue
Cleveland, OH 44195-5038
USA
Tel. +1 216 444 2843
Fax. +1 216 445 6967
levinh@ccf.org

Dr W. Marston LINEHAN
Urologic Oncology Branch
NCI Center for Cancer Research
National Institutes of Health
Building 10, Room 2B47
Bethesda, MD 20892
USA
Tel. +1 301 496 6353
Fax. +1 301 402 0922

Dr Leendert H.J. LOOIJENGA*
Dept. of Pathology, Rm. Be 430b
Erasmus University Med. Center
Josephine Nefkens Inst. / Univ. Hosp. Rotterdam
Laboratory for Experimental Patho-Oncology
P.O. Box 2040
3000 CA Rotterdam THE NETHERLANDS
Tel. +31 10 408 8329 / Fax. +31 10 408 8365
looijenga@leph.azr.nl

Dr Antonio LOPEZ-BELTRAN*
Unit of Anatomical Pathology
Cordoba University Medical School
Avenida Menendez Pidal s/n
14004 Cordoba
SPAIN
Tel. +34 957 218993
Fax. +34 957 218229
em1lobea@uco.es

Dr J. Carlos MANIVEL
Dept. of Laboratory Medicine & Pathology
University of Minnesota, Medical School
420 Delaware St. S.E. MMC 76
Minneapolis, MN 55455
USA
Tel. +1 612 273 5848
Fax. +1 612 273 1142
maniv001@umn.edu

Dr Guido MARTIGNONI*
Dipartimento di Patologia
Sezione Anatomia Patologica
Universita di Verona, Policlinico G.B. Rossi
P.LE L.A. Scuro 10
37134 Verona ITALY
Tel. +39 045 8074846
Fax. +39 045 8027136
guidomart@yahoo.com

Dr Alexander MARX
Department of Pathology
University of Wuerzburg
Josef-Schneider-Strasse 2
97080 Wuerzburg
GERMANY
Tel. +49 931 201 3776
Fax. +49 931 201 3440 / 3505
path062@mail.uni-wuerzburg.de

Dr David G. MCLEOD
Urology Services, Ward 56 (CPDR)
Walter Reed Army Medical Center
6900 Georgia Avenue, N.W.
Washington, DC 20307-5001
USA
Tel. +1 202 782 6408
Fax. +1 202 782 2310
david.mcleod@na.amedd.army.mil

Dr L. Jeffrey MEDEIROS
Division of Pathology & Laboratory Med.
M.D. Anderson Cancer Center
1515, Holcombe Boulevard Box 0072
Houston, TX 77030
USA
Tel. +1 713 794 5446
Fax. +1 713 745 0736
jmedeiro@mdanderson.org

Dr Maria J. MERINO
Department of Surgical Pathology
Building 10, Room 2N212
National Cancer Institute
9000, Rockville Pike
Bethesda, MD 20892 USA
Tel. +1 301 496 2441
Fax. +1 301 480 9488
mjmerino@mail.nih.gov

Dr Helen MICHAEL
Department of Pathology
Indiana University School of Medicine
Wishard Memorial Hospital
1001 West 10th Street
Indianapolis, IN 46202 USA
Tel. +1 317 630 7208
Fax. +1 317 630 7913
hmichael@iupui.edu

Dr Markku MIETTINEN
Department of Soft Tissue Pathology
Armed Forces Institute of Pathology
6825, 16th Street, N.W.
Washington, DC 20306-6000
USA
Tel. +1 202 782 2793
Fax. +1 202 782 9182
miettinen@afip.osd.mil

Dr Holger MOCH*
Institute for Pathology
University of Basel
Schönbeinstrasse, 40
CH 4003 Basel
SWITZERLAND
Tel. +41 61 265 2890
Fax. +41 61 265 31 94
hmoch@uhbs.ch

Dr Henrik MØLLER
Thames' Cancer Registry
Guy's, King's, & St Thomas' School of Med.
King's College London
1st Floor, Capital House
42 Weston Street
London SE1 3QD UNITED KINGDOM
Tel. +44 20 7378 7688 / Fax. +44 20 73789510
henrik.moller@kcl.ac.uk

Dr Rodolfo MONTIRONI*
Institute of Pathological Anatomy &
Histopathology
University of Ancona School of Med.
I-60020 Torrette, Ancona
ITALY
Tel. +39 071 5964830
Fax. +39 071 889985
r.montironi@popcsi.unian.it

Dr F. Kash MOSTOFI
Department of Genitourinary Pathology
Armed Forces Institute of Pathology
14th and Alaska Avenue, NW
Washington, DC 20306-6000
USA
(deceased)

Dr Hartmut P.H. NEUMANN
Dpt. of Nephrology and Hypertension
Albert-Ludwigs-University
Hugstetter Strasse 55
D-79106 Freiburg
GERMANY
Tel. +49 761 270 3578 / 3401
Fax. +49 761 270 3778
neumann@mm41.ukl.uni-freiburg.de

Dr Manuel NISTAL
Department of Morphology
Universidad Autonoma
de Madrid
c/ Arzobispo Morcillo s/n
28029 Madrid
SPAIN
Tel. +34 91 727 7300 / 397 5323
Fax. +34 91 397 5353

Dr Lucien NOCHOMOVITZ
Department of Pathology
North Shore University Hospital
300 Community Drive
Manhasset NY 11030
USA
Tel. +1 516 562-3249
Fax. +1 516 562-4591
lnochomo@nshs.edu

Dr Esther OLIVA
Pathology, Warren 2/Rm 251 A
Massachusetts General Hospital
55 Fruit Street
Boston, MA 02114
USA
Tel. +1 617 724 8272
Fax. +1 617 726 7474
eoliva@partners.org

Dr Tim D. OLIVER
Department of Medical Oncology
Saint Bartholomew's Hospital
1st Fl. KGV Building, West Smithfield
London, EC1A 7BE
UNITED KINGDOM
Tel. +44 20 7601 8522
Fax. +44 20 7796 0432
c.l.crickmore@gmul.ac.uk

Dr J. Wolter OOSTERHUIS
Department of Pathology, Room Be 200a
Erasmus Medical Center
Josephine Nefkens Institute
PO Box 1738
3000 DR Rotterdam THE NETHERLANDS
Tel. +31 10 40 88449
Fax. +31 10 40 88450
j.w.oosterhuis@erasmusmc.nl

Dr Attilio ORAZI
Department of Pathology
Indiana University School of Medicine
Riley Hospital, IU Medical Center
702 Barhhill Drive Room 0969
Indianapolis, IN 46202 USA
Tel. +1 317 274 7250
Fax. +1 317 274 0149
aorazi@iupui.edu

Dr Chin-Chen PAN
Department of Pathology
Veterans General Hospital-Taipei
No. 201, Sec. 2 Shih-Pai Road
11217 Taipei
TAIWAN R.O.C.
Tel. +886 2 28757449 ext. 213
Fax. +886 2 28757056
ccpan@vghtpe.gov.tw

Dr Ricardo PANIAGUA
Department of Cell Biology and Genetics
University of Alcala
28871 Alcala de Henares, Madrid
SPAIN
Tel. +34 1 885 47 51
Fax. + 34 91 885 47 99
ricardo.paniagua@uah.es
dep402@uah.es

Dr David M. PARHAM
Department of Pathology
Arkansas Children's Hospital
800, Marshall Street
Little Rock, AR 72202-3591
USA
Tel. +1 501 320 1307
Fax. +1 501 320 3912
parhamdavidm@uams.edu

Dr D. Max PARKIN
Unit of Descriptive Epidemiology
Intl. Agency for Research on Cancer (IARC)
World Health Organization (WHO)
150, Cours Albert Thomas
69008 Lyon FRANCE
Tel. +33 4 72 73 84 82
Fax. +33 4 72 73 86 50
parkin@iarc.fr

Dr M. Constance PARKINSON*
UCL Hospitals Trust & Institute of Urology
University College London
Rockefeller Building
University Street
London, WC1E 6JJ UNITED KINGDOM
Tel. +44 20 7679 6033
Fax. +44 20 7387 3674
rmkdhmp@ucl.ac.uk

Dr Christian P. Pavlovich
Assistant Professor of Urology
Director, Urologic Oncology
Johns Hopkins Bayview Medical Center
Brady Urological Institute, A-345
4940 Eastern Avenue
Baltimore, MD 21224 USA
Tel. +1 410-550-3506 / Fax. +1 410-550-3341
cpavlov2@jhmi.edu

Dr Elizabeth J. PERLMAN
Department of Pathology
Children's Memorial Hospital
2373 Lincoln N. A 203
Chicago, IL 60614
USA
Tel. +1 773 880 4306
Fax. +1 773 880 3858
eperlman@childrensmemorial.org

Dr Paola PISANI
Unit of Descriptive Epidemiology Office 519
Intl. Agency for Research on Cancer (IARC)
World Health Organization (WHO)
150, Cours Albert Thomas
69008 Lyon FRANCE
Tel. +33 4 72 73 85 22
Fax. +33 4 72 73 86 50
pisani@iarc.fr

Dr Andrew A. RENSHAW
Baptist Hospital
Department of Pathology
8900 N. Kendall Drive
Miami, FL 33176
USA
Tel. +1 305 5966525
Fax. +1 305 598 5986
AndrewR@bhssf.org

Dr Victor E. REUTER
Department of Pathology
Memorial Sloan Kettering Cancer Center
1275, York Avenue
New York, NY 10021
USA
Tel. +1 212 639 8225
Fax. +1 212 717 3203
reuterv@mskcc.org

Dr Jae Y. RO
Department of Pathology
Asan Medical Center
Ulsan University School of Medicine #3881
Pungnap-dong, Songpa-gu
138-736 Seoul KOREA
Tel. +82 2 3010 4550
Fax. +82 2 472 7898
jaero@www.amc.seoul.kr

Professor Mark A. RUBIN*
Department of Urologic Pathology
Brigham and Women's Hospital
Harvard Medical School
75 Francis Street
Boston, MA 02115 USA
Tel. +1 617 525 6747
Fax. +1 617 278 6950
marubin@partners.org

Dr H. Gil RUSHTON
Department of Pathology
Children's National Medical Center
111, Michigan Avenue N.W. Ste 500-3W
Washington, DC 20010-2916
USA
Tel. +1 202 884 5550 / 5042
Fax. +1 202 884 4739
hrushton@cnmc.org

Dr Wael A. SAKR*
Department of Pathology
Harper Hospital
3990, John R. Street
Detroit, MI 48201
USA
Tel. +1 313 745 2525
Fax. +1 313 745 9299
wsakr@dmc.org

Dr Hemamali SAMARATUNGA
Dept. of Pathology
Sullivan Nicolaides Pathology
134, Whitmore Street
Taringa, QLD 4068 AUSTRALIA
Tel. +61 07 33778666
Fax. +61 07 33783089 / 33778724
hemamali@medihesa.com
hema_samaratunga@snp.com.au

Dr Guido SAUTER*
Institute for Pathology
University of Basel
Schönbeinstrasse 40
4003 Basel
SWITZERLAND
Tel. +41 61 265 2889 / 2525
Fax. +41 61 265 2966
Guido.Sauter@unibas.ch

Dr Paul F. SCHELLHAMMER
Department of Urology
Eastern Virginia Graduate School of Medicine
6333 Center Drive Elizabeth Building #1
Norfolk, VA 23502
USA
Tel. +1 757 457 5175 / 5170
Fax. +1 757 627 3211
schellpf@evms.edu

Dr Bernd J. SCHMITZ-DRAGER
Department of Urology
Euromed-Clinic
Europa-Allee 1
D-90763 Fürth
GERMANY
Tel. +49 911 971 4531
Fax. +49 911 971 4532
bsd@euromed.de

Dr Mark Philip SCHOENBERG
Brady Urological Institute
Johns Hopkins Hospital
600 N Wolfe St. Marburg 150
Baltimore, MD 21287-2101
USA
Tel. +1 410 955 1039
Fax. +1 410 955 0833
mschoenberg@jhmi.edu

Dr Isabell A. SESTERHENN*
Department of Genitourinary Pathology
Armed Forces Institute of Pathology
14th and Alaska Avenue, NW Rm. 2088
Washington, DC 20306-6000 USA
Tel. +1 202 782 2756
Fax. +1 202 782 3056
Sesterhe@afip.osd.mil
TYREE@afip.osd.mil

Dr David SIDRANSKY
Dept. of Otolaryngology, Head & Neck
Surgery, Oncology, Pathology, Urology &
Cellular & Molecular Med.
The Johns Hopkins University School of Medicine
818 Ross Research Bldg, 720 Rutland Avenue
Baltimore, MD 21205-2196 USA
Tel. +1 410 502 5153 / Fax. +1 410 614 1411
dsidrans@jhmi.edu

Dr Ronald SIMON
Institut für Pathologie
Universität Basel
Schönbeinstrasse 40
4003 Basel
SWITZERLAND
Tel. +41 61 265 3152
Fax. +41 61 265 2966
ronald_simon_de@yahoo.de

Dr Leslie H. SOBIN
Dept. of Hepatic & Gastrointestinal Pathology
Armed Forces Institute of Pathology
14th Street and Alaska Avenue
Washington, DC 20306
USA
Tel. +1 202 782 2880
Fax. +1 202 782 9020
sobin@afip.osd.mil

Dr Poul H. B. SORENSEN
Depts. of Pathology and Pediatrics, BC Research
Institute for Children's & Women's Health
950 West 28th Avenue, Room 3082
Vancouver (BC) V5Z 4H4
CANADA
Tel. +1 604 875 2936
Fax. +1 604 875 3417
psor@interchange.ubc.ca

Dr John R. SRIGLEY*
Laboratory Medicine
The Credit Valley Hospital
2200, Eglinton Avenue, West
Mississauga (Ontario)
CANADA
Tel. +1 905 813 2696
Fax. +1 905 813 4132
jsrigley@cvh.on.ca

Dr Stephan STÖRKEL
Institute of Pathology
University of Witten / Herdecke
Helios-Klinikum Wuppertal
Heusnerstrasse, 40
42283 Wuppertal GERMANY
Tel. +49 202 896 2850
Fax. +49 202 896 2739
sstoerkel@wuppertal.helios-kliniken.de

Dr Aleksander TALERMAN
Department of Pathology
Thomas Jefferson University Hospital
Main Building 132 South 10th Street,
Room 285Q
Philadelphia, PA 19107-5244
USA
Tel. +1 215 955 2433
Fax. +1 215 923 1969

Dr Pheroze TAMBOLI
Department of Pathology
M.D. Anderson Cancer Center
1515, Holcombe Boulevard Box 0085
Houston, TX 77030
USA
Tel. +1 713 794 5445
Fax. +1 713 745 3740
ptamboli@mdanderson.org

Dr Puay H. TAN
Department of Pathology
Singapore General Hospital
1, Hospital Drive, Outram Road
169608 Singapore
SINGAPORE
Tel. +65 6321 4900
Fax. +65 6222 6826
gpttph@sgh.com.sg

Dr Bernard TÊTU
Service de Pathologie
CHUQ, L'Hôtel-Dieu de Québec
11, Côte du Palais
Québec, G1R 2J6
CANADA
Tel. +1 418 691-5233
Fax. +1 418 691 5226
bernard.tetu@crhdq.ulaval.ca

Dr Kaori TOGASHI
Dept. of Nuclear Medicine & Diagnostic Imaging
Graduate School of Medicine Kyoto University
54 Shogoin Kawahara-cho
Kyoto 606-8507
JAPAN
Tel. +81 75 751 3760
Fax. +81 75 771 9709
ktogashi@kuhp.kyoto-u.ac.jp

Dr Lawrence TRUE
Department of Pathology
University of Washington Medical Center
1959, NE Pacific Street
Seattle, WA 98195
USA
Tel. +1 206 598 6400 / +1 206 548 4027
Fax. +1 206 598 4928 / 3803
ltrue@u.washington.edu

Dr Jerzy E. TYCZYNSKI
Unit of Descriptive Epidemiology Office 518
Intl. Agency for Research on Cancer (IARC)
World Health Organization (WHO)
150, Cours Albert Thomas
69008 Lyon FRANCE
Tel. +33 4 72 73 84 97
Fax. +33 4 72 73 86 50
tyczynski@iarc.fr

Dr Thomas M. ULBRIGHT*
Department of Pathology and Laboratory
Medicine, Room 3465
Indiana University Hospital
550, N. University Boulevard
Indianapolis, IN 46202-5280 USA
Tel. +1 317 274 5786
Fax. +1 317 274 5346
tulbrigh@iupui.edu

Dr Eva VAN DEN BERG
Department of Clinical Genetics
Academic Hospital Groningen
Ant. Deusinglaan 4
NL-9713 AW Groningen
THE NETHERLANDS
Tel. +31 50 3632938 / 3632942
Fax. +31 50 3632457
e.van.den.berg-de.ruiter@medgen.azg.nl

Dr Theo H. VAN DER KWAST
Department of Pathology
Josephine Nefkens Institute Erasmus MC
Postbox 1738
3000 DR Rotterdam
THE NETHERLANDS
Tel. +31 10 4087924
Fax. +31 10 4088450
t.vanderkwast@erasmusmc.nl

Dr Annick VIEILLEFOND*
Service d'Anatomie & Cytologie Pathologiques
Hôpital COCHIN Cochin-St Vincent de
Paul-Laroche
27, rue du Faubourg Saint Jacques
75679 Paris Cedex 14 FRANCE
Tel. +33 1 58 41 14 65
Fax. +33 1 58 41 14 80
annick.vieillefond@cch.ap-hop-paris.fr

Dr Geo VON KROGH
Department of Medicine
Unit of Dermatology and Venereology B:3
Karolinska Hospital /Karolinska Sjukhuset
Hudkliniken B2:01
171 76 Stockholm   SWEDEN
Tel. +46 8 5177 5371
Fax. +46 8 714 9888 / +46 8 08 517 77851
Geo.von.Krogh@ood.ki.se

Dr Thomas WHEELER
Department of Pathology Room M227
The Methodist Hospital
6565 Fannin Street, MS 205
Houston, TX 77030
USA
Tel. +1 713 394 6475
Fax. +1 713 793 1603
twheeler@bcm.tmc.edu

Dr Paula J. WOODWARD
Department of Genitourinary Radiology
Armed Forces Institute of Pathology
6825 16th Street NW
Washington, DC 20306-6000
USA
Tel. +1 202 782 2161
Fax. +1 202 782 0768
woodwardp@afip.osd.mil

Dr Ximing J. YANG
Department of Pathology, Feinberg 7-334
Northwestern Memorial Hospital
Northwestern Univ., Feinberg School of Med.
251 E Huron Street
Chicago, IL 60611 USA
Tel. +1 312 926-0931
Fax. +1 312 926-3127
xyang@northwestern.edu

Dr Berton ZBAR
Laboratory of Immunology, National
Cancer Institute
Frederick Cancer Research & Dev. Center
Building 560, Room 12-68
Frederick, MD 21702 USA
Tel. +1 301 846 1557
Fax. +1 301 846 6145
zbarb@mail.ncifcrf.gov

Source of charts and photographs

1.

01.01	IARC (Dr P. Pisani)
01.02	Dr P. Pisani
01.03	IARC (Dr P. Pisani)
01.04-01.05	Dr M.J. Merino
01.06A,B	Dr G. Kovacs
01.07	Dr P. Kleihues
01.08	Dr F. Algaba
01.09	Dr W.M. Linehan/ Dr B. Zbar
01.10A,B	Dr M.J. Merino
01.11A-01.12A	Dr L.A. Aaltonen
01.12B	Dr M.J. Merino
01.13A-C	Dr D.M. Eccles
01.14A,B	Dr M.J. Merino
01.15	Dr A. Geurts van Kessel
01.16A-C	Dr S.M. Bonsib
01.17	Dr H. Moch
01.18A	Dr P. Argani
01.18B	Dr R.B. Shah, Dept. Pathology & Urology, University of Michigan Med. School, Ann Arbor MI, USA
01.19	Dr G. Kovacs
01.20	Dr J. Cheville
01.21-01.22	Dr H. Moch
01.23	Dr S.M. Bonsib
01.24A,B	Dr J.N. Eble
01.25A	Dr S.M. Bonsib
01.25B	Dr B. Delahunt
01.25C	Dr S.M. Bonsib
01.26A,B	Dr B. Delahunt
01.27A	Dr H. Moch
01.27B	Dr B. Delahunt
01.28	Dr H. Moch
01.29A	Dr B. Delahunt
01.29B	Dr J. Cheville
01.30	Dr A. Vieillefond
01.31A	Dr C.J. Davis
01.31B	Dr G. Kovacs
01.32A	Dr C.J. Davis
01.32B-01.33	Dr H. Moch
01.34A	Dr R.B. Shah (see 01.18B)
01.34B	Dr F. Algaba
01.35	Dr H. Moch
01.36	Dr E. van den Berg
01.37A,B	Dr S.M. Bonsib
01.38	Dr J. Cheville
01.39-01.41C	Dr J.R. Srigley
01.42-01.44C	Dr C.J. Davis
01.45-01.48	Dr P. Argani
01.49	Dr P. Argani/ Dr M. Ladanyi
01.50A-01.52C	Dr J.N. Eble
01.53	Dr H. Moch
01.54A,B	Dr J.N. Eble
01.55	Dr A. Vieillefond
01.56A	Dr R.B. Shah (see 01.18B)
01.56B,C	Dr C.J. Davis
01.57	Dr A. Vieillefond
01.58A	Dr R.B. Shah (see 01.18B)
01.58B-01.59A	Dr J.N. Eble
01.59B	Dr R.B. Shah (see 01.18B)
01.60A,B	Dr J.N. Eble
01.61-01.66B	Dr P. Argani
01.67	Dr J.L. Grosfeld
01.68A-01.72	Dr E.J. Perlman
01.73-01.74	Dr P. Argani
01.75A,B	Dr E.J. Perlman
01.76-01.77B	Dr J.N. Eble
01.78A-01.81	Dr P. Argani
01.82-01.84B	Dr B. Delahunt
01.85A	Dr P. Argani
01.85B	Dr B. Delahunt
01.86	Dr P. Argani
01.87A-01.88A	Dr B. Delahunt
01.88B	Dr S.M. Bonsib
01.89-01.90C	Dr P. Argani
01.91	Dr C.E. Keen
01.92	Dr A. Vieillefond
01.93	Dr F. Algaba
01.94	Dr G. Martignoni
01.95A	Dr F. Algaba
01.95B	Dr G. Martignoni
01.95C	Dr S.M. Bonsib
01.96A-01.101B	Dr G. Martignoni
01.102-01.104	Dr S.M. Bonsib
01.105A-01.106B	Dr J.R. Srigley
01.107	Dr P. Bruneval, Laboratoire d'Anatomie Pathologique, Hopital Européen G. Pompidou, Paris, France
01.108A	Dr S.M. Bonsib
01.108B	Dr B. Têtu
01.109	Dr H. Moch
01.110-01.111C	Dr J.N. Eble
01.112	Dr T. Hasegawa
01.113A	Dr S.M. Bonsib
01.113B	Dr B. Delahunt
01.114A	Dr S.M. Bonsib
01.114B	Dr R.B. Shah (see 01.18B)
01.115	Dr H. Moch
01.116A	Dr A. Vieillefond
01.116B	Dr H. Moch
01.117-01.118B	Dr J.N. Eble
01.119	Dr J.Y. Ro
01.120A-C	Dr P. Argani
01.121-01.122	Dr J.Y. Ro
01.123-01.125B	Dr L.R. Bégin
01.126A-C	Dr L. Guillou
01.127A	Dr A. Vieillefond
01.127B	Dr P. Argani
01.128	Dr H. Moch
01.129	Dr A. Vieillefond
01.130A-C	Dr A. Orazi
01.131-01.132	Dr S. Pileri, Istituto di Ematologia e Oncologia Medica, Policlinico S. Orsola, Universitá di Bologna, Bologna, Italy

2.

02.01-02.02	IARC (Dr J.E. Tyczynski)
02.03A-C	Dr T. Gasser
02.04A	Dr A. Vieillefond
02.04B,C	Dr G. Sauter
02.04D	Dr M.N. El-Bolkainy
02.05	Dr T. Gasser
02.06A,B	Dr A. Lopez-Beltran
02.07A-02.08B	Dr F. Algaba
02.09A	Dr M.N. El-Bolkainy
02.09B	Dr A. Lopez-Beltran
02.10A,B	Dr J.I. Epstein
02.11A	Dr F. Algaba
02.11B	Dr J.I. Epstein
02.12A	Dr A. Lopez-Beltran
02.12B	Dr F. Algaba
02.13A-C	Dr A.G. Ayala
02.14A,B	Dr A. Lopez-Beltran
02.15A	Dr F. Algaba
02.15B	Dr J.I. Epstein
02.16A	Dr F. Algaba
02.16B-02.17C	Dr A. Lopez-Beltran
02.17D	Dr F. Algaba
02.18A	Dr B. Helpap
02.18B-02.19A	Dr A. Lopez-Beltran
02.19B	Dr F. Algaba
02.19C	Dr A. Lopez-Beltran
02.20A	Dr M.B. Amin
02.20B	Dr J.I. Epstein
02.21A-D	Dr A. Lopez-Beltran
02.22	Dr R. Simon
02.23-02.27	Dr G. Sauter
02.28	Dr A. Lopez-Beltran
02.29A,B	Dr A. Hartmann/ Dr D. Zaak, Urologische Klinik und Poliklinik, Klinikum Großhadern der LMU München, München, Germany
02.29C	Dr T. Gasser
02.30	Dr A. Lopez-Beltran
02.31A	Dr I.A. Sesterhenn
02.31B	Dr A. Lopez-Beltran
02.32	Dr I.A. Sesterhenn
02.33	Dr C. Busch
02.34A	Dr G. Sauter
02.34B-02.35	Dr A. Lopez-Beltran
02.36	Dr C. Busch
02.37A	Dr I.A. Sesterhenn
02.37B	Dr C. Busch
02.38A	Dr I.A. Sesterhenn
02.38B	Dr C. Busch
02.39	Dr G. Sauter
02.40	Dr C. Busch
02.41A-C	Dr V.E. Reuter
02.42	Dr C. Busch
02.43	Dr M.B. Amin
02.44A,B	Dr I.A. Sesterhenn
02.45A	Dr F. Algaba
02.45B	Dr I.A. Sesterhenn
02.46A	Dr M.N. El-Bolkainy
02.46B	Dr M.C. Parkinson
02.47A,B	Dr M.N. El-Bolkainy
02.48	Dr A. Lopez-Beltran
02.49	Dr M.N. El-Bolkainy
02.50	Dr A. Lopez-Beltran
02.51	Dr F. Algaba
02.52-02.53	Dr A. Lopez-Beltran
02.54	Dr M.N. El-Bolkainy
02.55A-02.56A	Dr A.G. Ayala
02.56B-02.59B	Dr A. Lopez-Beltran
02.60	Dr F. Algaba
02.61A	Dr J.I. Epstein
02.61B	Dr I.A. Sesterhenn
02.62A-02.63B	Dr A.G. Ayala
02.64A-02.65	Dr A. Lopez-Beltran
02.66	Dr M.B. Amin
02.67-02.68B	Dr A. Lopez-Beltran
02.69A,B	Dr F. Algaba
02.70A,B	Dr Ph.U. Heitz
02.70C-02.71C	Dr C.J. Davis
02.72	Dr Ph.U. Heitz
02.73	Dr B. Delahunt
02.74-02.75	Dr J. Cheville
02.76	Dr M.C. Parkinson
02.77	Dr J.I. Epstein
02.78-02.79D	Dr A. Lopez-Beltran
02.80A,B	Dr B. Delahunt
02.81	Dr J.I. Epstein
02.82	Dr A. Lopez-Beltran
02.83-02.85B	Dr J.I. Epstein
02.86	Dr B. Helpap
02.87A-D	Dr J.I. Epstein
02.88	IARC (Dr J.E. Tyczynski)
02.89A,B	Dr T. Gasser
02.90-02.91	Dr M.C. Parkinson
02.92-02.95	Dr A. Hartmann
02.96	Dr R.J. Cohen, Urological Research Center, University of Western Australia, Nedland, Australia/ Dr B. Delahunt
02.97A-02.99	Dr A. Hartmann
02.100	Dr M.B. Amin

3.

03.01	Dr D.M. Parkin
03.02	WHO/NCHS
03.03	IARC (Dr D.M. Parkin)
03.04A	Dr J.I. Epstein
03.04B	Dr L. Egevad
03.05A-03.08	Dr J.I. Epstein
03.09	Dr L. Egevad
03.10A-C	Dr J.I. Epstein
03.11A,B	Dr L. Egevad
03.12A,B	Dr J.I. Epstein
03.13A,B	Dr P.A. Humphrey
03.14-03.16	Dr J.I. Epstein
03.17A	Dr L. Egevad
03.17B	Dr P.A. Humphrey
03.18-03.21B	Dr J.I. Epstein
03.22A	Dr P.A. Humphrey
03.22B-03.24A	Dr J.I. Epstein
03.24B	Dr L. Egevad
03.25A-C	Dr J.I. Epstein
03.26A	Dr L. Egevad
03.26B-03.28A	Dr J.I. Epstein
03.28B	Dr R.B. Shah (see 01.18B)
03.29	Dr J.I. Epstein
03.30A	Dr M.B. Amin/ Dr J.I. Epstein
03.30B-03.31A	Dr J.I. Epstein
03.31B	Dr M.B. Amin Dr J.I. Epstein
03.32A	Dr J.I. Epstein
03.32B	Dr P.A. Humphrey
03.33A	Dr I.A. Sesterhenn
03.33B	Dr J.I. Epstein
03.34A-C	Dr I.A. Sesterhenn
03.35A-03.37B	Dr J.I. Epstein
03.38A,B	Dr L. Egevad
03.39A	Dr J.I. Epstein
03.39B	Dr L. Egevad
03.40A	Dr J.I. Epstein
03.40B	Dr L. Egevad
03.41	Dr P.A. Humphrey
03.42	Dr J.I. Epstein
03.43A,B	Dr L. Egevad
03.44A-03.45A	Dr J.I. Epstein
03.45B	Dr L. Egevad
03.46A,B	Dr J.I. Epstein
03.47-03.48	Dr M.A. Rubin
03.49	Dr W.A. Sakr
03.50	Dr A.M. Chinnaiyan, Dept. of Pathology & Urology, University of Michigan Medical School, Ann Arbor MI, USA/ Dr M.A. Rubin
03.51-03.55	Dr M.A. Rubin
03.56	Dr W.A. Sakr
03.57A-03.59	Dr T. Wheeler

03.60-03.61A	Dr J.I. Epstein
03.61B	Dr W.A. Sakr
03.62A	Dr J.I. Epstein
03.62B	Dr F. Algaba
03.63A,B	Dr J.I. Epstein
03.64A,B	Dr P.A. Humphrey
03.65A,B	Dr J.I. Epstein
03.66A	Dr P.A. Humphrey
03.66B	Dr J.I. Epstein
03.67	Dr P.A. Humphrey
03.68A-03.72B	Dr J.I. Epstein
03.72C	Dr M.A. Rubin
03.73	Dr M.C. Parkinson
03.74A,B	Dr D.J. Grignon
03.75A-03.76A	Dr J.I. Epstein
03.76B-03.77A	Dr D.J. Grignon
03.77B	Dr I.A. Sesterhenn
03.77C	Dr P.A. Humphrey
03.78	Dr D.J. Grignon
03.79A-03.88A	Dr J.I. Epstein
03.88B	Dr B. Helpap
03.89	Dr M.C. Parkinson
03.90	Dr M. Hirsch, Dept. of Urologic Pathology, Brigham and Women's Hospital, Boston MA, USA
03.91-03.96B	Dr J.I. Epstein

4.

04.01	Dr H. Møller
04.02	IARC (Dr J. Ferlay)
04.03-04.09	Dr L.H.J. Looijenga
04.10A,B	Dr M.C. Parkinson
04.11A	Dr G.K. Jacobsen
04.11B,C	Dr I.A. Sesterhenn
04.12	Dr M.C. Parkinson
04.13A	Dr T.M. Ulbright
04.13B	Dr I.A. Sesterhenn
04.14A	Dr G.K. Jacobsen
04.14B	Dr M.C. Parkinson
04.15	Dr I.A. Sesterhenn
04.16A,B	Dr P.J. Woodward
04.17A,B	Dr M.C. Parkinson
04.18A-04.19A	Dr I.A. Sesterhenn
04.19B	Dr M.C. Parkinson
04.20A	Dr T.M. Ulbright
04.20B-04.22A	Dr I.A. Sesterhenn
04.22B,C	Dr T.M. Ulbright
04.22D	Dr G.K. Jacobsen
04.23	Dr I.A. Sesterhenn
04.24	Dr M.C. Parkinson
04.25	Dr I.A. Sesterhenn
04.26	Dr G.K. Jacobsen
04.27A,B	Dr I.A. Sesterhenn
04.28	Dr L. True
04.29A,B	Dr I.A. Sesterhenn

04.29C	Dr L. True
04.30	Dr P.J. Woodward
04.31-04.32A	Dr T.M. Ulbright
04.32B-04.33B	Dr G.K. Jacobsen
04.34A	Dr I.A. Sesterhenn
04.34B-04.35	Dr T.M. Ulbright
04.36	Dr G.K. Jacobsen
04.37A	Dr T.M. Ulbright
04.37B-04.38A	Dr I.A. Sesterhenn
04.38B	Dr G.K. Jacobsen
04.39A	Dr T.M. Ulbright
04.39B-04.41	Dr I.A. Sesterhenn
04.42A,B	Dr P.J. Woodward
04.43A,B	Dr I.A. Sesterhenn
04.43C	Dr T.M. Ulbright
04.43D	Dr G.K. Jacobsen
04.44A	Dr T.M. Ulbright
04.44B	Dr I.A. Sesterhenn
04.45	Dr J.C. Manivel
04.46A-04.47A	Dr P.J. Woodward
04.47B	Dr F. Algaba
04.48A	Dr M.C. Parkinson
04.48B-04.49D	Dr I.A. Sesterhenn
04.50	Dr G.K. Jacobsen
04.51A	Dr I.A. Sesterhenn
04.51B	Dr T.M. Ulbright
04.51C	Dr I.A. Sesterhenn
04.52A-04.53B	Dr H. Michael
04.54-04.55	Dr P.J. Woodward
04.56-04.57A	Dr M.C. Parkinson
04.57B	Dr G.K. Jacobsen
04.57C,D	Dr M.C. Parkinson
04.58A	Dr T.M. Ulbright
04.58B	Dr G.K. Jacobsen
04.59A,B	Dr T.M. Ulbright
04.60A	Dr G.K. Jacobsen
04.60B	Dr T.M. Ulbright
04.61	Dr M.C. Parkinson
04.62A,B	Dr I.A. Sesterhenn
04.63A,B	Dr T.M. Ulbright
04.64A,B	Dr I.A. Sesterhenn
04.64C	Dr T.M. Ulbright
04.65A	Dr R.B. Shah (see 01.18B)
04.65B	Dr T.M. Ulbright
04.66	Dr M.C. Parkinson
04.67A-C	Dr I.A. Sesterhenn
04.67D-04.68	Dr T.M. Ulbright
04.69A	Dr M.C. Parkinson
04.69B	Dr I.A. Sesterhenn
04.70	Dr P.J. Woodward
04.71	Dr M.A. Rubin
04.72A	Dr P.J. Woodward
04.72B	Dr T.M. Ulbright
04.73A	Dr I.A. Sesterhenn
04.73B-04.74A	Dr T.M. Ulbright
04.74B	Dr G.K. Jacobsen
04.75	Dr T.M. Ulbright
04.76-04.77B	Dr G.K. Jacobsen
04.78	Dr I.A. Sesterhenn

04.79	Dr T.M. Ulbright
04.80	Dr A. Vieillefond
04.81A,B	Dr I.A. Sesterhenn
04.82A-04.84A	Dr T.M. Ulbright
04.84B	Dr I.A. Sesterhenn
04.85A-04.86	Dr J.R. Srigley
04.87A,B	Dr P.J. Woodward
04.88A,B	Dr M.C. Parkinson
04.89-04.90	Dr I.A. Sesterhenn
04.91	Dr M.C. Parkinson
04.92A	Dr T.M. Ulbright
04.92B	Dr I.A. Sesterhenn
04.93A,B	Dr L. Nochomovitz
04.93C,D	Dr I.A. Sesterhenn
04.93E,F	Dr L. Nochomovitz
04.94A,B	Dr P.J. Woodward
04.95A,B	Dr B. Delahunt
04.96A-D	Dr C.J. Davis
04.97	Dr I.A. Sesterhenn
04.98-04.100B	Dr C.J. Davis
04.101-04.102	Dr I.A. Sesterhenn
04.103-04.104B	Dr C.J. Davis
04.105A,B	Dr J.R. Srigley
04.106-04.107	Dr I.A. Sesterhenn
04.108A	Dr T.M. Ulbright
04.108B	Dr I.A. Sesterhenn
04.109-04.110	Dr W.L. Gerald
04.111	Dr M. Miettinen
04.112	Dr P.J. Woodward
04.113	Dr M.C. Parkinson
04.114A,B	Dr M. Miettinen
04.115	Dr P.J. Woodward
04.116	Dr M. Miettinen
04.117	Dr M.C. Parkinson
04.118-04.119B	Dr M. Miettinen
04.120-04.121	Dr M.C. Parkinson
04.122A-04.123B	Dr C.J. Davis

5.

05.01	Dr A.L. Cubilla
05.02	IARC (Dr J. Ferlay)
05.03	Dr M.A. Rubin
05.04A,B	Dr A.L. Cubilla
05.05A	Dr S.M. Bonsib
05.05B-05.10B	Dr A.L. Cubilla
05.11A	Dr M.A. Rubin
05.11B-05.12A	Dr A.L. Cubilla
05.12B,C	Dr M.A. Rubin
05.13-05.19B	Dr A.L. Cubilla
05.20A-05.21	Dr G. von Krogh
05.22-05.24	Dr A.L. Cubilla
05.25-05.26B	Dr A.G. Ayala
05.27-05.34B	Dr J.F. Fetsch
05.35-05.36	Dr C.J. Davis

References

1. Anon. (1955). Case records of the Massachussets General Hospital (case no 41471). *N Engl J Med* 253: 926-931.

2. Anon. (1987). Revision of the CDC surveillance case definition for Acquired Immunodeficiency Syndrome. Council of state and territorial epidemiologists; AIDS program, Center for Infectious Diseases. *MMWR Morb Mortal Wkly Rep* 36 (Suppl 1): 1S-15S.

3. Anon. (1994). Aetiology of testicular cancer: association with congenital abnormalities, age at puberty, infertility, and exercise. United Kingdom Testicular Cancer Study Group. *BMJ* 308: 1393-1399.

4. Anon. (1994). Social, behavioural and medical factors in the aetiology of testicular cancer: results from the UK study. UK Testicular Cancer Study Group. *Br J Cancer* 70: 513-520.

5. Anon. (1997). International Germ Cell Consensus Classification: a prognostic factor-based staging system for metastatic germ cell cancers. International Germ Cell Cancer Collaborative Group. *J Clin Oncol* 15: 594-603.

6. Aaronson IA, Sinclair-Smith C (1980). Multiple cystic teratomas of the kidney. *Arch Pathol Lab Med* 104: 614.

7. Aass N, Klepp O, Cavallin-Stahl E, Dahl O, Wicklund H, Unsgaard B, Baldetorp L, Ahlstrom S, Fossa SD (1991). Prognostic factors in unselected patients with non-seminomatous metastatic testicular cancer: a multicenter experience. *J Clin Oncol* 9: 818-826.

8. Abbas F, Civantos F, Benedetto P, Soloway MS (1995). Small cell carcinoma of the bladder and prostate. *Urology* 46: 617-630.

9. Abdel-Tawab GA, el Zoghby SM, Abdel-Samie YM, Zaki A, Saad AA (1966). Studies on the aetiology of bilharzial carcinoma of the urinary bladder. VI. Beta-glucuronidases in urine. *Int J Cancer* 1: 383-389.

10. Abdel-Tawab GA, el Zoghby SM, Abdel-Samie YM, Zaki AM, Kholef IS, el Sewedi SM (1968). Urinary Beta-glucuronidase enzyme activity in some bilharzial urinary tract diseases. *Trans R Soc Trop Med Hyg* 62: 501-505.

11. Abdel-Tawab GA, Ibrahim EK, el Masri A, Al-Ghorab M, Makhyoun N (1968). Studies on tryptophan metabolism in bilharzial bladder cancer patients. *Invest Urol* 5: 591-601.

12. Abdel-Tawab GA, Kelada ES, Kelada NL, Abdel-Daim MH, Makhyoun N (1966). Studies on the aetiology of bilharzial carcinoma of the urinary bladder. V. Excretion of tryptophan metabolites in urine. *Int J Cancer* 1: 377-382.

13. Abdel Hamid AM, Rogers PB, Sibtain A, Plowman PN (1999). Bilateral renal cancer in children: a difficult, challenging and changing management problem. *Clin Oncol (R Coll Radiol)* 11: 200-204.

14. Abdel Mohsen MA, Hassan AA, el Sewedi SM, Aboul-Azm T, Magagnotti C, Fanelli R, Airoldi L (1999). Biomonitoring of n-nitroso compounds, nitrite and nitrate in the urine of Egyptian bladder cancer patients with or without Schistosoma haematobium infection. *Int J Cancer* 82: 789-794.

15. Abdul-Fadl MAM, Metwalli OM (1963). Studies on certain urinary blood serum enzymes in bilharziasis and their possible relation to bladder cancer in Egypt. *Br J Cancer* 15: 137-141.

16. Abdul M, Anezinis PE, Logothetis CJ, Hoosein NM (1994). Growth inhibition of human prostatic carcinoma cell lines by serotonin antagonists. *Anticancer Res* 14: 1215-1220.

17. Abdulkadir SA, Magee JA, Peters TJ, Kaleem Z, Naughton CK, Humphrey PA, Milbrandt J (2002). Conditional loss of Nkx3.1 in adult mice induces prostatic intraepithelial neoplasia. *Mol Cell Biol* 22: 1495-1503.

18. Abdulla M, Bui HX, del Rosario AD, Wolf BC, Ross JS (1994). Renal angiomyolipoma. DNA content and immunohistochemical study of classic and multicentric variants. *Arch Pathol Lab Med* 118: 735-739.

19. Abel PD, Henderson D, Bennett MK, Hall RR, Williams G (1988). Differing interpretations by pathologists of the pT category and grade of transitional cell cancer of the bladder. *Br J Urol* 62: 339-342.

20. Abell MR, Fayos JV, Lampe I (1965). Retroperitoneal germinomas (seminomas) without evidence of testicular involvement. *Cancer* 18: 273-290.

21. Aben KK, Cloos J, Koper NP, Braakhuis BJ, Witjes JA, Kiemeney LA (2000). Mutagen sensitivity in patients with familial and non-familial urothelial cell carcinoma. *Int J Cancer* 88: 493-496.

22. Aben KK, Macville MV, Smeets DF, Schoenberg MP, Witjes JA, Kiemeney LA (2001). Absence of karyotype abnormalities in patients with familial urothelial cell carcinoma. *Urology* 57: 266-269.

23. Aben KK, Witjes JA, Schoenberg MP, Hulsbergen-van de Kaa C, Verbeek AL, Kiemeney LA (2002). Familial aggregation of urothelial cell carcinoma. *Int J Cancer* 98: 274-278.

24. Abenoza P, Manivel C, Fraley EE (1987). Primary adenocarcinoma of urinary bladder. Clinicopathologic study of 16 cases. *Urology* 29: 9-14.

25. Abercrombie GF, Eardley I, Payne SR, Walmsley BH, Vinnicombe J (1988). Modified nephro-ureterectomy. Long-term follow-up with particular reference to subsequent bladder tumours. *Br J Urol* 61: 198-200.

26. Ablin RJ (1993). On the identification and characterization of prostate-specific antigen. *Hum Pathol* 24: 811-812.

27. Abraham NZJr, Maher TJ, Hutchison RE (1993). Extra-nodal monocytoid B-cell lymphoma of the urinary bladder. *Mod Pathol* 6: 145-149.

28. Abrahams JM, Pawel BR, Duhaime AC, Sutton LN, Schut L (1999). Extrarenal nephroblastic proliferation in spinal dysraphism. A report of 4 cases. *Pediatr Neurosurg* 31: 40-44.

29. Abrahamsson PA (1999). Neuroendocrine differentiation in prostatic carcinoma. *Prostate* 39: 135-148.

30. Abrahamsson PA, Cockett AT, di Sant'Agnese PA (1998). Prognostic significance of neuroendocrine differentiation in clinically localized prostatic carcinoma. *Prostate Suppl* 8: 37-42.

31. Abrahamsson PA, Wadstrom LB, Alumets J, Falkmer S, Grimelius L (1987). Peptide-hormone- and serotonin-immunoreactive tumour cells in carcinoma of the prostate. *Pathol Res Pract* 182: 298-307.

32. Accetta PA, Gardner WAJr (1983). Adenosquamous carcinoma of prostate. *Urology* 22: 73-75.

33. Adam BL, Qu Y, Davis JW, Ward MD, Clements MA, Cazares LH, Semmes OJ, Schellhammer PF, Yasui Y, Feng Z, Wright GLJr (2002). Serum protein fingerprinting coupled with a pattern-matching algorithm distinguishes prostate cancer from benign prostate hyperplasia and healthy men. *Cancer Res* 62: 3609-3614.

34. Adlakha K, Bostwick DG (1994). Lymphoepithelioma-like carcinoma of the prostate. *J Urol Pathol* 2: 319-325.

35. Adsay NV, Eble JN, Srigley JR, Jones EC, Grignon DJ (2000). Mixed epithelial and stromal tumor of the kidney. *Am J Surg Pathol* 24: 958-970.

36. Aggarwal M, Lakhar B, Shetty D, Ullal S (2000). Malignant peritoneal mesothelioma in an inguinal hernial sac: an unusual presentation. *Indian J Cancer* 37: 91-94.

37. Agoff SN, Lamps LW, Philip AT, Amin MB, Schmidt RA, True LD, Folpe AL (2000). Thyroid transcription factor-1 is expressed in extrapulmonary small cell carcinomas but not in other extrapulmonary neuroendocrine tumors. *Mod Pathol* 13: 238-242.

38. Aguirre P, Scully RE (1983). Primitive neuroectodermal tumor of the testis. Report of a case. *Arch Pathol Lab Med* 107: 643-645.

39. Ahlgren AD, Simrell CR, Triche TJ, Ozols R, Barsky SH (1984). Sarcoma arising in a residual testicular teratoma after cytoreductive chemotherapy. *Cancer* 54: 2015-2018.

40. Ahmed T, Bosl GJ, Hajdu SI (1985). Teratoma with malignant transformation in germ cell tumors in men. *Cancer* 56: 860-863.

41. Aihara M, Wheeler TM, Ohori M, Scardino PT (1994). Heterogeneity of prostate cancer in radical prostatectomy specimens. *Urology* 43: 60-66.

42. Akhtar M, Chantziantoniou N (1998). Flow cytometric and quantitative image cell analysis of DNA ploidy in renal chromophobe cell carcinoma. *Hum Pathol* 29: 1181-1188.

43. Akre O, Ekbom A, Hsieh CC, Trichopoulos D, Adami HO (1996). Testicular nonseminoma and seminoma in relation to perinatal characteristics. *J Natl Cancer Inst* 88: 883-889.

44. Al Adani MS (1985). Schistosomiasis, metaplasia and squamous cell carcinoma of the prostate: Histogenesis of squamous cancer cell determined by localization of specific markers. *Neoplasm* 32: 613-617.

45. Al Ali M, Samalia KP (2000). Genitourinary carcinoid tumors: initial report of ureteral carcinoid tumor. *J Urol* 163: 1864-1865.

46. Al Bozom IA, el Faqih SR, Hassan SH, el Tiraifi AE, Talic RF (2000). Granulosa cell tumor of the adult type: a case report and review of the literature of a very rare testicular tumor. *Arch Pathol Lab Med* 124: 1525-1528.

47. Al Maghrabi J, Kamel-Reid S, Jewett M, Gospodarowicz M, Wells W, Banerjee D (2001). Primary low-grade B-cell lymphoma of mucosa-associated lymphoid tissue type arising in the urinary bladder: report of 4 cases with molecular genetic analysis. *Arch Pathol Lab Med* 125: 332-336.

48. Al Maghrabi J, Vorobyova L, Chapman W, Jewett M, Zielenska M, Squire JA (2001). p53 Alteration and chromosomal instability in prostatic high-grade intraepithelial neoplasia and concurrent carcinoma: analysis by immunohistochemistry, interphase in situ hybridization, and sequencing of laser-captured microdissected specimens. *Mod Pathol* 14: 1252-1262.

49. Al Rikabi AC, Diab AR, Buckai A, Abdullah AI, Grech AB (1999). Primary synovial sarcoma of the penis—case report and literature review. *Scand J Urol Nephrol* 33: 413-415.

50. Al Saleem T, Wessner LL, Scheithauer BW, Patterson K, Roach ES, Dreyer SJ, Fujikawa K, Bjornsson J, Bernstein J, Henske EP (1998). Malignant tumors of the kidney, brain, and soft tissues in children and young adults with the tuberous sclerosis complex. *Cancer* 83: 2208-2216.

51. Alam NA, Bevan S, Churchman M, Barclay E, Barker K, Jaeger EE, Nelson HM, Healy E, Pembroke AC, Friedmann PS, Dalziel K, Calonje E, Anderson J, August PJ, Davies MG, Felix R, Munro CS, Murdoch M, Rendall J, Kennedy S, Leigh IM, Kelsell DP, Tomlinson IP, Houlston RS (2001). Localization of a gene (MCUL1) for multiple cutaneous leiomyomata and uterine fibroids to chromosome 1q42.3-q43. *Am J Hum Genet* 68: 1264-1269.

52. Alam NA, Rowan AJ, Wortham NC, Pollard PJ, Mitchell M, Tyrer JP, Barclay E, Calonje E, Manek S, Adams SJ, Bowers PW, Burrows NP, Charles-Holmes R, Cook LJ, Daly BM, Ford GP, Fuller LC, Hadfield-Jones SE, Hardwick N, Highet AS, Keefe M, MacDonald-Hull SP, Potts ED, Crone M, Wilkinson S, Camacho-Martinez F, Jablonska S, Ratnavel R, MacDonald A, Mann RJ, Grice K, Guillet G, Lewis-Jones MS, McGrath H, Seukeran DC, Morrison PJ, Fleming S, Rahman S, Kelsell D, Leigh I, Olpin S, Tomlinson IP (2003). Genetic and functional analyses of FH mutations in multiple cutaneous and uterine leiomyomatosis, hereditary leiomyomatosis and renal cancer, and fumarate hydratase deficiency. *Hum Mol Genet* 12: 1241-1252.
53. Albanell J, Bosl GJ, Reuter VE, Engelhardt M, Franco S, Moore MA, Dmitrovsky E (1999). Telomerase activity in germ cell cancers and mature teratomas. *J Natl Cancer Inst* 91: 1321-1326.
54. Albertsen PC, Fryback DG, Storer BE, Kolon TF, Fine J (1995). Long-term survival among men with conservatively treated localized prostate cancer. *JAMA* 274: 626-631.
55. Albores-Saavedra J, Huffman H, Alvarado-Cabrero I, Ayala AG (1996). Anaplastic variant of spermatocytic seminoma. *Hum Pathol* 27: 650-655.
56. Alexander AA (1995). To color Doppler image the prostate or not: that is the question. *Radiology* 195: 11-13.
57. Alexander EE, Qian J, Wollan PC, Myers RP, Bostwick DG (1996). Prostatic intraepithelial neoplasia does not appear to raise serum prostate-specific antigen concentration. *Urology* 47: 693-698.
58. Algaba F (1999). Evolution of isolated high-grade prostate intraepithelial neoplasia in a Mediterranean patient population. *Eur Urol* 35: 496-497.
59. Algaba F, Sole-Balcells FJ (1992). [Carcinosarcoma of the prostate. Immunophenotype, morphologic course and clinico-pathologic differential diagnosis]. *Arch Esp Urol* 45: 779-782.
60. Ali SZ, Reuter VE, Zakowski MF (1997). Small cell neuroendocrine carcinoma of the urinary bladder. A clinicopathologic study with emphasis on cytologic features. *Cancer* 79: 356-361.
61. Alikasifoglu A, Gonc EN, Akcoren Z, Kale G, Ciftci AO, Senocak ME, Yordam N (2002). Feminizing Sertoli cell tumor associated with Peutz-Jeghers syndrome. *J Pediatr Endocrinol Metab* 15: 449-452.
62. Allen EA, Brinker DA, Coppola D, Diaz JI, Epstein JI (2003). Multilocular prostatic cystadenoma with high-grade prostatic intraepithelial neoplasia. *Urology* 61: 644.
63. Allen FJ, Steenkamp JW (1992). Intravenous urography in patients with transitional cell carcinoma of the bladder. The incidence and implications of ureteral obstruction. *S Afr J Surg* 30: 28-32.
64. Allen PR, King AR, Sage MD, Sorrell VF (1990). A benign gonadal stromal tumor of the testis of spindle fibroblastic type. *Pathology* 22: 227-229.
65. Allen W, Parrott TS, Saripkin L, Allan C (1986). Chylous ascites following retroperitoneal lymphadenectomy for granulosa cell tumor of the testis. *J Urol* 135: 797-798.
66. Allsbrook WC, Pfeiffer EA (1998). Histochemistry of the prostate. In: *Pathology of the Prostate*, CS Foster, DG Bostwick, eds. W.B. Saunders Company: Philadelphia, pp. 282-303.
67. Allsbrook WCJr, Mangold KA, Johnson MH, Lane RB, Lane CG, Epstein JI (2001). Interobserver reproducibility of Gleason grading of prostatic carcinoma: general pathologist. *Hum Pathol* 32: 81-88.
68. Alroy J, Miller AW3rd, Coon JS, James KK, Gould VE (1980). Inverted papilloma of the urinary bladder: ultrastructural and immunologic studies. *Cancer* 46: 64-70.
69. Alsheikh A, Mohamedali Z, Jones E, Masterson J, Gilks CB (2001). Comparison of the WHO/ISUP classification and cytokeratin 20 expression in predicting the behavior of low-grade papillary urothelial tumors. *Mod Pathol* 14: 267-272.
70. Alsikafi NF, Brendler CB, Gerber GS, Yang XJ (2001). High-grade prostatic intraepithelial neoplasia with adjacent atypia is associated with a higher incidence of cancer on subsequent needle biopsy than high-grade prostatic intraepithelial neoplasia alone. *Urology* 57: 296-300.
71. Althausen AF, Prout GRJr, Daly JJ (1976). Non-invasive papillary carcinoma of the bladder associated with carcinoma in situ. *J Urol* 116: 575-580.
72. Alvarado-Cabrero I, Candanedo-Gonzalez F, Sosa-Romero A (2001). Leiomyoma of the urethra in a Mexican woman: a rare neoplasm associated with the expression of estrogen receptors by immunohistochemistry. *Arch Med Res* 32: 88-90.
73. Alvarado-Cabrero I, Folpe AL, Srigley JR, Gaudin P, Philip AT, Reuter VE, Amin MB (2000). Intrarenal schwannoma: a report of four cases including three cellular variants. *Mod Pathol* 13: 851-856.
74. Aly MS, Khaled HM (2002). Chromosomal aberrations in early-stage bilharzial bladder cancer. *Cancer Genet Cytogenet* 132: 41-45.
75. Amato RJ, Logothetis CJ, Hallinan R, Ro JY, Sella A, Dexeus FH (1992). Chemotherapy for small cell carcinoma of prostatic origin. *J Urol* 147: 935-937.
76. Amin MB, Corless CL, Renshaw AA, Tickoo SK, Kubus J, Schultz DS (1997). Papillary (chromophil) renal cell carcinoma: histomorphologic characteristics and evaluation of conventional pathologic prognostic parameters in 62 cases. *Am J Surg Pathol* 21: 621-635.
77. Amin MB, Crotty TB, Tickoo SK, Farrow GM (1997). Renal oncocytoma: a reappraisal of morphologic features with clinicopathologic findings in 80 cases. *Am J Surg Pathol* 21: 1-12.
78. Amin MB, Gomez JA, Young RH (1997). Urothelial transitional cell carcinoma with endophytic growth patterns: a discussion of patterns of invasion and problems associated with assessment of invasion in 18 cases. *Am J Surg Pathol* 21: 1057-1068.
79. Amin MB, McKenney JK (2002). An approach to the diagnosis of flat intraepithelial lesions of the urinary bladder using the World Health Organization/ International Society of Urological Pathology consensus classification system. *Adv Anat Pathol* 9: 222-232.
80. Amin MB, Murphy WM, Reuter VE, Ro JY, Ayala AG, Weiss MA, Eble JN, Young RH (1996). A symposium on controversies in the pathology of transitional cell carcinomas of the urinary bladder. Part I. *Anat Pathol* 1: 1-39.
81. Amin MB, Ro JY, el Sharkawy T, Lee KM, Troncoso P, Silva EG, Ordonez NG, Ayala AG (1994). Micropapillary variant of transitional cell carcinoma of the urinary bladder. Histologic pattern resembling ovarian papillary serous carcinoma. *Am J Surg Pathol* 18: 1224-1232.
82. Amin MB, Ro JY, Lee KM, Ordonez NG, Dinney CP, Gulley ML, Ayala AG (1994). Lymphoepithelioma-like carcinoma of the urinary bladder. *Am J Surg Pathol* 18: 466-473.
83. Amin MB, Tamboli P, Varma M, Srigley JR (1999). Postatrophic hyperplasia of the prostate gland: a detailed analysis of its morphology in needle biopsy specimens. *Am J Surg Pathol* 23: 925-931.
84. Amin MB, Young RH (1997). Intraepithelial lesions of the urinary bladder with a discussion of the histogenesis of urothelial neoplasia. *Semin Diagn Pathol* 14: 84-97.
85. Amin MB, Young RH (1997). Primary carcinomas of the urethra. *Semin Diagn Pathol* 14: 147-160.
86. Amin R (1995). Case report: primary non-Hodgkin's lymphoma of the bladder. *Br J Radiol* 68: 1257-1260.
87. Amirkhan RH, Molberg KH, Wiley EL, Nurenberg P, Sagalowsky AI (1994). Primary leiomyosarcoma of the seminal vesicle. *Urology* 44: 132-135.
88. Andersen R, Hoeg K (1961). Myoblastoma of the bladder neck: report of a case. *Br J Urol* 33: 76-79.
89. Anderson C, Knibbs DR, Ludwig ME, Ely MG3rd (1992). Lymphangioma of the kidney: a pathologic entity distinct from solitary multilocular cyst. *Hum Pathol* 23: 465-468.
90. Anderson CK (1973). Proceedings: Pyogenic granuloma of the urinary bladder. *J Clin Pathol* 26: 984.
91. Anderson JD, Scardino P, Smith RB (1977). Inflammatory fibrous histiocytoma presenting as a renal pelvic and bladder mass. *J Urol* 118: 470-471.
92. Anderson JR, Strickland D, Corbin D, Byrnes JA, Zweiback E (1995). Age-specific reference ranges for serum prostate-specific antigen. *Urology* 46: 54-57.
93. Anderson NE, Rosenblum MK, Graus F, Wiley RG, Posner JB (1988). Autoantibodies in paraneoplastic syndromes associated with small-cell lung cancer. *Neurology* 38: 1391-1398.
94. Anderstrom C, Johansson SL, Pettersson S, Wahlqvist L (1989). Carcinoma of the ureter: a clinicopathologic study of 49 cases. *J Urol* 142: 280-283.
95. Anderstrom C, Johansson SL, von Schultz L (1983). Primary adenocarcinoma of the urinary bladder. A clinicopathologic and prognostic study. *Cancer* 52: 1273-1280.
96. Andresen R, Wegner HE (1997). Intravenous urography revisited in the age of ultrasound and computerized tomography: diagnostic yield in cases of renal colic, suspected pelvic and abdominal malignancies, suspected renal mass, and acute pyelonephritis. *Urol Int* 58: 221-226.
97. Andrews PW, Banting G, Damjanov I, Arnaud D, Avner P (1984). Three monoclonal antibodies defining distinct differentiation antigens associated with different high molecular weight polypeptides on the surface of human embryonal carcinoma cells. *Hybridoma* 3: 347-361.
98. Anghel G, Petti N, Remotti D, Ruscio C, Blandino F, Majolino I (2002). Testicular plasmacytoma: Report of a case and review of the literature. *Am J Hematol* 71: 98-104.
99. Angulo J, Escribano J, Tamayo JC, Dehaini A, Guily M, Sanchez-Chapado M (1997). [Upper urinary tract and urethral tumors in patients with bladder carcinoma]. *Arch Esp Urol* 50: 115-120.
100. Angulo JC, Lopez JI, Sánchez-Chapado M, Sakr W, Montie JE, Pontes EJ, Redman B, Flaherty L, Grignon DJ (1996). Small cell carcinoma of the urinary bladder. A report of two cases with complete remission and a comprehensive literature review with emphasis on therapeutic decisions. *J Urol Pathol* 5: 1-19.
101. Antman K, Chang Y (2000). Kaposi's sarcoma. *N Engl J Med* 342: 1027-1038.
102. Antonescu CR, Gerald WL, Magid MS, Ladanyi M (1998). Molecular variants of the EWS-WT1 gene fusion in desmoplastic small round cell tumor. *Diagn Mol Pathol* 7: 24-28.
103. Antonini C, Zucconelli R, Forgiarini O, Chiara A, Briani G, Belmonte P, Fiaccavento G, Sacchi G (1997). Carcinosarcoma of penis. Case report and review of the literature. *Adv Clin Path* 1: 281-285.
104. Anwar WA (1994). Praziquantel (antischistosomal drug): is it clastogenic, co-clastogenic or anticlastogenic? *Mutat Res* 305: 165-173.
105. Applewhite JC, Matlaga BR, McCullough DL (2002). Results of the 5 region prostate biopsy method: the repeat biopsy population. *J Urol* 168: 500-503.
106. Arda K, Ozdemir G, Gunes Z, Ozdemir H (1997). Primary malignant lymphoma of the bladder. A case report and review of the literature. *Int Urol Nephrol* 29: 319-322.
107. Arena F, di Stefano C, Peracchia G, Barbieri A, Cortellini P (2001). Primary lymphoma of the penis: diagnosis and treatment. *Eur Urol* 39: 232-235.
108. Argani P, Antonescu CR, Couturier J, Fournet JC, Sciot R, Debiec-Rychter M, Hutchinson B, Reuter VE, Boccon-Gibod L, Timmons CF, Hafez N, Ladanyi M (2002). PRCC-TFE3 renal carcinomas: morphologic, immunohistochemical, ultrastructural, and molecular analysis of an entity associated with the t(X;1) (p11.2;q21). *Am J Surg Pathol* 26: 1553-1566.
109. Argani P, Antonescu CR, Illei PB, Lui MY, Timmons CF, Newbury R, Reuter VE, Garvin AJ, Perez-Atayde AR, Fletcher JA, Beckwith JB, Bridge JA, Ladanyi M (2001). Primary renal neoplasms with the ASPL-TFE3 gene fusion of alveolar soft part sarcoma: a distinctive tumor entity previously included among renal cell carcinomas of children and adolescents. *Am J Pathol* 159: 179-192.
110. Argani P, Beckwith JB (2000). Metanephric stromal tumor: report of 31 cases of a distinctive pediatric renal neoplasm. *Am J Surg Pathol* 24: 917-926.
111. Argani P, Epstein JI (2001). Inverted (Hobnail) high-grade prostatic intraepithelial neoplasia (PIN): report of 15 cases of a previously undescribed pattern of high-grade PIN. *Am J Surg Pathol* 25: 1534-1539.
112. Argani P, Faria PA, Epstein JI, Reuter VE, Perlman EJ, Beckwith JB, Ladanyi M (2000). Primary renal synovial sarcoma: molecular and morphologic delineation of an entity previously included among embryonal sarcomas of the kidney. *Am J Surg Pathol* 24: 1087-1096.
113. Argani P, Lal P, Hutchinson B, Lui MY, Reuter VE, Ladanyi M (2003). Aberrant nuclear immunoreactivity for TFE3 in neoplasms with TFE3 gene fusions: a sensitive and specific immunohistochemical assay. *Am J Surg Pathol* 27: 750-761.
114. Argani P, Perlman EJ, Breslow NE, Browning NG, Green DM, D'Angio GJ, Beckwith JB (2000). Clear cell sarcoma of the kidney: a review of 351 cases from the National Wilms Tumor Study Group Pathology Center. *Am J Surg Pathol* 24: 4-18.

115. Ariel I, Sughayer M, Fellig Y, Pizov G, Ayesh S, Podeh D, Libdeh BA, Levy C, Birman T, Tykocinski ML, de Groot N, Hochberg A (2000). The imprinted H19 gene is a marker of early recurrence in human bladder carcinoma. *Mol Pathol* 53: 320-323.

116. Arkovitz MS, Ginsburg HB, Eidelman J, Greco MA, Rauson A (1996). Primary extrarenal Wilms' tumor in the inguinal canal: case report and review of the literature. *J Pediatr Surg* 31: 957-959.

117. Armas OA, Aprikian AG, Melamed J, Cordon-Cardo C, Cohen DW, Erlandson R, Fair WR, Reuter VE (1994). Clinical and pathobiological effects of neoadjuvant total androgen ablation therapy on clinically localized prostatic adenocarcinoma. *Am J Surg Pathol* 18: 979-991.

118. Armstrong GR, Buckley CH, Kelsey AM (1991). Germ cell expression of placental alkaline phosphatase in male pseudohermaphroditism. *Histopathology* 18: 541-547.

119. Arrizabalaga M, Navarro J, Mora M, Castro M, Extramiana J, Manas A, Diez J, Paniagua P (1994). [Transitional carcinomas of the urinary tract: synchronous and metachronous lesions]. *Actas Urol Esp* 18: 782-796.

120. Arroyo MR, Green DM, Perlman EJ, Beckwith JB, Argani P (2001). The spectrum of metanephric adenofibroma and related lesions: clinicopathologic study of 25 cases from the National Wilms Tumor Study Group Pathology Center. *Am J Surg Pathol* 25: 433-444.

121. Artandi SE, Chang S, Lee SL, Alson S, Gottlieb GJ, Chin L, Depinho RA (2000). Telomere dysfunction promotes non-reciprocal translocations and epithelial cancers in mice. *Nature* 406: 641-645.

122. Arya M, Hayne D, Brown RS, O'Donnell PJ, Mundy AR (2001). Hemangiopericytoma of the seminal vesicle presenting with hypoglycemia. *J Urol* 166: 992.

123. Asakura H, Nakazono M, Masuda T, Yamamoto T, Tazaki H (1989). [Priapism with malignant lymphoma: a case report]. *Hinyokika Kiyo* 35: 1811-1814.

124. Ascoli V, Facciolo F, Rahimi S, Scalzo CC, Nardi F (1996). Concomitant malignant mesothelioma of the pleura, peritoneum, and tunica vaginalis testis. *Diagn Cytopathol* 14: 243-248.

125. Ashfaq R, Weinberg AG, Albores-Saavedra J (1993). Renal angiomyolipomas and HMB-45 reactivity. *Cancer* 71: 3091-3097.

126. Assaf G, Mosbah A, Homsy Y, Michaud J (1983). Dermoid cyst of testis in five-year-old-child. *Urology* 22: 432-434.

127. Atalay AC, Karaman MI, Basak T, Utkan G, Ergenekon E (1998). Non-Hodgkin's lymphoma of the female urethra presenting as a caruncle. *Int Urol Nephrol* 30: 609-610.

128. Atiyeh BA, Barakat AJ, Abumrad NN (1997). Extra-adrenal pheochromocytoma. *J Nephrol* 10: 25-29.

129. Atkin NB, Baker MC (1982). Specific chromosome change, i(12p), in testicular tumours? *Lancet* 2: 1349.

130. Atkin NB, Baker MC (1983). i(12p): specific chromosomal marker in seminoma and malignant teratoma of the testis? *Cancer Genet Cytogenet* 10: 199-204.

131. Atkin NB, Baker MC (1985). Cytogenetic study of ten carcinomas of the bladder: involvement of chromosomes 1 and 11. *Cancer Genet Cytogenet* 15: 253-268.

132. Atkin NB, Baker MC (1991). Numerical chromosome changes in 165 malignant tumors. Evidence for a nonrandom distribution of normal chromosomes. *Cancer Genet Cytogenet* 52: 113-121.

133. Atkin NB, Baker MC, Wilson GD (1995). Chromosome abnormalities and p53 expression in a small cell carcinoma of the bladder. *Cancer Genet Cytogenet* 79: 111-114.

134. Atkin NB, Fox MF (1990). 5q deletion. The sole chromosome change in a carcinoma of the bladder. *Cancer Genet Cytogenet* 46: 129-131.

135. Attanoos RL, Gibbs AR (2000). Primary malignant gonadal mesotheliomas and asbestos. *Histopathology* 37: 150-159.

136. Atuk NO, Stolle C, Owen JA, Carpenter JT, Vance ML (1998). Pheochromocytoma in von Hippel-Lindau disease: clinical presentation and mutation analysis in a large, multigenerational kindred. *J Clin Endocrinol Metab* 83: 117-120.

137. Au WY, Shek WH, Nicholls J, Tse KM, Todd D, Kwong YL (1997). T-cell intravascular lymphomatosis (angiotropic large cell lymphoma): association with Epstein-Barr viral infection. *Histopathology* 31: 563-567.

138. Aubert J, Casamayou J, Denis P, Hoppler A, Payen J (1978). Intrarenal teratoma in a newborn child. *Eur Urol* 4: 306-308.

139. Aus G, Bergdahl S, Frosing R, Lodding P, Pileblad E, Hugosson J (1996). Reference range of prostate-specific antigen after transurethral resection of the prostate. *Urology* 47: 529-531.

140. Avery AK, Beckstead J, Renshaw AA, Corless CL (2000). Use of antibodies to RCC and CD10 in the differential diagnosis of renal neoplasms. *Am J Surg Pathol* 24: 203-210.

141. Aveyard JS, Skilleter A, Habuchi T, Knowles MA (1999). Somatic mutation of PTEN in bladder carcinoma. *Br J Cancer* 80: 904-908.

142. Axelrod HR, Gilman SC, D'Aleo CJ, Petrylak D, Reuter V, Gulfo JV, Saad A, Cordon-Cardo C, Scher HI (1992). Preclinical results and human immunohistochemical studies with 90y-CYT-366: a new prostate cancer therapeutic agent. *J Urol* 147: 361A.

143. Ayala AG, Ro JY, Babaian R, Troncoso P, Grignon DJ (1989). The prostatic capsule: does it exist? Its importance in the staging and treatment of prostatic carcinoma. *Am J Surg Pathol* 13: 21-27.

144. Azzopardi JD, Mostofi FK, Theiss EA (1961). Lesions of testes observed in certain patients with widespread choriocarcinoma and related tumors; the significance and genesis of henatoxylin-staining bodies in human testes. *Am J Pathol* 38: 207-225.

145. Azzopardi JG, Hoffbrand AV (1965). Retrogression in testicular seminoma with viable metastases. *J Clin Pathol* 18: 135-141.

146. Babaian RJ, Johnson DE (1980). Primary carcinoma of the ureter. *J Urol* 123: 357-359.

147. Babaian RJ, Sayer J, Podoloff DA, Steelhammer LC, Bhadkamkar VA, Gulfo JV (1994). Radioimmunoscintigraphy of pelvic lymph nodes with 111indium-labeled monoclonal antibody CYT-356. *J Urol* 152: 1952-1955.

148. Babu VR, Lutz MD, Miles BJ, Farah RN, Weiss L, van Dyke DL (1987). Tumor behavior in transitional cell carcinoma of the bladder in relation to chromosomal markers and histopathology. *Cancer Res* 47: 6800-6805.

149. Badawi AF, Cooper DP, Mostafa MH, Aboul-Azm T, Barnard R, Margison GP, O'Connor PJ (1994). O6-alkylguanine-DNA alkyltransferase activity in schistosomiasis-associated human bladder cancer. *Eur J Cancer* 30A: 1314-1319.

150. Badawi AF, Mostafa MH, Aboul-Azm T, Haboubi NY, O'Connor PJ, Cooper DP (1992). Promutagenic methylation damage in bladder DNA from patients with bladder cancer associated with schistosomiasis and from normal individuals. *Carcinogenesis* 13: 877-881.

151. Badcock G, Pigott C, Goepel J, Andrews PW (1999). The human embryonal carcinoma marker antigen TRA-1-60 is a sialylated keratan sulfate proteoglycan. *Cancer Res* 59: 4715-4719.

152. Badoual C, Tissier F, Lagorce-Pages C, Delcourt A, Vieillefond A (2002). Pulmonary metastases from a chromophobe renal cell carcinoma: 10 years' evolution. *Histopathology* 40: 300-302.

153. Baer SC, Ro JY, Ordonez NG, Maiese RL, Loose JH, Grignon DJ, Ayala AG (1993). Sarcomatoid collecting duct carcinoma: a clinicopathologic and immunohistochemical study of five cases. *Hum Pathol* 24: 1017-1022.

154. Bagg MD, Wettlaufer JN, Willadsen DS, Ho V, Lane D, Thrasher JB (1994). Granulocytic sarcoma presenting as a diffuse renal mass before hematological manifestations of acute myelogenous leukemia. *J Urol* 152: 2092-2093.

155. Bahn DK, Brown RK, Shei KY, White DB (1990). Sonographic findings of leiomyoma in the seminal vesicle. *J Clin Ultrasound* 18: 517-519.

156. Bahnson RR, Dresner SM, Gooding W, Becich MJ (1989). Incidence and prognostic significance of lymphatic and vascular invasion in radical prostatectomy specimens. *Prostate* 15: 149-155.

157. Bailey D, Baumal R, Law J, Sheldon K, Kannampuzha P, Stratis M, Kahn H, Marks A (1986). Production of a monoclonal antibody specific for seminomas and dysgerminomas. *Proc Natl Acad Sci USA* 83: 5291-5295.

158. Bain GO, Danyluk JM, Shnitka TK, Jewell LD, Manickavel V (1985). Malignant fibrous histiocytoma of prostate gland. *Urology* 26: 89-91.

159. Bainbridge TC, Singh RR, Mentzel T, Katenkamp D (1997). Solitary fibrous tumor of urinary bladder: report of two cases. *Hum Pathol* 28: 1204-1206.

160. Baisden BL, Kahane H, Epstein JI (1999). Perineural invasion, mucinous fibroplasia, and glomerulations: diagnostic features of limited cancer on prostate needle biopsy. *Am J Surg Pathol* 23: 918-924.

161. Baker JM, Murty VV, Potla L, Mendola CE, Rodriguez E, Reuter VE, Bosl GG, Chaganti RS (1994). Loss of heterozygosity and decreased expression of NME genes correlate with teratomatous differentiation in human male germ cell tumors. *Biochem Biophys Res Commun* 202: 1096-1103.

162. Bala S, Oliver H, Renault B, Montgomery K, Dutta S, Rao P, Houldsworth J, Kucherlapati R, Wang X, Chaganti RS, Murty VV (2000). Genetic analysis of the APAF1 gene in male germ cell tumors. *Genes Chromosomes Cancer* 28: 258-268.

163. Balaji KC, McGuire M, Grotas J, Grimaldi G, Russo P (1999). Upper tract recurrences following radical cystectomy: an analysis of prognostic factors, recurrence pattern and stage at presentation. *J Urol* 162: 1603-1606.

164. Ballotta MR, Borghi L, Barucchello G (2000). Adenocarcinoma of the rete testis. Report of two cases. *Adv Clin Path* 4: 169-173.

165. Balsitis M, Sokol M (1990). Ossifying malignant Leydig (interstitial) cell tumour of the testis. *Histopathology* 16: 597-601.

166. Banks ER, Mills SE (1990). Histiocytoid (epithelioid) hemangioma of the testis. The so-called vascular variant of "adenomatoid tumor". *Am J Surg Pathol* 14: 584-589.

167. Bar W, Hedinger C (1976). Comparison of histologic types of primary testicular germ cell tumors with their metastases: consequences for the WHO and the British Nomenclatures? *Virchows Arch A Pathol Anat Histol* 370: 41-54.

168. Barentsz JO, Jager GJ, Witjes JA, Ruijs JH (1996). Primary staging of urinary bladder carcinoma: the role of MRI and a comparison with CT. *Eur Radiol* 6: 129-133.

169. Barker KT, Bevan S, Wang R, Lu YJ, Flanagan AM, Bridge JA, Fisher C, Finlayson CJ, Shipley J, Houlston RS (2002). Low frequency of somatic mutations in the FH/multiple cutaneous leiomyomatosis gene in sporadic leiomyosarcomas and uterine leiomyomas. *Br J Cancer* 87: 446-448.

170. Barocas DA, Han M, Epstein JI, Chan DY, Trock BJ, Walsh PC, Partin AW (2001). Does capsular incision at radical retropubic prostatectomy affect disease-free survival in otherwise organ-confined prostate cancer? *Urology* 58: 746-751.

171. Barreto J, Caballero C, Cubilla AL (1997). Penis. In: *Histology for Pathologists*, SS Sternberg, ed. Lippincott Raven Press: New York.

172. Barsky SH (1987). Germ cell tumors of the testis. In: *Surgical Pathology of Urologic Diseases*, N Javadpour, SH Barsky, eds. Williams and Wilkins: Baltimore, pp. 224-246.

173. Bartel F, Taubert H, Harris LC (2002). Alternative and aberrant splicing of MDM2 mRNA in human cancer. *Cancer Cell* 2: 9-15.

174. Bartkova J, Rajpert-de Meyts E, Skakkebaek NE, Bartek J (1999). D-type cyclins in adult human testis and testicular cancer: relation to cell type, proliferation, differentiation, and malignancy. *J Pathol* 187: 573-581.

175. Bartkova J, Thullberg M, Rajpert-de Meyts E, Skakkebaek NE, Bartek J (2000). Cell cycle regulators in testicular cancer: loss of p18INK4C marks progression from carcinoma in situ to invasive germ cell tumours. *Int J Cancer* 85: 370-375.

176. Bartkova J, Thullberg M, Rajpert-de Meyts E, Skakkebaek NE, Bartek J (2000). Lack of p19INK4d in human testicular germ-cell tumours contrasts with high expression during normal spermatogenesis. *Oncogene* 19: 4146-4150.

177. Baschinsky DY, Niemann TH, Maximo CB, Bahnson RR (1998). Seminal vesicle cystadenoma: a case report and literature review. *Urology* 51: 840-845.

178. Baserga R (2000). The contradictions of the insulin-like growth factor 1 receptor. *Oncogene* 19: 5574-5581.

179. Bassler TJJr, Orozco R, Bassler IC, Boyle LM, Bormes T (1999). Adenosquamous carcinoma of the prostate: case report with DNA analysis, immunohistochemistry, and literature review. *Urology* 53: 832-834.

180. Bastacky SI, Walsh PC, Epstein JI (1993). Relationship between perineural tumor invasion on needle biopsy and radical prostatectomy capsular penetration in clinical stage B adenocarcinoma of the prostate. *Am J Surg Pathol* 17: 336-341.

181. Bastacky SI, Wojno KJ, Walsh PC, Carmichael MJ, Epstein JI (1995). Pathological features of hereditary prostate cancer. *J Urol* 153: 987-992.
182. Bastus R, Caballero JM, Gonzalez G, Borrat P, Casalots J, Gomez de Segura G, Marti LI, Ristol J, Cirera L (1999). Small cell carcinoma of the urinary bladder treated with chemotherapy and radiotherapy: results in five cases. *Eur Urol* 35: 323-326.
183. Batata MA, Whitmore WF, Hilaris BS, Tokita N, Grabstald H (1975). Primary carcinoma of the ureter: a prognostic study. *Cancer* 35: 1626-1632.
184. Bates AW, Baithun SI (2000). Secondary neoplasms of the bladder are histological mimics of nontransitional cell primary tumours: clinicopathological and histological features of 282 cases. *Histopathology* 36: 32-40.
185. Bates AW, Baithun SI (2002). Secondary solid neoplasms of the prostate: a clinicopathological series of 51 cases. *Virchows Arch* 440: 392-396.
186. Batta AG, Engen DE, Reiman HM, Winkelmann RK (1990). Intravesical condyloma acuminatum with progression to verrucous carcinoma. *Urology* 36: 457-464.
187. Beach R, Gown AM, Peralta-Venturina MN, Folpe AL, Yaziji H, Salles PG, Grignon DJ, Fanger GR, Amin MB (2002). P504S immunohistochemical detection in 405 prostatic specimens including 376 18-gauge needle biopsies. *Am J Surg Pathol* 26: 1588-1596.
188. Beal K, Mears JG (2001). Short report: penile lymphoma following local injections for erectile dysfunction. *Leuk Lymphoma* 42: 247-249.
189. Beckstead JH (1983). Alkaline phosphatase histochemistry in human germ cell neoplasms. *Am J Surg Pathol* 7: 341-349.
190. Beckwith JB (1993). Precursor lesions of Wilms tumor: clinical and biological implications. *Med Pediatr Oncol* 21: 158-168.
191. Beckwith JB (1998). Children at increased risk for Wilms tumor: monitoring issues. *J Pediatr* 132: 377-379.
192. Beckwith JB (1998). Nephrogenic rests and the pathogenesis of Wilms tumor: developmental and clinical considerations. *Am J Med Genet* 79: 268-273.
193. Beckwith JB (1998). Renal tumors. In: *Pathology of Solid Tumors in Children*, JT Stocker, FB Askin, eds. Chapman and Hall Medical: New York, pp. 1-23.
194. Beckwith JB (2002). Revised SIOP working classification of renal tumors of childhood. *Med Pediatr Oncol* 38: 77-78.
195. Beckwith JB, Kiviat NB, Bonadio JF (1990). Nephrogenic rests, nephroblastomatosis, and the pathogenesis of Wilms' tumor. *Pediatr Pathol* 10: 1-36.
196. Beckwith JB, Palmer NF (1978). Histopathology and prognosis of Wilms tumors: results from the First National Wilms' Tumor Study. *Cancer* 41: 1937-1948.
197. Beckwith JB, Zuppan CE, Browning NG, Moksness J, Breslow NE (1996). Histological analysis of aggressiveness and responsiveness in Wilms' tumor. *Med Pediatr Oncol* 27: 422-428.
198. Beduschi MC, Beduschi R, Oesterling JE (1997). Stage T1c prostate cancer: defining the appropriate staging evaluation and the role for pelvic lymphadenectomy. *World J Urol* 15: 346-358.
199. Bedwani R, Renganathan E, el Kwhsky F, Braga C, Abu Seif HH, Abul Azm T, Zaki A, Franceschi S, Boffetta P, La Vecchia C (1998). Schistosomiasis and the risk of bladder cancer in Alexandria, Egypt. *Br J Cancer* 77: 1186-1189.
200. Begara Morillas F, Silmi Moyano A, Hermida Gutierrez J, Chicharro Almarza J, Fernandez Acenero MJ, Martin Rodilla C, Ramirez Fernandez JC, Rapariz Gonzalez M, Salinas Casado J, Resel Estevez L (1996). [Lymphoproliferative pathology of the genitourinary tract. Report of 6 cases and review of the literature]. *Arch Esp Urol* 49: 562-570.
201. Begg RC (1931). The colloid adenocarcinoma of the bladder vault arising from the epithelium of the urachal canal : with a critical survey of the tumours of the urachus. *Br J Surg* 18: 422-464.
202. Begin LR, Guy L, Jacobson SA, Aprikian AG (1998). Renal carcinoid and horseshoe kidney: a frequent association of two rare entities—a case report and review of the literature. *J Surg Oncol* 68: 113-119.
203. Begin LR, Jamison BM (1993). Renal carcinoid - A tumor of probable hindgut neuroendocrine phenotype. Report of a case and a literature review. *J Urol Pathol* 1: 269-282.
204. Beheshti B, Park PC, Sweet JM, Trachtenberg J, Jewett MA, Squire JA (2001). Evidence of chromosomal instability in prostate cancer determined by spectral karyotyping (SKY) and interphase fish analysis. *Neoplasia* 3: 62-69.
205. Beiko DT, Nickel JC, Boag AH, Srigley JR (2001). Benign mixed epithelial stromal tumor of the kidney of possible mullerian origin. *J Urol* 166: 1381-1382.
206. Ben-Izhak O (1997). Solitary papillary cystadenoma of the spermatic cord presenting as an inguinal mass. *J Urol Pathol* 7: 55-61.
207. Benchekroun A, Zannoud M, Ghadouane M, Alami M, Belahnech Z, Faik M (2001). [Sarcomatoid carcinoma of the prostate]. *Prog Urol* 11: 327-330.
208. Bennett CL, Price DK, Kim S, Liu D, Jovanovic BD, Nathan D, Johnson ME, Montgomery JS, Cude K, Brockbank JC, Sartor O, Figg WD (2002). Racial variation in CAG repeat lengths within the androgen receptor gene among prostate cancer patients of lower socioeconomic status. *J Clin Oncol* 20: 3599-3604.
209. Bennington JL (1987). Tumors of the kidney. In: *Surgical Pathology of Urologic Diseases*, N Javadpour, SH Barsky, eds. Williams and Wilkins: Baltimore, pp. 120-122.
210. Bennington JL, Beckwith JB (1975). *Tumours of the Kidney, Renal Pelvis and Ureter.* HI Firminger, ed. 2nd Edition. AFIP: Washington, DC.
211. Benson CB, Doubilet PM, Richie JP (1989). Sonography of the male genital tract. *AJR Am J Roentgenol* 153: 705-713.
212. Benson RCJr, Clark WR, Farrow GM (1984). Carcinoma of the seminal vesicle. *J Urol* 132: 483-485.
213. Bercovici JP, Nahoul K, Tater D, Charles JF, Scholler R (1984). Hormonal profile of Leydig cell tumors with gynecomastia. *J Clin Endocrinol Metab* 59: 625-630.
214. Berdjis CC, Mostofi FK (1977). Carcinoid tumors of the testis. *J Urol* 118: 777-782.
215. Berenson RJ, Flynn S, Freiha FS, Kempson RL, Torti FM (1986). Primary osteogenic sarcoma of the bladder. Case report and review of the literature. *Cancer* 57: 350-355.
216. Berger CS, Sandberg AA, Todd IA, Pennington RD, Haddad FS, Hecht BK, Hecht F (1986). Chromosomes in kidney, ureter, and bladder cancer. *Cancer Genet Cytogenet* 23: 1-24.
217. Berger MS, Greenfield C, Gullick WJ, Haley J, Downward J, Neal DE, Harris AL, Waterfield MD (1987). Evaluation of epidermal growth factor receptors in bladder tumours. *Br J Cancer* 56: 533-537.
218. Bergh A, Cajander S (1990). Immunohistochemical localization of inhibin-alpha in the testes of normal men and in men with testicular disorders. *Int J Androl* 13: 463-469.
219. Bergkvist A, Ljungqvist A, Moberger G (1965). Classification of bladder tumours based on the cellular pattern. Preliminary report of a clinical-pathological study of 300 cases with a minimum follow-up of eight years. *Acta Chir Scand* 130: 371-378.
220. Bergner DM, Duck GB, Rao M (1980). Bilateral sequential spermatocytic seminoma. *J Urol* 124: 565.
221. Bergstrom A, Lindblad P, Wolk A (2001). Birth weight and risk of renal cell cancer. *Kidney Int* 59: 1110-1113.
222. Bergstrom R, Adami HO, Mohner M, Zatonski W, Storm H, Ekbom A, Tretli S, Teppo L, Akre O, Hakulinen T (1996). Increase in testicular cancer incidence in six European countries: a birth cohort phenomenon. *J Natl Cancer Inst* 88: 727-733.
223. Berman DM, Yang J, Epstein JI (2000). Foamy gland high-grade prostatic intraepithelial neoplasia. *Am J Surg Pathol* 24: 140-144.
224. Bernardini S, Chabannes E, Algros MP, Billerey C, Bittard H (2002). Variants of renal angiomyolipoma closely simulating renal cell carcinoma: difficulties in the histological diagnosis. *Urol Int* 69: 78-81.
225. Berner A, Jacobsen AB, Fossa SD, Nesland JM (1993). Expression of c-erbB-2 protein, neuron-specific enolase and DNA flow cytometry in locally advanced transitional cell carcinoma of the urinary bladder. *Histopathology* 22: 327-333.
226. Beroud C, Fournet JC, Jeanpierre C, Droz D, Bouvier R, Froger D, Chretien Y, Marechal JM, Weissenbach J, Junien C (1996). Correlations of allelic imbalance of chromosome 14 with adverse prognostic parameters in 148 renal cell carcinomas. *Genes Chromosomes Cancer* 17: 215-224.
227. Berruti A, Dogliotti L, Mosca A, Bellina M, Mari M, Torta M, Tarabuzzi R, Bollito E, Fontana D, Angeli A (2000). Circulating neuroendocrine markers in patients with prostate carcinoma. *Cancer* 88: 2590-2597.
228. Berruti A, Dogliotti L, Mosca A, Tarabuzzi R, Torta M, Mari M, Gorzegno G, Fontana D, Angeli A (2001). Effects of the somatostatin analog lanreotide on the circulating levels of chromogranin-A, prostate-specific antigen, and insulin-like growth factor-1 in advanced prostate cancer patients. *Prostate* 47: 205-211.
229. Berry R, Schroeder JJ, French AJ, McDonnell SK, Peterson BJ, Cunningham JM, Thibodeau SN, Schaid DJ (2000). Evidence for a prostate cancer-susceptibility locus on chromosome 20. *Am J Hum Genet* 67: 82-91.
230. Berthon P, Valeri A, Cohen-Akenine A, Drelon E, Paiss T, Wohr G, Latil A, Millasseau P, Mellah I, Cohen N, Blanche H, Bellane-Chantelot C, Demenais F, Teillac P, Le Duc A, de Petriconi R, Hautmann R, Chumakov I, Bachner L, Maitland NJ, Lidereau R, Vogel W, Fournier G, Mangin P, Cohen D, Cussenot O (1998). Predisposing gene for early-onset prostate cancer, localized on chromosome 1q42.2-43. *Am J Hum Genet* 62: 1416-1424.
231. Bertrand G, Simard C (1970). [Ureteral metastasis disclosing a latent carcinoid tumor of the cecum]. *J Urol Nephrol (Paris)* 76: 576-581.
232. Bessette PL, Abell MR, Herwig KR (1974). A clinicopathologic study of squamous cell carcinoma of the bladder. *J Urol* 112: 66-67.
233. Bettocchi C, Coker CB, Deacon J, Parkinson C, Pryor JP (1994). A review of testicular intratubular germ cell neoplasia in infertile men. *J Androl* 15 Suppl: 14S-16S.
234. Beyersdorff D, Taupitz M, Giessing M, Turk I, Schnorr D, Loening S, Hamm B (2000). [The staging of bladder tumors in MRT: the value of the intravesical application of an iron oxide-containing contrast medium in combination with high-resolution T2-weighted imaging]. *Rofo Fortschr Geb Rontgenstr Neuen Bildgeb Verfahr* 172: 504-508.
235. Bezerra AL, Lopes A, Landman G, Alencar GN, Torloni H, Villa LL (2001). Clinicopathologic features and human papillomavirus DNA prevalence of warty and squamous cell carcinoma of the penis. *Am J Surg Pathol* 25: 673-678.
236. Bezerra AL, Lopes A, Santiago GH, Ribeiro KC, Latorre MR, Villa LL (2001). Human papillomavirus as a prognostic factor in carcinoma of the penis: analysis of 82 patients treated with amputation and bilateral lymphadenectomy. *Cancer* 91: 2315-2321.
237. Bhatia-Gaur R, Donjacour AA, Sciavolino PJ, Kim M, Desai N, Young P, Norton CR, Gridley T, Cardiff RD, Cunha GR, Abate-Shen C, Shen MM (1999). Roles for Nkx3.1 in prostate development and cancer. *Genes Dev* 13: 966-977.
238. Bhattachary V, Gammall MM (1995). Bilateral non-Hodgkin's intrinsic lymphoma of ureters. *Br J Urol* 75: 673-674.
239. Bhutani MS, Suryaprasad S, Moezzi J, Seabrook D (1999). Improved technique for performing endoscopic ultrasound guided fine needle aspiration of lymph nodes. *Endoscopy* 31: 550-553.
240. Biegel JA, Conard K, Brooks JJ (1993). Translocation (11;22)(p13;q12): primary change in intra-abdominal desmoplastic small round cell tumor. *Genes Chromosomes Cancer* 7: 119-121.
241. Biegel JA, Fogelgren B, Wainwright LM, Zhou JY, Bevan H, Rorke LB (2000). Germline INI1 mutation in a patient with a central nervous system atypical teratoid tumor and renal rhabdoid tumor. *Genes Chromosomes Cancer* 28: 31-37.
242. Biegel JA, Zhou JY, Rorke LB, Stenstrom C, Wainwright LM, Fogelgren B (1999). Germline and acquired mutations of INI1 in atypical teratoid and rhabdoid tumors. *Cancer Res* 59: 74-79.
243. Billerey C, Chopin D, Aubriot-Lorton MH, Ricol D, Gil Diez de Medina S, van Rhijn B, Bralet MP, Lefrere-Belda MA, Lahaye JB, Abbou CC, Bonaventure J, Zafrani ES, van der Kwast T, Thiery JP, Radvanyi F (2001). Frequent FGFR3 mutations in papillary non-invasive bladder (pTa) tumors. *Am J Pathol* 158: 1955-1959.
244. Billis A (1996). Age and race distribution of high grade prostatic intraepithelial neoplasia: An autopsy study in Brazil (South America). *J Urol Pathol* 5: 175-181.
245. Birkeland SA, Storm HH, Lamm LU, Barlow L, Blohme I, Forsberg B, Eklund B, Fjeldborg O, Friedberg M, Frodin L, Glattre E, Halvorsen S, Holm NV, Jakobsen A, Jorgensen HE, Ladefoged J, Lindholm T, Lundgren G, Pukkala E (1995). Cancer risk after renal transplantation in the Nordic countries, 1964-1986. *Int J Cancer* 60: 183-189.

246. Birt AR, Hogg GR, Dube WJ (1977). Hereditary multiple fibrofolliculomas with trichodiscomas and acrochordons. *Arch Dermatol* 113: 1674-1677.
247. Bissig H, Richter J, Desper R, Meier V, Schraml P, Schaffer AA, Sauter G, Mihatsch MJ, Moch H (1999). Evaluation of the clonal relationship between primary and metastatic renal cell carcinoma by comparative genomic hybridization. *Am J Pathol* 155: 267-274.
248. Blacher EJ, Johnson DE, Abdul-Karim FW, Ayala AG (1985). Squamous cell carcinoma of renal pelvis. *Urology* 25: 124-126.
249. Blanchet P, Droupy S, Eschwege P, Viellefond A, Paradis V, Pichon MF, Jardin A, Benoit G (2001). Prospective evaluation of Ki-67 labeling in predicting the recurrence and progression of superficial bladder transitional cell carcinoma. *Eur Urol* 40: 169-175.
250. Blasco MA, Lee HW, Hande MP, Samper E, Lansdorp PM, Depinho RA, Greider CW (1997). Telomere shortening and tumor formation by mouse cells lacking telomerase RNA. *Cell* 91: 25-34.
251. Blaszyk H, Wang L, Dietmaier W, Hofstadter F, Burgart LJ, Cheville JC, Hartmann A (2002). Upper tract urothelial carcinoma: a clinicopathologic study including microsatellite instability analysis. *Mod Pathol* 15: 790-797.
252. Blitzer PH, Dosoretz DE, Proppe KH, Shipley WU (1981). Treatment of malignant tumors of the spermatic cord: a study of 10 cases and a review of the literature. *J Urol* 126: 611-614.
253. Blohme I, Johansson S (1981). Renal pelvic neoplasms and atypical urothelium in patients with end-stage analgesic nephropathy. *Kidney Int* 20: 671-675.
254. Blomjous CE, Vos W, de Voogt HJ, van der Valk P, Meijer CJ (1989). Small cell carcinoma of the urinary bladder. A clinicopathologic, morphometric, immunohistochemical, and ultrastructural study of 18 cases. *Cancer* 64: 1347-1357.
255. Bluebond-Langner R, Pinto PA, Argani P, Chan TY, Halushka M, Jarrett TW (2002). Adult presentation of metanephric stromal tumor. *J Urol* 168: 1482-1483.
256. Bluestein DL, Bostwick DG, Bergstralh EJ, Oesterling JE (1994). Eliminating the need for bilateral pelvic lymphadenectomy in select patients with prostate cancer. *J Urol* 151: 1315-1320.
257. Blute ML, Engen DE, Travis WD, Kvols LK (1989). Primary signet ring cell adenocarcinoma of the bladder. *J Urol* 141: 17-21.
258. Bluth EI, Bush WHJr, Amis ESJr, Bigongiari LR, Choyke PL, Fritzsche PJ, Holder LE, Newhouse JH, Sandler CM, Segal AJ, Resnick MI, Rutsky EA (2000). Indeterminate renal masses. American College of Radiology. ACR Appropriateness Criteria. *Radiology* 215 Suppl: 747-752.
259. Boccon-Gibod L, Rey A, Sandstedt B, Delemarre J, Harms D, Vujanic G, de Kraker J, Weirich A, Tournade MF (2000). Complete necrosis induced by preoperative chemotherapy in Wilms tumor as an indicator of low risk: report of the International Society of Paediatric Oncology (SIOP) nephroblastoma trial and study 9. *Med Pediatr Oncol* 34: 183-190.
260. Bochner BH, Cote RJ, Weidner N, Groshen S, Chen SC, Skinner DG, Nichols PW (1995). Angiogenesis in bladder cancer: relationship between microvessel density and tumor prognosis. *J Natl Cancer Inst* 87: 1603-1612.
261. Bodner DR, Cohen JK, Resnick MI (1986). Primary transitional cell carcinoma of the prostate. *J Urol (Paris)* 92: 121-122.
262. Bohle A, Studer UE, Sonntag RW, Scheidegger JR (1986). Primary or secondary extragonadal germ cell tumors? *J Urol* 135: 939-943.
263. Bohm M, Kleine-Besten R, Wieland I (2000). Loss of heterozygosity analysis on chromosome 5p defines 5p13-12 as the critical region involved in tumor progression of bladder carcinomas. *Int J Cancer* 89: 194-197.
264. Boland CR, Thibodeau SN, Hamilton SR, Sidransky D, Eshleman JR, Burt RW, Meltzer SJ, Rodriguez-Bigas MA, Fodde R, Ranzani GN, Srivastava S (1998). A National Cancer Institute Workshop on Microsatellite Instability for cancer detection and familial predisposition: development of international criteria for the determination of microsatellite instability in colorectal cancer. *Cancer Res* 58: 5248-5257.
265. Bolande RP, Brough AJ, Izant RJJr (1967). Congenital mesoblastic nephroma of infancy. A report of eight cases and the relationship to Wilms' tumor. *Pediatrics* 40: 272-278.
266. Bolen JW (1981). Mixed germ cell-sex cord stromal tumor. A gonadal tumor distinct from gonadoblastoma. *Am J Clin Pathol* 75: 565-573.
267. Bollito E, Berruti A, Bellina M, Mosca A, Leonardo E, Tarabuzzi R, Cappia S, Ari MM, Tampellini M, Fontana D, Gubetta L, Angeli A, Dogliotti L (2001). Relationship between neuroendocrine features and prognostic parameters in human prostate adenocarcinoma. *Ann Oncol* 12 Suppl 2: S159-S164.
268. Bonetti F, Chiodera PL, Pea M, Martignoni G, Bosi F, Zamboni G, Mariuzzi GM (1993). Transbronchial biopsy in lymphangiomyomatosis of the lung. HMB45 for diagnosis. *Am J Surg Pathol* 17: 1092-1102.
269. Bonetti F, Pea M, Martignoni G, Doglioni C, Zamboni G, Capelli P, Rimondi P, Andrion A (1994). Clear cell ("sugar") tumor of the lung is a lesion strictly related to angiomyolipoma—the concept of a family of lesions characterized by the presence of the perivascular epithelioid cells (PEC). *Pathology* 26: 230-236.
270. Bonin SR, Hanlon AL, Lee WR, Movsas B, al Saleem TI, Hanks GE (1997). Evidence of increased failure in the treatment of prostate carcinoma patients who have perineural invasion treated with three-dimensional conformal radiation therapy. *Cancer* 79: 75-80.
271. Bonkhoff H (1996). Role of the basal cells in premalignant changes of the human prostate: a stem cell concept for the development of prostate cancer. *Eur Urol* 30: 201-205.
272. Bonkhoff H (2001). Neuroendocrine differentiation in human prostate cancer. Morphogenesis, proliferation and androgen receptor status. *Ann Oncol* 12 Suppl 2: S141-S144.
273. Bonsib SM (1996). HMB-45 reactivity in renal leiomyomas and leiomyosarcomas. *Mod Pathol* 9: 664-669.
274. Bonsib SM, Fischer J, Plattner S, Fallon B (1987). Sarcomatoid renal tumors. Clinicopathologic correlation of three cases. *Cancer* 59: 527-532.
275. Bonzanini M, Pea M, Martignoni G, Zamboni G, Capelli P, Bernardello F, Bonetti F (1994). Preoperative diagnosis of renal angiomyolipoma: fine needle aspiration cytology and immunocytochemical characterization. *Pathology* 26: 170-175.
276. Bookstein R (2001). Tumor suppressor genes in prostate cancer. In: *Prostate Cancer: Biology, Genetics, and the New Therapeutics*, LW Chung, WB Isaacs, JW Simons, eds. Humana press: Totowa, NJ, pp. 61-93.
277. Borboroglu PG, Sur RL, Roberts JL, Amling CL (2001). Repeat biopsy strategy in patients with atypical small acinar proliferation or high grade prostatic intraepithelial neoplasia on initial prostate needle biopsy. *J Urol* 166: 866-870.
278. Borge N, Fossa SD (1990). Late relapses of testicular cancer: a review. *Cancer J* 3: 53-55.
279. Bos JL (1989). ras oncogenes in human cancer: a review. *Cancer Res* 49: 4682-4689.
280. Bosch FX, Cardis E (1990). Cancer incidence correlations: genital, urinary and some tobacco-related cancers. *Int J Cancer* 46: 178-184.
281. Bosl GJ, Geller NL, Cirrincione C, Vogelzang NJ, Kennedy BJ, Whitmore WFJr, Vugrin D, Scher H, Nisselbaum J, Golbey RB (1983). Multivariate analysis of prognostic variables in patients with metastatic testicular cancer. *Cancer Res* 43: 3403-3407.
282. Bosl GJ, Sheinfeld J (1997). Cancer of the testis. In: *Cancer: Principles and Practice of Pediatric Oncology*, VT DeVita, S Hellman, S Rosenberg, eds. 5th Edition. JB Lippincott: Philadelphia, pp. 1397-1425.
283. Bosniak MA (1986). The current radiological approach to renal cysts. *Radiology* 158: 1-10.
284. Bosniak MA, Megibow AJ, Hulnick DH, Horii S, Raghavendra BN (1988). CT diagnosis of renal angiomyolipoma: the importance of detecting small amounts of fat. *AJR Am J Roentgenol* 151: 497-501.
285. Bostwick DG (1992). Natural history of early bladder cancer. *J Cell Biochem Suppl* 16I: 31-38.
286. Bostwick DG (1997). Neoplasm of the prostate. In: *Urologic Surgical Pathology*, DG Bostwick, JN Eble, eds. Mosby: St Louis, pp. 366-368.
287. Bostwick DG (1997). Spermatic cord and testicular adnexa. In: *Urologic Surgical Pathology*, DG Bostwick, JN Eble, eds. Mosby: St Louis, p. 661.
288. Bostwick DG, Amin MB, Dundore P, Marsh W, Schultz DS (1993). Architectural patterns of high-grade prostatic intraepithelial neoplasia. *Hum Pathol* 24: 298-310.
289. Bostwick DG, Foster CS (1997). Examination of radical prostatectomy specimens: therapeutic and prognostic significance. In: *Pathology of the Prostate*, CS Foster, DG Bostwick, eds. WB Saunders: Philadelphia, pp. 172-189.
290. Bostwick DG, Grignon DJ, Hammond ME, Amin MB, Cohen M, Crawford D, Gospodarowicz M, Kaplan RS, Miller DS, Montironi R, Pajak TF, Pollack A, Srigley JR, Yarbro JW (2000). Prognostic factors in prostate cancer. College of American Pathologists Consensus Statement 1999. *Arch Pathol Lab Med* 124: 995-1000.
291. Bostwick DG, Iczkowski KA, Amin MB, Discigil G, Osborne B (1998). Malignant lymphoma involving the prostate: report of 62 cases. *Cancer* 83: 732-738.
292. Bostwick DG, Kindrachuk RW, Rouse RV (1985). Prostatic adenocarcinoma with endometrioid features. Clinical, pathologic, and ultrastructural findings. *Am J Surg Pathol* 9: 595-609.
293. Bostwick DG, Lopez-Beltran A (1999). *Bladder Biopsy Interpretation.* United Pathologists Press: Washington, DC.
294. Bostwick DG, Norlen BJ, Denis L (2000). Prostatic intraepithelial neoplasia: the preinvasive stage of prostate cancer. Overview of the prostate committee report. *Scand J Urol Nephrol Suppl* 205: 1-2.
295. Bostwick DG, Pacelli A, Lopez-Beltran A (1996). Molecular biology of prostatic intraepithelial neoplasia. *Prostate* 29: 117-134.
296. Bostwick DG, Qian J, Frankel K (1995). The incidence of high grade prostatic intraepithelial neoplasia in needle biopsies. *J Urol* 154: 1791-1794.
297. Bouchardy C, Mirra AP, Khlat M, Parkin DM, de Souza JM, Gotlieb SL (1991). Ethnicity and cancer risk in Sao Paulo, Brazil. *Cancer Epidemiol Biomarkers Prev* 1: 21-27.
298. Boulanger P, Somma M, Chevalier S, Bleau G, Roberts KD, Chapdelaine A (1984). Elevated secretion of androstenedione in a patient with a Leydig cell tumour. *Acta Endocrinol (Copenh)* 107: 104-109.
299. Bouras M, Tabone E, Bertholon J, Sommer P, Bouvier R, Droz JP, Benahmed M (2000). A novel SMAD4 gene mutation in seminoma germ cell tumors. *Cancer Res* 60: 922-928.
300. Bourdon V, Naef F, Rao PH, Reuter V, Mok SC, Bosl GJ, Koul S, Murty VV, Kucherlapati RS, Chaganti RS (2002). Genomic and expression analysis of the 12p11-p12 amplicon using EST arrays identifies two novel amplified and overexpressed genes. *Cancer Res* 62: 6218-6223.
301. Bourque JL, Charghi A, Gauthier GE, Drouin G, Charbonneau J (1970). Primary carcinoma of Cowper's gland. *J Urol* 103: 758-761.
302. Bova GS, Partin AW, Isaacs SD, Carter BS, Beaty TL, Isaacs WB, Walsh PC (1998). Biological aggressiveness of hereditary prostate cancer: long-term evaluation following radical prostatectomy. *J Urol* 160: 660-663.
303. Bove KE, McAdams AJ (1976). The nephroblastomatosis complex and its relationship to Wilms' tumor: a clinicopathologic treatise. *Perspect Pediatr Pathol* 3: 185-223.
304. Bowen C, Bubendorf L, Voeller HJ, Slack R, Willi N, Sauter G, Gasser TC, Koivisto P, Lack EE, Kononen J, Kallioniemi OP, Gelmann EP (2000). Loss of NKX3.1 expression in human prostate cancers correlates with tumor progression. *Cancer Res* 60: 6111-6115.
305. Bower M, Rustin G (2000). Serum tumour markers and their role in monitoring germ cell cancers of the testis. In: *Comprehensive Textbook of Genitourinary Oncology*, NJ Vogelzang, WU Shipley, PT Scardino, DS Coffey, BJ Miles, eds. 2nd Edition. Lippincott Williams & Wilkins: New York, pp. 927-938.
306. Brandes SB, Chelsky MJ, Petersen RO, Greenberg RE (1996). Leiomyosarcoma of the renal vein. *J Surg Oncol* 63: 195-200.
307. Brauch H, Weirich G, Brieger J, Glavac D, Rodl H, Eichinger M, Feurer M, Weidt E, Puranakanitstha C, Neuhaus C, Pomer S, Brenner W, Schirmacher P, Storkel S, Rotter M, Masera A, Gugeler N, Decker HJ (2000). VHL alterations in human clear cell renal cell carcinoma: association with advanced tumor stage and a novel hot spot mutation. *Cancer Res* 60: 1942-1948.
308. Brawer MK, Meyer GE, Letran JL, Bankson DD, Morris DL, Yeung KK, Allard WJ (1998). Measurement of complexed PSA improves specificity for early detection of prostate cancer. *Urology* 52: 372-378.

309. Brawer MK, Peehl DM, Stamey TA, Bostwick DG (1985). Keratin immunoreactivity in the benign and neoplastic human prostate. *Cancer Res* 45: 3663-3667.
310. Brawley OW (1997). Prostate carcinoma incidence and patient mortality: the effects of screening and early detection. *Cancer* 80: 1857-1863.
311. Brawn PN (1987). The characteristics of embryonal carcinoma cells in teratocarcinomas. *Cancer* 59: 2042-2046.
312. Brennan MK, Srigley JR (1999). Brenner tumours of testis and the paratestis: case report and a literature review. *J Urol Pathol* 10: 219-228.
313. Brennan P, Bogillot O, Cordier S, Greiser E, Schill W, Vineis P, Lopez-Abente G, Tzonou A, Chang-Claude J, Bolm-Audorff U, Jockel KH, Donato F, Serra C, Wahrendorf J, Hours M, T'Mannetje A, Kogevinas M, Boffetta P (2000). Cigarette smoking and bladder cancer in men: a pooled analysis of 11 case-control studies. *Int J Cancer* 86: 289-294.
314. Brennick JB, O'Connell JX, Dickersin GR, Pilch BZ, Young RH (1994). Lipofuscin pigmentation (so-called "melanosis") of the prostate. *Am J Surg Pathol* 18: 446-454.
315. Breslow N, Beckwith JB, Ciol M, Sharples K (1988). Age distribution of Wilms' tumor: report from the National Wilms' Tumor Study. *Cancer Res* 48: 1653-1657.
316. Breslow N, Chan CW, Dhom G, Drury RA, Franks LM, Gellei B, Lee YS, Lundberg S, Sparke B, Sternby NH, Tulinius H (1977). Latent carcinoma of prostate at autopsy in seven areas. The International Agency for Research on Cancer, Lyons, France. *Int J Cancer* 20: 680-688.
317. Breslow N, Olshan A, Beckwith JB, Green DM (1993). Epidemiology of Wilms tumor. *Med Pediatr Oncol* 21: 172-181.
318. Breslow NE, Churchill G, Nesmith B, Thomas PR, Beckwith JB, Othersen HB, D'Angio GJ (1986). Clinicopathologic features and prognosis for Wilms' tumor patients with metastases at diagnosis. *Cancer* 58: 2501-2511.
319. Bretheau D, Lechevallier E, Jean F, Rampal M, Coulange C (1993). [Tumors of the superior urinary tract and associated bladder tumors: clinical and etiological aspects]. *Prog Urol* 3: 979-987.
320. Brieger J, Weidt EJ, Schirmacher P, Storkel S, Huber C, Decker HJ (1999). Inverse regulation of vascular endothelial growth factor and VHL tumor suppressor gene in sporadic renal cell carcinomas is correlated with vascular growth: an in vivo study on 29 tumors. *J Mol Med* 77: 505-510.
321. Bringuier PP, McCredie M, Sauter G, Bilous M, Stewart J, Mihatsch MJ, Kleihues P, Ohgaki H (1998). Carcinomas of the renal pelvis associated with smoking and phenacetin abuse: p53 mutations and polymorphism of carcinogen-metabolising enzymes. *Int J Cancer* 79: 531-536.
322. Bringuier PP, Tamimi Y, Schuuring E, Schalken J (1996). Expression of cyclin D1 and EMS1 in bladder tumours; relationship with chromosome 11q13 amplification. *Oncogene* 12: 1747-1753.
323. Brinker DA, Potter SR, Epstein JI (1999). Ductal adenocarcinoma of the prostate diagnosed on needle biopsy: correlation with clinical and radical prostatectomy findings and progression. *Am J Surg Pathol* 23: 1471-1479.
324. Broggi G, Appetito C, di Leone L, Ciprandi G, Menichella P, Broggi M, Boldrini R, Zaccara A (1991). Dermoid cyst in undescended testis in a 9-year-old boy. *Urol Int* 47: 110-112.
325. Brooks JD, Weinstein M, Lin X, Sun Y, Pin SS, Bova GS, Epstein JI, Isaacs WB, Nelson WG (1998). CG island methylation changes near the GSTP1 gene in prostatic intraepithelial neoplasia. *Cancer Epidemiol Biomarkers Prev* 7: 531-536.
326. Brosman SA (1979). Testicular tumors in prepubertal children. *Urology* 13: 581-588.
327. Brouland JP, Meeus F, Rossert J, Hernigou A, Gentric D, Jacquot C, Diebold J, Nochy D (1994). Primary bilateral B-cell renal lymphoma: a case report and review of the literature. *Am J Kidney Dis* 24: 586-589.
328. Brown DF, Chason DP, Schwartz LF, Coimbra CP, Rushing EJ (1998). Supratentorial giant cell ependymoma: a case report. *Mod Pathol* 11: 398-403.
329. Brown JM (1975). Cystic partially differentiated nephroblastoma. *J Pathol* 115: 175-178.
330. Brown NJ (1976). Teratomas and yolk-sac tumours. *J Clin Pathol* 29: 1021-1025.
331. Bruneton JN, Drouillard J, Normand F, Tavernier J, Thyss A, Schneider M (1987). Non-renal urological lymphomas. *ROFO Fortschr Geb Rontgenstr Nuklearmed* 146: 42-46.
332. Bryan GT (1969). Role of tryptophan metabolites in urinary bladder cancer. *Am Ind Hyg Assoc J* 30: 27-34.
333. Bryant J (1995). Granular cell tumor of penis and scrotum. *Urology* 45: 332-334.
334. Bubendorf L, Grilli B, Sauter G, Mihatsch MJ, Gasser TC, Dalquen P (2001). Multiprobe FISH for enhanced detection of bladder cancer in voided urine specimens and bladder washings. *Am J Clin Pathol* 116: 79-86.
335. Bubendorf L, Sauter G, Moch H, Schmid HP, Gasser TC, Jordan P, Mihatsch MJ (1996). Ki67 labelling index: an independent predictor of progression in prostate cancer treated by radical prostatectomy. *J Pathol* 178: 437-441.
336. Budia Alba A, Queipo Zaragoza JA, Perez Ebri ML, Fuster Escriva A, Vera Donoso DC, Vera Sempere FJ, Jimenez Cruz JF (1999). [Comparative study of pure epidermoid carcinoma of the bladder and transitional cell carcinoma with squamous or mixed differentiated foci]. *Actas Urol Esp* 23: 111-118.
337. Bue P, Wester K, Sjostrom A, Holmberg A, Nilsson S, Carlsson J, Westlin JE, Busch C, Malmstrom PU (1998). Expression of epidermal growth factor receptor in urinary bladder cancer metastases. *Int J Cancer* 76: 189-193.
338. Bugert P, Kovacs G (1996). Molecular differential diagnosis of renal cell carcinomas by microsatellite analysis. *Am J Pathol* 149: 2081-2088.
339. Bugert P, von Knobloch R, Kovacs G (1998). Duplication of two distinct regions on chromosome 5q in non-papillary renal-cell carcinomas. *Int J Cancer* 76: 337-340.
340. Bullock MJ, Srigley JR, Klotz LH, Goldenberg SL (2002). Pathologic effects of neoadjuvant cyproterone acetate on nonneoplastic prostate, prostatic intraepithelial neoplasia, and adenocarcinoma: a detailed analysis of radical prostatectomy specimens from a randomized trial. *Am J Surg Pathol* 26: 1400-1413.
341. Bullock PS, Thoni DE, Murphy WM (1987). The significance of colonic mucosa (intestinal metaplasia) involving the urinary tract. *Cancer* 59: 2086-2090.
342. Bunesch Villalba L, Bargallo Castello X, Vilana Puig R, Burrel Samaranch M, Bru Saumell C (2001). Lymphoma of the penis: sonographic findings. *J Ultrasound Med* 20: 929-931.
343. Burgess NA, Lewis DC, Matthews PN (1992). Primary carcinoid of the bladder. *Br J Urol* 69: 213-214.
344. Burgues O, Ferrer J, Navarro S, Ramos D, Botella E, Llombart-Bosch A (1999). Hepatoid adenocarcinoma of the urinary bladder. An unusual neoplasm. *Virchows Arch* 435: 71-75.
345. Burke AP, Mostofi FK (1988). Intratubular malignant germ cells in testicular biopsies: clinical course and identification by staining for placental alkaline phosphatase. *Mod Pathol* 1: 475-479.
346. Burke AP, Mostofi FK (1988). Placental alkaline phosphatase immunohistochemistry of intratubular malignant germ cells and associated testicular germ cell tumors. *Hum Pathol* 19: 663-670.
347. Burke AP, Mostofi FK (1993). Spermatocytic seminoma: A clinicopathologic study of 79 cases. *J Urol Pathol* 1: 21-32.
348. Burrig KF, Pfitzer P, Hort W (1990). Well-differentiated papillary mesothelioma of the peritoneum: a borderline mesothelioma. Report of two cases and review of literature. *Virchows Arch A Pathol Anat Histopathol* 417: 443-447.
349. Burt AD, Cooper G, MacKay C, Boyd JF (1987). Dermoid cyst of the testis. *Scott Med J* 32: 146-148.
350. Burt ME, Javadpour N (1981). Germ-cell tumors in patients with apparently normal testes. *Cancer* 47: 1911-1915.
351. Bussey KJ, Lawce HJ, Olson SB, Arthur DC, Kalousek DK, Krailo M, Giller R, Heifetz S, Womer R, Magenis RE (1999). Chromosome abnormalities of eighty-one pediatric germ cell tumors: sex-, age-, site-, and histopathology-related differences—A Children's Cancer Group study. *Genes Chromosomes Cancer* 25: 134-146.
352. Buszello H, Muller-Mattheis V, Ackermann R (1994). [Value of computerized tomography in detection of lymph node metastases in bladder cancer]. *Urologe A* 33: 243-246.
353. Butnor KJ, Sporn TA, Hammar SP, Roggli VL (2001). Well-differentiated papillary mesothelioma. *Am J Surg Pathol* 25: 1304-1309.
354. Byar DP, Mostofi FK (1972). Carcinoma of the prostate: prognostic evaluation of certain pathologic features in 208 radical prostatectomies. The Veterans Administrative Cooperative Urologic Research Groups. *Cancer* 30: 5-13.
355. Byard RW, Bell ME, Alkan MK (1987). Primary carcinosarcoma: a rare cause of unilateral ureteral obstruction. *J Urol* 137: 732-733.
356. Cabanas RM (1977). An approach for the treatment of penile carcinoma. *Cancer* 39: 456-466.
357. Caccamo D, Socias M, Truchet C (1991). Malignant Brenner tumor of the testis and epididymis. *Arch Pathol Lab Med* 115: 524-527.
358. Caduff RF, Schwobel MG, Willi UV, Briner J (1997). Lymphangioma of the right kidney in an infant boy. *Pediatr Pathol Lab Med* 17: 631-637.
359. Cairns P, Evron E, Okami K, Halachmi N, Esteller M, Herman JG, Bose S, Wang SI, Parsons R, Sidransky D (1998). Point mutation and homozygous deletion of PTEN/MMAC1 in primary bladder cancers. *Oncogene* 16: 3215-3218.
360. Cairns P, Proctor AJ, Knowles MA (1991). Loss of heterozygosity at the RB locus is frequent and correlates with muscle invasion in bladder carcinoma. *Oncogene* 6: 2305-2309.
361. Cairns P, Shaw ME, Knowles MA (1993). Initiation of bladder cancer may involve deletion of a tumour-suppressor gene on chromosome 9. *Oncogene* 8: 1083-1085.
362. Call KM, Glaser T, Ito CY, Buckler AJ, Pelletier J, Haber DA, Rose EA, Kral A, Yeger H, Lewis WH, Jones C, Housman DE (1990). Isolation and characterization of a zinc finger polypeptide gene at the human chromosome 11 Wilms' tumor locus. *Cell* 60: 509-520.
363. Cameron KM, Lupton CH (1976). Inverted papilloma of the lower urinary tract. *Br J Urol* 48: 567-577.
364. Campani R, Bottinelli O, Calliada F, Coscia D (1998). The latest in ultrasound: three-dimensional imaging. Part II. *Eur J Radiol* 27 Suppl 2: S183-S187.
365. Campo E, Algaba F, Palacin A, Germa R, Sole-Balcells FJ, Cardesa A (1989). Placental proteins in high-grade urothelial neoplasms. An immunohistochemical study of human chorionic gonadotropin, human placental lactogen, and pregnancy-specific beta-1-glycoprotein. *Cancer* 63: 2497-2504.
366. Cano-Valdez AM, Chanona-Vilchis J, Dominguez-Malagon H (1999). Large cell calcifying Sertoli cell tumor of the testis: a clinicopathological, immunohistochemical, and ultrastructural study of two cases. *Ultrastruct Pathol* 23: 259-265.
367. Cantor KP, Lynch CF, Hildesheim ME, Dosemeci M, Lubin J, Alavanja M, Craun G (1998). Drinking water source and chlorination byproducts. I. Risk of bladder cancer. *Epidemiology* 9: 21-28.
368. Capella C, Eusebi V, Rosai J (1984). Primary oat cell carcinoma of the kidney. *Am J Surg Pathol* 8: 855-861.
369. Cappellen D, de Oliveira C, Ricol D, de Medina S, Bourdin J, Sastre-Garau X, Chopin D, Thiery JP, Radvanyi F (1999). Frequent activating mutations of FGFR3 in human bladder and cervix carcinomas. *Nat Genet* 23: 18-20.
370. Carbonara C, Longa L, Grosso E, Mazzucco G, Borrone C, Garre ML, Brisigotti M, Filippi G, Scabar A, Giannotti A, Falzoni P, Monga G, Garini G, Gabrielli M, Riegler P, Danesino C, Ruggieri M, Magro G, Migone N (1996). Apparent preferential loss of heterozygosity at TSC2 over TSC1 chromosomal region in tuberous sclerosis hamartomas. *Genes Chromosomes Cancer* 15: 18-25.
371. Carcao MD, Taylor GP, Greenberg ML, Bernstein ML, Champagne M, Hershon L, Baruchel S (1998). Renal-cell carcinoma in children: a different disorder from its adult counterpart? *Med Pediatr Oncol* 31: 153-158.
372. Cardenosa G, Papanicolaou N, Fung CY, Tung GA, Yoder IC, Althausen AF, Shipley WU (1990). Spermatic cord sarcomas: sonographic and CT features. *Urol Radiol* 12: 163-167.
373. Cardillo MR, Castagna G, Memeo L, de Bernardinis E, di Silverio F (2000). Epidermal growth factor receptor, MUC-1 and MUC-2 in bladder cancer. *J Exp Clin Cancer Res* 19: 225-233.

374. Cardone G, Malventi M, Roffi M, Toscano S, Atzeni G, Marino G, Simi G, Tagliaferri D (1995). [Assessment of primary renal lymphoma with computerized tomography]. *Radiol Med (Torino)* 90: 75-79.

375. Carlson GD, Calvanese CB, Kahane H, Epstein JI (1998). Accuracy of biopsy Gleason scores from a large uropathology laboratory: use of a diagnostic protocol to minimize observer variability. *Urology* 51: 525-529.

376. Caro DJ, Tessler A (1978). Inverted papilloma of the bladder: a distinct urological lesion. *Cancer* 42: 708-713.

377. Carpten J, Nupponen N, Isaacs S, Sood R, Robbins C, Xu J, Faruque M, Moses T, Ewing C, Gillanders E, Hu P, Bujnovszky P, Makalowska I, Baffoe-Bonnie A, Faith D, Smith J, Stephan D, Wiley K, Brownstein M, Gildea D, Kelly B, Jenkins R, Hostetter G, Matikainen M, Schleutker J, Klinger K, Connors T, Xiang Y, Wang Z, de Marzo A, Papadopoulos N, Kallioniemi OP, Burk R, Meyers D, Gronberg H, Meltzer P, Silverman R, Bailey-Wilson J, Walsh P, Isaacs W, Trent J (2002). Germline mutations in the ribonuclease L gene in families showing linkage with HPC1. *Nat Genet* 30: 181-184.

378. Carroll BA, Gross DM (1983). High-frequency scrotal sonography. *AJR Am J Roentgenol* 140: 511-515.

379. Carstens PH (1980). Perineural glands in normal and hyperplastic prostates. *J Urol* 123: 686-688.

380. Carter HB, Morrell CH, Pearson JD, Brant LJ, Plato CC, Metter EJ, Chan DW, Fozard JL, Walsh PC (1992). Estimation of prostatic growth using serial prostate-specific antigen measurements in men with and without prostate disease. *Cancer Res* 52: 3323-3328.

381. Carter HB, Pearson JD, Metter EJ, Brant LJ, Chan DW, Andres R, Fozard JL, Walsh PC (1992). Longitudinal evaluation of prostate-specific antigen levels in men with and without prostate disease. *JAMA* 267: 2215-2220.

382. Casado M, Jimenez F, Borbujo J, Almagro M (1988). Spontaneous healing of Kaposi's angiosarcoma of the penis. *J Urol* 139: 1313-1315.

383. Casale AJ, Menashe DS (1989). Massive strawberry hemangioma of the male genitalia. *J Urol* 141: 593-594.

384. Casella R, Bubendorf L, Sauter G, Moch H, Mihatsch MJ, Gasser TC (1998). Focal neuroendocrine differentiation lacks prognostic significance in prostate core needle biopsies. *J Urol* 160: 406-410.

385. Casella R, Moch H, Rochlitz C, Meier V, Seifert B, Mihatsch MJ, Gasser TC (2001). Metastatic primitive neuroectodermal tumor of the kidney in adults. *Eur Urol* 39: 613-617.

386. Casiraghi O, Martinez-Madrigal F, Mostofi FK, Micheau C, Caillou B, Tursz T (1991). Primary prostatic Wilms' tumor. *Am J Surg Pathol* 15: 885-890.

387. Cassio A, Cacciari E, D'Errico A, Balsamo A, Grigioni FW, Pascucci MG, Bacci F, Tacconi M, Mancini AM (1990). Incidence of intratubular germ cell neoplasia in androgen insensitivity syndrome. *Acta Endocrinol (Copenh)* 123: 416-422.

388. Castedo SM, de Jong B, Oosterhuis JW, Seruca R, Buist J, Koops HS (1988). Cytogenetic study of a combined germ cell tumor of the testis. *Cancer Genet Cytogenet* 35: 159-165.

389. Castedo SM, de Jong B, Oosterhuis JW, Seruca R, Idenburg VJ, Dam A, te Meerman G, Koops HS, Sleijfer DT (1989). Chromosomal changes in human primary testicular nonseminomatous germ cell tumors. *Cancer Res* 49: 5696-5701.

390. Castedo SM, de Jong B, Oosterhuis JW, Seruca R, te Meerman GJ, Dam A, Schraffordt Koops H (1989). Cytogenetic analysis of ten human seminomas. *Cancer Res* 49: 439-443.

391. Castelao JE, Yuan JM, Skipper PL, Tannenbaum SR, Gago-Dominguez M, Crowder JS, Ross RK, Yu MC (2001). Gender- and smoking-related bladder cancer risk. *J Natl Cancer Inst* 93: 538-545.

392. Catalona WJ (1997). Clinical utility of measurements of free and total PSA: a review. In: *First International Consultation on Prostate Cancer*, G Murphy, L Denis, C Chatelain, K Griffiths, S Khoury, AT Cockett, eds. Scientific Communication International Ltd: London, pp. 104-111.

393. Catalona WJ, Smith DS (1998). Cancer recurrence and survival rates after anatomic radical retropubic prostatectomy for prostate cancer: intermediate-term results. *J Urol* 160: 2428-2434.

394. Caterino M, Giunta S, Finocchi V, Giglio L, Mainiero G, Carpanese L, Crecco M (2001). Primary cancer of the urinary bladder: CT evaluation of the T parameter with different techniques. *Abdom Imaging* 26: 433-438.

395. Cattan N, Saison-Behmoaras T, Mari B, Mazeau C, Amiel JL, Rossi B, Gioanni J (2000). Screening of human bladder carcinomas for the presence of Ha-ras codon 12 mutation. *Oncol Rep* 7: 497-500.

396. Cerilli LA, Huffman HT, Anand A (1998). Primary renal angiosarcoma: a case report with immunohistochemical, ultrastructural, and cytogenetic features and review of the literature. *Arch Pathol Lab Med* 122: 929-935.

397. Cervantes RB, Stringer JR, Shao C, Tischfield JA, Stambrook PJ (2002). Embryonic stem cells and somatic cells differ in mutation frequency and type. *Proc Natl Acad Sci USA* 99: 3586-3590.

398. Chaitin BA, Manning JT, Ordonez NG (1984). Hematologic neoplasms with initial manifestations in lower urinary tract. *Urology* 23: 35-42.

399. Chalik YN, Wieczorek R, Grasso M (1998). Lymphoepithelioma-like carcinoma of the ureter. *J Urol* 159: 503-504.

400. Chan JK, Chan VS, Mak KL (1990). Congenital juvenile granulosa cell tumour of the testis: report of a case showing extensive degenerative changes. *Histopathology* 17: 75-80.

401. Chan JK, Loo KT, Yau BK, Lam SY (1997). Nodular histiocytic/mesothelial hyperplasia: a lesion potentially mistaken for a neoplasm in transbronchial biopsy. *Am J Surg Pathol* 21: 658-663.

402. Chan JK, Sin VC, Wong KF, Ng CS, Tsang WY, Chan CH, Cheung MM, Lau WH (1997). Nonnasal lymphoma expressing the natural killer cell marker CD56: a clinicopathologic study of 49 cases of an uncommon aggressive neoplasm. *Blood* 89: 4501-4513.

403. Chan JM, Stampfer MJ, Giovannucci E, Gann PH, Ma J, Wilkinson P, Hennekens CH, Pollak M (1998). Plasma insulin-like growth factor-I and prostate cancer risk: a prospective study. *Science* 279: 563-566.

404. Chan JM, Stampfer MJ, Giovannucci EL (1998). What causes prostate cancer? A brief summary of the epidemiology. *Semin Cancer Biol* 8: 263-273.

405. Chan TY, Epstein JI (2001). In situ adenocarcinoma of the bladder. *Am J Surg Pathol* 25: 892-899.

406. Chan TY, Partin AW, Walsh PC, Epstein JI (2000). Prognostic significance of Gleason score 3+4 versus Gleason score 4+3 tumor at radical prostatectomy. *Urology* 56: 823-827.

407. Chan YF, Restall P, Kimble R (1997). Juvenile granulosa cell tumor of the testis: report of two cases in newborns. *J Pediatr Surg* 32: 752-753.

408. Chandra A, Baruah RK, Ramanujam, Rajalakshmi KR, Sagar G, Vishwanathan P, Raman (2001). Primary intratesticular sarcoma. *Indian J Med Sci* 55: 421-428.

409. Chang A, Yousef GM, Jung K, Rajpert-de Meyts E, Diamandis EP (2001). Identification and molecular characterization of five novel kallikrein gene 13 (KLK13; KLK-L4) splice variants: differential expression in the human testis and testicular cancer. *Anticancer Res* 21: 3147-3152.

410. Chang B, Borer JG, Tan PE, Diamond DA (1998). Large-cell calcifying Sertoli cell tumor of the testis: case report and review of the literature. *Urology* 52: 520-522.

411. Chang BS, Kim HL, Yang XJ, Steinberg GD (2001). Correlation between biopsy and radical cystectomy in assessing grade and depth of invasion in bladder urothelial carcinoma. *Urology* 57: 1063-1066.

412. Chang Y, Cesarman E, Pessin MS, Lee F, Culpepper J, Knowles DM, Moore PS (1994). Identification of herpesvirus-like DNA sequences in AIDS-associated Kaposi's sarcoma. *Science* 266: 1865-1869.

413. Chapman WH, Plymyer MR, Dresner ML (1990). Gonadoblastoma in an anatomically normal man: a case report and literature review. *J Urol* 144: 1472-1474.

414. Charles AK, Berry PJ, Joyce MR, Keen CE (1997). Ossifying renal tumor of infancy. *Pediatr Pathol Lab Med* 17: 332-334.

415. Charles AK, Mall S, Watson J, Berry PJ (1997). Expression of the Wilms' tumour gene WT1 in the developing human and in paediatric renal tumours: an immunohistochemical study. *Mol Pathol* 50: 138-144.

416. Charny CK, Glick RD, Genega EM, Meyers PA, Reuter VE, La Quaglia MP (2000). Ewing's sarcoma/primitive neuroectodermal tumor of the ureter: a case report and review of the literature. *J Pediatr Surg* 35: 1356-1358.

417. Chaubert P, Guillou L, Kurt AM, Bertholet MM, Metthez G, Leisinger HJ, Bosman F, Shaw P (1997). Frequent p16INK4 (MTS1) gene inactivation in testicular germ cell tumors. *Am J Pathol* 151: 859-865.

418. Chauhan RD, Gingrich JR, Eltorky M, Steiner MS (2001). The natural progression of adenocarcinoma of the epididymis. *J Urol* 166: 608-610.

419. Cheever AW (1978). Schistosomiasis and neoplasia. *J Natl Cancer Inst* 61: 13-18.

420. Chemeris GI (1989). [Effect of sex hormones on the induction of renal capsule angiosarcomas in mice]. *Eksp Onkol* 11: 71-72.

421. Chen F, Slife L, Kishida T, Mulvihill JJ, Tisherman SE, Zbar B (1996). Genotype-phenotype correlation in von Hippel-Lindau disease: identification of a mutation associated with VHL type 2A. *J Med Genet* 33: 716-717.

422. Chen YH, Wong TW, Lee JY (2001). Depigmented genital extramammary Paget's disease: a possible histogenetic link to Toker's clear cells and clear cell papulosis. *J Cutan Pathol* 28: 105-108.

423. Cheng L, Cheville JC, Neumann RM, Bostwick DG (1999). Natural history of urothelial dysplasia of the bladder. *Am J Surg Pathol* 23: 443-447.

424. Cheng L, Cheville JC, Neumann RM, Bostwick DG (2000). Flat intraepithelial lesions of the urinary bladder. *Cancer* 88: 625-631.

425. Cheng L, Cheville JC, Neumann RM, Leibovich BC, Egan KS, Spotts BE, Bostwick DG (1999). Survival of patients with carcinoma in situ of the urinary bladder. *Cancer* 85: 2469-2474.

426. Cheng L, Darson M, Cheville JC, Neumann RM, Zincke H, Nehra A, Bostwick DG (1999). Urothelial papilloma of the bladder. Clinical and biologic implications. *Cancer* 86: 2098-2101.

427. Cheng L, Henley JD, Cummings OW, Foster RS, Ulbright TM (2001). Cystic trophoblastic tumor: a favorable histologic lesion in post-chemotherapy resections of patients with testicular germ cell tumors. *Mod Pathol* 14: 104.

428. Cheng L, Leibovich BC, Cheville JC, Ramnani DM, Sebo TJ, Nehra A, Malek RS, Zincke H, Bostwick DG (2000). Squamous papilloma of the urinary tract is unrelated to condyloma acuminata. *Cancer* 88: 1679-1686.

429. Cheng L, Leibovich BC, Cheville JC, Ramnani DM, Sebo TJ, Neumann RM, Nascimento AG, Zincke H, Bostwick DG (2000). Paraganglioma of the urinary bladder: can biologic potential be predicted? *Cancer* 88: 844-852.

430. Cheng L, Montironi R, Bostwick DG (1999). Villous adenoma of the urinary tract: a report of 23 cases, including 8 with coexistent adenocarcinoma. *Am J Surg Pathol* 23: 764-771.

431. Cheng L, Nascimento AG, Neumann RM, Nehra A, Cheville JC, Ramnani DM, Leibovich BC, Bostwick DG (1999). Hemangioma of the urinary bladder. *Cancer* 86: 498-504.

432. Cheng L, Neumann RM, Bostwick DG (1999). Papillary urothelial neoplasms of low malignant potential. Clinical and biologic implications. *Cancer* 86: 2102-2108.

433. Cheng L, Neumann RM, Nehra A, Spotts BE, Weaver AL, Bostwick DG (2000). Cancer heterogeneity and its biologic implications in the grading of urothelial carcinoma. *Cancer* 88: 1663-1670.

434. Cheng L, Scheithauer BW, Leibovich BC, Ramnani DM, Cheville JC, Bostwick DG (1999). Neurofibroma of the urinary bladder. *Cancer* 86: 505-513.

435. Cheng L, Weaver AL, Neumann RM, Scherer BG, Bostwick DG (1999). Substaging of T1 bladder carcinoma based on the depth of invasion as measured by micrometer: A new proposal. *Cancer* 86: 1035-1043.

436. Cher ML, MacGrogan D, Bookstein R, Brown JA, Jenkins RB, Jensen RH (1994). Comparative genomic hybridization, allelic imbalance, and fluorescence in situ hybridization on chromosome 8 in prostate cancer. *Genes Chromosomes Cancer* 11: 153-162.

437. Chern HD, Becich MJ, Persad RA, Romkes M, Smith P, Collins C, Li YH, Branch RA (1996). Clonal analysis of human recurrent superficial bladder cancer by immunohistochemistry of P53 and retinoblastoma proteins. *J Urol* 156: 1846-1849.

438. Cherukuri SV, Johenning PW, Ram MD (1977). Systemic effects of hypernephroma. *Urology* 10: 93-97.

439. Cheung AN, Chan AC, Chung LP, Chan TM, Cheng IK, Chan KW (1998). Post-transplantation lymphoproliferative disorder of donor origin in a sex-mismatched renal allograft as proven by chromosome in situ hybridization. *Mod Pathol* 11: 99-102.

440. Cheville JC (1998). Urothelial carcinoma of the prostate: an immunohistochemical comparison with high grade prostatic adenocarcinoma and review of the literature. *J Urol Pathol* 9: 141-154.

441. Cheville JC, Blute ML, Zincke H, Lohse CM, Weaver AL (2001). Stage pT1 conventional (clear cell) renal cell carcinoma: pathological features associated with cancer specific survival. *J Urol* 166: 453-456.

442. Cheville JC, Dundore PA, Bostwick DG, Lieber MM, Batts KP, Sebo TJ, Farrow GM (1998). Transitional cell carcinoma of the prostate: clinicopathologic study of 50 cases. *Cancer* 82: 703-707.

443. Cheville JC, Dundore PA, Nascimento AG, Meneses M, Kleer E, Farrow GM, Bostwick DG (1995). Leiomyosarcoma of the prostate. Report of 23 cases. *Cancer* 76: 1422-1427.

444. Cheville JC, Rao S, Iczkowski KA, Lohse CM, Pankratz VS (2000). Cytokeratin expression in seminoma of the human testis. *Am J Clin Pathol* 113: 583-588.

445. Cheville JC, Sebo TJ, Lager DJ, Bostwick DG, Farrow GM (1998). Leydig cell tumor of the testis: a clinicopathologic, DNA content, and MIB-1 comparison of nonmetastasizing and metastasizing tumors. *Am J Surg Pathol* 22: 1361-1367.

446. Cheville JC, Tindall D, Boelter C, Jenkins R, Lohse CM, Pankratz VS, Sebo TJ, Davis B, Blute ML (2002). Metastatic prostate carcinoma to bone: clinical and pathologic features associated with cancer-specific survival. *Cancer* 95: 1028-1036.

447. Cheville JC, Wu K, Sebo TJ, Cheng L, Riehle D, Lohse CM, Shane V (2000). Inverted urothelial papilloma: is ploidy, MIB-1 proliferative activity, or p53 protein accumulation predictive of urothelial carcinoma? *Cancer* 88: 632-636.

448. Chin KC, Perry GJ, Dowling JP, Thomson NM (1999). Primary T-cell-rich B-cell lymphoma in the kidney presenting with acute renal failure and a second malignancy. *Pathology* 31: 325-327.

449. Chin NW, Marinescu AM, Fani K (1992). Composite adenocarcinoma and carcinoid tumor of urinary bladder. *Urology* 40: 249-252.

450. Chin W, Fay R, Ortega P (1986). Malignant fibrous histiocytoma of prostate. *Urology* 27: 363-365.

451. Chiou RK, Limas C, Lange PH (1985). Hemangiosarcoma of the seminal vesicle: case report and literature review. *J Urol* 134: 371-373.

452. Chiu TY, Huang HS, Lai MK, Chen J, Hsieh TS, Chueh SC (1998). Penile cancer in Taiwan—20 years' experience at National Taiwan University Hospital. *J Formos Med Assoc* 97: 673-678.

453. Choi H, Almagro UA, McManus JT, Norback DH, Jacobs SC (1983). Renal oncocytoma. A clinicopathologic study. *Cancer* 51: 1887-1896.

454. Choi H, Lamb S, Pintar K, Jacobs SC (1984). Primary signet-ring cell carcinoma of the urinary bladder. *Cancer* 53: 1985-1990.

455. Choi YL, Song SY (2001). Cytologic clue of so-called nodular histiocytic hyperplasia of the pleura. *Diagn Cytopathol* 24: 256-259.

456. Chor PJ, Gaum LD, Young RH (1993). Clear cell adenocarcinoma of the urinary bladder: report of a case of probable mullerian origin. *Mod Pathol* 6: 225-228.

457. Chow NH, Tzai TS, Lin SN, Chan SH, Tang MJ (1993). Reappraisal of the biological role of epidermal growth factor receptor in transitional cell carcinoma. *Eur Urol* 24: 140-143.

458. Chow WH, Gridley G, Fraumeni JFJr, Jarvholm B (2000). Obesity, hypertension, and the risk of kidney cancer in men. *N Engl J Med* 343: 1305-1311.

459. Chowdhury PR, Tsuda N, Anami M, Hayashi T, Iseki M, Kishikawa M, Matsuya F, Kanetake H, Saito Y (1996). A histopathologic and immunohistochemical study of small nodules of renal angiomyolipoma: a comparison of small nodules with angiomyolipoma. *Mod Pathol* 9: 1081-1088.

460. Christensen TE, Ladefoged J (1979). [Uroepithelial tumors in patients with contracted kidneys and massive abuse of analgesics (phenacetin)]. *Ugeskr Laeger* 141: 3522-3524.

461. Christensen WN, Partin AW, Walsh PC, Epstein JI (1990). Pathologic findings in clinical stage A2 prostate cancer. Relation of tumor volume, grade, and location to pathologic stage. *Cancer* 65: 1021-1027.

462. Christensen WN, Steinberg G, Walsh PC, Epstein JI (1991). Prostatic duct adenocarcinoma. Findings at radical prostatectomy. *Cancer* 67: 2118-2124.

463. Christiano AP, Yang X, Gerber GS (1999). Malignant transformation of renal angiomyolipoma. *J Urol* 161: 1900-1901.

464. Chu PG, Weiss LM (2001). Cytokeratin 14 immunoreactivity distinguishes oncocytic tumour from its renal mimics: an immunohistochemical study of 63 cases. *Histopathology* 39: 455-462.

465. Chuang GS, Martinez-Mir A, Horev L, Glaser B, Geyer A, Landau M, Waldman A, Gordon D, Spelman LJ, Hatzibougias I, Engler DE, Cserhalmi-Friedman PB, Green JS, Garcia Muret MP, Prieto Cid M, Brenner S, Sprecher E, Christiano AM, Zlotogorski A (2003). Germline fumarate hydratase mutations and evidence for a founder mutation underlying multiple cutaneous and uterine leiomyomata. *The American Journal of Human Genetics* 73 (Supplement): 577.

466. Cibas ES, Goss GA, Kulke MH, Demetri GD, Fletcher CD (2001). Malignant epithelioid angiomyolipoma ('sarcoma ex angiomyolipoma') of the kidney: a case report and review of the literature. *Am J Surg Pathol* 25: 121-126.

467. Cina SJ, Epstein JI (1997). Adenocarcinoma of the prostate with atrophic features. *Am J Surg Pathol* 21: 289-295.

468. Cina SJ, Epstein JI, Endrizzi JM, Harmon WJ, Seay TM, Schoenberg MP (2001). Correlation of cystoscopic impression with histologic diagnosis of biopsy specimens of the bladder. *Hum Pathol* 32: 630-637.

469. Cina SJ, Lancaster-Weiss KJ, Lecksell K, Epstein JI (2001). Correlation of Ki-67 and p53 with the new World Health Organization/International Society of Urological Pathology Classification System for Urothelial Neoplasia. *Arch Pathol Lab Med* 125: 646-651.

470. Civantos F, Marcial MA, Banks ER, Ho CK, Speights VO, Drew PA, Murphy WM, Soloway MS (1995). Pathology of androgen deprivation therapy in prostate carcinoma. A comparative study of 173 patients. *Cancer* 75: 1634-1641.

471. Clark J, Lu YJ, Sidhar SK, Parker C, Gill S, Smedley D, Hamoudi R, Linehan WM, Shipley J, Cooper CS (1997). Fusion of splicing factor genes PSF and NonO (p54nrb) to the TFE3 gene in papillary renal cell carcinoma. *Oncogene* 15: 2233-2239.

472. Clasen S, Schulz WA, Gerharz CD, Grimm MO, Christoph F, Schmitz-Drager BJ (1998). Frequent and heterogeneous expression of cyclin-dependent kinase inhibitor WAF1/p21 protein and mRNA in urothelial carcinoma. *Br J Cancer* 77: 515-521.

473. Clemente Ramos LM, Garcia Gonzalez R, Burgos Revilla FJ, Maganto Pavon E, Fernandez Canadas S, Blazquez Gomez J, Carrera Puerta C, Escudero Barrilero A (1998). [Hybrid tumor of the penis: is this denomination correct?]. *Arch Esp Urol* 51: 821-823.

474. Clifford SC, Prowse AH, Affara NA, Buys CH, Maher ER (1998). Inactivation of the von Hippel-Lindau (VHL) tumour suppressor gene and allelic losses at chromosome arm 3p in primary renal cell carcinoma: evidence for a VHL-independent pathway in clear cell renal tumourigenesis. *Genes Chromosomes Cancer* 22: 200-209.

475. Cochand-Priollet B, Molinie V, Bougaran J, Bouvier R, Dauge-Geffroy MC, Deslignieres S, Fournet JC, Gros P, Lesourd A, Saint-Andre JP, Toublanc M, Vieillefond A, Wassef M, Fontaine A, Groleau L (1997). Renal chromophobe cell carcinoma and oncocytoma. A comparative morphologic, histochemical, and immunohistochemical study of 124 cases. *Arch Pathol Lab Med* 121: 1081-1086.

476. Cohen AJ, Li FP, Berg S, Marchetto DJ, Tsai S, Jacobs SC, Brown RS (1979). Hereditary renal-cell carcinoma associated with a chromosomal translocation. *N Engl J Med* 301: 592-595.

477. Cohen J, Diamond J (1953). Leontiasis ossea, slipped epiphyses and granulosa cell tumor of the testis with renal disease: report of a case with autopsy findings. *Arch Pathol* 56: 488-500.

478. Cohen RJ, Glezerson G, Haffejee Z (1991). Neuro-endocrine cells—a new prognostic parameter in prostate cancer. *Br J Urol* 68: 258-262.

479. Cohen RJ, McNeal JE, Baillie T (2000). Patterns of differentiation and proliferation in intraductal carcinoma of the prostate: significance for cancer progression. *Prostate* 43: 11-19.

480. Colby TV (1980). Carcinoid tumor of the bladder. A case report. *Arch Pathol Lab Med* 104: 199-200.

481. Coleman MP, Esteve J, Damiecki P, Arslan A, Renard H (1993). Trends in cancer incidence and mortality. *IARC Sci Publ* 121 1-806.

482. Collins DH, Symington T (1964). Sertoli-cell tumor. *Br J Urol* 36: 52-61.

483. Collins GN, Lee RJ, McKelvie GB, Rogers AC, Hehir M (1993). Relationship between prostate specific antigen, prostate volume and age in the benign prostate. *Br J Urol* 71: 445-450.

484. Comiter CV, Kibel AS, Richie JP, Nucci MR, Renshaw AA (1998). Prognostic features of teratomas with malignant transformation: a clinicopathological study of 21 cases. *J Urol* 159: 859-863.

485. Congregado Ruiz B, Campoy Martinez P, Luque Barona R, Garcia Ramos JB, Perez Perez M, Soltero Gonzalez A (2001). [Fibroepithelial polyp of the urethra in a young woman]. *Actas Urol Esp* 25: 377-379.

486. Contractor H, Zariwala M, Bugert P, Zeisler J, Kovacs G (1997). Mutation of the p53 tumour suppressor gene occurs preferentially in the chromophobe type of renal cell tumour. *J Pathol* 181: 136-139.

487. Cook JA, Oliver K, Mueller RF, Sampson J (1996). A cross sectional study of renal involvement in tuberous sclerosis. *J Med Genet* 33: 480-484.

488. Cook PJ, Doll R, Fellingham SA (1969). A mathematical model for the age distribution of cancer in man. *Int J Cancer* 4: 93-112.

489. Coombs LM, Pigott DA, Sweeney E, Proctor AJ, Eydmann ME, Parkinson C, Knowles MA (1991). Amplification and over-expression of c-erbB-2 in transitional cell carcinoma of the urinary bladder. *Br J Cancer* 63: 601-608.

490. Coovadia YM (1978). Primary testicular tumours among White, Black and Indian patients. *S Afr Med J* 54: 351-352.

491. Copeland JN, Amin MB, Humphrey PA, Tamboli P, Ro JY, Gal AA (2002). The morphologic spectrum of metastatic prostatic adenocarcinoma to the lung: special emphasis on histologic features overlapping with other pulmonary neoplasms. *Am J Clin Pathol* 117: 552-557.

492. Coppes MJ, Arnold M, Beckwith JB, Ritchey ML, D'Angio GJ, Green DM, Breslow NE (1999). Factors affecting the risk of contralateral Wilms tumor development: a report from the National Wilms Tumor Study Group. *Cancer* 85: 1616-1625.

493. Coppes MJ, Haber DA, Grundy PE (1994). Genetic events in the development of Wilms' tumor. *N Engl J Med* 331: 586-590.

494. Cordon-Cardo C, Cote RJ, Sauter G (2000). Genetic and molecular markers of urothelial premalignancy and malignancy. *Scand J Urol Nephrol Suppl* 205: 82-93.

495. Cordon-Cardo C, Dalbagni G, Saez GT, Oliva MR, Zhang ZF, Rosai J, Reuter VE, Pellicer A (1994). p53 mutations in human bladder cancer: genotypic versus phenotypic patterns. *Int J Cancer* 56: 347-353.

496. Cordon-Cardo C, Koff A, Drobnjak M, Capodieci P, Osman I, Millard SS, Gaudin PB, Fazzari M, Zhang ZF, Massague J, Scher HI (1998). Distinct altered patterns of p27KIP1 gene expression in benign prostatic hyperplasia and prostatic carcinoma. *J Natl Cancer Inst* 90: 1284-1291.

497. Cordon-Cardo C, Reuter VE (1997). Alterations of tumor suppressor genes in bladder cancer. *Semin Diagn Pathol* 14: 123-132.

498. Cordon-Cardo C, Wartinger D, Petrylak D, Dalbagni G, Fair WR, Fuks Z, Reuter VE (1992). Altered expression of the retinoblastoma gene product: prognostic indicator in bladder cancer. *J Natl Cancer Inst* 84: 1251-1256.

499. Corica FA, Husmann DA, Churchill BM, Young RH, Pacelli A, Lopez-Beltran A, Bostwick DG (1997). Intestinal metaplasia is not a strong risk factor for bladder cancer: study of 53 cases with long-term follow-up. *Urology* 50: 427-431.

500. Corless CL, Kibel AS, Iliopoulos O, Kaelin WGJr (1997). Immunostaining of the von Hippel-Lindau gene product in normal and neoplastic human tissues. *Hum Pathol* 28: 459-464.

501. Cortes D, Visfeldt J, Moller H, Thorup J (1999). Testicular neoplasia in cryptorchid boys at primary surgery: case series. *BMJ* 319: 888-889.

502. Corti B, Carella R, Gabusi E, D'Errico A, Martorana G, Grigioni WF (2001). Solitary fibrous tumour of the urinary bladder with expression of bcl-2, CD34, and insulin-like growth factor type II. *Eur Urol* 39: 484-488.
503. Cosgrove DJ, Monga M (2000). Inverted papilloma as a cause of high-grade ureteral obstruction. *Urology* 56: 856.
504. Cote RJ, Dunn MD, Chatterjee SJ, Stein JP, Shi SR, Tran QC, Hu SX, Xu HJ, Groshen S, Taylor CR, Skinner DG, Benedict WF (1998). Elevated and absent pRb expression is associated with bladder cancer progression and has cooperative effects with p53. *Cancer Res* 58: 1090-1094.
505. Cote RJ, Esrig D, Groshen S, Jones PA, Skinner DG (1997). p53 and treatment of bladder cancer. *Nature* 385: 123-125.
506. Coup AJ (1988). Angiosarcoma of the ureter. *Br J Urol* 62: 275-276.
507. Cramer BM, Schlegel EA, Thueroff JW (1991). MR imaging in the differential diagnosis of scrotal and testicular disease. *Radiographics* 11: 9-21.
508. Creager AJ, Maia DM, Funkhouser WK (1998). Epstein-Barr virus-associated renal smooth muscle neoplasm: report of a case with review of the literature. *Arch Pathol Lab Med* 122: 277-281.
509. Crellin AM, Hudson BV, Bennett MH, Harland S, Hudson GV (1993). Non-Hodgkin's lymphoma of the testis. *Radiother Oncol* 27: 99-106.
510. Crist WM, Anderson JR, Meza JL, Fryer C, Raney RB, Ruymann FB, Breneman J, Qualman SJ, Wiener E, Wharam M, Lobe T, Webber B, Maurer HM, Donaldson SS (2001). Intergroup rhabdomyosarcoma study-IV: results for patients with nonmetastatic disease. *J Clin Oncol* 19: 3091-3102.
511. Crook J, Malone S, Perry G, Bahadur Y, Robertson S, Abdolell M (2000). Postradiotherapy prostate biopsies: what do they really mean? Results for 498 patients. *Int J Radiat Oncol Biol Phys* 48: 355-367.
512. Crotty TB, Farrow GM, Lieber MM (1995). Chromophobe cell renal carcinoma: clinicopathological features of 50 cases. *J Urol* 154: 964-967.
513. Crotty TB, Lawrence KM, Moertel CA, Bartelt DHJr, Batts KP, Dewald GW, Farrow GM, Jenkins RB (1992). Cytogenetic analysis of six renal oncocytomas and a chromophobe cell renal carcinoma. Evidence that -Y, -1 may be a characteristic anomaly in renal oncocytomas. *Cancer Genet Cytogenet* 61: 61-66.
514. Cubilla AL (1995). Carcinoma of the penis. *Mod Pathol* 8: 116-118.
515. Cubilla AL (2002). Caracteristicas clinicas y patologicas del carcinoma peneal: 10 años de estudios investigativos en el Paraguay. *Urol Integr y de Invest (Spain)* 7: 113-135.
516. Cubilla AL, Ayala MT, Barreto JE, Bellasai JG, Noel JC (1996). Surface adenosquamous carcinoma of the penis. A report of three cases. *Am J Surg Pathol* 20: 156-160.
517. Cubilla AL, Barreto J, Caballero C, Ayala G, Riveros M (1993). Pathologic features of epidermoid carcinoma of the penis. A prospective study of 66 cases. *Am J Surg Pathol* 17: 753-763.
518. Cubilla AL, Barreto JE, Ayala G (1999). Penis. In: *Diagnostic Surgical Pathology*, SS Sternberg, ed. 3rd Edition. Lippincott-Raven: New York.
519. Cubilla AL, Caballero C, Piris A, Reuter V, Alcabes P (2000). Prognostic Index (PI): A novel method to predict mortality in squamous cell carcinoma of the penis. *Lab Invest* 80: 97A.
520. Cubilla AL, Piris A, Pfannl R, Rodriguez I, Aguero F, Young RH (2001). Anatomic levels: important landmarks in penectomy specimens: a detailed anatomic and histologic study based on examination of 44 cases. *Am J Surg Pathol* 25: 1091-1094.
521. Cubilla AL, Reuter V, Velazquez E, Piris A, Saito S, Young RH (2001). Histologic classification of penile carcinoma and its relation to outcome in 61 patients with primary resection. *Int J Surg Pathol* 9: 111-120.
522. Cubilla AL, Reuter VE, Gregoire L, Ayala G, Ocampos S, Lancaster WD, Fair W (1998). Basaloid squamous cell carcinoma: a distinctive human papilloma virus-related penile neoplasm: a report of 20 cases. *Am J Surg Pathol* 22: 755-761.
523. Cubilla AL, Velazques EF, Reuter VE, Oliva E, Mihm MCJr, Young RH (2000). Warty (condylomatous) squamous cell carcinoma of the penis: a report of 11 cases and proposed classification of 'verruciform' penile tumors. *Am J Surg Pathol* 24: 505-512.
524. Cubilla AL, Velazquez EF (2001). Pseudohyperplastic superficial squamous cell carcinoma of the foreskin associated with lichen sclerosus: a distinctive clinico pathologic entity. Report of 10 cases. *Mod Pathol* 14: 105A.
525. Cuesta Alcala JA, Solchaga Martinez A, Caballero Martinez MC, Gomez Dorronsoro M, Pascual Piedrola I, Ripa Saldias L, Aldave Villanueva J, Arrondo Arrondo JL, Grasa Lanau V, Ponz Gonzalez M, Ipiens Aznar A (2001). [Primary neuroectodermal tumor (PNET) of the kidney: 26 cases. Current status of its diagnosis and treatment]. *Arch Esp Urol* 54: 1081-1093.
526. Cumming JA, Ritchie AW, Goodman CM, McIntyre MA, Chisholm GD (1990). De-differentiation with time in prostate cancer and the influence of treatment on the course of the disease. *Br J Urol* 65: 271-274.
527. Cummings OW, Ulbright TM, Eble JN, Roth LM (1994). Spermatocytic seminoma: an immunohistochemical study. *Hum Pathol* 25: 54-59.
528. Cummings OW, Ulbright TM, Young RH, del Tos AP, Fletcher CD, Hull MT (1997). Desmoplastic small round cell tumors of the paratesticular region. A report of six cases. *Am J Surg Pathol* 21: 219-225.
529. Cupp MR, Malek RS, Goellner JR, Espy MJ, Smith TF (1996). Detection of human papillomavirus DNA in primary squamous cell carcinoma of the male urethra. *Urology* 48: 551-555.
530. Curry NS, Chung CJ, Potts W, Bissada N (1993). Isolated lymphoma of genitourinary tract and adrenals. *Urology* 41: 494-498.
531. Cutler SJ, Henry NM, Friedell GH (1982). Longitudinal study of patients with bladder cancer: factors associated with disease recurrence and progression. In: *Bladder Cancer*, WW Bonney, GR Prout, eds. William and Wilkins: Baltimore, pp. 35-46.
532. Czene K, Lichtenstein P, Hemminki K (2002). Environmental and heritable causes of cancer among 9.6 million individuals in the Swedish Family-Cancer Database. *Int J Cancer* 99: 260-266.
533. Czerniak B, Cohen GL, Etkind P, Deitch D, Simmons H, Herz F, Koss LG (1992). Concurrent mutations of coding and regulatory sequences of the Ha-ras gene in urinary bladder carcinomas. *Hum Pathol* 23: 1199-1204.
534. Czerniak B, Li L, Chaturvedi V, Ro JY, Johnston DA, Hodges S, Benedict WF (2000). Genetic modeling of human urinary bladder carcinogenesis. *Genes Chromosomes Cancer* 27: 392-402.
535. Czernobilsky H, Czernobilsky B, Schneider HG, Franke WW, Ziegler R (1985). Characterization of a feminizing testicular Leydig cell tumor by hormonal profile, immunocytochemistry, and tissue culture. *Cancer* 56: 1667-1676.
536. D'Amico AV, Whittington R, Malkowicz SB, Schultz D, Schnall M, Tomaszewski JE, Wein A (1995). A multivariate analysis of clinical and pathological factors that predict for prostate specific antigen failure after radical prostatectomy for prostate cancer. *J Urol* 154: 131-138.
537. Da'as N, Polliack A, Cohen Y, Amir G, Darmon D, Kleinman Y, Goldfarb AW, Ben Yehuda D (2001). Kidney involvement and renal manifestations in non-Hodgkin's lymphoma and lymphocytic leukemia: a retrospective study in 700 patients. *Eur J Haematol* 67: 158-164.
538. Dahms SE, Hohenfellner M, Linn JF, Eggersmann C, Haupt G, Thuroff JW (1999). Retrovesical mass in men: pitfalls of differential diagnosis. *J Urol* 161: 1244-1248.
539. Dahnert WF, Hamper UM, Eggleston JC, Walsh PC, Sanders RC (1986). Prostatic evaluation by transrectal sonography with histopathologic correlation: the echopenic appearance of early carcinoma. *Radiology* 158: 97-102.
540. Dalbagni G, Herr HW, Reuter VE (2002). Impact of a second transurethral resection on the staging of T1 bladder cancer. *Urology* 60: 822-824.
541. Dalbagni G, Ren ZP, Herr H, Cordon-Cardo C, Reuter V (2001). Genetic alterations in tp53 in recurrent urothelial cancer: a longitudinal study. *Clin Cancer Res* 7: 2797-2801.
542. Dalbagni G, Zhang ZF, Lacombe L, Herr HW (1998). Female urethral carcinoma: an analysis of treatment outcome and a plea for a standardized management strategy. *Br J Urol* 82: 835-841.
543. Dalbagni G, Zhang ZF, Lacombe L, Herr HW (1999). Male urethral carcinoma: analysis of treatment outcome. *Urology* 53: 1126-1132.
544. Dalesio O, Schulman CC, Sylvester R, de Pauw M, Robinson M, Denis L, Smith P, Viggiano G (1983). Prognostic factors in superficial bladder tumors. A study of the European Organization for Research on Treatment of Cancer: Genitourinary Tract Cancer Cooperative Group. *J Urol* 129: 730-733.
545. Dalkin B, Zaontz MR (1989). Rhabdomyosarcoma of the penis in children. *J Urol* 141: 908-909.
546. Dalkin BL, Ahmann FR, Kopp JB (1993). Prostate specific antigen levels in men older than 50 years without clinical evidence of prostatic carcinoma. *J Urol* 150: 1837-1839.
547. Dalle JH, Mechinaud F, Michon J, Gentet JC, de Lumley L, Rubie H, Schmitt C, Patte C (2001). Testicular disease in childhood B-cell non-Hodgkin's lymphoma: the French Society of Pediatric Oncology experience. *J Clin Oncol* 19: 2397-2403.
548. Damjanov I (1997). Tumors of the testis and epididymis. In: *Urological Pathology*, WM Murphy, ed. 2nd Edition. WB Saunders: Philadelphia, pp. 385-386.
549. Damjanov I, Niejadlik DC, Rabuffo JV, Donadio JA (1980). Cribriform and sclerosing seminoma devoid of lymphoid infiltrates. *Arch Pathol Lab Med* 104: 527-530.
550. Damjanov I, Osborn M, Miettinen M (1990). Keratin 7 is a marker for a subset of trophoblastic cells in human germ cell tumors. *Arch Pathol Lab Med* 114: 81-83.
551. Dandekar NP, Dalal AV, Tongaonkar HB, Kamat MR (1997). Adenocarcinoma of bladder. *Eur J Surg Oncol* 23: 157-160.
552. Das AK, Carson CC, Bolick D, Paulson DF (1990). Primary carcinoma of the upper urinary tract. Effect of primary and secondary therapy on survival. *Cancer* 66: 1919-1923.
553. Dash A, Sanda MG, Yu M, Taylor JM, Fecko A, Rubin MA (2002). Prostate cancer involving the bladder neck: recurrence-free survival and implications for AJCC staging modification. American Joint Committee on Cancer. *Urology* 60: 276-280.
554. Datta SN, Allen GM, Evans R, Vaughton KC, Lucas MG (2002). Urinary tract ultrasonography in the evaluation of haematuria—a report of over 1,000 cases. *Ann R Coll Surg Engl* 84: 203-205.
555. Daugaard G, Rorth M, von der Maase H, Skakkebaek NE (1992). Management of extragonadal germ-cell tumors and the significance of bilateral testicular biopsies. *Ann Oncol* 3: 283-289.
556. Daugaard G, von der Maase H, Olsen J, Rorth M, Skakkebaek NE (1987). Carcinoma-in-situ testis in patients with assumed extragonadal germ-cell tumours. *Lancet* 2: 528-530.
557. Davidson AJ, Choyke PL, Hartman DS, Davis CJJr (1995). Renal medullary carcinoma associated with sickle cell trait: radiologic findings. *Radiology* 195: 83-85.
558. Davidson AJ, Hayes WS, Hartman DS, McCarthy WF, Davis CJJr (1993). Renal oncocytoma and carcinoma: failure of differentiation with CT. *Radiology* 186: 693-696.
559. Davidson D, Bostwick DG, Qian J, Wollan PC, Oesterling JE, Rudders RA, Siroky M, Stilmant M (1995). Prostatic intraepithelial neoplasia is a risk factor for adenocarcinoma: predictive accuracy in needle biopsies. *J Urol* 154: 1295-1299.
560. Davis CJ, Sesterhenn IA, Brinsko R (2002). Melanocytic clear cell neoplasms of the kidney. *Mod Pathol* 12: 93.
561. Davis CJJr, Barton JH, Sesterhenn IA, Mostofi FK (1995). Metanephric adenoma. Clinicopathological study of fifty patients. *Am J Surg Pathol* 19: 1101-1114.
562. Davis CJJr, Mostofi FK, Sesterhenn IA (1995). Renal medullary carcinoma. The seventh sickle cell nephropathy. *Am J Surg Pathol* 19: 1-11.
563. Davis CJJr, Mostofi FK, Sesterhenn IA, Ho CK (1991). Renal oncocytoma. Clinicopathological study of 166 patients. *J Urogen Pathol* 1: 41-52.
564. de Alava E, Ladanyi M, Rosai J, Gerald WL (1995). Detection of chimeric transcripts in desmoplastic small round cell tumor and related developmental tumors by reverse transcriptase polymerase chain reaction. A specific diagnostic assay. *Am J Pathol* 147: 1584-1591.
565. de Castro R, Campobasso P, Belloli G, Pavanello P (1993). Solitary polyp of posterior urethra in children: report on seventeen cases. *Eur J Pediatr Surg* 3: 92-96.

566. de Chiara A, van Tornout JM, Hachitanda Y, Ortega JA, Shimada H (1992). Melanotic neuroectodermal tumor of infancy. A case report of paratesticular primary with lymph node involvement. *Am J Pediatr Hematol Oncol* 14: 356-360.
567. de Graaff WE, Oosterhuis JW, de Jong B, Dam A, van Putten WL, Castedo SM, Sleijfer DT, Schraffordt Koops H (1992). Ploidy of testicular carcinoma in situ. *Lab Invest* 66: 166-168.
568. de la Torre M, Haggman MJ, Brandstedt S, Busch C (1993). Prostatic intraepithelial neoplasia and invasive carcinoma in total prostatectomy specimens: distribution, volumes and DNA ploidy. *Br J Urol* 72: 207-213.
569. de Marzo AM, Nelson WG, Meeker AK, Coffey DS (1998). Stem cell features of benign and malignant prostate epithelial cells. *J Urol* 160: 2381-2392.
570. de Nictolis M, Tommasoni S, Fabris G, Prat J (1993). Intratesticular serous cystadenoma of borderline malignancy. A pathological, histochemical and DNA content study of a case with long-term follow-up. *Virchows Arch A Pathol Anat Histopathol* 423: 221-225.
571. de Pinieux G, Glaser C, Chatelain D, Perie G, Flam T, Vieillefond A (1999). Testicular fibroma of gonadal stromal origin with minor sex cord elements: clinicopathologic and immunohistochemical study of 2 cases. *Arch Pathol Lab Med* 123: 391-394.
572. de Silva MV, Fernando MS, Abeygunasekera AM, Serozsha Goonewardene SA (1998). Prevalence of prostatic intraepithelial (PIN) in surgical resections. *Indian J Cancer* 35: 137-141.
573. de Vere White RW, Deitch AD, Daneshmand S, Blumenstein B, Lowe BA, Sagalowsky AI, Smith JAJr, Schellhammer PF, Stanisic TH, Grossman HB, Messing E, Crissman JD, Crawford ED (2000). The prognostic significance of S-phase analysis in stage Ta/T1 bladder cancer. A Southwest Oncology Group Study. *Eur Urol* 37: 595-600.
574. de Villiers EM (2001). Taxonomic classification of papillomaviruses. *Papillomavirus Report* 12: 57-63.
575. de Wit R, Sylvester R, Tsitsa C, de Mulder PH, Sleyfer DT, Bokkel Huinink WW, Kaye SB, van Oosterom AT, Boven E, Vermeylen K, Stoter G (1997). Tumour marker concentration at the start of chemotherapy is a stronger predictor of treatment failure than marker half-life: a study in patients with disseminated non-seminomatous testicular cancer. *Br J Cancer* 75: 432-435.
576. DeAntoni EP, Crawford ED, Oesterling JE, Ross CA, Berger ER, McLeod DG, Staggers F, Stone NN (1996). Age- and race-specific reference ranges for prostate-specific antigen from a large community-based study. *Urology* 48: 234-239.
577. DeBaun MR, Niemitz EL, McNeil DE, Brandenburg SA, Lee MP, Feinberg AP (2002). Epigenetic alterations of H19 and LIT1 distinguish patients with Beckwith-Wiedemann syndrome with cancer and birth defects. *Am J Hum Genet* 70: 604-611.
578. Debiec-Rychter M, Kaluzewski B, Saryusz-Wolska H, Jankowska J (1990). A case of renal lymphangioma with a karyotype 45,X,-X,i dic(7q). *Cancer Genet Cytogenet* 46: 29-33.
579. Debras B, Guillonneau B, Bougaran J, Chambon E, Vallancien G (1998). Prognostic significance of seminal vesicle invasion on the radical prostatectomy specimen. Rationale for seminal vesicle biopsies. *Eur Urol* 33: 271-277.
580. Dehner LP (1973). Intrarenal teratoma occurring in infancy: report of a case with discussion of extragonodal germ cell tumors in infancy. *J Pediatr Surg* 8: 369-378.
581. Dehner LP, Smith BH (1970). Soft tissue tumors of the penis. A clinicopathologic study of 46 cases. *Cancer* 25: 1431-1447.
582. Dekker I, Rozeboom T, Delemarre J, Dam A, Oosterhuis JW (1992). Placental-like alkaline phosphatase and DNA flow cytometry in spermatocytic seminoma. *Cancer* 69: 993-996.
583. del Mistro A, Braunstein JD, Halwer M, Koss LG (1987). Identification of human papillomavirus types in male urethral condylomata acuminata by in situ hybridization. *Hum Pathol* 18: 936-940.
584. del Vecchio MT, Lazzi S, Bruni A, Mangiavacchi P, Cevenini G, Luzi P (1998). DNA ploidy pattern in papillary renal cell carcinoma. Correlation with clinicopathological parameters and survival. *Pathol Res Pract* 194: 325-333.
585. Delahunt B, Eble JN (1997). Papillary renal cell carcinoma: a clinicopathologic and immunohistochemical study of 105 tumors. *Mod Pathol* 10: 537-544.
586. Delahunt B, Eble JN, King D, Bethwaite PB, Nacey JN, Thornton A (2000). Immunohistochemical evidence for mesothelial origin of paratesticular adenomatoid tumour. *Histopathology* 36: 109-115.
587. Delahunt B, Eble JN, McCredie MR, Bethwaite PB, Stewart JH, Bilous AM (2001). Morphologic typing of papillary renal cell carcinoma: comparison of growth kinetics and patient survival in 66 cases. *Hum Pathol* 32: 590-595.
588. Delahunt B, Eble JN, Nacey JN, Grebe SK (1999). Sarcomatoid carcinoma of the prostate: progression from adenocarcinoma is associated with p53 over-expression. *Anticancer Res* 19: 4279-4283.
589. Delahunt B, Eble JN, Nacey JN, Thornton A (2001). Immunohistochemical evidence for mesothelial origin of paratesticular adenomatoid tumour. *Histopathology* 38: 479.
590. Delahunt B, Nacey JN, Meffan PJ, Clark MG (1991). Signet ring cell adenocarcinoma of the ureter. *Br J Urol* 68: 555-556.
591. Delbello MW, Dick WH, Carter CB, Butler FO (1991). Polyclonal B cell lymphoma of renal transplant ureter induced by cyclosporine: case report. *J Urol* 146: 1613-1614.
592. Delemarre JF, Sandstedt B, Tournade MF (1984). Nephroblastoma with fibroadenomatous-like structures. *Histopathology* 8: 55-62.
593. Delgado R, de Leon Bojorge B, Albores-Saavedra J (1998). Atypical angiomyolipoma of the kidney: a distinct morphologic variant that is easily confused with a variety of malignant neoplasms. *Cancer* 83: 1581-1592.
594. Deliveliotis C, Louras G, Raptidis G, Giannakopoulos S, Kastriotis J, Kostakopoulos A (1998). Evaluation of needle biopsy in the diagnosis of prostatic carcinoma in men with prostatic intraepithelial neoplasia. *Scand J Urol Nephrol* 32: 107-110.
595. Dembitzer F, Greenebaum E (1993). Fine Needle Aspiration or Renal Paraganglioma: An Unusual Location for a Rare Tumor. *Mod Pathol* 6: 29A.
596. Demeester LJ, Farrow GM, Utz DC (1975). Inverted papillomas of the urinary bladder. *Cancer* 36: 505-513.
597. Denholm SW, Webb JN, Howard GC, Chisholm GD (1992). Basaloid carcinoma of the prostate gland: histogenesis and review of the literature. *Histopathology* 20: 151-155.
598. Denkhaus H, Crone-Munzebrock W, Huland H (1985). Noninvasive ultrasound in detecting and staging bladder carcinoma. *Urol Radiol* 7: 121-131.
599. Dennis PJ, Lewandowski AE, Rohner TJJr, Weidner WA, Mamourian AC, Stern DR (1989). Pheochromocytoma of the prostate: an unusual location. *J Urol* 141: 130-132.
600. Desai S, Lim SD, Jimenez RE, Chun T, Keane TE, McKenney JK, Zavala-Pompa A, Cohen C, Young RH, Amin MB (2000). Relationship of cytokeratin 20 and CD44 protein expression with WHO/ISUP grade in pTa and pT1 papillary urothelial neoplasia. *Mod Pathol* 13: 1315-1323.
601. Deveci MS, Deveci G, Onguru O, Kilciler M, Celasun B (2002). Testicular (gonadal stromal) fibroma: Case report and review of the literature. *Pathol Int* 52: 326-330.
602. Devesa SS, Silverman DT, McLaughlin JK, Brown CC, Connelly RR, Fraumeni JFJr (1990). Comparison of the descriptive epidemiology of urinary tract cancers. *Cancer Causes Control* 1: 133-141.
603. Devouassoux-Shisheboran M (2001). Expression of hMLH1 hMSH2 and assessment of microsatellite instability in testicular and mediastinal germ cell tumors. *Mol Hum Reprod* 7: 1099-1105.
604. Dhanasekaran SM, Barrette TR, Ghosh D, Shah R, Varambally S, Kurachi K, Pienta KJ, Rubin MA, Chinnaiyan AM (2001). Delineation of prognostic biomarkers in prostate cancer. *Nature* 412: 822-826.
605. Dharkar D, Kraft JR (1994). Paraganglioma of the spermatic cord. An incidental finding. *J Urol Pathol* 2: 89-93.
606. Dhom G (1985). Histopathology of prostate carcinoma. Diagnosis and differential diagnosis. *Pathol Res Pract* 179: 277-303.
607. Dhom G, Degro S (1982). Therapy of prostatic cancer and histopathologic follow-up. *Prostate* 3: 531-542.
608. di Pietro M, Zeman RK, Keohane M, Rosenfield AT (1983). Oat cell carcinoma metastatic to ureter. *Urology* 22: 419-420.
609. di Sant'Agnese PA (1992). Neuroendocrine differentiation in carcinoma of the prostate. Diagnostic, prognostic, and therapeutic implications. *Cancer* 70: 254-268.
610. di Sant'Agnese PA (2001). Neuroendocrine differentiation in prostatic carcinoma: an update on recent developments. *Ann Oncol* 12 Suppl 2: S135-S140.
611. di Sant'Agnese PA, Mesy Jensen KL (1987). Neuroendocrine differentiation in prostatic carcinoma. *Hum Pathol* 18: 849-856.
612. Dias P, Chen B, Dilday B, Palmer H, Hosoi H, Singh S, Wu C, Li X, Thompson J, Parham D, Qualman S, Houghton P (2000). Strong immunostaining for myogenin in rhabdomyosarcoma is significantly associated with tumors of the alveolar subclass. *Am J Pathol* 156: 399-408.
613. Dieckmann KP, Loy V (1996). Prevalence of contralateral testicular intraepithelial neoplasia in patients with testicular germ cell neoplasms. *J Clin Oncol* 14: 3126-3132.
614. Dieckmann KP, Loy V (1998). The value of the biopsy of the contralateral testis in patients with testicular germ cell cancer: the recent German experience. *APMIS* 106: 13-20.
615. Dieckmann KP, Loy V, Buttner P (1993). Prevalence of bilateral testicular germ cell tumours and early detection based on contralateral testicular intra-epithelial neoplasia. *Br J Urol* 71: 340-345.
616. Dieckmann KP, Skakkebaek NE (1999). Carcinoma in situ of the testis: review of biological and clinical features. *Int J Cancer* 83: 815-822.
617. Dietrich H, Dietrich B (2001). Ludwig Rehn (1849-1930)—pioneering findings on the aetiology of bladder tumours. *World J Urol* 19: 151-153.
618. Dijkhuizen T, van den Berg E, van den Berg A, Storkel S, de Jong B, Seitz G, Henn W (1996). Chromosomal findings and p53-mutation analysis in chromophilic renal-cell carcinomas. *Int J Cancer* 68: 47-50.
619. Dillner J, Meijer CJ, von Krogh G, Horenblas S (2000). Epidemiology of human papillomavirus infection. *Scand J Urol Nephrol Suppl* 205: 194-200.
620. Dillner J, von Krogh G, Horenblas S, Meijer CJ (2000). Etiology of squamous cell carcinoma of the penis. *Scand J Urol Nephrol Suppl* 205: 189-193.
621. Dimitriou RJ, Gattuso P, Coogan CL (2000). Carcinosarcoma of the renal pelvis. *Urology* 56: 508.
622. Dimopoulos MA, Moulopoulos LA, Costantinides C, Deliveliotis C, Pantazopoulos D, Dimopoulos C (1996). Primary renal lymphoma: a clinical and radiological study. *J Urol* 155: 1865-1867.
623. Dinney CP, Ro JY, Babaian RJ, Johnson DE (1993). Lymphoepithelioma of the bladder: a clinicopathological study of 3 cases. *J Urol* 149: 840-841.
624. Dittrich A, Vandendris M (1990). Giant leiomyoma of the kidney. *Eur Urol* 17: 93-94.
625. Djavan B, Zlotta A, Kratzik C, Remzi M, Seitz C, Schulman CC, Marberger M (1999). PSA, PSA density, PSA density of transition zone, free/total PSA ratio, and PSA velocity for early detection of prostate cancer in men with serum PSA 2.5 to 4.0 ng/mL. *Urology* 54: 517-522.
626. Dobkin SF, Brem AS, Caldamone AA (1991). Primary renal lymphoma. *J Urol* 146: 1588-1590.
627. Dobos N, Nisenbaum HL, Axel L, van Arsdalen K, Tomaszewski JE (2001). Penile leiomyosarcoma: sonographic and magnetic resonance imaging findings. *J Ultrasound Med* 20: 553-557.
628. Docimo SG, Chow NH, Steiner G, Silver RI, Rodriguez R, Kinsman S, Sidransky D, Schoenberg M (1999). Detection of adenocarcinoma by urinary microsatellite analysis after augmentation cystoplasty. *Urology* 54: 561.
629. Dockerty MD, Priestley JT (2002). Dermoid cysts of testis. *J Urol* 48: 392-400.
630. Doerfler O, Reittner P, Groell R, Ratscheck M, Trummer H, Szolar D (2001). Peripheral primitive neuroectodermal tumour of the kidney: CT findings. *Pediatr Radiol* 31: 117-119.
631. Dogra PN, Aron M, Rajeev TP, Pawar R, Nair M (1999). Primary chondrosarcoma of the prostate. *BJU Int* 83: 150-151.
632. Dominguez G, Carballido J, Silva J, Silva JM, Garcia JM, Menendez J, Provencio M, Espana P, Bonilla F (2002). p14ARF promoter hypermethylation in plasma DNA as an indicator of disease recurrence in bladder cancer patients. *Clin Cancer Res* 8: 980-985.

633. Donhuijsen K, Schmidt U, Richter HJ, Leder LD (1992). Mucoid cytoplasmic inclusions in urothelial carcinomas. *Hum Pathol* 23: 860-864.

634. Donmez T, Kale M, Ozyurek Y, Atalay H (1992). Erythrocyte sedimentation rates in patients with renal cell carcinoma. *Eur Urol* 21 Suppl 1: 51-52.

635. Douglas TH, Connelly RR, McLeod DG, Erickson SJ, Barren R3rd, Murphy GP (1995). Effect of exogenous testosterone replacement on prostate-specific antigen and prostate-specific membrane antigen levels in hypogonadal men. *J Surg Oncol* 59: 246-250.

636. Dow JA, Young JDJr (1968). Mesonephric adenocarcinoma of the bladder. *J Urol* 100: 466-469.

637. Downs TM, Kibel AS, de Wolf WC (1997). Primary lymphoma of the bladder: a unique cystoscopic appearance. *Urology* 49: 276-278.

638. Drago JR, Mostofi FK, Lee F (1992). Introductory remarks and workshop summary. *Urology* 39: 2-8.

639. Drew PA, Furman J, Civantos F, Murphy WM (1996). The nested variant of transitional cell carcinoma: an aggressive neoplasm with innocuous histology. *Mod Pathol* 9: 989-994.

640. Drew PA, Murphy WM, Civantos F, Speights VO (1996). The histogenesis of clear cell adenocarcinoma of the lower urinary tract. Case series and review of the literature. *Hum Pathol* 27: 248-252.

641. Dry SM, Renshaw AA (1998). Extensive calcium oxalate crystal deposition in papillary renal cell carcinoma: report of two cases. *Arch Pathol Lab Med* 122: 260-261.

642. Duan DR, Pause A, Burgess WH, Aso T, Chen DY, Garrett KP, Conaway RC, Conaway JW, Linehan WM, Klausner RD (1995). Inhibition of transcription elongation by the VHL tumor suppressor protein. *Science* 269: 1402-1406.

643. Duncan PR, Checa F, Gowing NF, McElwain TJ, Peckham MJ (1980). Extranodal non-Hodgkin's lymphoma presenting in the testicle: a clinical and pathologic study of 24 cases. *Cancer* 45: 1578-1584.

644. Dundore PA, Cheville JC, Nascimento AG, Farrow GM, Bostwick DG (1995). Carcinosarcoma of the prostate. Report of 21 cases. *Cancer* 76: 1035-1042.

645. Dutta SC, Smith JAJr, Shappell SB, Coffey CS, Chang SS, Cookson MS (2001). Clinical under staging of high risk nonmuscle invasive urothelial carcinoma treated with radical cystectomy. *J Urol* 166: 490-493.

646. Eble JN (1994). Cystic nephroma and cystic partially differentiated nephroblastoma: two entities or one? *Adv Anat Pathol* 1: 99-102.

647. Eble JN (1994). Spermatocytic seminoma. *Hum Pathol* 25: 1035-1042.

648. Eble JN (1996). Renal medullary carcinoma: a distinct entity emerges from the confusion of collecting duct carcinoma. *Advances Anat Pathol* 3: 233-238.

649. Eble JN (1998). Angiomyolipoma of kidney. *Semin Diagn Pathol* 15: 21-40.

650. Eble JN, Bonsib SM (1998). Extensively cystic renal neoplasms: cystic nephroma, cystic partially differentiated nephroblastoma, multilocular cystic renal cell carcinoma, and cystic hamartoma of renal pelvis. *Semin Diagn Pathol* 15: 2-20.

651. Eble JN, Epstein JI (1990). Stage A carcinoma of the prostate. In: *Pathology of the Prostate, Seminal Vesicles, and Male Urethra*, DG Bostwick, LM Roth, eds. Churchill Livingstone: New York, pp. 61-82.

652. Eble JN, Hull MT, Warfel KA, Donohue JP (1984). Malignant sex cord-stromal tumor of testis. *J Urol* 131: 546-550.

653. Eble JN, Warfel K (1991). Early human renal cortical epithelial neoplasia. *Mod Pathol* 4: 45A.

654. Eble JN, Young RH (1989). Benign and low-grade papillary lesions of the urinary bladder: a review of the papilloma-papillary carcinoma controversy, and a report of five typical papillomas. *Semin Diagn Pathol* 6: 351-371.

655. Eble JN, Young RH (1991). Stromal osseous metaplasia in carcinoma of the bladder. *J Urol* 145: 823-825.

656. Eble JN, Young RH (1997). Carcinoma of the urinary bladder: a review of its diverse morphology. *Semin Diagn Pathol* 14: 98-108.

657. Eble JN, Young RH, Storkel S, Thoenes W (1991). Osteosarcoma of the kidney: a report of three cases. *J Urogen Pathol* 1: 99-104.

658. Eckersley RJ, Sedelaar JP, Blomley MJ, Wijkstra H, de Souza NM, Cosgrove DO, de la Rosette JJ (2002). Quantitative microbubble enhanced transrectal ultrasound as a tool for monitoring hormonal treatment of prostate carcinoma. *Prostate* 51: 256-267.

659. Edelstein RA, Zietman AL, de las Morenas A, Krane RJ, Babayan RK, Dallow KC, Traish A, Moreland RB (1996). Implications of prostate micrometastases in pelvic lymph nodes: an archival tissue study. *Urology* 47: 370-375.

660. Edwards PD, Hurm RA, Jaeschke WH (1972). Conversion of cystitis glandularis to adenocarcinoma. *J Urol* 108: 568-570.

661. Edwards YH, Hopkinson DA (1979). Further characterization of the human fumarase variant, FH 2—1. *Ann Hum Genet* 43: 103-108.

662. Edwards YH, Hopkinson DA (1979). The genetic determination of fumarase isozymes in human tissues. *Ann Hum Genet* 42: 303-313.

663. Egan AJ, Bostwick DG (1997). Prediction of extraprostatic extension of prostate cancer based on needle biopsy findings: perineural invasion lacks significance on multivariate analysis. *Am J Surg Pathol* 21: 1496-1500.

664. Egan AJ, Lopez-Beltran A, Bostwick DG (1997). Prostatic adenocarcinoma with atrophic features: malignancy mimicking a benign process. *Am J Surg Pathol* 21: 931-935.

665. Egevad L (2001). Reproducibility of Gleason grading of prostate cancer can be improved by the use of reference images. *Urology* 57: 291-295.

666. Egevad L, Granfors T, Karlberg L, Bergh A, Stattin P (2002). Percent Gleason grade 4/5 as prognostic factor in prostate cancer diagnosed at transurethral resection. *J Urol* 168: 509-513.

667. Egevad L, Granfors T, Karlberg L, Bergh A, Stattin P (2002). Prognostic value of the Gleason score in prostate cancer. *BJU Int* 89: 538-542.

668. Egevad L, Norlen BJ, Norberg M (2001). The value of multiple core biopsies for predicting the Gleason score of prostate cancer. *BJU Int* 88: 716-721.

669. Ehara H, Takahashi Y, Saitoh A, Kawada Y, Shimokawa K, Kanemura T (1997). Clear cell melanoma of the renal pelvis presenting as a primary tumor. *J Urol* 157: 634.

670. Einstein MH (2001). Persistent human papillomavirus infection: definitions and clinical implications. *Papillomavirus Report* 12: 119-123.

671. Eisenmenger M, Lang S, Donner G, Kratzik C, Marberger M (1993). Epidermoid cysts of the testis: organ-preserving surgery following diagnosis by ultrasonography. *Br J Urol* 72: 955-957.

672. Ejeskar K, Sjoberg RM, Abel F, Kogner P, Ambros PF, Martinsson T (2001). Fine mapping of a tumour suppressor candidate gene region in 1p36.2-3, commonly deleted in neuroblastomas and germ cell tumours. *Med Pediatr Oncol* 36: 61-66.

673. Ekfors TO, Aho HJ, Kekomaki M (1985). Malignant rhabdoid tumor of the prostatic region. Immunohistological and ultrastructural evidence for epithelial origin. *Virchows Arch A Pathol Anat Histopathol* 406: 381-388.

674. el-Naggar AK, Batsakis JG, Wang G, Lee MS (1993). PCR-based RFLP screening of the commonly deleted 3p loci in renal cortical neoplasms. *Diagn Mol Pathol* 2: 269-276.

675. el-Naggar AK, Ro JY, Ensign LG (1993). Papillary renal cell carcinoma: clinical implication of DNA content analysis. *Hum Pathol* 24: 316-321.

676. el-Naggar AK, Ro JY, McLemore D, Ayala AG, Batsakis JG (1992). DNA ploidy in testicular germ cell neoplasms. Histogenetic and clinical implications. *Am J Surg Pathol* 16: 611-618.

677. el-Naggar AK, Troncoso P, Ordonez NG (1995). Primary renal carcinoid tumor with molecular abnormality characteristic of conventional renal cell neoplasms. *Diagn Mol Pathol* 4: 48-53.

678. el Aaser AA, el Merzabani MM, Higgy NA, el Habet AE (1982). A study on the etiological factors of bilharzial bladder cancer in Egypt. 6. The possible role of urinary bacteria. *Tumori* 68: 23-28.

679. el Aaser AA, el Merzabani MM, Higgy NA, Kader MM (1979). A study on the aetiological factors of bilharzial bladder cancer in Egypt. 3. Urinary beta-glucuronidase. *Eur J Cancer* 15: 573-583.

680. el Bolkainy MN, Mokhtar NM, Ghoneim MA, Hussein MH (1981). The impact of schistosomiasis on the pathology of bladder carcinoma. *Cancer* 48: 2643-2648.

681. el Rifai W, Kamel D, Larramendy ML, Shoman S, Gad Y, Baithun S, el Awady M, Eissa S, Khaled H, Soloneski S, Sheaff M, Knuutila S (2000). DNA copy number changes in Schistosoma-associated and non-Schistosoma-associated bladder cancer. *Am J Pathol* 156: 871-878.

682. el Sebai I, Sherif M, el Bolkainy MN, Mansour MA, Ghoneim MA (1974). Verrucose squamous carcinoma of bladder. *Urology* 4: 407-410.

683. el Sewedi SM, Arafa A, Abdel-Aal G, Mostafa MH (1978). The activities of urinary alpha-esterases in bilharziasis and their possible role in the diagnosis of bilharzial bladder cancer in Egypt. *Trans R Soc Trop Med Hyg* 72: 525-528.

684. el Sharkawi A, Murphy J (1996). Primary penile lymphoma: the case for combined modality therapy. *Clin Oncol (R Coll Radiol)* 8: 334-335.

685. Elbadawi A, Batchvarov MM, Linke CA (1979). Intratesticular papillary mucinous cystadenocarcinoma. *Urology* 14: 280-284.

686. Elbahnasy AM, Hoenig DM, Shalhav A, McDougall EM, Clayman RV (1998). Laparoscopic staging of bladder tumor: concerns about port site metastases. *J Endourol* 12: 55-59.

687. Elem B, Purohit R (1983). Carcinoma of the urinary bladder in Zambia. A quantitative estimation of Schistosoma haematobium infection. *Br J Urol* 55: 275-278.

688. Elliott GB, Moloney PJ, Anderson GH (1973). "Denuding cystitis" and in situ urothelial carcinoma. *Arch Pathol* 96: 91-94.

689. Ellis WJ, Chetner MP, Preston SD, Brawer MK (1994). Diagnosis of prostatic carcinoma: the yield of serum prostate specific antigen, digital rectal examination and transrectal ultrasonography. *J Urol* 152: 1520-1525.

690. Ellison DA, Silverman JF, Strausbauch PH, Wakely PE, Holbrook CT, Joshi VV (1996). Role of immunocytochemistry, electron microscopy, and DNA analysis in fine-needle aspiration biopsy diagnosis of Wilms' tumor. *Diagn Cytopathol* 14: 101-107.

691. Ellsworth PI, Schned AR, Heaney JA, Snyder PM (1995). Surgical treatment of verrucous carcinoma of the bladder unassociated with bilharzial cystitis: case report and literature review. *J Urol* 153: 411-414.

692. Elsobky E, el Baz M, Gomha M, Abol-Enein H, Shaaban AA (2002). Prognostic value of angiogenesis in schistosoma-associated squamous cell carcinoma of the urinary bladder. *Urology* 60: 69-73.

693. Emerson RE, Ulbright TM, Eble JN, Geary WA, Eckert GJ, Cheng L (2001). Predicting cancer progression in patients with penile squamous cell carcinoma: the importance of depth of invasion and vascular invasion. *Mod Pathol* 14: 963-968.

694. Emmert-Buck MR, Vocke CD, Pozzatti RO, Duray PH, Jennings SB, Florence CD, Zhuang Z, Bostwick DG, Liotta LA, Linehan WM (1995). Allelic loss on chromosome 8p12-21 in microdissected prostatic intraepithelial neoplasia. *Cancer Res* 55: 2959-2962.

695. Emmert GKJr, Bissada NK (1994). Primary neoplasms of the penile shaft. *South Med J* 87: 848-850.

696. Ende N, Woods LP, Shelley H.S. (1963). Carcinoma originating in ducts surrounding the prostatic urethra. *Am J Clin Pathol* 40: 183-189.

697. Eng C, Kiuru M, Fernandez MJ, Aaltonen LA (2003). A role for mitochondrial enzymes in inherited neoplasia and beyond. *Nat Rev Cancer* 3: 193-202.

698. Engel F, McPherson HT, Petter BF (1964). Clinical, morphological, and biochemical studies on a malignant testicular tumor. *J Clin Endocrinol Metab* 24: 528-542.

699. Engel JD, Kuzel TM, Moceanu MC, Oefelein MG, Schaeffer AJ (1998). Angiosarcoma of the bladder: a review. *Urology* 52: 778-784.

700. Engel LS, Taioli E, Pfeiffer R, Garcia-Closas M, Marcus PM, Lan Q, Boffetta P, Vineis P, Autrup H, Bell DA, Branch RA, Brockmoller J, Daly AK, Heckbert SR, Kalina I, Kang D, Katoh T, Lafuente A, Lin HJ, Romkes M, Taylor JA, Rothman N (2002). Pooled analysis and meta-analysis of glutathione S-transferase M1 and bladder cancer: a HuGE review. *Am J Epidemiol* 156: 95-109.

701. Epstein JI (1991). The evaluation of radical prostatectomy specimens. Therapeutic and prognostic implications. *Pathol Annu* 26 Pt 1: 159-210.

702. Epstein JI (1993). PSA and PAP as immunohistochemical markers in prostate cancer. *Urol Clin North Am* 20: 757-770.

703. Epstein JI (1995). Diagnostic criteria of limited adenocarcinoma of the prostate on needle biopsy. *Hum Pathol* 26: 223-229.

704. Epstein JI (2000). Gleason score 2-4 adenocarcinoma of the prostate on needle biopsy: a diagnosis that should not be made. *Am J Surg Pathol* 24: 477-478.

705. Epstein JI (2001). Pathological assessment of the surgical specimen. *Urol Clin North Am* 28: 567-594.

706. Epstein JI, Amin MB, Reuter VR, Mostofi FK (1998). The World Health Organization/International Society of Urological Pathology consensus classification of urothelial (transitional cell) neoplasms of the urinary bladder. Bladder Consensus Conference Committee. *Am J Surg Pathol* 22: 1435-1448.

707. Epstein JI, Carmichael MJ, Partin AW, Walsh PC (1994). Small high grade adenocarcinoma of the prostate in radical prostatectomy specimens performed for nonpalpable disease: pathogenetic and clinical implications. *J Urol* 151: 1587-1592.

708. Epstein JI, Cho KR, Quinn BD (1990). Relationship of severe dysplasia to stage A (incidental) adenocarcinoma of the prostate. *Cancer* 65: 2321-2327.

709. Epstein JI, Grignon DJ, Humphrey PA, McNeal JE, Sesterhenn IA, Troncoso P, Wheeler TM (1995). Interobserver reproducibility in the diagnosis of prostatic intraepithelial neoplasia. *Am J Surg Pathol* 19: 873-886.

710. Epstein JI, Lieberman PH (1985). Mucinous adenocarcinoma of the prostate gland. *Am J Surg Pathol* 9: 299-308.

711. Epstein JI, Oesterling JE, Walsh PC (1988). The volume and anatomical location of residual tumor in radical prostatectomy specimens removed for stage A1 prostate cancer. *J Urol* 139: 975-979.

712. Epstein JI, Partin AW, Potter SR, Walsh PC (2000). Adenocarcinoma of the prostate invading the seminal vesicle: prognostic stratification based on pathologic parameters. *Urology* 56: 283-288.

713. Epstein JI, Partin AW, Sauvageot J, Walsh PC (1996). Prediction of progression following radical prostatectomy. A multivariate analysis of 721 men with long-term follow-up. *Am J Surg Pathol* 20: 286-292.

714. Epstein JI, Pizov G, Walsh PC (1993). Correlation of pathologic findings with progression after radical retropubic prostatectomy. *Cancer* 71: 3582-3593.

715. Epstein JI, Potter SR (2001). The pathological interpretation and significance of prostate needle biopsy findings: implications and current controversies. *J Urol* 166: 402-410.

716. Epstein JI, Walsh PC, Carmichael M, Brendler CB (1994). Pathologic and clinical findings to predict tumor extent of nonpalpable (stage T1c) prostate cancer. *JAMA* 271: 368-374.

717. Epstein JI, Walsh PC, Carter HB (2001). Dedifferentiation of prostate cancer grade with time in men followed expectantly for stage T1c disease. *J Urol* 166: 1688-1691.

718. Epstein JI, Woodruff JM (1986). Adenocarcinoma of the prostate with endometrioid features. A light microscopic and immunohistochemical study of ten cases. *Cancer* 57: 111-119.

719. Epstein JI, Yang XJ (2002). *Prostate Biopsy Interpretation.* 3rd Edition. Lippincott Williams and Wilkins: Philadelphia, PA.

720. Epstein JI, Yang XJ (2002). Prostatic duct adenocarcinoma. In: *Prostate Biopsy Interpretation*, Lippincott Williams and Wilkins: Philadelphia, PA, pp. 185-197.

721. Erbersdobler A, Gurses N, Henke RP (1996). Numerical chromosomal changes in high-grade prostatic intraepithelial neoplasia (PIN) and concomitant invasive carcinoma. *Pathol Res Pract* 192: 418-427.

722. Erlandson RA, Shek TW, Reuter VE (1997). Diagnostic significance of mitochondria in four types of renal epithelial neoplasms: an ultrastructural study of 60 tumors. *Ultrastruct Pathol* 21: 409-417.

723. Erlandson RA, Woodruff JM (1982). Peripheral nerve sheath tumors: an electron microscopic study of 43 cases. *Cancer* 49: 273-287.

724. Eskew LA, Bare RL, McCullough DL (1997). Systematic 5 region prostate biopsy is superior to sextant method for diagnosing carcinoma of the prostate. *J Urol* 157: 199-202.

725. Esrig D, Elmajian D, Groshen S, Freeman JA, Stein JP, Chen SC, Nichols PW, Skinner DG, Jones PA, Cote RJ (1994). Accumulation of nuclear p53 and tumor progression in bladder cancer. *N Engl J Med* 331: 1259-1264.

726. Esrig D, Freeman JA, Elmajian DA, Stein JP, Chen SC, Groshen S, Simoneau A, Skinner EC, Lieskovsky G, Boyd SD, Cote RJ, Skinner DG (1996). Transitional cell carcinoma involving the prostate with a proposed staging classification for stromal invasion. *J Urol* 156: 1071-1076.

727. Essenfeld H, Manivel JC, Benedetto P, Albores-Saavedra J (1990). Small cell carcinoma of the renal pelvis: a clinicopathological, morphological and immunohistochemical study of 2 cases. *J Urol* 144: 344-347.

728. Etzioni R, Legler JM, Feuer EJ, Merrill RM, Cronin KA, Hankey BF (1999). Cancer surveillance series: interpreting trends in prostate cancer—part III: Quantifying the link between population prostate-specific antigen testing and recent declines in prostate cancer mortality. *J Natl Cancer Inst* 91: 1033-1039.

729. Eusebi V, Massarelli G (1971). Phaeochromocytoma of the spermatic cord: report of a case. *J Pathol* 105: 283-284.

730. Evans RW (1957). Developmental stages of embryo-like bodies in teratoma testis. *J Clin Pathol* 10: 31-39.

731. Fadl-Elmula I, Gorunova L, Lundgren R, Mandahl N, Forsby N, Mitelman F, Heim S (1998). Chromosomal abnormalities in two bladder carcinomas with secondary squamous cell differentiation. *Cancer Genet Cytogenet* 102: 125-130.

732. Fadl-Elmula I, Gorunova L, Mandahl N, Elfving P, Heim S (1998). Chromosome abnormalities in squamous cell carcinoma of the urethra. *Genes Chromosomes Cancer* 23: 72-73.

733. Fadl-Elmula I, Gorunova L, Mandahl N, Elfving P, Lundgren R, Mitelman F, Heim S (1999). Cytogenetic monoclonality in multifocal uroepithelial carcinomas: evidence of intraluminal tumour seeding. *Br J Cancer* 81: 6-12.

734. Fadl-Elmula I, Gorunova L, Mandahl N, Elfving P, Lundgren R, Rademark C, Heim S (1999). Cytogenetic analysis of upper urinary tract transitional cell carcinomas. *Cancer Genet Cytogenet* 115: 123-127.

735. Fadl-Elmula I, Kytola S, Leithy ME, Abdel-Hameed M, Mandahl N, Elagib A, Ibrahim M, Larsson C, Heim S (2002). Chromosomal aberrations in benign and malignant bilharzia-associated bladder lesions analyzed by comparative genomic hybridization. *BMC Cancer* 2: 5.

736. Fahn HJ, Lee YH, Chen MT, Huang JK, Chen KK, Chang LS (1991). The incidence and prognostic significance of humoral hypercalcemia in renal cell carcinoma. *J Urol* 145: 248-250.

737. Fain JS, Cosnow I, King BF, Zincke H, Bostwick DG (1993). Cystosarcoma phyllodes of the seminal vesicle. *Cancer* 71: 2055-2061.

738. Fairey AE, Mead GM, Murphy D, Theaker J (1993). Primary seminal vesicle choriocarcinoma. *Br J Urol* 71: 756-757.

739. Fairfax CA, Hammer CJ3rd, Dana BW, Hanifin JM, Barry JM (1995). Primary penile lymphoma presenting as a penile ulcer. *J Urol* 153: 1051-1052.

740. Fakruddin JM, Chaganti RS, Murty VV (1999). Lack of BCL10 mutations in germ cell tumors and B cell lymphomas. *Cell* 97: 683-684.

741. Fam A, Ishak KG (1958). Androblastoma of the testicle: report of a case in an infant 3 and a half months old. *J Urol* 79: 859-862.

742. Faria P, Beckwith JB, Mishra K, Zuppan C, Weeks DA, Breslow N, Green DM (1996). Focal versus diffuse anaplasia in Wilms tumor—new definitions with prognostic significance: a report from the National Wilms Tumor Study Group. *Am J Surg Pathol* 20: 909-920.

743. Farrow GM (1992). Pathology of carcinoma in situ of the urinary bladder and related lesions. *J Cell Biochem Suppl* 16I: 39-43.

744. Farrow GM, Utz DC, Rife CC (1976). Morphological and clinical observations of patients with early bladder cancer treated with total cystectomy. *Cancer Res* 36: 2495-2501.

745. Faysal MH (1981). Squamous cell carcinoma of the bladder. *J Urol* 126: 598-599.

746. Fein RL, Hamm FC (1965). Malignant schwannoma of the renal pelvis: a review of the literature and a case report. *J Urol* 94: 356-361.

747. Feinberg AP (1996). Multiple genetic abnormalities of 11p15 in Wilms' tumor. *Med Pediatr Oncol* 27: 484-489.

748. Ferdinandusse S, Denis S, IJlst L, Dacremont G, Waterham HR, Wanders RJ (2000). Subcellular localization and physiological role of alpha-methylacyl-CoA racemase. *J Lipid Res* 41: 1890-1896.

749. Ferlay J, Bray F, Pisani P, Parkin DM (2001). *GLOBOCAN 2000: Cancer Incidence, Mortality and Prevalence Worldwide.* IARC Press: Lyon.

750. Fernandez Acenero MJ, Galindo M, Bengoechea O, Borrega P, Reina JJ, Carapeto R (1998). Primary malignant lymphoma of the kidney: case report and literature review. *Gen Diagn Pathol* 143: 317-320.

751. Fernandez Gomez JM, Rodriguez Martinez JJ, Escaf Barmadah S, Perez Garcia J, Garcia J, Casasola Chamorro J (2000). [Significance of random biopsies of healthy mucosa in superficial bladder tumor]. *Arch Esp Urol* 53: 785-797.

752. Fernandez PL, Arce Y, Farre X, Martinez A, Nadal A, Rey MJ, Peiro N, Campo E, Cardesa A (1999). Expression of p27/Kip1 is down-regulated in human prostate carcinoma progression. *J Pathol* 187: 563-566.

753. Ferrari A, Bisogno G, Casanova M, Meazza C, Piva L, Cecchetto G, Zanetti I, Pilz T, Mattke A, Treuner J, Carli M (2002). Paratesticular rhabdomyosarcoma: report from the Italian and German Cooperative Group. *J Clin Oncol* 20: 449-455.

754. Ferrie BG, Imrie JE, Paterson PJ (1984). Osteosarcoma of bladder 27 years after local radiotherapy. *J R Soc Med* 77: 962-963.

755. Ferry JA, Harris NL, Papanicolaou N, Young RH (1995). Lymphoma of the kidney. A report of 11 cases. *Am J Surg Pathol* 19: 134-144.

756. Ferry JA, Harris NL, Young RH, Coen J, Zietman A, Scully RE (1994). Malignant lymphoma of the testis, epididymis, and spermatic cord. A clinicopathologic study of 69 cases with immunophenotypic analysis. *Am J Surg Pathol* 18: 376-390.

757. Ferry JA, Malt RA, Young RH (1991). Renal angiomyolipoma with sarcomatous transformation and pulmonary metastases. *Am J Surg Pathol* 15: 1083-1088.

758. Ferry JA, Young RH, Scully RE (1997). Testicular and epididymal plasmacytoma: a report of 7 cases, including three that were the initial manifestation of plasma cell myeloma. *Am J Surg Pathol* 21: 590-598.

759. Fetissof F, Benatre A, Dubois MP, Lanson Y, Arbeille-Brassart B, Jobard P (1984). Carcinoid tumor occurring in a teratoid malformation of the kidney. An immunohistochemical study. *Cancer* 54: 2305-2308.

760. Fetsch JF, Brinsko RW, Davis CJJr, Mostofi FK, Sesterhenn IA (2000). A distinctive myointimal proliferation ('myointimoma') involving the corpus spongiosum of the glans penis: a clinicopathologic and immunohistochemical analysis of 10 cases. *Am J Surg Pathol* 24: 1524-1530.

761. Fetsch JF, Weiss SW (1991). Observations concerning the pathogenesis of epithelioid hemangioma (angiolymphoid hyperplasia). *Mod Pathol* 4: 449-455.

762. Fetsch PA, Fetsch JF, Marincola FM, Travis W, Batts KP, Abati A (1998). Comparison of melanoma antigen recognized by T cells (MART-1) to HMB-45: additional evidence to support a common lineage for angiomyolipoma, lymphangiomyomatosis, and clear cell sugar tumor. *Mod Pathol* 11: 699-703.

763. Feuer EJ, Merrill RM, Hankey BF (1999). Cancer surveillance series: interpreting trends in prostate cancer—part II: Cause of death misclassification and the recent rise and fall in prostate cancer mortality. *J Natl Cancer Inst* 91: 1025-1032.

764. Ficarra V, Righetti R, Martignoni G, D'Amico A, Pilloni S, Rubilotta E, Malossini G, Mobilio G (2001). Prognostic value of renal cell carcinoma nuclear grading: multivariate analysis of 333 cases. *Urol Int* 67: 130-134.

765. Fielding JR, Hoyte LX, Okon SA, Schreyer A, Lee J, Zou KH, Warfield S, Richie JP, Loughlin KR, O'Leary MP, Doyle CJ, Kikinis R (2002). Tumor detection by virtual cystoscopy with color mapping of bladder wall thickness. *J Urol* 167: 559-562.

766. Finci R, Gunhan O, Celasun B, Gungor S (1987). Carcinoid tumor of undescended testis. *J Urol* 137: 301-302.

767. Finn LS, Viswanatha DS, Belasco JB, Snyder H, Huebner D, Sorbara L, Raffeld M, Jaffe ES, Salhany KE (1999). Primary follicular lymphoma of the testis in childhood. *Cancer* 85: 1626-1635.

768. Fischer J, Palmedo G, von Knobloch R, Bugert P, Prayer-Galetti T, Pagano F, Kovacs G (1998). Duplication and overexpression of the mutant allele of the MET proto-oncogene in multiple hereditary papillary renal cell tumours. *Oncogene* 17: 733-739.
769. Fisher C, Goldblum JR, Epstein JI, Montgomery E (2001). Leiomyosarcoma of the paratesticular region: a clinicopathologic study. *Am J Surg Pathol* 25: 1143-1149.
770. Fisher ER, Klieger H (1966). Epididymal carcinoma (malignant adenomatoid tumor, mesonephric, mesodermal carcinoma of epididymis). *J Urol* 95: 568-572.
771. Fisher M, Hricak H, Reinhold C, Proctor E, Williams R (1985). Female urethral carcinoma: MRI staging. *AJR Am J Roentgenol* 144: 603-604.
772. Fitzgerald JM, Ramchurren N, Rieger K, Levesque P, Silverman M, Libertino JA, Summerhayes IC (1995). Identification of H-ras mutations in urine sediments complements cytology in the detection of bladder tumors. *J Natl Cancer Inst* 87: 129-133.
773. Fitzpatrick JM, West AB, Butler MR, Lane V, O'Flynn JD (1986). Superficial bladder tumors (stage pTa, grades 1 and 2): the importance of recurrence pattern following initial resection. *J Urol* 135: 920-922.
774. Fleming S (1987). Carcinosarcoma (mixed mesodermal tumor) of the ureter. *J Urol* 138: 1234-1235.
775. Fleming S, Lewi HJ (1986). Collecting duct carcinoma of the kidney. *Histopathology* 10: 1131-1141.
776. Fleming S, Lindop GB, Gibson AA (1985). The distribution of epithelial membrane antigen in the kidney and its tumours. *Histopathology* 9: 729-739.
777. Fleshner N, Kapusta L, Ezer D, Herschorn S, Klotz L (2000). p53 nuclear accumulation is not associated with decreased disease-free survival in patients with node positive transitional cell carcinoma of the bladder. *J Urol* 164: 1177-1182.
778. Fleshner NE, Fair WR (1997). Indications for transition zone biopsy in the detection of prostatic carcinoma. *J Urol* 157: 556-558.
779. Fletcher MS, Aker M, Hill JT, Pryor JP, Whimster WF (1985). Granular cell myoblastoma of the bladder. *Br J Urol* 57: 109-110.
780. Florentine BD, Roscher AA, Garrett J, Warner NE (2002). Necrotic seminoma of the testis: establishing the diagnosis with Masson trichrome stain and immunostains. *Arch Pathol Lab Med* 126: 205-206.
781. Florine BL, Simonton SC, Sane SM, Stickel FR, Singher LJ, Dehner LP (1988). Clear cell sarcoma of the kidney: report of a case with mandibular metastasis simulating a benign myxomatous tumor. *Oral Surg Oral Med Oral Pathol* 65: 567-574.
782. Flotte TJ, Bell DA, Sidhu GS, Plair CM (1981). Leiomyosarcoma of the dartos muscle. *J Cutan Pathol* 8: 69-74.
783. Floyd C, Ayala AG, Logothetis CJ, Silva EG (1988). Spermatocytic seminoma with associated sarcoma of the testis. *Cancer* 61: 409-414.
784. Fogel M, Lifschitz-Mercer B, Moll R, Kushnir I, Jacob N, Waldherr R, Livoff A, Franke WW, Czernobilsky B (1990). Heterogeneity of intermediate filament expression in human testicular seminomas. *Differentiation* 45: 242-249.
785. Folpe AL, Goodman ZD, Ishak KG, Paulino AF, Taboada EM, Meehan SA, Weiss SW (2000). Clear cell myomelanocytic tumor of the falciform ligament/ligamentum teres: a novel member of the perivascular epithelioid clear cell family of tumors with a predilection for children and young adults. *Am J Surg Pathol* 24: 1239-1246.
786. Folpe AL, Patterson K, Gown AM (1997). Antibodies to desmin identify the blastemal component of nephroblastoma. *Mod Pathol* 10: 895-900.
787. Ford TF, Parkinson MC, Pryor JP (1985). The undescended testis in adult life. *Br J Urol* 57: 181-184.
788. Fornaro R, Terrizzi A, Secco GB, Canaletti M, Baldi E, Bonfante P, Sticchi C, Baccini P, Cittadini GJr, Fiorini G, Ferraris R (1999). [Renal hemangiopericytoma. Anatomo-pathologic and clinico-therapeutic considerations. A case report]. *G Chir* 20: 20-24.
789. Forstner R, Hricak H, Kalbhen CL, Kogan BA, McAninch JW (1995). Magnetic resonance imaging of vascular lesions of the scrotum and penis. *Urology* 46: 581-583.
790. Fort DW, Tonk VS, Tomlinson GE, Timmons CF, Schneider NR (1994). Rhabdoid tumor of the kidney with primitive neuroectodermal tumor of the central nervous system: associated tumors with different histologic, cytogenetic, and molecular findings. *Genes Chromosomes Cancer* 11: 146-152.
791. Fortuny J, Kogevinas M, Chang-Claude J, Gonzalez CA, Hours M, Jockel KH, Bolm-Audorff U, Lynge E, 't Mannetje A, Porru S, Ranft U, Serra C, Tzonou A, Wahrendorf J, Boffetta P (1999). Tobacco, occupation and non-transitional-cell carcinoma of the bladder: an international case-control study. *Int J Cancer* 80: 44-46.
792. Foster K, Prowse A, van den Berg A, Fleming S, Hulsbeek MM, Crossey PA, Richards FM, Cairns P, Affara NA, Ferguson-Smith MA (1994). Somatic mutations of the von Hippel-Lindau disease tumour suppressor gene in non-familial clear cell renal carcinoma. *Hum Mol Genet* 3: 2169-2173.
793. Foster RS, Baniel J, Leibovitch I, Curran M, Bihrle R, Rowland R, Donohue JP (1996). Teratoma in the orchiectomy specimen and volume of metastasis are predictors of retroperitoneal teratoma in low stage nonseminomatous testis cancer. *J Urol* 155: 1943-1945.
794. Fox JM (1966). Basal cell epithelioma of the glans penis. *Arch Dermatol* 94: 807-809.
795. Fralick RA, Malek RS, Goellner JR, Hyland KM (1994). Urethroscopy and urethral cytology in men with external genital condyloma. *Urology* 43: 361-364.
796. Francis NJ, Kingston RE (2001). Mechanisms of transcriptional memory. *Nat Rev Mol Cell Biol* 2: 409-421.
797. Franke KH, Miklosi M, Goebell P, Clasen S, Steinhoff C, Anastasiadis AG, Gerharz C, Schulz WA (2000). Cyclin-dependent kinase inhibitor P27(KIP1) is expressed preferentially in early stages of urothelial carcinoma. *Urology* 56: 689-695.
798. Franks LM, Chesterman FC (1956). Intra-epithelial carcinoma of prostatic urethra, peri-urethral glands and prostatic ducts (Bowen's disease of urinary epithelium). *Br J Cancer* 10: 223-235.
799. Franksson C, Bergstrand A, Ljungdahl I, Magnusson G, Nordenstam H (1972). Renal carcinoma (hypernephroma) occurring in 5 siblings. *J Urol* 108: 58-61.
800. Frasier BL, Wachs BH, Watson LR, Tomasulo JP (1988). Malignant melanoma of the renal pelvis presenting as a primary tumor. *J Urol* 140: 812-814.
801. Frates MC, Benson CB, di Salvo DN, Brown DL, Laing FC, Doubilet PM (1997). Solid extratesticular masses evaluated with sonography: pathologic correlation. *Radiology* 204: 43-46.
802. Freedman LS, Parkinson MC, Jones WG, Oliver RT, Peckham MJ, Read G, Newlands ES, Williams CJ (1987). Histopathology in the prediction of relapse of patients with stage I testicular teratoma treated by orchidectomy alone. *Lancet* 2: 294-298.
803. Frese R, Doehn C, Baumgartel M, Holl-Ulrich K, Jocham D (2001). Carcinoid tumor in an ileal neobladder. *J Urol* 165: 522-523.
804. Friedman NB, Moore RA (1946). Tumors of the testis: a report on 922 cases. *Milit Surgeon* 99: 573-593.
805. Fripp PJ (1965). The origin of urinary beta-glucuronidase. *Br J Cancer* 19: 330-335.
806. Fripp PJ, Keen P (1980). Bladder cancer in an endemic *Schistosoma Haematobium* area. The excretion patterns of 3-hydroxanthranilic acid and kyurenine. *S Afr J Sci* 76: 212-215.
807. Frisch SM, Francis H (1994). Disruption of epithelial cell-matrix interactions induces apoptosis. *J Cell Biol* 124: 619-626.
808. Fritz A, Percy C, Jack A, Shanmugaratnam K, Sobin L, Parkin DM, Whelan S (2000). *International Classification of Diseases for Oncology.* 3rd Edition. WHO: Geneva.
809. Froehner M, Manseck A, Haase M, Hakenberg OW, Wirth MP (1999). Locally recurrent malignant fibrous histiocytoma: a rare and aggressive genitourinary malignancy. *Urol Int* 62: 164-170.
810. Froehner M, Schobl R, Wirth MP (2000). Mucoepidermoid penile carcinoma: clinical, histologic, and immunohistochemical characterization of an uncommon neoplasm. *Urology* 56: 154.
811. Froehner M, Tsatalpas P, Wirth MP (1999). Giant penile cavernous hemangioma with intrapelvic extension. *Urology* 53: 414-415.
812. Frydenberg M, Eckstein RP, Saalfield JA, Breslin FH, Alexander JH, Roche J (1991). Renal oncocytomas—an Australian experience. *Br J Urol* 67: 352-357.
813. Fu YT, Wang HH, Yang TH, Chang SY, Ma CP (1996). Epidermoid cysts of the testis: diagnosis by ultrasonography and magnetic resonance imaging resulting in organ-preserving surgery. *Br J Urol* 78: 116-118.
814. Fuglsang F, Ohlse NS (1957). Androblastoma predominantly feminizing. With report of a case. *Acta Chir Scand* 112: 405-410.
815. Fuhrman SA, Lasky LC, Limas C (1982). Prognostic significance of morphologic parameters in renal cell carcinoma. *Am J Surg Pathol* 6: 655-663.
816. Fujii Y, Ajima J, Oka K, Tosaka A, Takehara Y (1995). Benign renal tumors detected among healthy adults by abdominal ultrasonography. *Eur Urol* 27: 124-127.
817. Fujikawa K, Matsui Y, Oka H, Fukuzawa S, Sasaki M, Takeuchi H (2000). Prognosis of primary testicular seminoma: a report on 57 new cases. *Cancer Res* 60: 2152-2154.
818. Fujimoto K, Yamada Y, Okajima E, Kakizoe T, Sasaki H, Sugimura T, Terada M (1992). Frequent association of p53 gene mutation in invasive bladder cancer. *Cancer Res* 52: 1393-1398.
819. Fujisaki M, Tokuda Y, Sato S, Fujiyama C, Matsuo Y, Sugihara H, Masaki Z (2000). Case of mesothelioma of the tunica vaginalis testis with characteristic findings on ultrasonography and magnetic resonance imaging. *Int J Urol* 7: 427-430.
820. Fukunaga M, Ushigome S (1998). Lymphoepithelioma-like carcinoma of the renal pelvis: a case report with immunohistochemical analysis and in situ hybridization for the Epstein-Barr viral genome. *Mod Pathol* 11: 1252-1256.
821. Fukunaga M, Yokoi K, Miyazawa Y, Harada T, Ushigome S (1994). Penile verrucous carcinoma with anaplastic transformation following radiotherapy. A case report with human papillomavirus typing and flow cytometric DNA studies. *Am J Surg Pathol* 18: 501-505.
822. Fukuoka T, Honda M, Namiki M, Tada Y, Matsuda M, Sonoda T (1987). Renal cell carcinoma with heterotopic bone formation. Case report and review of the Japanese literature. *Urol Int* 42: 458-460.
823. Fung CY, Kalish LA, Brodsky GL, Richie JP, Garnick MB (1988). Stage I nonseminomatous germ cell testicular tumor: prediction of metastatic potential by primary histopathology. *J Clin Oncol* 6: 1467-1473.
824. Furihata M, Sonobe H, Iwata J, Ido E, Ohtsuki Y, Kuwahara M, Fujisaki N (1996). Granular cell tumor expressing myogenic markers in the prostate. *Pathol Int* 46: 298-300.
825. Furuya S, Ogura H, Tanaka Y, Tsukamoto T, Isomura H (1997). Hemangioma of the prostatic urethra: hematospermia and massive postejaculation hematuria with clot retention. *Int J Urol* 4: 524-526.
826. Fuzesi L, Gunawan B, Braun S, Bergmann F, Brauers A, Effert P, Mittermayer C (1998). Cytogenetic analysis of 11 renal oncocytomas: further evidence of structural rearrangements of 11q13 as a characteristic chromosomal anomaly. *Cancer Genet Cytogenet* 107: 1-6.
827. Gabrilove JL, Freiberg EK, Leiter E, Nicolis GL (1980). Feminizing and non-feminizing Sertoli cell tumors. *J Urol* 124: 757-767.
828. Gabrilove JL, Nicolis GL, Mitty HA, Sohval AR (1975). Feminizing interstitial cell tumor of the testis: personal observations and a review of the literature. *Cancer* 35: 1184-1202.
829. Gago-Dominguez M, Yuan JM, Castelao JE, Ross RK, Yu MC (2001). Family history and risk of renal cell carcinoma. *Cancer Epidemiol Biomarkers Prev* 10: 1001-1004.
830. Galanis E, Frytak S, Lloyd RV (1997). Extrapulmonary small cell carcinoma. *Cancer* 79: 1729-1736.
831. Galatica Z, Kovatich A, Miettinen M (1995). Consistent expression of cytokeratin 7 in papillary renal cell carcinoma. *J Urol Pathol* 3: 205-211.
832. Gandour-Edwards R, Lara PNJr, Folkins AK, LaSalle JM, Beckett L, Li Y, Meyers FJ, de Vere White R (2002). Does HER2/neu expression provide prognostic information in patients with advanced urothelial carcinoma? *Cancer* 95: 1009-1015.
833. Ganem JP, Jhaveri FM, Marroum MC (1998). Primary adenocarcinoma of the epididymis: case report and review of the literature. *Urology* 52: 904-908.
834. Ganguly S, Murty VV, Samaniego F, Reuter VE, Bosl GJ, Chaganti RS (1990). Detection of preferential NRAS mutations in human male germ cell tumors by the polymerase chain reaction. *Genes Chromosomes Cancer* 1: 228-232.

835. Gao CL, Dean RC, Pinto A, Mooneyhan R, Connelly RR, McLeod DG, Srivastava S, Moul JW (1999). Detection of circulating prostate specific antigen expressing prostatic cells in the bone marrow of radical prostatectomy patients by sensitive reverse transcriptase polymerase chain reaction. *J Urol* 161: 1070-1076.

836. Gardiner RA, Samaratunga ML, Walsh MD, Seymour GJ, Lavin MF (1992). An immunohistological demonstration of c-erbB-2 oncoprotein expression in primary urothelial bladder cancer. *Urol Res* 20: 117-120.

837. Garrett JE, Cartwright PC, Snow BW, Coffin CM (2000). Cystic testicular lesions in the pediatric population. *J Urol* 163: 928-936.

838. Garufi A, Priolo GD, Coppolino F, Giammusso B, Materazzo S (1993). [Computed tomography evaluation of urothelial carcinomas of the upper urinary tract]. *Radiol Med (Torino)* 86: 489-495.

839. Gassel AM, Westphal E, Hansmann ML, Leimenstoll G, Gassel HJ (1991). Malignant lymphoma of donor origin after renal transplantation: a case report. *Hum Pathol* 22: 1291-1293.

840. Gatalica Z, Grujic S, Kovatich A, Petersen RO (1996). Metanephric adenoma: histology, immunophenotype, cytogenetics, ultrastructure. *Mod Pathol* 9: 329-333.

841. Gattuso P, Carson HJ, Candel A, Castelli MJ (1995). Adenosquamous carcinoma of the prostate. *Hum Pathol* 26: 123-126.

842. Gaudin PB (1998). Histopathologic effects of radiation and hormonal therapies on benign and malignant prostate tissue. *J Urol Pathol* 8: 55-67.

843. Gaudin PB, Epstein JI (1994). Adenosis of the prostate. Histologic features in transurethral resection specimens. *Am J Surg Pathol* 18: 863-870.

844. Gaudin PB, Rosai J, Epstein JI (1998). Sarcomas and related proliferative lesions of specialized prostatic stroma: a clinicopathologic study of 22 cases. *Am J Surg Pathol* 22: 148-162.

845. Gaudin PB, Sesterhenn IA, Wojno KJ, Mostofi FK, Epstein JI (1997). Incidence and clinical significance of high-grade prostatic intraepithelial neoplasia in TURP specimens. *Urology* 49: 558-563.

846. Gelfand M, Weinberg RW, Castle WM (1967). Relation between carcinoma of the bladder and infestation with Schistosoma haematobium. *Lancet* 1: 1249-1251.

847. Gelmann EP (2002). Molecular biology of the androgen receptor. *J Clin Oncol* 20: 3001-3015.

848. Gels ME, Hoekstra HJ, Sleijfer DT, Marrink J, de Bruijn HW, Molenaar WM, Freling NJ, Droste JH, Schraffordt Koops H (1995). Detection of recurrence in patients with clinical stage I nonseminomatous testicular germ cell tumors and consequences for further follow-up: a single-center 10-year experience. *J Clin Oncol* 13: 1188-1194.

849. Genega EM, Hutchinson B, Reuter VE, Gaudin PB (2000). Immunophenotype of high-grade prostatic adenocarcinoma and urothelial carcinoma. *Mod Pathol* 13: 1186-1191.

850. Gentile AT, Moseley HS, Quinn SF, Franzini D, Pitre TM (1994). Leiomyoma of the seminal vesicle. *J Urol* 151: 1027-1029.

851. Gentile JM (1985). Schistosome related cancers: a possible role for genotoxins. *Environ Mutagen* 7: 775-785.

852. Gentile JM (1991). A possible role for genotoxins in parasite-associated cancers. *Rev Latinoam Genet* 1: 239-248.

853. Gentile JM, Brown S, Aardema M, Clark D, Blankespoor H (1985). Modified mutagen metabolism in Schistosoma hematobium-infested organisms. *Arch Environ Health* 40: 5-12.

854. Gentile JM, Gentile GJ (1994). Implications for the involvement of the immune system in parasite-associated cancers. *Mutat Res* 305: 315-320.

855. George DJ, Kaelin WGJr (2003). The von Hippel-Lindau protein, vascular endothelial growth factor, and kidney cancer. *N Engl J Med* 349: 419-421.

856. Gerald WL, Ladanyi M, de Alava E, Cuatrecasas M, Kushner BH, LaQuaglia MP, Rosai J (1998). Clinical, pathologic, and molecular spectrum of tumors associated with t(11;22)(p13;q12): desmoplastic small round-cell tumor and its variants. *J Clin Oncol* 16: 3028-3036.

857. Gerald WL, Miller HK, Battifora H, Miettinen M, Silva EG, Rosai J (1991). Intra-abdominal desmoplastic small round-cell tumor. Report of 19 cases of a distinctive type of high-grade polyphenotypic malignancy affecting young individuals. *Am J Surg Pathol* 15: 499-513.

858. Gerald WL, Rosai J, Ladanyi M (1995). Characterization of the genomic breakpoint and chimeric transcripts in the EWS-WT1 gene fusion of desmoplastic small round cell tumor. *Proc Natl Acad Sci USA* 92: 1028-1032.

859. Gervasi LA, Mata J, Easley JD, Wilbanks JH, Seale-Hawkins C, Carlton CEJr, Scardino PT (1989). Prognostic significance of lymph nodal metastases in prostate cancer. *J Urol* 142: 332-336.

860. Gessler M, Poustka A, Cavenee W, Neve RL, Orkin SH, Bruns GA (1990). Homozygous deletion in Wilms tumours of a zinc-finger gene identified by chromosome jumping. *Nature* 343: 774-778.

861. Geurts van Kessel A, Suijkerbuijk RF, Sinke RJ, Looijenga LH, Oosterhuis JW, de Jong B (1993). Molecular cytogenetics of human germ cell tumours: i(12p) and related chromosomal anomalies. *Eur Urol* 23: 23-28.

862. Geurts van Kessel A, Wijnhoven H, Bodmer D, Eleveld M, Kiemeney L, Mulders P, Weterman M, Ligtenberg M, Smeets D, Smits A (1999). Renal cell cancer: chromosome 3 translocations as risk factors. *J Natl Cancer Inst* 91: 1159-1160.

863. Ghalayini IF, Bani-Hani IH, Almasri NM (2001). Osteosarcoma of the urinary bladder occurring simultaneously with prostate and bowel carcinomas: report of a case and review of the literature. *Arch Pathol Lab Med* 125: 793-795.

864. Ghandur-Mnaymneh L, Gonzalez MS (1981). Angiosarcoma of the penis with hepatic angiomas in a patient with low vinyl chloride exposure. *Cancer* 47: 1318-1324.

865. Gheiler EL, Tefilli MV, Tiguert R, de Oliveira JG, Pontes JE, Wood DPJr (1998). Management of primary urethral cancer. *Urology* 52: 487-493.

866. Ghoneim MA, Ashamallah AK, Awaad HK, Whitmore WFJr (1985). Randomized trial of cystectomy with or without preoperative radiotherapy for carcinoma of the bilharzial bladder. *J Urol* 134: 266-268.

867. Gibas Z, Griffin CA, Emanuel BS (1987). Trisomy 7 and i(5p) in a transitional cell carcinoma of the ureter. *Cancer Genet Cytogenet* 25: 369-370.

868. Gibas Z, Prout GR, Pontes JE, Connolly JG, Sandberg AA (1986). A possible specific chromosome change in transitional cell carcinoma of the bladder. *Cancer Genet Cytogenet* 19: 229-238.

869. Gibas Z, Prout GRJr, Connolly JG, Pontes JE, Sandberg AA (1984). Nonrandom chromosomal changes in transitional cell carcinoma of the bladder. *Cancer Res* 44: 1257-1264.

870. Gibbons RP, Monte JE, Correa RJJr, Mason JT (1976). Manifestations of renal cell carcinoma. *Urology* 8: 201-206.

871. Gibbs M, Stanford JL, McIndoe RA, Jarvik GP, Kolb S, Goode EL, Chakrabarti L, Schuster EF, Buckley VA, Miller EL, Brandzel S, Li S, Hood L, Ostrander EA (1999). Evidence for a rare prostate cancer-susceptibility locus at chromosome 1p36. *Am J Hum Genet* 64: 776-787.

872. Gibson GE, Ahmed I (2001). Perianal and genital basal cell carcinoma: A clinicopathologic review of 51 cases. *J Am Acad Dermatol* 45: 68-71.

873. Gierke CL, King BF, Bostwick DG, Choyke PL, Hattery RR (1994). Large-cell calcifying Sertoli cell tumor of the testis: appearance at sonography. *AJR Am J Roentgenol* 163: 373-375.

874. Gilbert RF, Ibarra J, Tansey LA, Shanberg AM (1992). Adenocarcinoma in a mullerian duct cyst. *J Urol* 148: 1262-1264.

875. Gilcrease MZ, Delgado R, Albores-Saavedra J (1998). Testicular Sertoli cell tumor with a heterologous sarcomatous component: immunohistochemical assessment of Sertoli cell differentiation. *Arch Pathol Lab Med* 122: 907-911.

876. Gilcrease MZ, Delgado R, Vuitch F, Albores-Saavedra J (1998). Clear cell adenocarcinoma and nephrogenic adenoma of the urethra and urinary bladder: a histopathologic and immunohistochemical comparison. *Hum Pathol* 29: 1451-1456.

877. Gilcrease MZ, Schmidt L, Zbar B, Truong L, Rutledge M, Wheeler TM (1995). Somatic von Hippel-Lindau mutation in clear cell papillary cystadenoma of the epididymis. *Hum Pathol* 26: 1341-1346.

878. Gill HS, Dhillon HK, Woodhouse CR (1989). Adenocarcinoma of the urinary bladder. *Br J Urol* 64: 138-142.

879. Gill IS, Sung GT, Hobart MG, Savage SJ, Meraney AM, Schweizer DK, Klein EA, Novick AC (2000). Laparoscopic radical nephroureterectomy for upper tract transitional cell carcinoma: the Cleveland Clinic experience. *J Urol* 164: 1513-1522.

880. Gillis AJ, Looijenga LH, de Jong B, Oosterhuis JW (1994). Clonality of combined testicular germ cell tumors of adults. *Lab Invest* 71: 874-878.

881. Gillis AJ, Oosterhuis JW, Schipper ME, Barten EJ, van Berlo R, van Gurp RJ, Abraham M, Saunders GF, Looijenga LH (1994). Origin and biology of a testicular Wilms' tumor. *Genes Chromosomes Cancer* 11: 126-135.

882. Gillis AJ, Verkerk AJ, Dekker MC, van Gurp RJ, Oosterhuis JW, Looijenga LH (1997). Methylation similarities of two CpG sites within exon 5 of human H19 between normal tissues and testicular germ cell tumours of adolescents and adults, without correlation with allelic and total level of expression. *Br J Cancer* 76: 725-733.

883. Gilman PA (1983). The epidemiology of human teratomas. In: *The Human Teratomas: Experimental and Clinical Biology*, I Damjavov, BB Knowles, D Solter, eds. Humana Press: Clifton, NJ, pp. 81-104.

884. Giovannucci E, Stampfer MJ, Krithivas K, Brown M, Dahl D, Brufsky A, Talcott J, Hennekens CH, Kantoff PW (1997). The CAG repeat within the androgen receptor gene and its relationship to prostate cancer. *Proc Natl Acad Sci USA* 94: 3320-3323.

885. Givler RL (1971). Involvement of the bladder in leukemia and lymphoma. *J Urol* 105: 667-670.

886. Giwercman A, Andrews PW, Jorgensen N, Muller J, Graem N, Skakkebaek NE (1993). Immunohistochemical expression of embryonal marker TRA-1-60 in carcinoma in situ and germ cell tumors of the testis. *Cancer* 72: 1308-1314.

887. Giwercman A, Bruun E, Frimodt-Moller C, Skakkebaek NE (1989). Prevalence of carcinoma in situ and other histopathological abnormalities in testes of men with a history of cryptorchidism. *J Urol* 142: 998-1001.

888. Giwercman A, Cantell L, Marks A (1991). Placental-like alkaline phosphatase as a marker of carcinoma-in-situ of the testis. Comparison with monoclonal antibodies M2A and 43-9F. *APMIS* 99: 586-594.

889. Giwercman A, Lindenberg S, Kimber SJ, Andersson T, Muller J, Skakkebaek NE (1990). Monoclonal antibody 43-9F as a sensitive immunohistochemical marker of carcinoma in situ of human testis. *Cancer* 65: 1135-1142.

890. Giwercman A, Marks A, Bailey D, Baumal R, Skakkebaek NE (1988). A monoclonal antibody as a marker for carcinoma in situ germ cells of the human adult testis. *APMIS* 96: 667-670.

891. Giwercman A, Muller J, Skakkebaek NE (1991). Prevalence of carcinoma in situ and other histopathological abnormalities in testes from 399 men who died suddenly and unexpectedly. *J Urol* 145: 77-80.

892. Giwercman A, von der Maase H, Skakkebaek NE (1993). Epidemiological and clinical aspects of carcinoma in situ of the testis. *Eur Urol* 23: 104-110.

893. Glavac D, Neumann HP, Wittke C, Jaenig H, Masek O, Streicher T, Pausch F, Engelhardt D, Plate KH, Hofler H, Chen F, Zbar B, Brauch H (1996). Mutations in the VHL tumor suppressor gene and associated lesions in families with von Hippel-Lindau disease from central Europe. *Hum Genet* 98: 271-280.

894. Gleason DF (1966). Classification of prostatic carcinomas. *Cancer Chemother Rep* 50: 125-128.

895. Gleason DF (1977). Histologic grading and clinical staging of prostatic carcinoma. In: *Urologic Pathology: The Prostate*, M Tannenbaum, ed. Lea and Feibiger: Philadelphia.

896. Glover SD, Buck AC (1982). Renal medullary fibroma: a case report. *J Urol* 127: 758-760.

897. Gnarra JR, Tory K, Weng Y, Schmidt L, Wei MH, Li H, Latif F, Liu S, Chen F, Duh FM, Lubensky I, Duan DR, Florence CD, Pozzatti RO, Walther MM, Bander NH, Grossman HB, Brauch H, Pomer S, Brooks JD, Isaacs WB, Lerman MI, Zbar B, Linehan WM (1994). Mutations of the VHL tumour suppressor gene in renal carcinoma. *Nat Genet* 7: 85-90.

898. Goddard JC, Sutton CD, Jones JL, O'Byrne KJ, Kockelbergh RC (2002). Reduced thrombospondin-1 at presentation predicts disease progression in superficial bladder cancer. *Eur Urol* 42: 464-468.

899. Goebbels R, Amberger L, Wernert N, Dhom G (1985). Urothelial carcinoma of the prostate. *Appl Pathol* 3: 242-254.

900. Goedert JJ, Cote TR, Virgo P, Scoppa SM, Kingma DW, Gail MH, Jaffe ES, Biggar RJ (1998). Spectrum of AIDS-associated malignant disorders. *Lancet* 351: 1833-1839.
901. Goessl C, Knispel HH, Miller K, Klan R (1997). Is routine excretory urography necessary at first diagnosis of bladder cancer? *J Urol* 157: 480-481.
902. Gold PJ, Fefer A, Thompson JA (1996). Paraneoplastic manifestations of renal cell carcinoma. *Semin Urol Oncol* 14: 216-222.
903. Goldblum JR, Lloyd RV (1993). Primary renal carcinoid. Case report and literature review. *Arch Pathol Lab Med* 117: 855-858.
904. Golde DW, Schambelan M, Weintraub BD, Rosen SW (1974). Gonadotropin-secreting renal carcinoma. *Cancer* 33: 1048-1053.
905. Goldgar DE, Easton DF, Cannon-Albright LA, Skolnick MH (1994). Systematic population-based assessment of cancer risk in first-degree relatives of cancer probands. *J Natl Cancer Inst* 86: 1600-1608.
906. Goldstein NS (2002). Immunophenotypic characterization of 225 prostate adenocarcinomas with intermediate or high Gleason scores. *Am J Clin Pathol* 117: 471-477.
907. Golub TR, Slonim DK, Tamayo P, Huard C, Gaasenbeek M, Mesirov JP, Coller H, Loh ML, Downing JR, Caligiuri MA, Bloomfield CD, Lander ES (1999). Molecular classification of cancer: class discovery and class prediction by gene expression monitoring. *Science* 286: 531-537.
908. Goluboff ET, O'Toole K, Sawczuk IS (1994). Leiomyoma of bladder: report of case and review of literature. *Urology* 43: 238-241.
909. Gomez CA, Soloway MS, Civantos F, Hachiya T (1993). Bladder neck preservation and its impact on positive surgical margins during radical prostatectomy. *Urology* 42: 689-693.
910. Gomez MR (1999). Definition and criteria for diagnosis. In: *Tuberous Sclerosis Complex*, MR Gomez, ed. Oxford University Press: Oxford, pp. 10-23.
911. Gondos B (1993). Ultrastructure of developing and malignant germ cells. *Eur Urol* 23: 68-74.
912. Gonzalez-Zulueta M, Shibata A, Ohneseit PF, Spruck CH3rd, Busch C, Shamaa M, el Baz M, Nichols PW, Gonzalgo ML, Malmstrom PU, Jones PA (1995). High frequency of chromosome 9p allelic loss and CDKN2 tumor suppressor gene alterations in squamous cell carcinoma of the bladder. *J Natl Cancer Inst* 87: 1383-1393.
913. Goodman JD, Carr L, Ostrovsky PD, Sunshine R, Yeh HC, Cohen EL (1985). Testicular lymphoma: sonographic findings. *Urol Radiol* 7: 25-27.
914. Gorgoulis VG, Barbatis C, Poulias I, Karameris AM (1995). Molecular and immunohistochemical evaluation of epidermal growth factor receptor and c-erb-B-2 gene product in transitional cell carcinomas of the urinary bladder: a study in Greek patients. *Mod Pathol* 8: 758-764.
915. Goto K, Konomoto T, Hayashi K, Kinukawa N, Naito S, Kumazawa J, Tsuneyoshi M (1997). p53 mutations in multiple urothelial carcinomas: a molecular analysis of the development of multiple carcinomas. *Mod Pathol* 10: 428-437.
916. Govender D, Nteene LM, Chetty R, Hadley GP (2001). Mature renal teratoma and a synchronous malignant neuroepithelial tumour of the ipsilateral adrenal gland. *J Clin Pathol* 54: 253-254.
917. Govender D, Sabaratnam RM, Essa AS (2002). Clear cell 'sugar' tumor of the breast: another extrapulmonary site and review of the literature. *Am J Surg Pathol* 26: 670-675.
918. Gown AM, Vogel AM (1984). Monoclonal antibodies to human intermediate filament proteins. II. Distribution of filament proteins in normal human tissues. *Am J Pathol* 114: 309-321.
919. Goyanna R, Emmet JL, McDonald JR (1951). Exstrophy of the bladder complicated by adenocarcinoma. *J Urol* 65: 391-400.
920. Grabstald H (1973). Proceedings: Tumors of the urethra in men and women. *Cancer* 32: 1236-1255.
921. Grabstald H (1984). Prostatic biopsy in selected patients with carcinoma in situ of the bladder: preliminary report. *J Urol* 132: 1117-1118.
922. Grabstald H, Whitmore WF, Melamed MR (1971). Renal pelvic tumors. *JAMA* 218: 845-854.
923. Grace DA, Winter CC (1968). Mixed differentiation of primary carcinoma of the urinary bladder. *Cancer* 21: 1239-1243.
924. Grady RW, Ross JH, Kay R (1997). Epidemiological features of testicular teratoma in a prepubertal population. *J Urol* 158: 1191-1192.
925. Grammatico D, Grignon DJ, Eberwein P, Shepherd RR, Hearn SA, Walton JC (1993). Transitional cell carcinoma of the renal pelvis with choriocarcinomatous differentiation. Immunohistochemical and immunoelectron microscopic assessment of human chorionic gonadotropin production by transitional cell carcinoma of the urinary bladder. *Cancer* 71: 1835-1841.
926. Granter SR, Fletcher JA, Renshaw AA (1997). Cytologic and cytogenetic analysis of metanephric adenoma of the kidney: a report of two cases. *Am J Clin Pathol* 108: 544-549.
927. Grantham JG, Charboneau JW, James EM, Kirschling RJ, Kvols LK, Segura JW, Wold LE (1985). Testicular neoplasms: 29 tumors studied by high-resolution US. *Radiology* 157: 775-780.
928. Grasso M, Blanco S, Franzoso F, Lania C, di Bella C, Crippa S (2002). Solitary fibrous tumor of the prostate. *J Urol* 168: 1100.
929. Gravas S, Papadimitriou K, Kyriakidis A (1999). Sclerosing sertoli cell tumor of the testis—a case report and review of the literature. *Scand J Urol Nephrol* 33: 197-199.
930. Gravholt CH, Fedder J, Naeraa RW, Muller J (2000). Occurrence of gonadoblastoma in females with Turner syndrome and Y chromosome material: a population study. *J Clin Endocrinol Metab* 85: 3199-3202.
931. Gray GFJr, Marshall VF (1975). Squamous carcinoma of the prostate. *J Urol* 113: 736-738.
932. Greco MA, Feiner HD, Theil KS, Mufarrij AA (1984). Testicular stromal tumor with myofilaments: ultrastructural comparison with normal gonadal stroma. *Hum Pathol* 15: 238-243.
933. Green AJ, Sepp T, Yates JR (1996). Clonality of tuberous sclerosis harmatomas shown by non-random X-chromosome inactivation. *Hum Genet* 97: 240-243.
934. Green DM, Beckwith JB, Breslow NE, Faria P, Moksness J, Finklestein JZ, Grundy P, Thomas PR, Kim T, Shochat S, Haase G, Ritchey ML, Kelalis PP, Dangio GJ (1994). Treatment of children with stages II to IV anaplastic Wilms' tumor: a report from the National Wilms' Tumor Study Group. *J Clin Oncol* 12: 2126-2131.
935. Green DM, Breslow NE, Beckwith JB, Moksness J, Finklestein JZ, D'Angio GJ (1994). Treatment of children with clear-cell sarcoma of the kidney: a report from the National Wilms' Tumor Study Group. *J Clin Oncol* 12: 2132-2137.
936. Green DM, Breslow NE, Beckwith JB, Norkool P (1993). Screening of children with hemihypertrophy, aniridia, and Beckwith-Wiedemann syndrome in patients with Wilms tumor: a report from the National Wilms Tumor Study. *Med Pediatr Oncol* 21: 188-192.
937. Green GA, Hanlon AL, Al Saleem T, Hanks GE (1998). A Gleason score of 7 predicts a worse outcome for prostate carcinoma patients treated with radiotherapy. *Cancer* 83: 971-976.
938. Green LF, Farrow GM, Ravits JM (1979). Prostatic adenocarcinoma of ductal origin. *J Urol* 121: 303-305.
939. Green R, Epstein JI (1999). Use of intervening unstained slides for immunohistochemical stains for high molecular weight cytokeratin on prostate needle biopsies. *Am J Surg Pathol* 23: 567-570.
940. Greene DR, Wheeler TM, Egawa S, Dunn JK, Scardino PT (1991). A comparison of the morphological features of cancer arising in the transition zone and in the peripheral zone of the prostate. *J Urol* 146: 1069-1076.
941. Greene DR, Wheeler TM, Egawa S, Weaver RP, Scardino PT (1991). Relationship between clinical stage and histological zone of origin in early prostate cancer: morphometric analysis. *Br J Urol* 68: 499-509.
942. Greene LF, Mulcahy JJ, Warren MM, Dockerty MB (1973). Primary transitional cell carcinoma of the prostate. *J Urol* 110: 235-237.
943. Greene LF, O'Dea MJ, Dockerty MB (1976). Primary transitional cell carcinoma of the prostate. *J Urol* 116: 761-763.
944. Greene LF, Page DL, Fleming D, Firtz A, Batch M, Haller DG, Morrow M (2002). *American Joint Committee on Cancer (AJCC) Cancer Staging Manual.* 6th Edition. Springer-Verlag: New York.
945. Gregoire L, Cubilla AL, Reuter VE, Haas GP, Lancaster WD (1995). Preferential association of human papillomavirus with high-grade histologic variants of penile-invasive squamous cell carcinoma. *J Natl Cancer Inst* 87: 1705-1709.
946. Griebling TL, Ozkutlu D, See WA, Cohen MB (1997). Prognostic implications of extracapsular extension of lymph node metastases in prostate cancer. *Mod Pathol* 10: 804-809.
947. Griffin JH, Waters WB (1996). Primary leiomyosarcoma of the ureter. *J Surg Oncol* 62: 148-152.
948. Grignon DJ (1997). Neoplasms of the urinary bladder. In: *Urologic Surgical Pathology*, DG Bostwick, JN Eble, eds. Mosby: St Louis, pp. 269-270.
949. Grignon DJ, Ayala AG, el-Naggar A, Wishnow KI, Ro JY, Swanson DA, McLemore D, Giacco GG, Guinee VF (1989). Renal cell carcinoma. A clinicopathologic and DNA flow cytometric analysis of 103 cases. *Cancer* 64: 2133-2140.
950. Grignon DJ, Ayala AG, Ro JY, el-Naggar A, Papadopoulos NJ (1990). Primary sarcomas of the kidney. A clinicopathologic and DNA flow cytometric study of 17 cases. *Cancer* 65: 1611-1618.
951. Grignon DJ, Eble JN (1998). Papillary and metanephric adenomas of the kidney. *Semin Diagn Pathol* 15: 41-53.
952. Grignon DJ, Ro JY, Ayala AG, Johnson DE (1991). Primary signet-ring cell carcinoma of the urinary bladder. *Am J Clin Pathol* 95: 13-20.
953. Grignon DJ, Ro JY, Ayala AG, Johnson DE, Ordonez NG (1991). Primary adenocarcinoma of the urinary bladder. A clinicopathologic analysis of 72 cases. *Cancer* 67: 2165-2172.
954. Grignon DJ, Ro JY, Ordonez NG, Ayala AG, Cleary KR (1988). Basal cell hyperplasia, adenoid basal cell tumor, and adenoid cystic carcinoma of the prostate gland: an immunohistochemical study. *Hum Pathol* 19: 1425-1433.
955. Groeneveld AE, Marszalek WW, Heyns CF (1996). Bladder cancer in various population groups in the greater Durban area of KwaZulu-Natal, South Africa. *Br J Urol* 78: 205-208.
956. Groisman GM, Dische MR, Fine EM, Unger PD (1993). Juvenile granulosa cell tumor of the testis: a comparative immunohistochemical study with normal infantile gonads. *Pediatr Pathol* 13: 389-400.
957. Gronau S, Menz CK, Melzner I, Hautmann R, Moller P, Barth TF (2002). Immunohistomorphologic and molecular cytogenetic analysis of a carcinosarcoma of the urinary bladder. *Virchows Arch* 440: 436-440.
958. Gronwald J, Storkel S, Holtgreve-Grez H, Hadaczek P, Brinkschmidt C, Jauch A, Lubinski J, Cremer T (1997). Comparison of DNA gains and losses in primary renal clear cell carcinomas and metastatic sites: importance of 1q and 3p copy number changes in metastatic events. *Cancer Res* 57: 481-487.
959. Grosfeld JL (1999). Risk-based management: current concepts of treating malignant solid tumors of childhood. *J Am Coll Surg* 189: 407-425.
960. Grossfeld GD, Ginsberg DA, Stein JP, Bochner BH, Esrig D, Groshen S, Dunn M, Nichols PW, Taylor CR, Skinner DG, Cote RJ (1997). Thrombospondin-1 expression in bladder cancer: association with p53 alterations, tumor angiogenesis, and tumor progression. *J Natl Cancer Inst* 89: 219-227.
961. Grossfeld GD, Shi SR, Ginsberg DA, Rich KA, Skinner DG, Taylor CR, Cote RJ (1996). Immunohistochemical detection of thrombospondin-1 in formalin-fixed, paraffin-embedded tissue. *J Histochem Cytochem* 44: 761-766.
962. Grossman E, Messerli FH, Boyko V, Goldbourt U (2002). Is there an association between hypertension and cancer mortality? *Am J Med* 112: 479-486.
963. Grossman HB, Liebert M, Antelo M, Dinney CP, Hu SX, Palmer JL, Benedict WF (1998). p53 and RB expression predict progression in T1 bladder cancer. *Clin Cancer Res* 4: 829-834.
964. Grossman HB, Schmitz-Drager B, Fradet Y, Tribukait B (2000). Use of markers in defining urothelial premalignant and malignant conditions. *Scand J Urol Nephrol Suppl* 205: 94-104.
965. Grubb GR, Yun K, Williams BR, Eccles MR, Reeve AE (1994). Expression of WT1 protein in fetal kidneys and Wilms tumors. *Lab Invest* 71: 472-479.

966. Grulich AE, Swerdlow AJ, Head J, Marmot MG (1992). Cancer mortality in African and Caribbean migrants to England and Wales. Br J Cancer 66: 905-911.

967. Grundy P, Koufos A, Morgan K, Li FP, Meadows AT, Cavenee WK (1988). Familial predisposition to Wilms' tumour does not map to the short arm of chromosome 11. Nature 336: 374-376.

968. Grussendorf-Conen EI (1997). Anogenital premalignant and malignant tumors (including Buschke-Lowenstein tumors). Clin Dermatol 15: 377-388.

969. Guillem P, Delcambre F, Cohen-Solal L, Triboulet JP, Antignac C, Heidet L, Quandalle P (2001). Diffuse esophageal leiomyomatosis with perirectal involvement mimicking Hirschsprung disease. Gastroenterology 120: 216-220.

970. Guillou L, Coindre JM, Bonichon F, Nguyen BB, Terrier P, Collin F, Vilain MO, Mandard AM, Le Doussal V, Leroux A, Jacquemier J, Duplay H, Sastre-Garau X, Costa J (1997). Comparative study of the National Cancer Institute and French Federation of Cancer Centers Sarcoma Group grading systems in a population of 410 adult patients with soft tissue sarcoma. J Clin Oncol 15: 350-362.

971. Guillou L, Duvoisin B, Chobaz C, Chapuis G, Costa J (1993). Combined small-cell and transitional cell carcinoma of the renal pelvis. A light microscopic, immunohistochemical, and ultrastructural study of a case with literature review. Arch Pathol Lab Med 117: 239-243.

972. Guillou L, Wadden C, Coindre JM, Krausz T, Fletcher CD (1997). "Proximal-type" epithelioid sarcoma, a distinctive aggressive neoplasm showing rhabdoid features. Clinicopathologic, immunohistochemical, and ultrastructural study of a series. Am J Surg Pathol 21: 130-146.

973. Gulley ML, Amin MB, Nicholls JM, Banks PM, Ayala AG, Srigley JR, Eagan PA, Ro JY (1995). Epstein-Barr virus is detected in undifferentiated nasopharyngeal carcinoma but not in lymphoepithelioma-like carcinoma of the urinary bladder. Hum Pathol 26: 1207-1214.

974. Gulmez I, Dogan A, Balkanli S, Yilmaz U, Karacagil M, Tatlisen A (1997). The first case of periureteric hibernoma. Case report. Scand J Urol Nephrol 31: 203-204.

975. Guo Y, Sklar GN, Borkowski A, Kyprianou N (1997). Loss of the cyclin-dependent kinase inhibitor p27(Kip1) protein in human prostate cancer correlates with tumor grade. Clin Cancer Res 3: 2269-2274.

976. Gupta AK, Gupta MK, Gupta K (1986). Dermoid cyst of the testis (a case report). Indian J Cancer 23: 21-23.

977. Gustafson H, Tribukait B, Esposti PL (1982). The prognostic value of DNA analysis in primary carcinoma in situ of the urinary bladder. Scand J Urol Nephrol 16: 141-146.

978. Haab F, Duclos JM, Guyenne T, Plouin PF, Corvol P (1995). Renin secreting tumors: diagnosis, conservative surgical approach and long-term results. J Urol 153: 1781-1784.

979. Haas GP, Pittaluga S, Gomella L, Travis WD, Sherins RJ, Doppman JL, Linehan WM, Robertson C (1989). Clinically occult Leydig cell tumor presenting with gynecomastia. J Urol 142: 1325-1327.

980. Haas JE, Bonadio JF, Beckwith JB (1984). Clear cell sarcoma of the kidney with emphasis on ultrastructural studies. Cancer 54: 2978-2987.

981. Haber DA, Englert C, Maheswaran S (1996). Functional properties of WT1. Med Pediatr Oncol 27: 453-455.

982. Habuchi T, Devlin J, Elder PA, Knowles MA (1995). Detailed deletion mapping of chromosome 9q in bladder cancer: evidence for two tumour suppressor loci. Oncogene 11: 1671-1674.

983. Habuchi T, Kinoshita H, Yamada H, Kakehi Y, Ogawa O, Wu WJ, Takahashi R, Sugiyama T, Yoshida O (1994). Oncogene amplification in urothelial cancers with p53 gene mutation or MDM2 amplification. J Natl Cancer Inst 86: 1331-1335.

984. Habuchi T, Luscombe M, Elder PA, Knowles MA (1998). Structure and methylation-based silencing of a gene (DBCCR1) within a candidate bladder cancer tumor suppressor region at 9q32-q33. Genomics 48: 277-288.

985. Habuchi T, Ogawa O, Kakehi Y, Ogura K, Koshiba M, Hamazaki S, Takahashi R, Sugiyama T, Yoshida O (1993). Accumulated allelic losses in the development of invasive urothelial cancer. Int J Cancer 53: 579-584.

986. Habuchi T, Takahashi R, Yamada H, Kakehi Y, Sugiyama T, Yoshida O (1993). Metachronous multifocal development of urothelial cancers by intraluminal seeding. Lancet 342: 1087-1088.

987. Habuchi T, Takahashi R, Yamada H, Ogawa O, Kakehi Y, Ogura K, Hamazaki S, Toguchida J, Ishizaki K, Fujita J, Sugiyama T, Yoshida O (1993). Influence of cigarette smoking and schistosomiasis on p53 gene mutation in urothelial cancer. Cancer Res 53: 3795-3799.

988. Habuchi T, Yoshida O, Knowles MA (1997). A novel candidate tumour suppressor locus at 9q32-33 in bladder cancer: localization of the candidate region within a single 840 kb YAC. Hum Mol Genet 6: 913-919.

989. Hachicha J, Ben Moussa F, Kolsi R, Ben Maiz H, Ben Ayed H, Jarraya A (1989). [Acute renal insufficiency revealing an acute lymphoblastic leukemia (apropos of a case)]. Nephrologie 10: 83-85.

990. Hadaczek P, Podolski J, Toloczko A, Kurzawski G, Sikorski A, Rabbitts P, Huebner K, Lubinski J (1996). Losses at 3p common deletion sites in subtypes of kidney tumours: histopathological correlations. Virchows Arch 429: 37-42.

991. Haddad FS, Shah IA, Manne RK, Costantino JM, Somsin AA (1993). Renal cell carcinoma insulated in the renal capsule with calcification and ossification. Urol Int 51: 97-101.

992. Hafner C, Knuechel R, Stoehr R, Hartmann A (2002). Clonality of multifocal urothelial carcinomas: 10 years of molecular genetic studies. Int J Cancer 101: 1-6.

993. Hafner C, Knuechel R, Zanardo L, Dietmaier W, Blaszyk H, Cheville J, Hofstaedter F, Hartmann A (2001). Evidence for oligoclonality and tumor spread by intraluminal seeding in multifocal urothelial carcinomas of the upper and lower urinary tract. Oncogene 20: 4910-4915.

994. Haggman MJ, Adolfsson J, Khoury S, Montie JE, Norlen J (2000). Clinical management of premalignant lesions of the prostate. WHO Collaborative Project and Consensus Conference on public health and clinical significance of premalignant alterations in the genitourinary tract. Scand J Urol Nephrol Suppl 205: 44-49.

995. Haggman MJ, Nordin B, Mattson S, Busch C (1997). Morphometric studies of intra-prostatic volume relationships in localized prostatic cancer. Br J Urol 80: 612-617.

996. Hailemariam S, Engeler DS, Bannwart F (1998). Significance of Intratubular Germ Cell Neoplasia (ITGCN) in prepubertal testes of patients with cryptorchidism (CO): correlation with clinical reappraisal after two decades. Mod Pathol 11: 84A.

997. Hailemariam S, Engeler DS, Bannwart F, Amin MB (1997). Primary mediastinal germ cell tumor with intratubular germ cell neoplasia of the testis—further support for germ cell origin of these tumors: a case report. Cancer 79: 1031-1036.

998. Haines IE, Schwarz MA, Westmore DD, Sutherland RC (1985). Rhabdomyosarcoma in a patient treated for metastatic germ cell tumour of the testis containing teratoma—a case report. Aust N Z J Surg 55: 141-143.

999. Haleblian GE, Skinner EC, Dickinson MG, Lieskovsky G, Boyd SD, Skinner DG (1998). Hydronephrosis as a prognostic indicator in bladder cancer patients. J Urol 160: 2011-2014.

1000. Hall BD (1971). Bladder hemangiomas in Klippel-Trenaunay-Weber syndrome. N Engl J Med 285: 1032-1033.

1001. Hall GS, Kramer CE, Epstein JI (1992). Evaluation of radical prostatectomy specimens. A comparative analysis of sampling methods. Am J Surg Pathol 16: 315-324.

1002. Hall MC, Sanders JS, Vuitch F, Ramirez E, Pettaway CA (1998). Deoxyribonucleic acid flow cytometry and traditional pathologic variables in invasive penile carcinoma: assessment of prognostic significance. Urology 52: 111-116.

1003. Hall MC, Womack S, Sagalowsky AI, Carmody T, Erickstad MD, Roehrborn CG (1998). Prognostic factors, recurrence, and survival in transitional cell carcinoma of the upper urinary tract: a 30-year experience in 252 patients. Urology 52: 594-601.

1004. Hamers A, de Jong B, Suijkerbuijk RF, Geurts van Kessel A, Oosterhuis JW, van Echten J, Evers J, Bosman F (1991). A 46,XY female with mixed gonadal dysgenesis and a 48,XY, +7, +i(12p) chromosome pattern in a primary gonadal tumor. Cancer Genet Cytogenet 57: 219-224.

1005. Hamilton DL, Dare AJ, Chilton CP (1996). Multiple neurilemmomas of the penis. Br J Urol 78: 468-469.

1006. Hamilton I, Reis L, Bilimoria S, Long RG (1980). A renal vipoma. Br Med J 281: 1323-1324.

1007. Hamm B (1997). Differential diagnosis of scrotal masses by ultrasound. Eur Radiol 7: 668-679.

1008. Hammerer P, Huland H (1994). Systematic sextant biopsies in 651 patients referred for prostate evaluation. J Urol 151: 99-102.

1009. Hammerer PG, McNeal JE, Stamey TA (1995). Correlation between serum prostate specific antigen levels and the volume of the individual glandular zones of the human prostate. J Urol 153: 111-114.

1010. Hamper UM, Sheth S, Walsh PC, Epstein JI (1990). Bright echogenic foci in early prostatic carcinoma: sonographic and pathologic correlation. Radiology 176: 339-343.

1011. Hamper UM, Sheth S, Walsh PC, Holtz PM, Epstein JI (1990). Carcinoma of the prostate: value of transrectal sonography in detecting extension into the neurovascular bundle. AJR Am J Roentgenol 155: 1015-1019.

1012. Hamper UM, Sheth S, Walsh PC, Holtz PM, Epstein JI (1991). Stage B adenocarcinoma of the prostate: transrectal US and pathologic correlation of nonmalignant hypoechoic peripheral zone lesions. Radiology 180: 101-104.

1013. Hamper UM, Trapanotto V, Dejong MR, Sheth S, Caskey CI (1999). Three-dimensional US of the prostate: early experience. Radiology 212: 719-723.

1014. Han S, Peschel RE (2000). Father-son testicular tumors: evidence for genetic anticipation? A case report and review of the literature. Cancer 88: 2319-2325.

1015. Hankey BF, Feuer EJ, Clegg LX, Hayes RB, Legler JM, Prorok PC, Ries LA, Merrill RM, Kaplan RS (1999). Cancer surveillance series: interpreting trends in prostate cancer—part I: Evidence of the effects of screening in recent prostate cancer incidence, mortality, and survival rates. J Natl Cancer Inst 91: 1017-1024.

1016. Hansson J, Abrahamsson PA (2001). Neuroendocrine pathogenesis in adenocarcinoma of the prostate. Ann Oncol 12 Suppl 2: S145-S152.

1017. Hansson J, Bjartell A, Gadaleanu V, Dizeyi N, Abrahamsson PA (2002). Expression of somatostatin receptor subtypes 2 and 4 in human benign prostatic hyperplasia and prostatic cancer. Prostate 53: 50-59.

1018. Hara M, Satake M, Ogino H, Itoh M, Miyagawa H, Hashimoto Y, Okabe M, Inagaki H (2002). Primary ureteral mucosa-associated lymphoid tissue (MALT) lymphoma—pathological and radiological findings. Radiat Med 20: 41-44.

1019. Hara S, Ito K, Nagata H, Tachibana M, Murai M, Hata J (2000). [Choriocarcinoma of the renal pelvis: a case report]. Hinyokika Kiyo 46: 117-121.

1020. Harland SJ, Cook PA, Fossa SD, Horwich A, Mead GM, Parkinson MC, Roberts JT, Stenning SP (1998). Intratubular germ cell neoplasia of the contralateral testis in testicular cancer: defining a high risk group. J Urol 160: 1353-1357.

1021. Harms D, Janig U (1986). Germ cell tumours of childhood. Report of 170 cases including 59 pure and partial yolk-sac tumours. Virchows Arch A Pathol Anat Histopathol 409: 223-239.

1022. Harms D, Kock LR (1997). Testicular juvenile granulosa cell and Sertoli cell tumours: a clinicopathological study of 29 cases from the Kiel Paediatric Tumour Registry. Virchows Arch 430: 301-309.

1023. Harnden P, Eardley I, Joyce AD, Southgate J (1996). Cytokeratin 20 as an objective marker of urothelial dysplasia. Br J Urol 78: 870-875.

1024. Harnden P, Mahmood N, Southgate J (1999). Expression of cytokeratin 20 redefines urothelial papillomas of the bladder. Lancet 353: 974-977.

1025. Harnden P, Southgate J (1997). Cytokeratin 14 as a marker of squamous differentiation in transitional cell carcinomas. J Clin Pathol 50: 1032-1033.

1026. Harper ME, Glynne-Jones E, Goddard L, Thurston VJ, Griffiths K (1996). Vascular endothelial growth factor (VEGF) expression in prostatic tumours and its relationship to neuroendocrine cells. Br J Cancer 74: 910-916.

1027. Hartge P, Hoover R, West DW, Lyon JL (1983). Coffee drinking and risk of bladder cancer. J Natl Cancer Inst 70: 1021-1026.

1028. Hartmann A, Dietmaier W, Hofstadter F, Burghart LJ, Cheville JC, Blaszyk H (2003). Urothelial carcinoma of the upper urinary tract: inverted growth pattern is predictive of microsatellite instability. *Hum Pathol* 34: 222-227.
1029. Hartmann A, Moser K, Kriegmair M, Hofstetter A, Hofstaedter F, Knuechel R (1999). Frequent genetic alterations in simple urothelial hyperplasias of the bladder in patients with papillary urothelial carcinoma. *Am J Pathol* 154: 721-727.
1030. Hartmann A, Rosner U, Schlake G, Dietmaier W, Zaak D, Hofstaedter F, Knuechel R (2000). Clonality and genetic divergence in multifocal low-grade superficial urothelial carcinoma as determined by chromosome 9 and p53 deletion analysis. *Lab Invest* 80: 709-718.
1031. Hartmann A, Schlake G, Zaak D, Hungerhuber E, Hofstetter A, Hofstaedter F, Knuechel R (2002). Occurrence of chromosome 9 and p53 alterations in multifocal dysplasia and carcinoma in situ of human urinary bladder. *Cancer Res* 62: 809-818.
1032. Hartmann A, Zanardo L, Bocker-Edmonston T, Blaszyk H, Dietmaier W, Stoehr R, Cheville JC, Junker K, Wieland W, Knuechel R, Rueschoff J, Hofstaedter F, Fishel R (2002). Frequent microsatellite instability in sporadic tumors of the upper urinary tract. *Cancer Res* 62: 6796-6802.
1033. Hartmann M, Pottek T, Bussar-Maatz R, Weissbach L (1997). Elevated human chorionic gonadotropin concentrations in the testicular vein and in peripheral venous blood in seminoma patients. An analysis of various parameters. *Eur Urol* 31: 408-413.
1034. Harvei S, Skjorten FJ, Robsahm TE, Berner A, Tretli S (1998). Is prostatic intraepithelial neoplasia in the transition/central zone a true precursor of cancer? A long-term retrospective study in Norway. *Br J Cancer* 78: 46-49.
1035. Hashimoto H, Tsugawa M, Nasu Y, Tsushima T, Kumon H (1999). Primary non-Hodgkin lymphoma of the ureter. *BJU Int* 83: 148-149.
1036. Hashine K, Akiyama M, Sumiyoshi Y (1994). Primary diffuse large cell lymphoma of the penis. *Int J Urol* 1: 189-190.
1037. Hasselstrom K (1975). [Inverted papilloma of the bladder]. *Ugeskr Laeger* 137: 2834-2835.
1038. Hasui Y, Nishi S, Kitada S, Osada Y, Sumiyoshi A (1991). Comparative immunohistochemistry of malignant fibrous histiocytoma and sarcomatoid carcinoma of the urinary tract. *Urol Res* 19: 69-72.
1039. Hasui Y, Osada Y, Kitada S, Nishi S (1994). Significance of invasion to the muscularis mucosae on the progression of superficial bladder cancer. *Urology* 43: 782-786.
1040. Hatcher PA, Wilson DD (1997). Primary lymphoma of the male urethra. *Urology* 49: 142-144.
1041. Hatta Y, Hirama T, Takeuchi S, Lee E, Pham E, Miller CW, Strohmeyer T, Wilczynski SP, Melmed S, Koeffler HP (1995). Alterations of the p16 (MTS1) gene in testicular, ovarian, and endometrial malignancies. *J Urol* 154: 1954-1957.
1042. Haupt HM, Mann RB, Trump DL, Abeloff MD (1984). Metastatic carcinoma involving the testis. Clinical and pathologic distinction from primary testicular neoplasms. *Cancer* 54: 709-714.
1043. Hautmann RE, Bachor R (1993). Juvenile xanthogranuloma of the penis. *J Urol* 150: 456-457.
1044. Hayami S, Sasagawa I, Suzuki H, Kubota Y, Nakada T, Endo Y (1998). Juxtaglomerular cell tumor without hypertension. *Scand J Urol Nephrol* 32: 231-233.
1045. Hayashi T, Iida S, Taguchi J, Miyajima J, Matsuo M, Tomiyasu K, Matsuoka K, Noda S (2001). Primary carcinoid of the testis associated with carcinoid syndrome. *Int J Urol* 8: 522-524.
1046. Hayman R, Patel A, Fisher C, Hendry WF (1995). Primary seminoma of the prostate. *Br J Urol* 76: 273-274.
1047. He WW, Sciavolino PJ, Wing J, Augustus M, Hudson P, Meissner PS, Curtis RT, Shell BK, Bostwick DG, Tindall DJ, Gelmann EP, Abate-Shen C, Carter KC (1997). A novel human prostate-specific, androgen-regulated homeobox gene (NKX3.1) that maps to 8p21, a region frequently deleted in prostate cancer. *Genomics* 43: 69-77.
1048. Hedrick L, Epstein JI (1989). Use of keratin 903 as an adjunct in the diagnosis of prostate carcinoma. *Am J Surg Pathol* 13: 389-396.
1049. Hefter LG, Young IS (1975). Inverted papilloma of bladder. *Urology* 5: 688-690.
1050. Heicappell R, Muller-Mattheis V, Reinhardt M, Vosberg H, Gerharz CD, Muller-Gartner H, Ackermann R (1999). Staging of pelvic lymph nodes in neoplasms of the bladder and prostate by positron emission tomography with 2-[(18)F]-2-deoxy-D-glucose. *Eur Urol* 36: 582-587.
1051. Heidelberger KP, Ritchey ML, Dauser RC, McKeever PE, Beckwith JB (1993). Congenital mesoblastic nephroma metastatic to the brain. *Cancer* 72: 2499-2502.
1052. Heidenberg HB, Sesterhenn IA, Gaddipati JP, Weghorst CM, Buzard GS, Moul JW, Srivastava S (1995). Alteration of the tumor suppressor gene p53 in a high fraction of hormone refractory prostate cancer. *J Urol* 154: 414-421.
1053. Heidenreich A, Gaddipati JP, Moul JW, Srivastava S (1998). Molecular analysis of P16(Ink4)/CDKN2 and P15(INK4B)/MTS2 genes in primary human testicular germ cell tumors. *J Urol* 159: 1725-1730.
1054. Heidenreich A, Sesterhenn IA, Mostofi FK, Moul JW (1998). Immunohistochemical expression of monoclonal antibody 43-9F in testicular germ cell tumours. *Int J Androl* 21: 283-288.
1055. Heimann P, Devalck C, Debusscher C, Sariban E, Vamos E (1998). Alveolar soft-part sarcoma: further evidence by FISH for the involvement of chromosome band 17q25. *Genes Chromosomes Cancer* 23: 194-197.
1056. Heimann P, el Housni, Ogur G, Weterman MA, Petty EM, Vassart G (2001). Fusion of a novel gene, RCC17, to the TFE3 gene in t(X;17)(p11.2;q25.3)-bearing papillary renal cell carcinomas. *Cancer Res* 61: 4130-4135.
1057. Hejka AG, England DM (1989). Signet ring cell carcinoma of prostate. Immunohistochemical and ultrastructural study of a case. *Urology* 34: 155-158.
1058. Hellberg D, Valentin J, Eklund T, Nilsson S (1987). Penile cancer: is there an epidemiological role for smoking and sexual behaviour? *Br Med J (Clin Res Ed)* 295: 1306-1308.
1059. Hellstrom M, Haggman MJ, Brandstedt S, de la Torre M, Pedersen K, Jarlsfeldt I, Wijkstrom H, Busch C (1993). Histopathological changes in androgen-deprived localized prostatic cancer. A study in total prostatectomy specimens. *Eur Urol* 24: 461-465.
1060. Helpap B (1985). Treated prostatic carcinoma. Histological, immunohistochemical and cell kinetic studies. *Appl Pathol* 3: 230-241.
1061. Helpap B (2002). Fundamentals on the pathology of prostatic carcinoma after brachytherapy. *World J Urol* 20: 207-212.
1062. Helpap B (2002). Morphology and therapeutic strategies for neuroendocrine tumors of the genitourinary tract. *Cancer* 95: 1415-1420.
1063. Helpap B (2002). Nonepithelial tumor-like lesions of the prostate: a never-ending diagnostic problem. *Virchows Arch* 441: 231-237.
1064. Helpap B, Kloppel G (2002). Neuroendocrine carcinomas of the prostate and urinary bladder: a diagnostic and therapeutic challenge. *Virchows Arch* 440: 241-248.
1065. Helpap B, Koch V (1991). Histological and immunohistochemical findings of prostatic carcinoma after external or interstitial radiotherapy. *J Cancer Res Clin Oncol* 117: 608-614.
1066. Helpap B, Kollermann J (2001). Immunohistochemical analysis of the proliferative activity of neuroendocrine tumors from various organs. Are there indications for a neuroendocrine tumor-carcinoma sequence? *Virchows Arch* 438: 86-91.
1067. Helwig EB, Graham GH (1963). Anogenital extramammary Pagets disease. A clinicopathologic study. *Cancer* 16: 387-403.
1068. Hemal AK, Singh I, Pawar R, Kumar M, Taneja P (2000). Primary malignant bladder carcinoid—a diagnostic and management dilemma. *Urology* 55: 949.
1069. Hemminki K, Dong C (2000). Cancer in husbands of cervical cancer patients. *Epidemiology* 11: 347-349.
1070. Henderson BE, Benton B, Jing J, Yu MC, Pike MC (1979). Risk factors for cancer of the testis in young men. *Int J Cancer* 23: 598-602.
1071. Henderson DW, Allen PW, Bourne AJ (1975). Inverted urinary papilloma: report of five cases and review of the literature. *Virchows Arch A Pathol Anat Histol* 366: 177-186.
1072. Heney NM, Ahmed S, Flanagan MJ, Frable W, Corder MP, Hafermann MD, Hawkins IR (1983). Superficial bladder cancer: progression and recurrence. *J Urol* 130: 1083-1086.
1073. Henley JD, Ferry J, Ulbright TM (2000). Miscellaneous rare paratesticular tumors. *Semin Diagn Pathol* 17: 319-339.
1074. Henley JD, Young RH, Ulbright TM (2002). Malignant Sertoli cell tumors of the testis: a study of 13 examples of a neoplasm frequently misinterpreted as seminoma. *Am J Surg Pathol* 26: 541-550.
1075. Hennigar RA, Beckwith JB (1992). Nephrogenic adenofibroma. A novel kidney tumor of young people. *Am J Surg Pathol* 16: 325-334.
1076. Henricks WH, Chu YC, Goldblum JR, Weiss SW (1997). Dedifferentiated liposarcoma: a clinicopathological analysis of 155 cases with a proposal for an expanded definition of dedifferentiation. *Am J Surg Pathol* 21: 271-281.
1077. Henske EP, Ao X, Short MP, Greenberg R, Neumann HP, Kwiatkowski DJ, Russo I (1998). Frequent progesterone receptor immunoreactivity in tuberous sclerosis-associated renal angiomyolipomas. *Mod Pathol* 11: 665-668.
1078. Henske EP, Neumann HP, Scheithauer BW, Herbst EW, Short MP, Kwiatkowski DJ (1995). Loss of heterozygosity in the tuberous sclerosis (TSC2) region of chromosome band 16p13 occurs in sporadic as well as TSC-associated renal angiomyolipomas. *Genes Chromosomes Cancer* 13: 295-298.
1079. Herbers J, Schullerus D, Chudek J, Bugert P, Kanamaru H, Zeisler J, Ljungberg B, Akhtar M, Kovacs G (1998). Lack of genetic changes at specific genomic sites separates renal oncocytomas from renal cell carcinomas. *J Pathol* 184: 58-62.
1080. Herbers J, Schullerus D, Muller H, Kenck C, Chudek J, Weimer J, Bugert P, Kovacs G (1997). Significance of chromosome arm 14q loss in nonpapillary renal cell carcinomas. *Genes Chromosomes Cancer* 19: 29-35.
1081. Herman CM, Wilcox GE, Kattan MW, Scardino PT, Wheeler TM (2000). Lymphovascular invasion as a predictor of disease progression in prostate cancer. *Am J Surg Pathol* 24: 859-863.
1082. Herman JG, Latif F, Weng Y, Lerman MI, Zbar B, Liu S, Samid D, Duan DS, Gnarra JR, Linehan WM, Baylin SB (1994). Silencing of the VHL tumor-suppressor gene by DNA methylation in renal carcinoma. *Proc Natl Acad Sci USA* 91: 9700-9704.
1083. Hermans BP, Sweeney CJ, Foster RS, Einhorn LE, Donohue JP (2000). Risk of systemic metastases in clinical stage I nonseminoma germ cell testis tumor managed by retroperitoneal lymph node dissection. *J Urol* 163: 1721-1724.
1084. Hernandez-Marti MJ, Orellana-Alonso C, Badia-Garrabou L, Verdeguer Miralles A, Paradis-Alos A (1995). Renal adenocarcinoma in an 8-year-old child, with a t(X;17)(p11.2;q25). *Cancer Genet Cytogenet* 83: 82-83.
1085. Herr HW, Donat SM, Dalbagni G (2002). Correlation of cystoscopy with histology of recurrent papillary tumors of the bladder. *J Urol* 168: 978-980.
1086. Herr HW, Whitmore WFJr (1982). Significance of prostatic biopsies after radiation therapy for carcinoma of the prostate. *Prostate* 3: 339-350.
1087. Hesketh PJ, Krane RJ (1990). Prognostic assessment in nonseminomatous testicular cancer: implications for therapy. *J Urol* 144: 1-9.
1088. Heyns CF, de Kock ML, Kirsten PH, van Velden DJ (1991). Pelvic lipomatosis associated with cystitis glandularis and adenocarcinoma of the bladder. *J Urol* 145: 364-366.
1089. Hickman ES, Moroni MC, Helin K (2002). The role of p53 and pRB in apoptosis and cancer. *Curr Opin Genet Dev* 12: 60-66.
1090. Hicks RM, Gough TA, Walters CL (1978). Demonstration of the presence of nitrosamines in human urine: preliminary observations on a possible etiology for bladder cancer in association with chronic urinary tract infection. *IARC Sci Publ* 19: 465-475.
1091. Hicks RM, Ismail MM, Walters CL, Beecham PT, Rabie MF, el Alamy MA (1982). Association of bacteriuria and urinary nitrosamine formation with Schistosoma haematobium infection in the Qalyub area of Egypt. *Trans R Soc Trop Med Hyg* 76: 519-527.
1092. Hicks RM, Walters CL, Elsebai I, Aasser AB, Merzabani ME, Gough TA (1977). Demonstration of nitrosamines in human urine: preliminary observations on a possible etiology for bladder cancer in association with chronic urinary tract infections. *Proc R Soc Med* 70: 413-417.

1093. Hill MJ (1979). Role of bacteria in human carcinogenesis. *J Hum Nutr* 33: 416-426.
1094. Hilton S (2000). Imaging of renal cell carcinoma. *Semin Oncol* 27: 150-159.
1095. Hinman F, Gibson T.E. (1924). Tumors of the epididymis, spermatic cord and testicular tunics. A review of the literature and a report of three new cases. *Arch Surg* 8: 100-137.
1096. Hiratsuka Y, Nishimura H, Kajiwara I, Matsuoka H, Kawamura K (1997). Renal angiosarcoma: a case report. *Int J Urol* 4: 90-93.
1097. Hirose M, Arakawa K, Kikuchi M, Kawasaki T, Omoto T (1974). Primary reninism with renal hamartomatous alteration. *JAMA* 230: 1288-1292.
1098. Hockley NM, Bihrle R, Bennett RM3rd, Curry JM (1989). Congenital genitourinary hemangiomas in a patient with the Klippel-Trenaunay syndrome: management with the neodymium:YAG laser. *J Urol* 141: 940-941.
1099. Hodge KK, McNeal JE, Terris MK, Stamey TA (1989). Random systematic versus directed ultrasound guided transrectal core biopsies of the prostate. *J Urol* 142: 71-74.
1100. Hofmann MC, Jeltsch W, Brecher J, Walt H (1989). Alkaline phosphatase isozymes in human testicular germ cell tumors, their precancerous stage, and three related cell lines. *Cancer Res* 49: 4696-4700.
1101. Hoglund M, Sall T, Heim S, Mitelman F, Mandahl N, Fadl-Elmula I (2001). Identification of cytogenetic subgroups and karyotypic pathways in transitional cell carcinoma. *Cancer Res* 61: 8241-8246.
1102. Holck S, Jorgensen L (1983). Verrucous carcinoma of urinary bladder. *Urology* 22: 435-437.
1103. Holm-Nielsen P, Sorensen FB (1988). Renal angiomyolipoma: an ultrastructural investigation of three cases with histogenetic considerations. *APMIS Suppl* 4: 37-47.
1104. Holmang S, Andius P, Hedelin H, Wester K, Busch C, Johansson SL (2001). Stage progression in Ta papillary urothelial tumors: relationship to grade, immunohistochemical expression of tumor markers, mitotic frequency and DNA ploidy. *J Urol* 165: 1124-1128.
1105. Holmang S, Borghede G, Johansson SL (1995). Primary small cell carcinoma of the bladder: a report of 25 cases. *J Urol* 153: 1820-1822.
1106. Holmang S, Borghede G, Johansson SL (1998). Bladder carcinoma with lymphoepithelioma-like differentiation: a report of 9 cases. *J Urol* 159: 779-782.
1107. Holmang S, Hedelin H, Anderstrom C, Holmberg E, Busch C, Johansson SL (1999). Recurrence and progression in low grade papillary urothelial tumors. *J Urol* 162: 702-707.
1108. Holmang S, Hedelin H, Anderstrom C, Holmberg E, Johansson SL (2000). Prospective registration of all patients in a geographical region with newly diagnosed bladder carcinomas during a two-year period. *Scand J Urol Nephrol* 34: 95-101.
1109. Holmang S, Johansson SL (2001). The nested variant of transitional cell carcinoma—a rare neoplasm with poor prognosis. *Scand J Urol Nephrol* 35: 102-105.
1110. Holmang S, Johansson SL (2002). Stage Ta-T1 bladder cancer: the relationship between findings at first followup cystoscopy and subsequent recurrence and progression. *J Urol* 167: 1634-1637.
1111. Holmes EJ (1977). Crystalloids of prostatic carcinoma: relationship to Bence-Jones crystals. *Cancer* 39: 2073-2080.
1112. Holtl W, Hruby W, Redtenbacher M (1982). Cavernous hemangioma originating from prostatic plexus. *Urology* 20: 184-185.
1113. Holzmann K, Blin N, Welter C, Zang KD, Seitz G, Henn W (1993). Telomeric associations and loss of telomeric DNA repeats in renal tumors. *Genes Chromosomes Cancer* 6: 178-181.
1114. Honda A, Shima M, Onoe S, Hanada M, Nagai T, Nakajima S, Okada S (2000). Botryoid Wilms tumor: case report and review of literature. *Pediatr Nephrol* 14: 59-61.
1115. Honma K (1994). Paraganglia of the urinary bladder. An autopsy study. *Zentralbl Pathol* 139: 465-469.
1116. Hooper JD, Nicol DL, Dickinson JL, Eyre HJ, Scarman AL, Normyle JF, Stuttgen MA, Douglas ML, Loveland KA, Sutherland GR, Antalis TM (1999). Testisin, a new human serine proteinase expressed by premeiotic testicular germ cells and lost in testicular germ cell tumors. *Cancer Res* 59: 3199-3205.
1117. Hopenhayn-Rich C, Biggs ML, Fuchs A, Bergoglio R, Tello EE, Nicolli H, Smith AH (1996). Bladder cancer mortality associated with arsenic in drinking water in Argentina. *Epidemiology* 7: 117-124.
1118. Hopkins SC, Nag SK, Soloway MS (1984). Primary carcinoma of male urethra. *Urology* 23: 128-133.
1119. Hopman AH, Kamps MA, Speel EJ, Schapers RF, Sauter G, Ramaekers FC (2002). Identification of chromosome 9 alterations and p53 accumulation in isolated carcinoma in situ of the urinary bladder versus carcinoma in situ associated with carcinoma. *Am J Pathol* 161: 1119-1125.
1120. Hopman AH, Poddighe PJ, Smeets AW, Moesker O, Beck JL, Vooijs GP, Ramaekers FC (1989). Detection of numerical chromosome aberrations in bladder cancer by in situ hybridization. *Am J Pathol* 135: 1105-1117.
1121. Horenblas S, van Tinteren H (1994). Squamous cell carcinoma of the penis. IV. Prognostic factors of survival: analysis of tumor, nodes and metastasis classification system. *J Urol* 151: 1239-1243.
1122. Hori K, Uematsu K, Yasoshima H, Sakurai K, Yamada A (1997). Contribution of cell proliferative activity to malignancy potential in testicular seminoma. *Pathol Int* 47: 282-287.
1123. Hori K, Uematsu K, Yasoshima H, Yamada A, Sakurai K, Ohya M (1997). Testicular seminoma with human chorionic gonadotropin production. *Pathol Int* 47: 592-599.
1124. Hornak M, Pauer M, Bardos AJr, Ondrus D (1987). The incidence of carcinoma in situ in postpubertal undescended testis. *Int Urol Nephrol* 19: 321-325.
1125. Horoszewicz JS, Kawinski E, Murphy GP (1987). Monoclonal antibodies to a new antigenic marker in epithelial prostatic cells and serum of prostatic cancer patients. *Anticancer Res* 7: 927-935.
1126. Horstman WG, Melson GL, Middleton WD, Andriole GL (1992). Testicular tumors: findings with color Doppler US. *Radiology* 185: 733-737.
1127. Hosking DH, Bowman DM, McMorris SL, Ramsey EW (1981). Primary carcinoid of the testis with metastases. *J Urol* 125: 255-256.
1128. Houldsworth J, Reuter V, Bosl GJ, Chaganti RS (1997). Aberrant expression of cyclin D2 is an early event in human male germ cell tumorigenesis. *Cell Growth Differ* 8: 293-299.
1129. Houldsworth J, Xiao H, Murty VV, Chen W, Ray B, Reuter VE, Bosl GJ, Chaganti RS (1998). Human male germ cell tumor resistance to cisplatin is linked to TP53 gene mutation. *Oncogene* 16: 2345-2349.
1130. Hsing AW, Tsao L, Devesa SS (2000). International trends and patterns of prostate cancer incidence and mortality. *Int J Cancer* 85: 60-67.
1131. Hsueh C, Gonzalez-Crussi F, Murphy SB (1993). Testicular angiocentric lymphoma of postthymic T-cell type in a child with T-cell acute lymphoblastic leukemia in remission. *Cancer* 72: 1801-1805.
1132. Hsueh SF, Lai MT, Yang CC, Chung YC, Hsu CP, Peng CC, Fu HH, Cheng YM, Chang KJ, Yang SD (2002). Association of overexpressed proline-directed protein kinase F(A) with chemoresistance, invasion, and recurrence in patients with bladder carcinoma. *Cancer* 95: 775-783.
1133. Hu JC, Palapattu GS, Kattan MW, Scardino PT, Wheeler TM (1998). The association of selected pathological features with prostate cancer in a single-needle biopsy accession. *Hum Pathol* 29: 1536-1538.
1134. Hu LM, Phillipson J, Barsky SH (1992). Intratubular germ cell neoplasia in infantile yolk sac tumor. Verification by tandem repeat sequence in situ hybridization. *Diagn Mol Pathol* 1: 118-128.
1135. Huang CH, Chen L, Hsieh HH (1992). Choriocarcinoma presenting as a unilateral renal mass and gross hematuria in a male: report of a case. *J Formos Med Assoc* 91: 922-925.
1136. Huang DJ, Stanisic TH, Hansen KK (1992). Epithelioid sarcoma of the penis. *J Urol* 147: 1370-1372.
1137. Huben RP, Mounzer AM, Murphy GP (1988). Tumor grade and stage as prognostic variables in upper tract urothelial tumors. *Cancer* 62: 2016-2020.
1138. Huddart RA, Rajan B, Law M, Meyer L, Dearnaley DP (1997). Spinal cord compression in prostate cancer: treatment outcome and prognostic factors. *Radiother Oncol* 44: 229-236.
1139. Hudson DL, Guy AT, Fry P, O'Hare MJ, Watt FM, Masters JR (2001). Epithelial cell differentiation pathways in the human prostate: identification of intermediate phenotypes by keratin expression. *J Histochem Cytochem* 49: 271-278.
1140. Huff V, Amos CI, Douglass EC, Fisher R, Geiser CF, Krill CE, Li FP, Strong LC, McDonald JM (1997). Evidence for genetic heterogeneity in familial Wilms' tumor. *Cancer Res* 57: 1859-1862.
1141. Huff V, Compton DA, Chao LY, Strong LC, Geiser CF, Saunders GF (1988). Lack of linkage of familial Wilms' tumour to chromosomal band 11p13. *Nature* 336: 377-378.
1142. Huff V, Reeve AE, Leppert M, Strong LC, Douglass EC, Geiser CF, Li FP, Meadows A, Callen DF, Lenoir G, Saunders GF (1992). Nonlinkage of 16q markers to familial predisposition to Wilms' tumor. *Cancer Res* 52: 6117-6120.
1143. Hughson MD, Buchwald D, Fox M (1986). Renal neoplasia and acquired cystic kidney disease in patients receiving long-term dialysis. *Arch Pathol Lab Med* 110: 592-601.
1144. Hull GW, Rabbani F, Abbas F, Wheeler TM, Kattan MW, Scardino PT (2002). Cancer control with radical prostatectomy alone in 1,000 consecutive patients. *J Urol* 167: 528-534.
1145. Hull GW3rd, Genega EM, Sogani PC (1999). Intravascular capillary hemangioma presenting as a solid renal mass. *J Urol* 162: 784-785.
1146. Humphrey PA, Kaleem Z, Swanson PE, Vollmer RT (1998). Pseudohyperplastic prostatic adenocarcinoma. *Am J Surg Pathol* 22: 1239-1246.
1147. Humphrey PA, Vollmer RT (1990). Intraglandular tumor extent and prognosis in prostatic carcinoma: application of a grid method to prostatectomy specimens. *Hum Pathol* 21: 799-804.
1148. Huser J, Grignon DJ, Ro JY, Ayala AG, Shannon RL, Papadopoulos NJ (1990). Adult Wilms' tumor: a clinicopathologic study of 11 cases. *Mod Pathol* 3: 321-326.
1149. Hussong J, Crussi FG, Chou PM (1997). Gonadoblastoma: immunohistochemical localization of Mullerian-inhibiting substance, inhibin, WT-1, and p53. *Mod Pathol* 10: 1101-1105.
1150. IARC (1987). *IARC Monographs on the Evaluation of Carcinogenic Risks to Humans. Overall evaluations of carcinogenicity: an updating of IARC Monographs volumes 1 to 42.* IARC Press: Lyon.
1151. IARC (1991). *IARC Monographs on the Evaluation of Carcinogenic Risks to Humans. Coffee, tea, mate, methylxanthines and methylglyoxal.* IARC Press: Lyon.
1152. IARC (1994). *IARC Monographs on the Evaluation of Carcinogenic Risks to Humans. Schistosomes, Liver Flukes, and Helicobacter Pylori.* IARC Press: Lyon.
1153. IARC (1995). *IARC Monographs on the Evaluation of Carcinogenic Risks to Humans. Human papillomaviruses.* IARC Press: Lyon.
1154. IARC (1999). *IARC Monographs on the Evaluation of Carcinogenic Risks to Humans. Hormonal contraception and post-menopausal hormonal therapy.* IARC Press: Lyon.
1155. IARC (1999). *IARC Monographs on the Evaluation of Carcinogenic Risks to Humans. Some chemicals that cause tumours of the kidney or urinary bladder in rodents, and some other substances.* IARC Press: Lyon.
1156. IARC (2002). *IARC Handbooks of Cancer Prevention. Weight control and physical activity.* IARC Press: Lyon.
1157. IARC (2004). *IARC Monographs on the Evaluation of Carcinogenic Risks to Humans. Some Drinking-water Disinfectants and Contaminants, including Arsenic.* IARC Press: Lyon (in press).
1158. IARC (2004). *IARC Monographs on the Evaluation of Carcinogenic Risks to Humans. Tobacco smoke and involuntary smoking.* IARC Press: Lyon (in press).
1159. Iczkowski KA, Bostwick DG, Roche PC, Cheville JC (1998). Inhibin A is a sensitive and specific marker for testicular sex cord-stromal tumors. *Mod Pathol* 11: 774-779.
1160. Iczkowski KA, Ferguson KL, Grier DD, Hossain D, Banerjee SS, McNeal JE, Bostwick DG (2003). Adenoid cystic/basal cell carcinoma of the prostate: clinicopathologic findings in 19 cases. *Am J Surg Pathol* 27: 1523-1529.
1161. Iczkowski KA, Shanks JH, Gadaleanu V, Cheng L, Jones EC, Neumann R, Nascimento AG, Bostwick DG (2001). Inflammatory pseudotumor and sarcoma of urinary bladder: differential diagnosis and outcome in thirty-eight spindle cell neoplasms. *Mod Pathol* 14: 1043-1051.

1162. Iezzoni JC, Fechner RE, Wong LS, Rosai J (1995). Aggressive angiomyxoma in males. A report of four cases. *Am J Clin Pathol* 104: 391-396.
1163. Iezzoni JC, Kap-Herr C, Golden WL, Gaffey MJ (1997). Gonadoblastomas in 45,X/46,XY mosaicism: analysis of Y chromosome distribution by fluorescence in situ hybridization. *Am J Clin Pathol* 108: 197-201.
1164. Igawa M, Urakami S, Shirakawa H, Shiina H, Ishibe T, Usui T, Moriyama H (1995). A mapping of histology and cell proliferation in human bladder cancer: an immunohistochemical study. *Hiroshima J Med Sci* 44: 93-97.
1165. Igel TC, Engen DE, Banks PM, Keeney GL (1991). Renal plasmacytoma: Mayo Clinic experience and review of the literature. *Urology* 37: 385-389.
1166. Iizumi T, Shinohara S, Amemiya H, Tomomasa H, Yazaki T, Umeda T, Tanaka F, Imamura T (1995). Plasmacytoma of the testis. *Urol Int* 55: 218-221.
1167. Ikeda I, Miura T, Kondo I, Kameda Y (1996). Neurilemmoma of the kidney. *Br J Urol* 78: 469-470.
1168. Ikeda I, Miura T, Kondo I, Kimura A (1996). Metastatic choriocarcinoma of the kidney discovered by refractory hematuria. *Hinyokika Kiyo* 42: 447-449.
1169. Ingles SA, Coetzee GA, Ross RK, Henderson BE, Kolonel LN, Crocitto L, Wang W, Haile RW (1998). Association of prostate cancer with vitamin D receptor haplotypes in African-Americans. *Cancer Res* 58: 1620-1623.
1170. Ingles SA, Ross RK, Yu MC, Irvine RA, La Pera G, Haile RW, Coetzee GA (1997). Association of prostate cancer risk with genetic polymorphisms in vitamin D receptor and androgen receptor. *J Natl Cancer Inst* 89: 166-170.
1171. Insabato L, de Rosa G, Terracciano LM, Fazioli F, di Santo F, Rosai J (2002). Primary monotypic epithelioid angiomyolipoma of bone. *Histopathology* 40: 286-290.
1172. Ioachim E, Charchanti A, Stavropoulos NE, Skopelitou A, Athanassiou ED, Agnantis NJ (2000). Immunohistochemical expression of retinoblastoma gene product (Rb), p53 protein, MDM2, c-erbB-2, HLA-DR and proliferation indices in human urinary bladder carcinoma. *Histol Histopathol* 15: 721-727.
1173. Isa SS, Almaraz R, Magovern J (1984). Leiomyosarcoma of the penis. Case report and review of the literature. *Cancer* 54: 939-942.
1174. Isaacson PG, Norton AJ (1994). *Extranodal Lymphomas*. Churchill Livingstone: Edinburgh.
1175. Ishida Y, Kato K, Kigasawa H, Ohama Y, Ijiri R, Tanaka Y (2000). Synchronous occurrence of pleuropulmonary blastoma and cystic nephroma: possible genetic link in cystic lesions of the lung and the kidney. *Med Pediatr Oncol* 35: 85-87.
1176. Ishigooka M, Yaguchi H, Tomaru M, Sasagawa I, Nakada T, Mitobe K (1994). Mixed prostatic carcinoma containing malignant squamous element. Reports of two cases. *Scand J Urol Nephrol* 28: 425-427.
1177. Ishikawa J, Xu HJ, Hu SX, Yandell DW, Maeda S, Kamidono S, Benedict WF, Takahashi R (1991). Inactivation of the retinoblastoma gene in human bladder and renal cell carcinomas. *Cancer Res* 51: 5736-5743.
1178. Ishimaru H, Kageyama Y, Hayashi T, Nemoto T, Eishi Y, Kihara K (2002). Expression of matrix metalloproteinase-9 and bombesin/gastrin-releasing peptide in human prostate cancers and their lymph node metastases. *Acta Oncol* 41: 289-296.
1179. Ishiwata S, Takahashi S, Homma Y, Tanaka Y, Kameyama S, Hosaka Y, Kitamura T (2001). Noninvasive detection and prediction of bladder cancer by fluorescence in situ hybridization analysis of exfoliated urothelial cells in voided urine. *Urology* 57: 811-815.
1180. Isobe H, Takashima H, Higashi N, Murakami Y, Fujita K, Hanazawa K, Fujime M, Matsumoto T (2000). Primary carcinoid tumor in a horseshoe kidney. *Int J Urol* 7: 184-188.
1181. Israeli RS, Wise GJ, Bansal S, Gerard PS, Castella A (1995). Bilateral renal oncocytomatosis in a patient with renal failure. *Urology* 46: 873-875.
1182. Issa MM, Yagol R, Tsang D (1993). Intrascrotal neurofibromas. *Urology* 41: 350-352.
1183. Isshiki S, Akakura K, Komiya A, Suzuki H, Kamiya N, Ito H (2002). Chromogranin a concentration as a serum marker to predict prognosis after endocrine therapy for prostate cancer. *J Urol* 167: 512-515.
1184. Ito J, Shinohara N, Koyanagi T, Hanioka K (1998). Ossifying renal tumor of infancy: the first Japanese case with long-term follow-up. *Pathol Int* 48: 151-159.
1185. Ito T, Yamamoto S, Ohno Y, Namiki K, Aizawa T, Akiyama A, Tachibana M (2001). Up-regulation of neuroendocrine differentiation in prostate cancer after androgen deprivation therapy, degree and androgen independence. *Oncol Rep* 8: 1221-1224.
1186. Ivanov SV, Kuzmin I, Wei MH, Pack S, Geil L, Johnson BE, Stanbridge EJ, Lerman MI (1998). Down-regulation of transmembrane carbonic anhydrases in renal cell carcinoma cell lines by wild-type von Hippel-Lindau transgenes. *Proc Natl Acad Sci USA* 95: 12596-12601.
1187. Iversen T, Tretli S, Johansen A, Holte T (1997). Squamous cell carcinoma of the penis and of the cervix, vulva and vagina in spouses: is there any relationship? An epidemiological study from Norway, 1960-92. *Br J Cancer* 76: 658-660.
1188. Iwai K, Yamanaka K, Kamura T, Minato N, Conaway RC, Conaway JW, Klausner RD, Pause A (1999). Identification of the von Hippel-Lindau tumor-suppressor protein as part of an active E3 ubiquitin ligase complex. *Proc Natl Acad Sci USA* 96: 12436-12441.
1189. Iwasaki H, Ishiguro M, Ohjimi Y, Ikegami H, Takeuchi T, Kikuchi M, Kaneko Y, Ariyoshi A (1999). Synovial sarcoma of the prostate with t(X;18)(p11.2;q11.2). *Am J Surg Pathol* 23: 220-226.
1190. Iwata H, Yokoyama M, Morita M, Bekku T, Ochi K, Takeuchi M (1982). Inverted papilloma of urinary bladder. Scanning and transmission electron microscopic observation. *Urology* 19: 322-324.
1191. Izquierdo MA, van der Valk P, van Ark-Otte J, Rubio G, Germa-Lluch JR, Ueda R, Scheper RJ, Takahashi T, Giaccone G (1995). Differential expression of the c-kit proto-oncogene in germ cell tumours. *J Pathol* 177: 253-258.
1192. Jacobo E, Loening S, Schmidt JD, Culp DA (1977). Primary adenocarcinoma of the bladder: a retrospective study of 20 patients. *J Urol* 117: 54-56.
1193. Jacobs SC, Berg SI, Lawson RK (1980). Synchronous bilateral renal cell carcinoma: total surgical excision. *Cancer* 46: 2341-2345.
1194. Jacobsen GK (1993). Malignant Sertoli cell tumors of the testis. *J Urol Pathol* 1: 233-255.
1195. Jacobsen GK, Barlebo H, Olsen J (1984). Testicular germ cell tumors in Denmark 1976-1980: pathology of 1058 consecutive cases. *Acta Radiol Oncol* 23: 293-347.
1196. Jacobsen GK, Jacobsen M (1983). Alpha-fetoprotein (AFP) and human chorionic gonadotropin (HCG) in testicular germ cell tumours. A prospective immunohistochemical study. *Acta Pathol Microbiol Immunol Scand [A]* 91: 165-176.
1197. Jacobsen GK, Jacobsen M (1983). Possible liver cell differentiation in testicular germ cell tumours. *Histopathology* 7: 537-548.
1198. Jacobsen GK, Jacobsen M, Clausen PP (1981). Distribution of tumor-associated antigens in the various histologic components of germ cell tumors of the testis. *Am J Surg Pathol* 5: 257-266.
1199. Jacobsen GK, Norgaard-Pedersen B (1984). Placental alkaline phosphatase in testicular germ cell tumours and in carcinoma-in-situ of the testis. An immunohistochemical study. *Acta Pathol Microbiol Immunol Scand [A]* 92: 323-329.
1200. Jacobsen GK, Rorth M, Osterlind K, von der Maase H, Jacobsen A, Madsen EL, Pedersen M, Schultz H (1990). Histopathological features in stage I nonseminomatous testicular germ cell tumours correlated to relapse. Danish Testicular Cancer Study Group. *APMIS* 98: 377-382.
1201. Jacobsen GK, Talerman A (1989). *Atlas of Germ Cell Tumours*. Munksgaard: Copenhagen.
1202. Jacobsen GK, von der Maase H, Specht L (1995). Histopathological features of stage I seminoma treated with orchidectomy only. *J Urol Pathol* 3: 85-94.
1203. Jacobsen R, Bostofte E, Engholm G, Hansen J, Olsen JH, Skakkebaek NE, Moller H (2000). Risk of testicular cancer in men with abnormal semen characteristics: cohort study. *BMJ* 321: 789-792.
1204. Jaeger N, Weissbach L, Bussar-Maatz R (1994). Size and status of metastases after inductive chemotherapy of germ-cell tumors. Indication for salvage operation. *World J Urol* 12: 196-199.
1205. Jahn H, Nissen HM (1991). Haemangioma of the urinary tract: review of the literature. *Br J Urol* 68: 113-117.
1206. Jahnson S, Karlsson MG (2000). Tumor mapping of regional immunostaining for p21, p53, and mdm2 in locally advanced bladder carcinoma. *Cancer* 89: 619-629.
1207. Jahnson S, Risberg B, Karlsson MG, Westman G, Bergstrom R, Pedersen J (1995). p53 and Rb immunostaining in locally advanced bladder cancer: relation to prognostic variables and predictive value for the local response to radical radiotherapy. *Eur Urol* 28: 135-142.
1208. Jamieson NV, Bullock KN, Barker TH (1986). Adenosquamous carcinoma of the penis associated with balanitis xerotica obliterans. *Br J Urol* 58: 730-731.
1209. Jarvinen TA, Tanner M, Barlund M, Borg A, Isola J (1999). Characterization of topoisomerase II alpha gene amplification and deletion in breast cancer. *Genes Chromosomes Cancer* 26: 142-150.
1210. Jarvinen TA, Tanner M, Rantanen V, Barlund M, Borg A, Grenman S, Isola J (2000). Amplification and deletion of topoisomerase IIalpha associate with ErbB-2 amplification and affect sensitivity to topoisomerase II inhibitor doxorubicin in breast cancer. *Am J Pathol* 156: 839-847.
1211. Javadpour N (1986). Misconceptions and source of errors in interpretation of cellular and serum markers in testicular cancer. *J Urol* 135: 879.
1212. Jeffers M, Fiscella M, Webb CP, Anver M, Koochekpour S, Vande Woude GF (1998). The mutationally activated Met receptor mediates motility and metastasis. *Proc Natl Acad Sci USA* 95: 14417-14422.
1213. Jeffers M, Schmidt L, Nakaigawa N, Webb CP, Weirich G, Kishida T, Zbar B, Vande Woude GF (1997). Activating mutations for the met tyrosine kinase receptor in human cancer. *Proc Natl Acad Sci USA* 94: 11445-11450.
1214. Jenkins RB, Qian J, Lieber MM, Bostwick DG (1997). Detection of c-myc oncogene amplification and chromosomal anomalies in metastatic prostatic carcinoma by fluorescence in situ hybridization. *Cancer Res* 57: 524-531.
1215. Jensen OM, Knudsen JB, McLaughlin JK, Sorensen BL (1988). The Copenhagen case-control study of renal pelvis and ureter cancer: role of smoking and occupational exposures. *Int J Cancer* 41: 557-561.
1216. Jhavar S, Agarwal JP, Naresh KN, Shrivastava SK, Borges AM, Dinshaw KA (2001). Primary extranodal mucosa associated lymphoid tissue (MALT) lymphoma of the prostate. *Leuk Lymphoma* 41: 445-449.
1217. Ji X, Li W (1994). Primary carcinoid of the renal pelvis. *J Environ Pathol Toxicol Oncol* 13: 269-271.
1218. Jiang F, Desper R, Papadimitriou CH, Schaffer AA, Kallioniemi OP, Richter J, Schraml P, Sauter G, Mihatsch MJ, Moch H (2000). Construction of evolutionary tree models for renal cell carcinoma from comparative genomic hybridization data. *Cancer Res* 60: 6503-6509.
1219. Jiang F, Richter J, Schraml P, Bubendorf L, Gasser T, Sauter G, Mihatsch MJ, Moch H (1998). Chromosomal imbalances in papillary renal cell carcinoma: genetic differences between histological subtypes. *Am J Pathol* 153: 1467-1473.
1220. Jiang Z, Woda BA, Rock KL, Xu Y, Savas L, Khan A, Pihan G, Cai F, Babcook JS, Rathanaswami P, Reed SG, Xu J, Fanger GR (2001). P504S: a new molecular marker for the detection of prostate carcinoma. *Am J Surg Pathol* 25: 1397-1404.
1221. Jiang Z, Wu CL, Woda BA, Dresser K, Xu J, Fanger GR, Yang XJ (2002). P504S/alpha-methylacyl-CoA racemase: a useful marker for diagnosis of small foci of prostatic carcinoma on needle biopsy. *Am J Surg Pathol* 26: 1169-1174.
1222. Jiborn T, Bjartell A, Abrahamsson PA (1998). Neuroendocrine differentiation in prostatic carcinoma during hormonal treatment. *Urology* 51: 585-589.
1223. Jimenez-Quintero LP, Ro JY, Zavala-Pompa A, Amin MB, Tetu B, Ordonez NG, Ayala AG (1993). Granulosa cell tumor of the adult testis: a clinicopathologic study of seven cases and a review of the literature. *Hum Pathol* 24: 1120-1125.
1224. Jimenez RE, Eble JN, Reuter VE, Epstein JI, Folpe AL, Peralta-Venturina M, Tamboli P, Ansell ID, Grignon DJ, Young RH, Amin MB (2001). Concurrent angiomyolipoma and renal cell neoplasia: a study of 36 cases. *Mod Pathol* 14: 157-163.

1225. Jimenez RE, Folpe AL, Lapham RL, Ro JY, O'Shea PA, Weiss SW, Amin MB (2002). Primary Ewing's sarcoma/primitive neuroectodermal tumor of the kidney: a clinicopathologic and immunohistochemical analysis of 11 cases. *Am J Surg Pathol* 26: 320-327.
1226. Jimenez RE, Gheiler E, Oskanian P, Tiguert R, Sakr W, Wood DPJr, Pontes JE, Grignon DJ (2000). Grading the invasive component of urothelial carcinoma of the bladder and its relationship with progression-free survival. *Am J Surg Pathol* 24: 980-987.
1227. Johansson S, Angervall L, Bengtsson U, Wahlqvist L (1974). Uroepithelial tumors of the renal pelvis associated with abuse of phenacetin-containing analgesics. *Cancer* 33: 743-753.
1228. Johansson SL, Borghede G, Holmang S (1999). Micropapillary bladder carcinoma: a clinicopathological study of 20 cases. *J Urol* 161: 1798-1802.
1229. Johnson DE, Ayala AG (1973). Primary melanoma of penis. *Urology* 2: 174-177.
1230. Johnson DE, Hodge GB, Abdul-Karim FW, Ayala AG (1985). Urachal carcinoma. *Urology* 26: 218-221.
1231. Johnson DE, Hogan JM, Ayala AG (1972). Transitional cell carcinoma of the prostate. A clinical morphological study. *Cancer* 29: 287-293.
1232. Johnson DE, Lo RK, Srigley J, Ayala AG (1985). Verrucous carcinoma of the penis. *J Urol* 133: 216-218.
1233. Johnson DE, Schoenwald MB, Ayala AG, Miller LS (1976). Squamous cell carcinoma of the bladder. *J Urol* 115: 542-544.
1234. Johnson RE, Scheithauer B (1982). Massive hyperplasia of testicular adrenal rests in a patient with Nelson's syndrome. *Am J Clin Pathol* 77: 501-507.
1235. Johnson RE, Scheithauer BW, Dahlin DC (1983). Melanotic neuroectodermal tumor of infancy. A review of seven cases. *Cancer* 52: 661-666.
1236. Jones EC, Murray SK, Young RH (2000). Cysts and epithelial proliferations of the testicular collecting system (including rete testis). *Semin Diagn Pathol* 17: 270-293.
1237. Jones EC, Pins M, Dickersin GR, Young RH (1995). Metanephric adenoma of the kidney. A clinicopathological, immunohistochemical, flow cytometric, cytogenetic, and electron microscopic study of seven cases. *Am J Surg Pathol* 19: 615-626.
1238. Jones EC, Young RH (1997). Myxoid and sclerosing sarcomatoid transitional cell carcinoma of the urinary bladder: a clinicopathologic and immunohistochemical study of 25 cases. *Mod Pathol* 10: 908-916.
1239. Jones MA, Young RH, Scully RE (1995). Malignant mesothelioma of the tunica vaginalis. A clinicopathologic analysis of 11 cases with review of the literature. *Am J Surg Pathol* 19: 815-825.
1240. Jones MA, Young RH, Scully RE (1997). Adenocarcinoma of the epididymis: a report of four cases and review of the literature. *Am J Surg Pathol* 21: 1474-1480.
1241. Jones MA, Young RH, Scully RE (1997). Benign fibromatous tumors of the testis and paratesticular region: a report of 9 cases with a proposed classification of fibromatous tumors and tumor-like lesions. *Am J Surg Pathol* 21: 296-305.
1242. Jones MA, Young RH, Srigley JR, Scully RE (1995). Paratesticular serous papillary carcinoma. A report of six cases. *Am J Surg Pathol* 19: 1359-1365.
1243. Jones MW (1989). Primary Hodgkin's disease of the urinary bladder. *Br J Urol* 63: 438.
1244. Jones VS, Chandra S, Smile SR, Narasimhan R (2000). A unique case of metastatic penile basal cell carcinoma. *Indian J Pathol Microbiol* 43: 465-466.
1245. Jones WA, Gibbons RP, Correa RJJr, Cummings KB, Mason JT (1980). Primary adenocarcinoma of bladder. *Urology* 15: 119-122.
1246. Joos S, Bergerheim US, Pan Y, Matsuyama H, Bentz M, du Manoir S, Lichter P (1995). Mapping of chromosomal gains and losses in prostate cancer by comparative genomic hybridization. *Genes Chromosomes Cancer* 14: 267-276.
1247. Jordan AM, Weingarten J, Murphy WM (1987). Transitional cell neoplasms of the urinary bladder. Can biologic potential be predicted from histologic grading? *Cancer* 60: 2766-2774.
1248. Jorgensen N, Muller J, Jaubert F, Clausen OP, Skakkebaek NE (1997). Heterogeneity of gonadoblastoma germ cells: similarities with immature germ cells, spermatogonia and testicular carcinoma in situ cells. *Histopathology* 30: 177-186.
1249. Joshi VV, Banerjee AK, Yadav K, Pathak IC (1977). Cystic partially differentiated nephroblastoma: a clinicopathologic entity in the spectrum of infantile renal neoplasia. *Cancer* 40: 789-795.
1250. Joshi VV, Beckwith JB (1989). Multilocular cyst of the kidney (cystic nephroma) and cystic, partially differentiated nephroblastoma. Terminology and criteria for diagnosis. *Cancer* 64: 466-479.
1251. Joshi VV, Beckwith JB (1990). Pathologic delineation of the papillonodular type of cystic partially differentiated nephroblastoma. A review of 11 cases. *Cancer* 66: 1568-1577.
1252. Juhasz J, Kiss P (1978). A hitherto undescribed case of "collision" tumour: liposarcoma of the seminal vesicle and prostatic carcinoma. *Int Urol Nephrol* 10: 185-193.
1253. Jun SY, Choi J, Kang GH, Park SH, Kim HW, Ro JY (2003). Synovial sarcomas of kidney with rhabdoid features. *Mod Pathol* 16: 155A.
1254. Jungbluth AA, Busam KJ, Gerald WL, Stockert E, Coplan KA, Iversen K, MacGregor DP, Old LJ, Chen YT (1998). A103: An anti-melan-a monoclonal antibody for the detection of malignant melanoma in paraffin-embedded tissues. *Am J Surg Pathol* 22: 595-602.
1255. Kabalin JN, Freiha FS, Niebel JD (1990). Leiomyoma of bladder. Report of 2 cases and demonstration of ultrasonic appearance. *Urology* 35: 210-212.
1256. Kagan J, Liu J, Stein JD, Wagner SS, Babkowski R, Grossman BH, Katz RL (1998). Cluster of allele losses within a 2.5 cM region of chromosome 10 in high-grade invasive bladder cancer. *Oncogene* 16: 909-913.
1257. Kahn DG, Rothman PJ, Weisman JD (1991). Urethral T-cell lymphoma as the initial manifestation of the acquired immune deficiency syndrome. *Arch Pathol Lab Med* 115: 1169-1170.
1258. Kaiserling E, Krober S, Xiao JC, Schaumburg-Lever G (1994). Angiomyolipoma of the kidney. Immunoreactivity with HMB-45. Light- and electron-microscopic findings. *Histopathology* 25: 41-48.
1259. Kakizaki H, Nakada T, Sugano O, Kato H, Yamakawa M (1994). Malignant lymphoma in the female urethra. *Int J Urol* 1: 281-282.
1260. Kakizoe T, Fujita J, Murase T, Matsumoto K, Kishi K (1980). Transitional cell carcinoma of the bladder in patients with renal pelvic and ureteral cancer. *J Urol* 124: 17-19.
1261. Kakizoe T, Matsumoto K, Andoh M, Nishio Y, Kishi K (1983). Adenocarcinoma of urachus. Report of 7 cases and review of literature. *Urology* 21: 360-366.
1262. Kamai T, Arai K, Sumi S, Tsujii T, Honda M, Yamanishi T, Yoshida KI (2002). The rho/rho-kinase pathway is involved in the progression of testicular germ cell tumour. *BJU Int* 89: 449-453.
1263. Kamat MR, Kulkarni JN, Tongaonkar HB (1991). Adenocarcinoma of the bladder: study of 14 cases and review of the literature. *Br J Urol* 68: 254-257.
1264. Kamura T, Koepp DM, Conrad MN, Skowyra D, Moreland RJ, Iliopoulos O, Lane WS, Kaelin WGJr, Elledge SJ, Conaway RC, Harper JW, Conaway JW (1999). Rbx1, a component of the VHL tumor suppressor complex and SCF ubiquitin ligase. *Science* 284: 657-661.
1265. Kanayama H, Lui WO, Takahashi M, Naroda T, Kedra D, Wong FK, Kuroki Y, Nakahori Y, Larsson C, Kagawa S, Teh BT (2001). Association of a novel constitutional translocation t(1q;3q) with familial renal cell carcinoma. *J Med Genet* 38: 165-170.
1266. Kandel LB, Harrison LH, Woodruff RD, Williams CD, Ahl ETJr (1984). Renal plasmacytoma: a case report and summary of reported cases. *J Urol* 132: 1167-1169.
1267. Kandel LB, McCullough DL, Harrison LH, Woodruff RD, Ahl ETJr, Munitz HA (1987). Primary renal lymphoma. Does it exist? *Cancer* 60: 386-391.
1268. Kanno H, Kondo K, Ito S, Yamamoto I, Fujii S, Torigoe S, Sakai N, Hosaka M, Shuin T, Yao M (1994). Somatic mutations of the von Hippel-Lindau tumor suppressor gene in sporadic central nervous system hemangioblastomas. *Cancer Res* 54: 4845-4847.
1269. Kanno T, Kamoto T, Terai A, Kakehi Y, Terachi T, Ogawa O (2001). [A case of malignant fibrous histiocytoma arising from the renal capsule]. *Hinyokika Kiyo* 47: 95-98.
1270. Kanoe H, Nakayama T, Murakami H, Hosaka T, Yamamoto H, Nakashima Y, Tsuboyama T, Nakamura T, Sasaki MS, Toguchida J (1998). Amplification of the CDK4 gene in sarcomas: tumor specificity and relationship with the RB gene mutation. *Anticancer Res* 18: 2317-2321.
1271. Kantor AF, Hartge P, Hoover RN, Fraumeni JFJr (1988). Epidemiological characteristics of squamous cell carcinoma and adenocarcinoma of the bladder. *Cancer Res* 48: 3853-3855.
1272. Kao J, Upton M, Zhang P, Rosen S (2002). Individual prostate biopsy core embedding facilitates maximal tissue representation. *J Urol* 168: 496-499.
1273. Kapadia SB, Frisman DM, Hitchcock CL, Ellis GL, Popek EJ (1993). Melanotic neuroectodermal tumor of infancy. Clinicopathological, immunohistochemical, and flow cytometric study. *Am J Surg Pathol* 17: 566-573.
1274. Kaplan GW, Cromie WC, Kelalis PP, Silber I, Tank ESJr (1988). Prepubertal yolk sac testicular tumors—report of the testicular tumor registry. *J Urol* 140: 1109-1112.
1275. Kaplan GW, Cromie WJ, Kelalis PP, Silber I, Tank ESJr (1986). Gonadal stromal tumors: a report of the Prepubertal Testicular Tumor Registry. *J Urol* 136: 300-302.
1276. Karamehmedovic O, Woodtli W, Pluss HJ (1975). Testicular tumors in childhood. *J Pediatr Surg* 10: 109-114.
1277. Karolyi P, Endes P, Krasznai G, Tonkol I (1988). Bizarre leiomyoma of the prostate. *Virchows Arch A Pathol Anat Histopathol* 412: 383-386.
1278. Karpas CM, Moumgis B (1969). Primary transitional cell carcinoma of prostate gland: possible pathogenesis and relationship to reserve cell hyperplasia of prostatic periurethral ducts. *J Urol* 101: 201-205.
1279. Karsdorp N, Elderson A, Wittebol-Post D, Hene RJ, Vos J, Feldberg MA, van Gils AP, Jansen-Schillhorn van Veen JM, Vroom TM, Hoppener JW, Lips CJ (1994). Von Hippel-Lindau disease: new strategies in early detection and treatment. *Am J Med* 97: 158-168.
1280. Kato H, Suzuki M, Mukai M, Aizawa S (1999). Clinicopathological study of pheochromocytoma of the urinary bladder: immunohistochemical, flow cytometric and ultrastructural findings with review of the literature. *Pathol Int* 49: 1093-1099.
1281. Kato K, Ijiri R, Tanaka Y, Kigasawa H, Toyoda Y, Senga Y (1999). Metachronous renal cell carcinoma in a child cured of neuroblastoma. *Med Pediatr Oncol* 33: 432-433.
1282. Kato K, Ijiri R, Tanaka Y, Toyoda Y, Chiba K, Kitami K (2000). Testicular immature teratoma with primitive neuroectodermal tumor in early childhood. *J Urol* 164: 2068-2069.
1283. Kattan J, Culine S, Terrier-Lacombe MJ, Theodore C, Droz JP (1993). Paratesticular rhabdomyosarcoma in adult patients: 16-year experience at Institut Gustave-Roussy. *Ann Oncol* 4: 871-875.
1284. Kattan MW, Wheeler TM, Scardino PT (1999). Postoperative nomogram for disease recurrence after radical prostatectomy for prostate cancer. *J Clin Oncol* 17: 1499-1507.
1285. Kaufman JJ, Waisman J (1985). Primary carcinoid tumor of testis with metastasis. *Urology* 25: 534-536.
1286. Kaufmann O, Fietze E, Mengs J, Dietel M (2001). Value of p63 and cytokeratin 5/6 as immunohistochemical markers for the differential diagnosis of poorly differentiated and undifferentiated carcinomas. *Am J Clin Pathol* 116: 823-830.
1287. Kausch I, Bohle A (2002). Molecular aspects of bladder cancer III. Prognostic markers of bladder cancer. *Eur Urol* 41: 15-29.
1288. Kausch I, Doehn C, Buttner H, Fornara P, Jocham D (1998). Primary lymphoma of the epididymis. *J Urol* 160: 1801-1802.
1289. Kawaguchi K, Oda Y, Nakanishi K, Saito T, Tamiya S, Nakahara K, Matsuoka H, Tsuneyoshi M (2002). Malignant transformation of renal angiomyolipoma: a case report. *Am J Surg Pathol* 26: 523-529.
1290. Kay S, Fu Y, Koontz WW, Chen AT (1975). Interstitial-cell tumor of the testis. Tissue culture and ultrastructural studies. *Am J Clin Pathol* 63: 366-376.
1291. Keen AJ, Knowles MA (1994). Definition of two regions of deletion on chromosome 9 in carcinoma of the bladder. *Oncogene* 9: 2083-2088.
1292. Keen MR, Golden RL, Richardson JF, Melicow MM (1970). Carcinoma of Cowper's gland treated with chemotherapy. *J Urol* 104: 854-859.

1293. Keetch DW, Catalona WJ (1995). Prostatic transition zone biopsies in men with previous negative biopsies and persistently elevated serum prostate specific antigen values. *J Urol* 154: 1795-1797.

1294. Keetch DW, Humphrey P, Stahl D, Smith DS, Catalona WJ (1995). Morphometric analysis and clinical followup of isolated prostatic intraepithelial neoplasia in needle biopsy of the prostate. *J Urol* 154: 347-351.

1295. Kellert E (1959). An ovarian type pseudomucinous cystadenoma in the scrotum. *Cancer* 12: 187-190.

1296. Kellie SJ, Pui CH, Murphy SB (1989). Childhood non-Hodgkin's lymphoma involving the testis: clinical features and treatment outcome. *J Clin Oncol* 7: 1066-1070.

1297. Kempton CL, Kurtin PJ, Inwards DJ, Wollan P, Bostwick DG (1997). Malignant lymphoma of the bladder: evidence from 36 cases that low-grade lymphoma of the MALT-type is the most common primary bladder lymphoma. *Am J Surg Pathol* 21: 1324-1333.

1298. Kennedy SM, Merino MJ, Linehan WM, Roberts JR, Robertson CN, Neumann RD (1990). Collecting duct carcinoma of the kidney. *Hum Pathol* 21: 449-456.

1299. Kennelly MJ, Grossman HB, Cho KJ (1994). Outcome analysis of 42 cases of renal angiomyolipoma. *J Urol* 152: 1988-1991.

1300. Kerley SW, Blute ML, Keeney GL (1991). Multifocal malignant melanoma arising in vesicovaginal melanosis. *Arch Pathol Lab Med* 115: 950-952.

1301. Kersemaekers AM, Mayer F, Molier M, van Weeren PC, Oosterhuis JW, Bokemeyer C, Looijenga LH (2002). Role of P53 and MDM2 in treatment response of human germ cell tumors. *J Clin Oncol* 20: 1551-1561.

1302. Keshet E, Lyman SD, Williams DE, Anderson DM, Jenkins NA, Copeland NG, Parada LF (1991). Embryonic RNA expression patterns of the c-kit receptor and its cognate ligand suggest multiple functional roles in mouse development. *EMBO J* 10: 2425-2435.

1303. Khalbuss WE, Hossain M, Elhosseiny A (2001). Primary malignant melanoma of the urinary bladder diagnosed by urine cytology: a case report. *Acta Cytol* 45: 631-635.

1304. Khan A, Thomas N, Costello B, Jobling L, de Kretser D, Broadfield E, O'Shea S (2000). Renal medullary carcinoma: sonographic, computed tomography, magnetic resonance and angiographic findings. *Eur J Radiol* 35: 1-7.

1305. Khanna S (1991). Cavernous haemangioma of the glans penis. *Br J Urol* 67: 332.

1306. Khoo SK, Bradley M, Wong FK, Hedblad MA, Nordenskjold M, Teh BT (2001). Birt-Hogg-Dube syndrome: mapping of a novel hereditary neoplasia gene to chromosome 17p12-q11.2. *Oncogene* 20: 5239-5242.

1307. Khoo SK, Giraud S, Kahnoski K, Chen J, Motorna O, Nickolov R, Binet O, Lambert D, Friedel J, Levy R, Ferlicot S, Wolkenstein P, Hammel P, Bergerheim U, Hedblad MA, Bradley M, Teh BT, Nordenskjold M, Richard S (2002). Clinical and genetic studies of Birt-Hogg-Dube syndrome. *J Med Genet* 39: 906-912.

1308. Khoo SK, Kahnoski K, Sugimura J, Petillo D, Chen J, Shockley K, Ludlow J, Knapp R, Giraud S, Richard S, Nordenskjold M, Teh BT (2003). Inactivation of BHD in sporadic renal tumors. *Cancer Res* 63: 4583-4587.

1309. Khoury JM, Stutzman RE, Sepulveda RA (1985). Inverted papilloma of the bladder with focal transitional cell carcinoma: a case report. *Mil Med* 150: 562-563.

1310. Kibel A, Iliopoulos O, Decaprio JA, Kaelin WGJr (1995). Binding of the von Hippel-Lindau tumor suppressor protein to Elongin B and C. *Science* 269: 1444-1446.

1311. Kidd JM (1970). Exclusion of certain renal neoplasms from the category of Wilms tumor. *Am J Pathol* 58: 16A.

1312. Kiemeney LA, Moret NC, Witjes JA, Schoenberg MP, Tulinius H (1997). Familial transitional cell carcinoma among the population of Iceland. *J Urol* 157: 1649-1651.

1313. Kiemeney LA, Schoenberg M (1996). Familial transitional cell carcinoma. *J Urol* 156: 867-872.

1314. Kiemeney LA, Witjes JA, Heijbroek RP, Verbeek AL, Debruyne FM (1993). Predictability of recurrent and progressive disease in individual patients with primary superficial bladder cancer. *J Urol* 150: 60-64.

1315. Kilicaslan I, Gulluoglu MG, Dogan O, Uysal V (2000). Intraglomerular microlesions in renal angiomyolipoma. *Hum Pathol* 31: 1325-1328.

1316. Kim DH, Sohn JH, Lee MC, Lee G, Yoon GS, Hashimoto H, Sonobe H, Ro JY (2000). Primary synovial sarcoma of the kidney. *Am J Surg Pathol* 24: 1097-1104.

1317. Kim ED, Kroft S, Dalton DP (1994). Basal cell carcinoma of the penis: case report and review of the literature. *J Urol* 152: 1557-1559.

1318. Kim I, Young RH, Scully RE (1985). Leydig cell tumors of the testis. A clinicopathological analysis of 40 cases and review of the literature. *Am J Surg Pathol* 9: 177-192.

1319. Kim MJ, Bhatia-Gaur R, Banach-Petrosky WA, Desai N, Wang Y, Hayward SW, Cunha GR, Cardiff RD, Shen MM, Abate-Shen C (2002). Nkx3.1 mutant mice recapitulate early stages of prostate carcinogenesis. *Cancer Res* 62: 2999-3004.

1320. Kim SI, Kwon SM, Kim YS, Hong SJ (2002). Association of cyclooxygenase-2 expression with prognosis of stage T1 grade 3 bladder cancer. *Urology* 60: 816-821.

1321. Kim TS, Seong DH, Ro JY (2001). Small cell carcinoma of the ureter with squamous cell and transitional cell carcinomatous components associated with ureteral stone. *J Korean Med Sci* 16: 796-800.

1322. Kindblom LG, Pettersson G (1976). Primary carcinoma of the seminal vesicle. Case report. *Acta Pathol Microbiol Scand [A]* 84: 301-305.

1323. Kirkland KL, Bale PM (1967). A cystic adenoma of the prostate. *J Urol* 97: 324-327.

1324. Kirsch AJ, Newhouse J, Hibshoosh H, O'Toole K, Ritter J, Benson MC (1996). Giant multilocular cystadenoma of the prostate. *Urology* 48: 303-305.

1325. Kitamura H, Umehara T, Miyake M, Shimizu T, Kohda K, Ando M (1996). NonHodgkin's lymphoma arising in the urethra of a man. *J Urol* 156: 175-176.

1326. Kitamura M, Miyanaga T, Hamada M, Nakata Y, Satoh Y, Terakawa T (1997). Small cell carcinoma of the kidney: case report. *Int J Urol* 4: 422-424.

1327. Kittredge WE, Collett AJ, Morgan C (1964). Adenocarcinoma of the bladder associated with cystitis glandularis. A case report. *J Urol* 91: 145-150.

1328. Kiuru M (2002). Molecular basis of hereditary leiomyomatosis and renal cell cancer (HLRCC).

1329. Kiuru M, Launonen V, Hietala M, Aittomaki K, Vierimaa O, Salovaara R, Arola J, Pukkala E, Sistonen P, Herva R, Aaltonen LA (2001). Familial cutaneous leiomyomatosis is a two-hit condition associated with renal cell cancer of characteristic histopathology. *Am J Pathol* 159: 825-829.

1330. Kiuru M, Lehtonen R, Arola J, Salovaara R, Jarvinen H, Aittomaki K, Sjoberg J, Visakorpi T, Knuutila S, Isola J, Delahunt B, Herva R, Launonen V, Karhu A, Aaltonen LA (2002). Few FH mutations in sporadic counterparts of tumor types observed in hereditary leiomyomatosis and renal cell cancer families. *Cancer Res* 62: 4554-4557.

1331. Kiyosawa T, Umebayashi Y, Nakayama Y, Soeda S (1995). Hereditary multiple glomus tumors involving the glans penis. A case report and review of the literature. *Dermatol Surg* 21: 895-899.

1332. Klan R, Loy V, Huland H (1991). Residual tumor discovered in routine second transurethral resection in patients with stage T1 transitional cell carcinoma of the bladder. *J Urol* 146: 316-318.

1333. Klein EA (1993). Tumor markers in testis cancer. *Urol Clin North Am* 20: 67-73.

1334. Klein FA, Herr HW, Vugrin D (1983). Fibrosarcoma associated with intensive chemotherapy for advanced germ cell testicular tumor. *J Surg Oncol* 23: 5-7.

1335. Klein MJ, Valensi QJ (1976). Proximal tubular adenomas of kidney with so-called oncocytic features. A clinicopathologic study of 13 cases of a rarely reported neoplasm. *Cancer* 38: 906-914.

1336. Knezevich SR, Garnett MJ, Pysher TJ, Beckwith JB, Grundy PE, Sorensen PH (1998). ETV6-NTRK3 gene fusions and trisomy 11 establish a histogenetic link between mesoblastic nephroma and congenital fibrosarcoma. *Cancer Res* 58: 5046-5048.

1337. Knezevich SR, McFadden DE, Tao W, Lim JF, Sorensen PH (1998). A novel ETV6-NTRK3 gene fusion in congenital fibrosarcoma. *Nat Genet* 18: 184-187.

1338. Knoll LD, Segura JW, Scheithauer BW (1986). Leiomyoma of the bladder. *J Urol* 136: 906-908.

1339. Knowles MA (1995). Molecular genetics of bladder cancer. *Br J Urol* 75 Suppl 1: 57-66.

1340. Knowles MA (2001). What we could do now: molecular pathology of bladder cancer. *Mol Pathol* 54: 215-221.

1341. Knowles MA, Williamson M (1993). Mutation of H-ras is infrequent in bladder cancer: confirmation by single-strand conformation polymorphism analysis, designed restriction fragment length polymorphisms, and direct sequencing. *Cancer Res* 53: 133-139.

1342. Koberle B, Masters JR, Hartley JA, Wood RD (1999). Defective repair of cisplatin-induced DNA damage caused by reduced XPA protein in testicular germ cell tumours. *Curr Biol* 9: 273-276.

1343. Kochevar J (1984). Adenocarcinoid tumor, goblet cell type, arising in a ureteroileal conduit: a case report. *J Urol* 131: 957-959.

1344. Koeneman KS, Pan CX, Jin JK, Pyle JM3rd, Flanigan RC, Shankey TV, Diaz MO (1998). Telomerase activity, telomere length, and DNA ploidy in prostatic intraepithelial neoplasia (PIN). *J Urol* 160: 1533-1539.

1345. Koide O, Iwai S, Baba K, Iri H (1987). Identification of testicular atypical germ cells by an immunohistochemical technique for placental alkaline phosphatase. *Cancer* 60: 1325-1330.

1346. Koide O, Matsuzaka K, Tanaka Y (1998). Multiple giant angiomyolipomas with a polygonal epithelioid cell component in tuberous sclerosis: an autopsy case report. *Pathol Int* 48: 998-1002.

1347. Kojima S, Mine M, Sekine H (1998). [Small cell carcinoma of the kidney. A case report]. *Nippon Hinyokika Gakkai Zasshi* 89: 614-617.

1348. Kolonel LN (1996). Nutrition and prostate cancer. *Cancer Causes Control* 7: 83-94.

1349. Komatsu H, Tanabe N, Kubodera S, Maezawa H, Ueno A (1997). The role of lymphadenectomy in the treatment of transitional cell carcinoma of the upper urinary tract. *J Urol* 157: 1622-1624.

1350. Kommoss F, Bibbo M, Talerman A (1990). Nuclear deoxyribonucleic acid content (ploidy) of endodermal sinus (yolk sac) tumor. *Lab Invest* 62: 223-231.

1351. Kondoh G, Murata Y, Aozasa K, Yutsudo M, Hakura A (1991). Very high incidence of germ cell tumorigenesis (seminomagenesis) in human papillomavirus type 16 transgenic mice. *J Virol* 65: 3335-3339.

1352. Konno N, Mori M, Kurooka Y, Kameyama S, Homma Y, Moriyama N, Tajima A, Murayama T, Kawabe K (1997). Carcinosarcoma in the region of the female urethra. *Int J Urol* 4: 229-231.

1353. Koochekpour S, Jeffers M, Wang PH, Gong C, Taylor GA, Roessler LM, Stearman R, Vasselli JR, Stetler-Stevenson WG, Kaelin WGJr, Linehan WM, Klausner RD, Gnarra JR, Vande Woude GF (1999). The von Hippel-Lindau tumor suppressor gene inhibits hepatocyte growth factor/scatter factor-induced invasion and branching morphogenesis in renal carcinoma cells. *Mol Cell Biol* 19: 5902-5912.

1354. Koolen MI, Schipper P, Liebergen FJ, Kurstjens RM, Unnik AJ, Bogman MJ (1988). Non-Hodgkin lymphoma with unique localization in the kidneys presenting with acute renal failure. *Clin Nephrol* 29: 41-46.

1355. Koolen MI, van der Meyden AP, Bodmer D, Eleveld M, van der Looij E, Brunner H, Smits A, van den Berg E, Smeets D, Geurts van Kessel A (1998). A familial case of renal cell carcinoma and a t(2;3) chromosome translocation. *Kidney Int* 53: 273-275.

1356. Kopf AW, Bart RS (1981). Tumor conference #38. Lymphangioma of the scrotum and penis. *J Dermatol Surg Oncol* 7: 870-872.

1357. Koraitim M, Kamal B, Metwalli N, Zaky Y (1995). Transurethral ultrasonographic assessment of bladder carcinoma: its value and limitation. *J Urol* 154: 375-378.

1358. Korkolopoulou P, Christodoulou P, Kapralos P, Exarchakos M, Bisbiroula A, Hadjiyannakis M, Georgountzos C, Thomas-Tsagli E (1997). The role of p53, MDM2 and c-erb B-2 oncoproteins, epidermal growth factor receptor and proliferation markers in the prognosis of urinary bladder cancer. *Pathol Res Pract* 193: 767-775.

1359. Korkolopoulou P, Christodoulou P, Konstantinidou AE, Thomas-Tsagli E, Kapralos P, Davaris P (2000). Cell cycle regulators in bladder cancer: a multivariate survival study with emphasis on p27Kip1. *Hum Pathol* 31: 751-760.

1360. Korn WM, Oide Weghuis DE, Suijkerbuijk RF, Schmidt U, Otto T, du Manoir S, Geurts van Kessel A, Harstrick A, Seeber S, Becher R (1996). Detection of chromosomal DNA gains and losses in testicular germ cell tumors by comparative genomic hybridization. *Genes Chromosomes Cancer* 17: 78-87.
1361. Koss LG (1975). *Tumours of the Urinary Bladder.* 2nd Edition. AFIP: Washington, DC.
1362. Koss LG (1979). Mapping of the urinary bladder: its impact on the concepts of bladder cancer. *Hum Pathol* 10: 533-548.
1363. Koss LG (1998). Natural history and patterns of invasive cancer of the bladder. *Eur Urol* 33 Suppl 4: 2-4.
1364. Kothari PS, Scardino PT, Ohori M, Kattan MW, Wheeler TM (2001). Incidence, location, and significance of periprostatic and periseminal vesicle lymph nodes in prostate cancer. *Am J Surg Pathol* 25: 1429-1432.
1365. Kotliar SN, Wood CG, Schaeffer AJ, Oyasu R (1995). Transitional cell carcinoma exhibiting clear cell features. A differential diagnosis for clear cell adenocarcinoma of the urinary tract. *Arch Pathol Lab Med* 119: 79-81.
1366. Kotti TJ, Savolainen K, Helander HM, Yagi A, Novikov DK, Kalkkinen N, Conzelmann E, Hiltunen JK, Schmitz W (2000). In mouse alpha-methylacyl-CoA racemase, the same gene product is simultaneously located in mitochondria and peroxisomes. *J Biol Chem* 275: 20887-20895.
1367. Kousseff BG, Hoover DL (1999). Penile neurofibromas. *Am J Med Genet* 87: 1-5.
1368. Kovacs G (1985). Serial cytogenetic analysis in a patient with pseudodiploid bladder cancer. *J Cancer Res Clin Oncol* 110: 249-251.
1369. Kovacs G (1993). Molecular differential pathology of renal cell tumours. *Histopathology* 22: 1-8.
1370. Kovacs G, Akhtar M, Beckwith BJ, Bugert P, Cooper CS, Delahunt B, Eble JN, Fleming S, Ljungberg B, Medeiros LJ, Moch H, Reuter VE, Ritz E, Roos G, Schmidt D, Srigley JR, Storkel S, van den Berg E, Zbar B (1997). The Heidelberg classification of renal cell tumours. *J Pathol* 183: 131-133.
1371. Kovacs G, Brusa P, de Riese W (1989). Tissue-specific expression of a constitutional 3;6 translocation: development of multiple bilateral renal-cell carcinomas. *Int J Cancer* 43: 422-427.
1372. Kovacs G, Frisch S (1989). Clonal chromosome abnormalities in tumor cells from patients with sporadic renal cell carcinomas. *Cancer Res* 49: 651-659.
1373. Kovacs G, Fuzesi L, Emanual A, Kung HF (1991). Cytogenetics of papillary renal cell tumors. *Genes Chromosomes Cancer* 3: 249-255.
1374. Kovacs G, Hoene E (1988). Loss of der(3) in renal carcinoma cells of a patient with constitutional t(3;12). *Hum Genet* 78: 148-150.
1375. Kovacs G, Soudah B, Hoene E (1988). Binucleated cells in a human renal cell carcinoma with 34 chromosomes. *Cancer Genet Cytogenet* 31: 211-215.
1376. Kovacs G, Szucs S, Eichner W, Maschek HJ, Wahnschaffe U, de Riese W (1987). Renal oncocytoma. A cytogenetic and morphologic study. *Cancer* 59: 2071-2077.
1377. Kovacs G, Szucs S, Maschek H (1987). Two chromosomally different cell populations in a partly cellular congenital mesoblastic nephroma. *Arch Pathol Lab Med* 111: 383-385.
1378. Kovacs G, Welter C, Wilkens L, Blin N, Deriese W (1989). Renal oncocytoma. A phenotypic and genotypic entity of renal parenchymal tumors. *Am J Pathol* 134: 967-971.
1379. Koyama S, Morimitsu Y, Morokuma F, Hashimoto H (2001). Primary synovial sarcoma of the kidney: Report of a case confirmed by molecular detection of the SYT-SSX2 fusion transcripts. *Pathol Int* 51: 385-391.
1380. Koyle MA, Hatch DA, Furness PD3rd, Lovell MA, Odom LF, Kurzrock EA (2001). Long-term urological complications in survivors younger than 15 months of advanced stage abdominal neuroblastoma. *J Urol* 166: 1455-1458.
1381. Krabbe S, Skakkebaek NE, Berthelsen JG, Eyben FV, Volsted P, Mauritzen K, Eldrup J, Nielsen AH (1979). High incidence of undetected neoplasia in maldescended testes. *Lancet* 1: 999-1000.
1382. Krag Jacobsen G, Barlebo H, Olsen J, Schultz HP, Starklint H, Sogaard H, Vaeth M (1984). Testicular germ cell tumours in Denmark 1976-1980. Pathology of 1058 consecutive cases. *Acta Radiol Oncol* 23: 239-247.
1383. Kragel PJ, Toker C (1985). Infiltrating recurrent renal angiomyolipoma with fatal outcome. *J Urol* 133: 90-91.
1384. Kraggerud SM, Aman P, Holm R, Stenwig AE, Fossa SD, Nesland JM, Lothe RA (2002). Alterations of the fragile histidine triad gene, FHIT, and its encoded products contribute to testicular germ cell tumorigenesis. *Cancer Res* 62: 512-517.
1385. Kraggerud SM, Berner A, Bryne M, Pettersen EO, Fossa SD (1999). Spermatocytic seminoma as compared to classical seminoma: an immunohistochemical and DNA flow cytometric study. *APMIS* 107: 297-302.
1386. Kraggerud SM, Skotheim RI, Szymanska J, Eknaes M, Fossa SD, Stenwig AE, Peltomaki P, Lothe RA (2002). Genome profiles of familial/bilateral and sporadic testicular germ cell tumors. *Genes Chromosomes Cancer* 34: 168-174.
1387. Kramer AA, Graham S, Burnett WS, Nasca P (1991). Familial aggregation of bladder cancer stratified by smoking status. *Epidemiology* 2: 145-148.
1388. Kramer SA, Bredael J, Croker BP, Paulson DF, Glenn JF (1979). Primary non-urachal adenocarcinoma of the bladder. *J Urol* 121: 278-281.
1389. Krasna IH, Lee M, Sciorra L, Salas M, Smilow P (1985). The importance of surgical evaluation of patients with "Turner-like" sex chromosomal abnormalities. *J Pediatr Surg* 20: 61-64.
1390. Krasna IH, Lee ML, Smilow P, Sciorra L, Eierman L (1992). Risk of malignancy in bilateral streak gonads: the role of the Y chromosome. *J Pediatr Surg* 27: 1376-1380.
1391. Kratzer SS, Ulbright TM, Talerman A, Srigley JR, Roth LM, Wahle GR, Moussa M, Stephens JK, Millos A, Young RH (1997). Large cell calcifying Sertoli cell tumor of the testis: contrasting features of six malignant and six benign tumors and a review of the literature. *Am J Surg Pathol* 21: 1271-1280.
1392. Kressel K, Schnell D, Thon WF, Heymer B, Hartmann M, Altwein JE (1988). Benign testicular tumors: a case for testis preservation? *Eur Urol* 15: 200-204.
1393. Krieger DT, Samojlik E, Bardin CW (1978). Cortisol and androgen secretion in a case of Nelson's syndrome with paratesticular tumors: response to cyproheptadine therapy. *J Clin Endocrinol Metab* 47: 837-844.
1394. Krigman HR, Bentley RC, Strickland DK, Miller CR, Dehner LP, Washington K (1995). Anaplastic renal cell carcinoma following neuroblastoma. *Med Pediatr Oncol* 25: 52-59.
1395. Krijnen JL, Bogdanowicz JF, Seldenrijk CA, Mulder PG, van der Kwast TH (1997). The prognostic value of neuroendocrine differentiation in adenocarcinoma of the prostate in relation to progression of disease after endocrine therapy. *J Urol* 158: 171-174.
1396. Krober SM, Aepinus C, Ruck P, Muller-Hermelink HK, Horny HP, Kaiserling E (2002). Extranodal marginal zone B cell lymphoma of MALT type involving the mucosa of both the urinary bladder and stomach. *J Clin Pathol* 55: 554-557.
1397. Kroft SH, Oyasu R (1994). Urinary bladder cancer: mechanisms of development and progression. *Lab Invest* 71: 158-174.
1398. Kronz JD, Allan CH, Shaikh AA, Epstein JI (2001). Predicting cancer following a diagnosis of high-grade prostatic intraepithelial neoplasia on needle biopsy: data on men with more than one follow-up biopsy. *Am J Surg Pathol* 25: 1079-1085.
1399. Kronz JD, Shaikh AA, Epstein JI (2001). High-grade prostatic intraepithelial neoplasia with adjacent small atypical glands on prostate biopsy. *Hum Pathol* 32: 389-395.
1400. Kronz JD, Silberman MA, Allsbrook WC, Epstein JI (2000). A web-based tutorial improves practicing pathologists' Gleason grading of images of prostate carcinoma specimens obtained by needle biopsy: validation of a new medical education paradigm. *Cancer* 89: 1818-1823.
1401. Kuan SF, Montag AG, Hart J, Krausz T, Recant W (2001). Differential expression of mucin genes in mammary and extramammary Paget's disease. *Am J Surg Pathol* 25: 1469-1477.
1402. Kuhara H, Tamura Z, Suchi T, Hattori R, Kinukawa T (1990). Primary malignant lymphoma of the urinary bladder. A case report. *Acta Pathol Jpn* 40: 764-769.
1403. Kulmala RV, Seppanen JH, Vaajalahti PJ, Tammela TL (1994). Malignant fibrous histiocytoma of the prostate. Case report. *Scand J Urol Nephrol* 28: 429-431.
1404. Kumar S, Perlman E, Harris CA, Raffeld M, Tsokos M (2000). Myogenin is a specific marker for rhabdomyosarcoma: an immunohistochemical study in paraffin-embedded tissues. *Mod Pathol* 13: 988-993.
1405. Kumon H, Tsugawa M, Matsumura Y, Ohmori H (1990). Endoscopic diagnosis and treatment of chronic unilateral hematuria of uncertain etiology. *J Urol* 143: 554-558.
1406. Kunimi K, Uchibayashi T, Hasegawa T, Lee SW, Ohkawa M (1994). Nuclear deoxyribonucleic acid content in inverted papilloma of the urothelium. *Eur Urol* 26: 149-152.
1407. Kunz GMJr, Epstein JI (2003). Should each core with prostate cancer be assigned a separate gleason score? *Hum Pathol* 34: 911-914.
1408. Kunze E, Francksen B, Schulz H (2001). Expression of MUC5AC apomucin in transitional cell carcinomas of the urinary bladder and its possible role in the development of mucus-secreting adenocarcinomas. *Virchows Arch* 439: 609-615.
1409. Kunze E, Schauer A, Schmitt M (1983). Histology and histogenesis of two different types of inverted urothelial papillomas. *Cancer* 51: 348-358.
1410. Kunze E, Theuring F, Kruger G (1994). Primary mesenchymal tumors of the urinary bladder. A histological and immunohistochemical study of 30 cases. *Pathol Res Pract* 190: 311-332.
1411. Kural AR, Obek C, Ozbay G, Onder AU (1998). Multilocular cystic nephroma: an unusual localization. *Urology* 52: 897-899.
1412. Kurhanewicz J, Vigneron DB, Males RG, Swanson MG, Yu KK, Hricak H (2000). The prostate: MR imaging and spectroscopy. Present and future. *Radiol Clin North Am* 38: 115-138.
1413. Kuroda N, Moriki T, Komatsu F, Miyazaki E, Hayashi Y, Naruse K, Nakayama H, Kiyoku H, Hiroi M, Shuin T, Enzan H (2000). Adult-onset giant juxtaglomerular cell tumor of the kidney. *Pathol Int* 50: 249-254.
1414. Kurtman C, Andrieu MN, Baltaci S, Gogus C, Akfirat C (2001). Conformal radiotherapy in primary non-Hodgkin's lymphoma of the male urethra. *Int Urol Nephrol* 33: 537-539.
1415. Kusser WC, Miao X, Glickman BW, Friedland JM, Rothman N, Hemstreet GP, Mellot J, Swan DC, Schulte PA, Hayes RB (1994). p53 mutations in human bladder cancer. *Environ Mol Mutagen* 24: 156-160.
1416. Kuwahara Y, Kubota Y, Hibi H, Yanaoka Y, Okishio N, Hoshinaga K, Naide Y, Kasahara M (1997). [Malignant lymphoma of the penis: report of two cases]. *Hinyokika Kiyo* 43: 371-374.
1417. Kvist E, Osmundsen PE, Sjolin KE (1992). Primary Paget's disease of the penis. Case report. *Scand J Urol Nephrol* 26: 187-190.
1418. Kwabi-Addo B, Giri D, Schmidt K, Podsypanina K, Parsons R, Greenberg N, Ittmann M (2001). Haploinsufficiency of the Pten tumor suppressor gene promotes prostate cancer progression. *Proc Natl Acad Sci USA* 98: 11563-11568.
1419. L'Hostis H, Deminiere C, Ferriere JM, Coindre JM (1999). Renal angiomyolipoma: a clinicopathologic, immunohistochemical, and follow-up study of 46 cases. *Am J Surg Pathol* 23: 1011-1020.
1420. Lack EE (1997). *Tumours of the Adrenal Gland and Extra-adrenal Paraganglia.* 3rd Edition. AFIP: Washington, DC.
1421. Lacombe L, Dalbagni G, Zhang ZF, Cordon-Cardo C, Fair WR, Herr HW, Reuter VE (1996). Overexpression of p53 protein in a high-risk population of patients with superficial bladder cancer before and after bacillus Calmette-Guerin therapy: correlation to clinical outcome. *J Clin Oncol* 14: 2646-2652.
1422. Ladanyi M, Antonescu CR, Leung DH, Woodruff JM, Kawai A, Healey JH, Brennan MF, Bridge JA, Neff JR, Barr FG, Goldsmith JD, Brooks JS, Goldblum JR, Ali SZ, Shipley J, Cooper CS, Fisher C, Skytting B, Larsson O (2002). Impact of SYT-SSX fusion type on the clinical behavior of synovial sarcoma: a multi-institutional retrospective study of 243 patients. *Cancer Res* 62: 135-140.
1423. Ladanyi M, Gerald W (1994). Fusion of the EWS and WT1 genes in the desmoplastic small round cell tumor. *Cancer Res* 54: 2837-2840.

1424. Ladanyi M, Lui MY, Antonescu CR, Krause-Boehm A, Meindl A, Argani P, Healey JH, Ueda T, Yoshikawa H, Meloni-Ehrig A, Sorensen PH, Mertens F, Mandahl N, van den Berghe H, Sciot R, Cin PD, Bridge J (2001). The der(17)t(X;17)(p11;q25) of human alveolar soft part sarcoma fuses the TFE3 transcription factor gene to ASPL, a novel gene at 17q25. *Oncogene* 20: 48-57.
1425. Ladocsi LT, Siebert CFJr, Rickert RR, Fletcher HS (1998). Basal cell carcinoma of the penis. *Cutis* 61: 25-27.
1426. Lagace R, Tremblay M (1968). Non-chromaffin paraganglioma of the kidney with distant metastases. *Can Med Assoc J* 99: 1095-1098.
1427. Lagalla R, Zappasodi F, Lo Casto A, Zenico T (1993). Cystadenoma of the seminal vesicle: US and CT findings. *Abdom Imaging* 18: 298-300.
1428. Lager DJ, Huston BJ, Timmerman TG, Bonsib SM (1995). Papillary renal tumors. Morphologic, cytochemical, and genotypic features. *Cancer* 76: 669-673.
1429. Lagrange JL, Ramaioli A, Theodore CH, Terrier-Lacombe MJ, Beckendorf V, Biron P, Chevreau CH, Chinet-Charrot P, Dumont J, Delobel-Deroide A, D'Anjou J, Chassagne C, Parache RM, Karsenty JM, Mercier J, Droz JP (2001). Non-Hodgkin's lymphoma of the testis: a retrospective study of 84 patients treated in the French anticancer centres. *Ann Oncol* 12: 1313-1319.
1430. Lambe M, Lindblad P, Wuu J, Remler R, Hsieh CC (2002). Pregnancy and risk of renal cell cancer: a population-based study in Sweden. *Br J Cancer* 86: 1425-1429.
1431. Lamiell JM, Salazar FG, Hsia YE (1989). von Hippel-Lindau disease affecting 43 members of a single kindred. *Medicine (Baltimore)* 68: 1-29.
1432. Lamont JS, Hesketh PJ, de las Morenas A, Babayan RK (1991). Primary angiosarcoma of the seminal vesicle. *J Urol* 146: 165-167.
1433. Lane AH, Lee MM, Fuller AFJr, Kehas DJ, Donahoe PK, MacLaughlin DT (1999). Diagnostic utility of Mullerian inhibiting substance determination in patients with primary and recurrent granulosa cell tumors. *Gynecol Oncol* 73: 51-55.
1434. Lane TM, Wilde M, Schofield J, Trotter GA (2001). Benign cystic mesothelioma of the tunica vaginalis. *BJU Int* 87: 415.
1435. Langer JE, Rovner ES, Coleman BG, Yin D, Arger PH, Malkowicz SB, Nisenbaum HL, Rowling SE, Tomaszewski JE, Wein AJ, Jacobs JE (1996). Strategy for repeat biopsy of patients with prostatic intraepithelial neoplasia detected by prostate needle biopsy. *J Urol* 155: 228-231.
1436. Lapham RL, Grignon DJ, Ro JY (1997). Pathologic prognostic parameters in bladder urothelial biopsy, transurethral resection, and cystectomy specimens. *Semin Diagn Pathol* 14: 109-122.
1437. Laplante M, Brice M (1973). The upper limits of hopeful application of radical cystectomy for vesical carcinoma: does nodal metastasis always indicate incurability? *J Urol* 109: 261-264.
1438. Lapointe A, Cain A (1923). Epithelioma de l'epidydime. *Bull Mem Soc Chir* 49: 701-705.
1439. Larsson KB, Shaw HM, Thompson JF, Harman RC, McCarthy WH (1999). Primary mucosal and glans penis melanomas: the Sydney Melanoma Unit experience. *Aust N Z J Surg* 69: 121-126.
1440. Larsson P, Wijkstrom H, Thorstenson A, Adolfsson J, Norming U, Wiklund P, Onelow E, Steineck G (2003). A population-based study of 538 patients with newly detected urinary bladder neoplasms followed during 5 years. *Scand J Urol Nephrol* 37: 195-201.
1441. Laski ME, Vugrin D (1987). Paraneoplastic syndromes in hypernephroma. *Semin Nephrol* 7: 123-130.
1442. Laskin WB, Fetsch JF, Mostofi FK (1998). Angiomyofibroblastomalike tumor of the male genital tract: analysis of 11 cases with comparison to female angiomyofibroblastoma and spindle cell lipoma. *Am J Surg Pathol* 22: 6-16.
1443. Laskowski J (1952). Feminizing tumors of the testis: a general review with case report of granulosa cell tumor of the testis. *Endokrynol Pol* 3: 337-343.
1444. Lasota J (2003). Genetics of soft tissue tumors. In: *Diagnostic Soft Tissue Pathology*, M Miettinen, ed. Churchill Livingstone: Philadelphia, PA, pp. 99-142.
1445. Latif F, Tory K, Gnarra J, Yao M, Duh FM, Orcutt ML, Stackhouse T, Kuzmin I, Modi W, Geil L, Schmidt L, Zhou FW, Li H, Wei MH, Chen F, Glenn G, Choyke P, Walther MM, Weng YK, Duan DS, Dean M, Glavac D, Richards FM, Crossey PA, Ferguson-Smith MA, Lepaslier D, Chumakov I, Cohen D, Chinault AC, Maher ER, Linehan WM, Zbar B, Lerman MI (1993). Identification of the von Hippel-Lindau disease tumor suppressor gene. *Science* 260: 1317-1320.
1446. Lau WK, Bergstralh EJ, Blute ML, Slezak JM, Zincke H (2002). Radical prostatectomy for pathological Gleason 8 or greater prostate cancer: influence of concomitant pathological variables. *J Urol* 167: 117-122.
1447. Lau WK, Blute ML, Bostwick DG, Weaver AL, Sebo TJ, Zincke H (2001). Prognostic factors for survival of patients with pathological Gleason score 7 prostate cancer: differences in outcome between primary Gleason grades 3 and 4. *J Urol* 166: 1692-1697.
1448. Lau Y, Chou P, Iezzoni J, Alonzo J, Komuves L (2000). Expression of a candidate gene for the gonadoblastoma locus in gonadoblastoma and testicular seminoma. *Cytogenet Cell Genet* 91: 160-164.
1449. Laughlin LW, Farid Z, Mansour N, Edman DC, Higashi GI (1978). Bacteriuria in urinary schistosomiasis in Egypt a prevalence survey. *Am J Trop Med Hyg* 27: 916-918.
1450. Launonen V, Vierimaa O, Kiuru M, Isola J, Roth S, Pukkala E, Sistonen P, Herva R, Aaltonen LA (2001). Inherited susceptibility to uterine leiomyomas and renal cell cancer. *Proc Natl Acad Sci USA* 98: 3387-3392.
1451. Laurila P, Leivo I, Makisalo H, Ruutu M, Miettinen M (1992). Mullerian adenosarcomalike tumor of the seminal vesicle. A case report with immunohistochemical and ultrastructural observations. *Arch Pathol Lab Med* 116: 1072-1076.
1452. Lavezzi AM, Biondo B, Cazzullo A, Giordano F, Pallotti F, Turconi P, Matturri L (2001). The role of different biomarkers (DNA, PCNA, apoptosis and karyotype) in prognostic evaluation of superficial transitional cell bladder carcinoma. *Anticancer Res* 21: 1279-1284.
1453. Lawrence WD, Young RH, Scully RE (1985). Juvenile granulosa cell tumor of the infantile testis. A report of 14 cases. *Am J Surg Pathol* 9: 87-94.
1454. Lawrence WD, Young RH, Scully RE (1986). Sex cord-stromal tumors. In: *Pathology of the Testis and its Adnexal*, A Talerman, LM Roth, eds. Churchill Livingston: New York.
1455. Layfield LJ, Liu K (2000). Mucoepidermoid carcinoma arising in the glans penis. *Arch Pathol Lab Med* 124: 148-151.
1456. Le Cheong L, Khan AN, Bisset RA (1990). Sonographic features of a renal pelvic neurofibroma. *J Clin Ultrasound* 18: 129-131.
1457. Leahy MG, Tonks S, Moses JH, Brett AR, Huddart R, Forman D, Oliver RT, Bishop DT, Bodmer JG (1995). Candidate regions for a testicular cancer susceptibility gene. *Hum Mol Genet* 4: 1551-1555.
1458. Leaute-Labreze C, Bioulac-Sage P, Belleannee G, Merlio JP, Vergnes P, Maleville J, Taieb A (1995). [Lymphomatoid papulosis in a child]. *Arch Pediatr* 2: 984-987.
1459. Lebe B, Koyuncuoglu M, Tuna B, Tuncer C (2001). Epithelioid angiomyolipoma: a case report. *Tumori* 87: 196-199.
1460. Leblanc B, Duclos AJ, Benard F, Cote J, Valiquette L, Paquin JM, Mauffette F, Faucher R, Perreault JP (1999). Long-term followup of initial Ta grade 1 transitional cell carcinoma of the bladder. *J Urol* 162: 1946-1950.
1461. Lebret T, Bohin D, Kassardjian Z, Herve JM, Molinie V, Barre P, Lugagne PM, Botto H (2000). Recurrence, progression and success in stage Ta grade 3 bladder tumors treated with low dose bacillus Calmette-Guerin instillations. *J Urol* 163: 63-67.
1462. Leder RA (1995). Genitourinary case of the day. Renal lymphangiomatosis. *AJR Am J Roentgenol* 165: 197-198.
1463. Lee AH, Mead GM, Theaker JM (1999). The value of central histopathological review of testicular tumours before treatment. *BJU Int* 84: 75-78.
1464. Lee CC, Yamamoto S, Morimura K, Wanibuchi H, Nishisaka N, Ikemoto S, Nakatani T, Wada S, Kishimoto T, Fukushima S (1997). Significance of cyclin D1 overexpression in transitional cell carcinomas of the urinary bladder and its correlation with histopathologic features. *Cancer* 79: 780-789.
1465. Lee WH, Morton RA, Epstein JI, Brooks JD, Campbell PA, Bova GS, Hsieh WS, Isaacs WB, Nelson WG (1994). Cytidine methylation of regulatory sequences near the pi-class glutathione S-transferase gene accompanies human prostatic carcinogenesis. *Proc Natl Acad Sci USA* 91: 11733-11737.
1466. Leestma JE, Price EBJr (1971). Paraganglioma of the urinary bladder. *Cancer* 28: 1063-1073.
1467. Legler JM, Feuer EJ, Potosky AL, Merrill RM, Kramer BS (1998). The role of prostate-specific antigen (PSA) testing patterns in the recent prostate cancer incidence decline in the United States. *Cancer Causes Control* 9: 519-527.
1468. Lehman JSJr, Farid Z, Smith JH, Bassily S, el Masry NA (1973). Urinary schistosomiasis in Egypt: clinical, radiological, bacteriological and parasitological correlations. *Trans R Soc Trop Med Hyg* 67: 384-399.
1469. Lehtonen R, Kiuru M, Vanharanta S, Sjoberg J, Aaltonen LM, Aittomaki K, Arola J, Butzow R, Eng C, Husgafvel-Pursiainen K, Isola J, Jarvinen H, Koivisto P, Mecklin JP, Peltomaki P, Salovaara R, Wasenius VM, Karhu A, Launonen V, Nupponen NN, Aaltonen LA (2003). Biallelic inactivation of *fumarate hydratase (FH)* occurs in non-syndromic uterine leiomyomas but is rare in other tumors. *Am J Pathol* (in press).
1470. Leibman BD, Dillioglugil O, Scardino PT, Abbas F, Rogers E, Wolfinger RD, Kattan MW (1998). Prostate-specific antigen doubling times are similar in patients with recurrence after radical prostatectomy or radiotherapy: a novel analysis. *J Clin Oncol* 16: 2267-2271.
1471. Leibovitch I, Foster RS, Ulbright TM, Donohue JP (1995). Adult primary pure teratoma of the testis. The Indiana experience. *Cancer* 75: 2244-2250.
1472. Lein M, Jung K, Laube C, Hubner T, Winkelmann B, Stephan C, Hauptmann S, Rudolph B, Schnorr D, Loening SA (2000). Matrix-metalloproteinases and their inhibitors in plasma and tumor tissue of patients with renal cell carcinoma. *Int J Cancer* 85: 801-804.
1473. Lemos N, Melo CR, Soares IC, Lemos RR, Lemos FR (2000). Plasmacytoma of the urethra treated by excisional biopsy. *Scand J Urol Nephrol* 34: 75-76.
1474. Leonard MP, Nickel JC, Morales A (1988). Cavernous hemangiomas of the bladder in the pediatric age group. *J Urol* 140: 1503-1504.
1475. Leonhardt WC, Gooding GA (1992). Sonography of intrascrotal adenomatoid tumor. *Urology* 39: 90-92.
1476. Lepor H, Wang B, Shapiro E (1994). Relationship between prostatic epithelial volume and serum prostate-specific antigen levels. *Urology* 44: 199-205.
1477. Lerner SP, Seale-Hawkins C, Carlton CEJr, Scardino PT (1991). The risk of dying of prostate cancer in patients with clinically localized disease. *J Urol* 146: 1040-1045.
1478. Leroy X, Augusto D, Leteurtre E, Gosselin B (2002). CD30 and CD117 (c-kit) used in combination are useful for distinguishing embryonal carcinoma from seminoma. *J Histochem Cytochem* 50: 283-285.
1479. Leroy X, Copin MC, Devisme L, Buisine MP, Aubert JP, Gosselin B, Porchet N (2002). Expression of human mucin genes in normal kidney and renal cell carcinoma. *Histopathology* 40: 450-457.
1480. Leroy X, Leteurtre E, de La Taille A, Augusto D, Biserte J, Gosselin B (2002). Microcystic transitional cell carcinoma: a report of 2 cases arising in the renal pelvis. *Arch Pathol Lab Med* 126: 859-861.
1481. Letocha H, Ahlstrom H, Malmstrom PU, Westlin JE, Fasth KJ, Nilsson S (1994). Positron emission tomography with L-methyl-11C-methionine in the monitoring of therapy response in muscle-invasive transitional cell carcinoma of the urinary bladder. *Br J Urol* 74: 767-774.
1482. Leuschner I, Harms D, Mattke A, Koscielniak E, Treuner J (2001). Rhabdomyosarcoma of the urinary bladder and vagina: a clinicopathologic study with emphasis on recurrent disease: a report from the Kiel Pediatric Tumor Registry and the German CWS Study. *Am J Surg Pathol* 25: 856-864.
1483. Leuschner I, Newton WAJr, Schmidt D, Sachs N, Asmar L, Hamoudi A, Harms D, Maurer HM (1993). Spindle cell variants of embryonal rhabdomyosarcoma in the paratesticular region. A report of the Intergroup Rhabdomyosarcoma Study. *Am J Surg Pathol* 17: 221-230.
1484. Levesque P, Ramchurren N, Saini K, Joyce A, Libertino J, Summerhayes IC (1993). Screening of human bladder tumors and urine sediments for the presence of H-ras mutations. *Int J Cancer* 55: 785-790.
1485. Levi AW, Epstein JI (2000). Pseudohyperplastic prostatic adenocarcinoma on needle biopsy and simple prostatectomy. *Am J Surg Pathol* 24: 1039-1046.

1486. Levin HS, Mostofi FK (1970). Symptomatic plasmacytoma of the testis. *Cancer* 25: 1193-1203.

1487. Levine RL (1980). Urethral cancer. *Cancer* 45: 1965-1972.

1488. Li B, Kanamaru H, Noriki S, Yamaguchi T, Fukuda M, Okada K (1998). Reciprocal expression of bcl-2 and p53 oncoproteins in urothelial dysplasia and carcinoma of the urinary bladder. *Urol Res* 26: 235-241.

1489. Li FP, Cassady JR, Jaffe N (1975). Risk of second tumors in survivors of childhood cancer. *Cancer* 35: 1230-1235.

1490. Li FP, Fraumeni JF (1972). Testicular cancers in children: epidemiologic characteristics. *J Natl Cancer Inst* 48: 1575-1581.

1491. Li J, Yen C, Liaw D, Podsypanina K, Bose S, Wang SI, Puc J, Miliaresis C, Rodgers L, McCombie R, Bigner SH, Giovanella BC, Ittmann M, Tycko B, Hibshoosh H, Wigler MH, Parsons R (1997). PTEN, a putative protein tyrosine phosphatase gene mutated in human brain, breast, and prostate cancer. *Science* 275: 1943-1947.

1492. Li M, Cannizzaro LA (1999). Identical clonal origin of synchronous and metachronous low-grade, noninvasive papillary transitional cell carcinomas of the urinary tract. *Hum Pathol* 30: 1197-1200.

1493. Li M, Squire JA, Weksberg R (1998). Molecular genetics of Wiedemann-Beckwith syndrome. *Am J Med Genet* 79: 253-259.

1494. Lianes P, Charytonowicz E, Cordon-Cardo C, Fradet Y, Grossman HB, Hemstreet GP, Waldman FM, Chew K, Wheeless LL, Faraggi D (1998). Biomarker study of primary nonmetastatic versus metastatic invasive bladder cancer. National Cancer Institute Bladder Tumor Marker Network. *Clin Cancer Res* 4: 1267-1271.

1495. Lianes P, Orlow I, Zhang ZF, Oliva MR, Sarkis AS, Reuter VE, Cordon-Cardo C (1994). Altered patterns of MDM2 and TP53 expression in human bladder cancer. *J Natl Cancer Inst* 86: 1325-1330.

1496. Lichtenstein P, Holm NV, Verkasalo PK, Iliadou A, Kaprio J, Koskenvuo M, Pukkala E, Skytthe A, Hemminki K (2000). Environmental and heritable factors in the causation of cancer—analyses of cohorts of twins from Sweden, Denmark, and Finland. *N Engl J Med* 343: 78-85.

1497. Lieber MM, Tomera KM, Farrow GM (1981). Renal oncocytoma. *J Urol* 125: 481-485.

1498. Lilja H (1993). Significance of different molecular forms of serum PSA. The free, noncomplexed form of PSA versus that complexed to alpha 1-antichymotrypsin. *Urol Clin North Am* 20: 681-686.

1499. Lilja H, Christensson A, Dahlen U, Matikainen MT, Nilsson O, Pettersson K, Lovgren T (1991). Prostate-specific antigen in serum occurs predominantly in complex with alpha 1-antichymotrypsin. *Clin Chem* 37: 1618-1625.

1500. Lilleby W, Paus E, Skovlund E, Fossa SD (2001). Prognostic value of neuroendocrine serum markers and PSA in irradiated patients with pN0 localized prostate cancer. *Prostate* 46: 126-133.

1501. Lim DJ, Hayden RT, Murad T, Nemcek AAJr, Dalton DP (1993). Multilocular prostatic cystadenoma presenting as a large complex pelvic cystic mass. *J Urol* 149: 856-859.

1502. Limmer S, Wagner T, Leipprand E, Arnholdt H (2001). [Primary renal hemangiosarcoma. Case report and review of the literature]. *Pathologe* 22: 343-348.

1503. Lin DW, Thorning DR, Krieger JN (1999). Primary penile lymphoma: diagnostic difficulties and management options. *Urology* 54: 366.

1504. Lin JI, Yong HS, Tseng CH, Marsidi PS, Choy C, Pilloff B (1980). Diffuse cystitis glandularis. Associated with adenocarcinomatous change. *Urology* 15: 411-415.

1505. Lin X, Tascilar M, Lee WH, Vles WJ, Lee BH, Veeraswamy R, Asgari K, Freije D, van Rees B, Gage WR, Bova GS, Isaacs WB, Brooks JD, de Weese TL, de Marzo AM, Nelson WG (2001). GSTP1 CpG island hypermethylation is responsible for the absence of GSTP1 expression in human prostate cancer cells. *Am J Pathol* 159: 1815-1826.

1506. Lindau A (1926). Studien uber Kleinhirncysten. Bau, Pathogenese und Beziehungen zur Angiomatosis Retinae. *Acta Pathol Microbiol Scand* Suppl 1.

1507. Linnenbach AJ, Robbins SL, Seng BA, Tomaszewski JE, Pressler LB, Malkowicz SB (1994). Urothelial carcinogenesis. *Nature* 367: 419-420.

1508. Linnoila RI, Keiser HR, Steinberg SM, Lack EE (1990). Histopathology of benign versus malignant sympathoadrenal paragangliomas: clinicopathologic study of 120 cases including unusual histologic features. *Hum Pathol* 21: 1168-1180.

1509. Lipponen P (1993). Expression of c-erbB-2 oncoprotein in transitional cell bladder cancer. *Eur J Cancer* 29A: 749-753.

1510. Lipponen P, Eskelinen M (1994). Expression of epidermal growth factor receptor in bladder cancer as related to established prognostic factors, oncoprotein (c-erbB-2, p53) expression and long-term prognosis. *Br J Cancer* 69: 1120-1125.

1511. Lipponen PK, Eskelinen MJ (1995). Reduced expression of E-cadherin is related to invasive disease and frequent recurrence in bladder cancer. *J Cancer Res Clin Oncol* 121: 303-308.

1512. Lipponen PK, Nordling S, Eskelinen MJ, Jauhiainen K, Terho R, Harju E (1993). Flow cytometry in comparison with mitotic index in predicting disease outcome in transitional-cell bladder cancer. *Int J Cancer* 53: 42-47.

1513. Little NA, Wiener JS, Walther PJ, Paulson DF, Anderson EE (1993). Squamous cell carcinoma of the prostate: 2 cases of a rare malignancy and review of the literature. *J Urol* 149: 137-139.

1514. Litton M, Bergeron C (1987). [Primary lymphoma of the penis]. *J Urol (Paris)* 93: 99-101.

1515. Liu JB, Bagley DH, Conlin MJ, Merton DA, Alexander AA, Goldberg BB (1997). Endoluminal sonographic evaluation of ureteral and renal pelvic neoplasms. *J Ultrasound Med* 16: 515-521.

1516. Liu Q, Schwaller J, Kutok J, Cain D, Aster JC, Williams IR, Gilliland DG (2000). Signal transduction and transforming properties of the TEL-TRKC fusions associated with t(12;15)(p13;q25) in congenital fibrosarcoma and acute myelogenous leukemia. *EMBO J* 19: 1827-1838.

1517. Liukkonen T, Lipponen P, Raitanen M, Kaasinen E, Ala-Opas M, Rajala P, Kosma VM (2000). Evaluation of p21WAF1/CIP1 and cyclin D1 expression in the progression of superficial bladder cancer. Finbladder Group. *Urol Res* 28: 285-292.

1518. Liukkonen T, Rajala P, Raitanen M, Rintala E, Kaasinen E, Lipponen P (1999). Prognostic value of MIB-1 score, p53, EGFr, mitotic index and papillary status in primary superficial (Stage pTa/T1) bladder cancer: a prospective comparative study. The Finnbladder Group. *Eur Urol* 36: 393-400.

1519. Lloyd DA, Rintala RJ (1998). Inguinal hernia and hydrocele. In: *Pediatric Surgery*, JA O'Neill, MI Rowe, JL Grosfeld, EW Fonkalsrud, AG Coran, eds. 5th Edition. Mosby: St Louis, p. 1071.

1520. Lloyd RV, Erickson LA, Jin L, Kulig E, Qian X, Cheville JC, Scheithauer BW (1999). p27kip1: a multifunctional cyclin-dependent kinase inhibitor with prognostic significance in human cancers. *Am J Pathol* 154: 313-323.

1521. Lloyd SN, Collins GN, McKelvie GB, Hehir M, Rogers AC (1994). Predicted and actual change in serum PSA following prostatectomy for BPH. *Urology* 43: 472-479.

1522. Lobe TE, Wiener E, Andrassy RJ, Bagwell CE, Hays D, Crist WM, Webber B, Breneman JC, Reed MM, Tefft MC, Heyn R (1996). The argument for conservative, delayed surgery in the management of prostatic rhabdomyosarcoma. *J Pediatr Surg* 31: 1084-1087.

1523. Lodato RF, Zentner GJ, Gomez CA, Nochomovitz LE (1991). Scrotal carcinoid. Presenting manifestation of multiple lesions in the small intestine. *Am J Clin Pathol* 96: 664-668.

1524. Loeb LA (2001). A mutator phenotype in cancer. *Cancer Res* 61: 3230-3239.

1525. Loehrer PJSr, Hui S, Clark S, Seal M, Einhorn LH, Williams SD, Ulbright T, Mandelbaum I, Rowland R, Donohue JP (1986). Teratoma following cisplatin-based combination chemotherapy for nonseminomatous germ cell tumors: a clinicopathological correlation. *J Urol* 135: 1183-1189.

1526. Loening SA, Jacobo E, Hawtrey CE, Culp DA (1978). Adenocarcinoma of the urachus. *J Urol* 119: 68-71.

1527. Lofts FJ, Gullick WJ (1992). c-erbB2 amplification and overexpression in human tumors. *Cancer Treat Res* 61: 161-179.

1528. Logothetis CJ, Dexeus FH, Chong C, Sella A, Ayala AG, Ro JY, Pilat S (1989). Cisplatin, cyclophosphamide and doxorubicin chemotherapy for unresectable urothelial tumors: the M.D. Anderson experience. *J Urol* 141: 33-37.

1529. Logothetis CJ, Samuels ML, Selig DE, Ogden S, Dexeus F, Swanson D, Johnson D, von Eschenbach A (1986). Cyclic chemotherapy with cyclophosphamide, doxorubicin, and cisplatin plus vinblastine and bleomycin in advanced germinal tumors. Results with 100 patients. *Am J Med* 81: 219-228.

1530. Logothetis CJ, Xu HJ, Ro JY, Hu SX, Sahin A, Ordonez N, Benedict WF (1992). Altered expression of retinoblastoma protein and known prognostic variables in locally advanced bladder cancer. *J Natl Cancer Inst* 84: 1256-1261.

1531. Lohrisch C, Murray N, Pickles T, Sullivan L (1999). Small cell carcinoma of the bladder: long term outcome with integrated chemoradiation. *Cancer* 86: 2346-2352.

1532. Lohse CM, Blute ML, Zincke H, Weaver AL, Cheville JC (2002). Comparison of standardized and nonstandardized nuclear grade of renal cell carcinoma to predict outcome among 2,042 patients. *Am J Clin Pathol* 118: 877-886.

1533. Lonergan KM, Iliopoulos O, Ohh M, Kamura T, Conaway RC, Conaway JW, Kaelin WGJr (1998). Regulation of hypoxia-inducible mRNAs by the von Hippel-Lindau tumor suppressor protein requires binding to complexes containing elongins B/C and Cul2. *Mol Cell Biol* 18: 732-741.

1534. Lonn U, Lonn S, Friberg S, Nilsson B, Silfversward C, Stenkvist B (1995). Prognostic value of amplification of c-erb-B2 in bladder carcinoma. *Clin Cancer Res* 1: 1189-1194.

1535. Lont AP, Besnard APE, Gallee MP, van Tinteren H, Horenblas S (2003). A comparison of physical examination and imaging in determining the extent of primary penile carcinoma. *BJU Int* 91: 493-495.

1536. Looijenga LH, Abraham M, Gillis AJ, Saunders GF, Oosterhuis JW (1994). Testicular germ cell tumors of adults show deletions of chromosomal bands 11p13 and 11p15.5, but no abnormalities within the zinc-finger regions and exons 2 and 6 of the Wilms' tumor 1 gene. *Genes Chromosomes Cancer* 9: 153-160.

1537. Looijenga LH, de Munnik H, Oosterhuis JW (1999). A molecular model for the development of germ cell cancer. *Int J Cancer* 83: 809-814.

1538. Looijenga LH, Gillis AJ, van Gurp RJ, Verkerk AJ, Oosterhuis JW (1997). X inactivation in human testicular tumors. XIST expression and androgen receptor methylation status. *Am J Pathol* 151: 581-590.

1539. Looijenga LH, Olie RA, van der Gaag I, van Sluijs FJ, Matoska J, Ploem-Zaaijer J, Knepfle C, Oosterhuis JW (1994). Seminomas of the canine testis. Counterpart of spermatocytic seminoma of men? *Lab Invest* 71: 490-496.

1540. Looijenga LH, Oosterhuis JW (1999). Pathogenesis of testicular germ cell tumours. *Rev Reprod* 4: 90-100.

1541. Looijenga LH, Oosterhuis JW (2002). Pathobiology of testicular germ cell tumors: views and news. *Anal Quant Cytol Histol* 24: 263-279.

1542. Looijenga LH, Oosterhuis JW, Ramaekers FC, de Jong B, Dam A, Beck JL, Sleijfer DT, Schraffordt Koops H (1991). Dual parameter flow cytometry for deoxyribonucleic acid and intermediate filament proteins of residual mature teratoma. All tumor cells are aneuploid. *Lab Invest* 64: 113-117.

1543. Looijenga LH, Rosenberg C, van Gurp RJ, Geelen E, Echten-Arends J, de Jong B, Mostert M, Oosterhuis WJ (2000). Comparative genomic hybridization of microdissected samples from different stages in the development of a seminoma and a non-seminoma. *J Pathol* 191: 187-192.

1544. Looijenga LH, Verkerk AJ, de Groot N, Hochberg AA, Oosterhuis JW (1997). H19 in normal development and neoplasia. *Mol Reprod Dev* 46: 419-439.

1545. Looijenga LH, Zafarana G, Grygalewitcz B, Summersgill B, Debiec-Rychter M, Veltman J, Shoenmakers EFPM, Rodriguez S, Jafer O, Clark J, Geurts van Kessel A, Shipley J, van Gurp RJ, Gillis AJM, Oosterhuis JW (2003). Role of gain of 12p in germ cell tumour development. *APMIS* 111: 161-171.

1546. Lopes A, Bezerra AL, Pinto CA, Serrano SV, de Mello CA, Villa LL (2002). p53 as a new prognostic factor for lymph node metastasis in penile carcinoma: analysis of 82 patients treated with amputation and bilateral lymphadenectomy. *J Urol* 168: 81-86.

1547. Lopez-Beltran A, Cheng L, Andersson L, Brausi M, de Matteis A, Montironi R, Sesterhenn I, van der Kwast T, Mazerolles C (2002). Preneoplastic non-papillary lesions and conditions of the urinary bladder: an update based on the Ancona International Consultation. *Virchows Arch* 440: 3-11.

1548. Lopez-Beltran A, Croghan GA, Croghan I, Matilla A, Gaeta JF (1994). Prognostic factors in bladder cancer. A pathologic, immunohistochemical, and DNA flow-cytometric study. *Am J Clin Pathol* 102: 109-114.
1549. Lopez-Beltran A, Escudero AL, Cavazzana AO, Spagnoli LG, Vicioso-Recio L (1996). Sarcomatoid transitional cell carcinoma of the renal pelvis. A report of five cases with clinical, pathological, immunohistochemical and DNA ploidy analysis. *Pathol Res Pract* 192: 1218-1224.
1550. Lopez-Beltran A, Lopez-Ruiz J, Vicioso L (1995). Inflammatory pseudotumor of the urinary bladder. A clinicopathological analysis of two cases. *Urol Int* 55: 173-176.
1551. Lopez-Beltran A, Luque RJ, Mazzucchelli R, Scarpelli M, Montironi R (2002). Changes produced in the urothelium by traditional and newer therapeutic procedures for bladder cancer. *J Clin Pathol* 55: 641-647.
1552. Lopez-Beltran A, Luque RJ, Moreno A, Bollito E, Carmona E, Montironi R (2002). The pagetoid variant of bladder urothelial carcinoma in situ. A clinicopathological study of 11 cases. *Virchows Arch* 441: 148-153.
1553. Lopez-Beltran A, Luque RJ, Vicioso L, Anglada F, Requena MJ, Quintero A, Montironi R (2001). Lymphoepithelioma-like carcinoma of the urinary bladder: a clinicopathologic study of 13 cases. *Virchows Arch* 438: 552-557.
1554. Lopez-Beltran A, Martin J, Garcia J, Toro M (1988). Squamous and glandular differentiation in urothelial bladder carcinomas. Histopathology, histochemistry and immunohistochemical expression of carcinoembryonic antigen. *Histol Histopathol* 3: 63-68.
1555. Lopez-Beltran A, Pacelli A, Rothenberg HJ, Wollan PC, Zincke H, Blute ML, Bostwick DG (1998). Carcinosarcoma and sarcomatoid carcinoma of the bladder: clinicopathological study of 41 cases. *J Urol* 159: 1497-1503.
1556. Lopez JI, Angulo JC (1994). Burned-out tumour of the testis presenting as retroperitoneal choriocarcinoma. *Int Urol Nephrol* 26: 549-553.
1557. Lopez JI, Angulo JC, Ibanez T (1993). Primary malignant melanoma mimicking urethral caruncle. Case report. *Scand J Urol Nephrol* 27: 125-126.
1558. Lopez JI, Elorriaga K, Imaz I, Bilbao FJ (1999). Micropapillary transitional cell carcinoma of the urinary bladder. *Histopathology* 34: 561-562.
1559. Los M, Jansen GH, Kaelin WG, Lips CJ, Blijham GH, Voest EE (1996). Expression pattern of the von Hippel-Lindau protein in human tissues. *Lab Invest* 75: 231-238.
1560. Lothe RA, Hastie N, Heimdal K, Fossa SD, Stenwig AE, Borresen AL (1993). Frequent loss of 11p13 and 11p15 loci in male germ cell tumours. *Genes Chromosomes Cancer* 7: 96-101.
1561. Lothe RA, Peltomaki P, Tommerup N, Fossa SD, Stenwig AE, Borresen AL, Nesland JM (1995). Molecular genetic changes in human male germ cell tumors. *Lab Invest* 73: 606-614.
1562. Lott ST, Lovell M, Naylor SL, Killary AM (1998). Physical and functional mapping of a tumor suppressor locus for renal cell carcinoma within chromosome 3p12. *Cancer Res* 58: 3533-3537.
1563. Loughlin KR, Retik AB, Weinstein HJ, Colodny AH, Shamberger RC, Delorey M, Tarbell N, Cassady JR, Hendren WH (1989). Genitourinary rhabdomyosarcoma in children. *Cancer* 63: 1600-1606.
1564. Louhelainen J, Wijkstrom H, Hemminki K (2000). Allelic losses demonstrate monoclonality of multifocal bladder tumors. *Int J Cancer* 87: 522-527.
1565. Lowe BA, Brewer J, Houghton DC, Jacobson E, Pitre T (1992). Malignant transformation of angiomyolipoma. *J Urol* 147: 1356-1358.
1566. Lowe FC, Lattimer DG, Metroka CE (1989). Kaposi's sarcoma of the penis in patients with acquired immunodeficiency syndrome. *J Urol* 142: 1475-1477.
1567. Lowe LH, Isuani BH, Heller RM, Stein SM, Johnson JE, Navarro OM, Hernanz-Schulman M (2000). Pediatric renal masses: Wilms tumor and beyond. *Radiographics* 20: 1585-1603.
1568. Lu D, Medeiros LJ, Eskenazi AE, Abruzzo LV (2001). Primary follicular large cell lymphoma of the testis in a child. *Arch Pathol Lab Med* 125: 551-554.
1569. Lu ML, Wikman F, Orntoft TF, Charytonowicz E, Rabbani F, Zhang Z, Dalbagni G, Pohar KS, Yu G, Cordon-Cardo C (2002). Impact of alterations affecting the p53 pathway in bladder cancer on clinical outcome, assessed by conventional and array-based methods. *Clin Cancer Res* 8: 171-179.
1570. Lubensky IA, Schmidt L, Zhuang Z, Weirich G, Pack S, Zambrano N, Walther MM, Choyke P, Linehan WM, Zbar B (1999). Hereditary and sporadic papillary renal carcinomas with c-met mutations share a distinct morphological phenotype. *Am J Pathol* 155: 517-526.
1571. Lucas DR, Lawrence WD, McDewitt WJ (1994). Mucinous papillary adenocarcinoma of the bladder arising within a villous adenoma urachal remnant: an immunohistochemical and ultrastructural study. *J Urol Pathol* 2: 173-182.
1572. Lundgren L, Aldenborg F, Angervall L, Kindblom LG (1994). Pseudomalignant spindle cell proliferations of the urinary bladder. *Hum Pathol* 25: 181-191.
1573. Lundgren R, Elfving P, Heim S, Kristoffersson U, Mandahl N, Mitelman F (1989). A squamous cell bladder carcinoma with karyotypic abnormalities reminiscent of transitional cell carcinoma. *J Urol* 142: 374-376.
1574. Luo J, Duggan DJ, Chen Y, Sauvageot J, Ewing CM, Bittner ML, Trent JM, Isaacs WB (2001). Human prostate cancer and benign prostatic hyperplasia: molecular dissection by gene expression profiling. *Cancer Res* 61: 4683-4688.
1575. Luo J, Zha S, Gage WR, Dunn TA, Hicks JL, Bennett CJ, Ewing CM, Platz EA, Ferdinandusse S, Wanders RJ, Trent JM, Isaacs WB, de Marzo AM (2002). Alpha-methylacyl-CoA racemase: a new molecular marker for prostate cancer. *Cancer Res* 62: 2220-2226.
1576. Luo JH, Yu YP, Cieply K, Lin F, Deflavia P, Dhir R, Finkelstein S, Michalopoulos G, Becich M (2002). Gene expression analysis of prostate cancers. *Mol Carcinog* 33: 25-35.
1577. Luo LY, Rajpert-De Meyts ER, Jung K, Diamandis EP (2001). Expression of the normal epithelial cell-specific 1 (NES1; KLK10) candidate tumour suppressor gene in normal and malignant testicular tissue. *Br J Cancer* 85: 220-224.
1578. Luque Barona RJ, Gonzalez Campora R, Vicioso-Recio L, Requena Tapias MJ, Lopez-Beltran A (2000). [Synchronous prostatic carcinosarcoma: report of 2 cases and review of the literature]. *Actas Urol Esp* 24: 173-178.
1579. Lutzeyer W, Rubben H, Dahm H (1982). Prognostic parameters in superficial bladder cancer: an analysis of 315 cases. *J Urol* 127: 250-252.
1580. Lutzker SG, Levine AJ (1996). A functionally inactive p53 protein in teratocarcinoma cells is activated by either DNA damage or cellular differentiation. *Nat Med* 2: 804-810.
1581. Lutzker SG, Mathew R, Taller DR (2001). A p53 dose-response relationship for sensitivity to DNA damage in isogenic teratocarcinoma cells. *Oncogene* 20: 2982-2986.
1582. Lynch CF, Cohen MB (1995). Urinary system. *Cancer* 75: 316-329.
1583. Lynch HT, Ens JA, Lynch JF (1990). The Lynch syndrome II and urological malignancies. *J Urol* 143: 24-28.
1584. Lytton B, Collins JT, Weiss RM, Schiff MJr, McGuire EJ, LiVolsi VA (1979). Results of biopsy after early stage prostatic cancer treatment by implantation of 125I seeds. *J Urol* 121: 306-309.
1585. Ma KF, Tse CH, Tsui MS (1990). Neurilemmoma of kidney—a rare occurrence. *Histopathology* 17: 378-380.
1586. Macedo AJr, Fichtner J, Hohenfellner R (1997). Extramammary Paget's disease of the penis. *Eur Urol* 31: 382-384.
1587. Mackey JR, Au HJ, Hugh J, Venner P (1998). Genitourinary small cell carcinoma: determination of clinical and therapeutic factors associated with survival. *J Urol* 159: 1624-1629.
1588. Macoska JA, Micale MA, Sakr WA, Benson PD, Wolman SR (1993). Extensive genetic alterations in prostate cancer revealed by dual PCR and FISH analysis. *Genes Chromosomes Cancer* 8: 88-97.
1589. Maddock IR, Moran A, Maher ER, Teare MD, Norman A, Payne SJ, Whitehouse R, Dodd C, Lavin M, Hartley N, Super M, Evans DG (1996). A genetic register for von Hippel-Lindau disease. *J Med Genet* 33: 120-127.
1590. Maden C, Sherman KJ, Beckmann AM, Hislop TG, Teh CZ, Ashley RL, Daling JR (1993). History of circumcision, medical conditions, and sexual activity and risk of penile cancer. *J Natl Cancer Inst* 85: 19-24.
1591. Magee JA, Araki T, Patil S, Ehrig T, True L, Humphrey PA, Catalona WJ, Watson MA, Milbrandt J (2001). Expression profiling reveals hepsin overexpression in prostate cancer. *Cancer Res* 61: 5692-5696.
1592. Magi-Galluzi C, Xu X, Hlatky L, Hahnfeldt P, Kaplan I, Hsiao P, Chang C, Loda M (1997). Heterogeneity of androgen receptor content in advanced prostate cancer. *Mod Pathol* 10: 839-845.
1593. Magi-Galluzzi C, Luo J, Isaacs WB, Hicks JL, de Marzo AM, Epstein JI (2003). Alpha-methylacyl-CoA racemase: a variably sensitive immunohistochemical marker for the diagnosis of small prostate cancer foci on needle biopsy. *Am J Surg Pathol* 27: 1128-1133.
1594. Magri J (1960). Cysts of the prostate gland. *Br J Urol* 32: 295-301.
1595. Magro G, Cavallaro V, Torrisi A, Lopes M, Dell'Albani M, Lanzafame S (2002). Intrarenal solitary fibrous tumor of the kidney report of a case with emphasis on the differential diagnosis in the wide spectrum of monomorphous spindle cell tumors of the kidney. *Pathol Res Pract* 198: 37-43.
1596. Mahadevia PS, Koss LG, Tar IJ (1986). Prostatic involvement in bladder cancer. Prostate mapping in 20 cystoprostatectomy specimens. *Cancer* 58: 2096-2102.
1597. Maher ER, Kaelin WGJr (1997). von Hippel-Lindau disease. *Medicine (Baltimore)* 76: 381-391.
1598. Maher ER, Yates JR, Ferguson-Smith MA (1990). Statistical analysis of the two stage mutation model in von Hippel-Lindau disease, and in sporadic cerebellar haemangioblastoma and renal cell carcinoma. *J Med Genet* 27: 311-314.
1599. Maher JD, Thompson GM, Loening S, Platz CE (1988). Penile plexiform neurofibroma: case report and review of the literature. *J Urol* 139: 1310-1312.
1600. Maheshkumar P, Harper C, Sunderland GT, Conn IG (2000). Cystic epithelial stromal tumour of the seminal vesicle. *BJU Int* 85: 1154.
1601. Mahmoudi T, Verrijzer CP (2001). Chromatin silencing and activation by Polycomb and trithorax group proteins. *Oncogene* 20: 3055-3066.
1602. Mahoney JP, Saffos RO (1981). Fetal rhabdomyomatous nephroblastoma with a renal pelvic mass simulating sarcoma botryoides. *Am J Surg Pathol* 5: 297-306.
1603. Mahran MR, el Baz M (1993). Verrucous carcinoma of the bilharzial bladder. Impact of invasiveness on survival. *Scand J Urol Nephrol* 27: 189-192.
1604. Mai KT (1994). Giant renomedullary interstitial cell tumor. *J Urol* 151: 986-988.
1605. Mai KT, Isotalo PA, Green J, Perkins DG, Morash C, Collins JP (2000). Incidental prostatic adenocarcinomas and putative premalignant lesions in TURP specimens collected before and after the introduction of prostrate-specific antigen screening. *Arch Pathol Lab Med* 124: 1454-1456.
1606. Mai KT, Perkins DG, Collins JP (1996). Epithelioid cell variant of renal angiomyolipoma. *Histopathology* 28: 277-280.
1607. Maiche AG (1992). Epidemiological aspects of cancer of the penis in Finland. *Eur J Cancer Prev* 1: 153-158.
1608. Maiche AG, Pyrhonen S, Karkinen M (1991). Histological grading of squamous cell carcinoma of the penis: a new scoring system. *Br J Urol* 67: 522-526.
1609. Maiti S, Chatterjee G, Pal SN, Mukherjee DR (1990). Benign cystic teratoma of the testis. *J Indian Med Assoc* 88: 287-288.
1610. Malmstrom PU, Busch C, Norlen BJ (1987). Recurrence, progression and survival in bladder cancer. A retrospective analysis of 232 patients with greater than or equal to 5-year follow-up. *Scand J Urol Nephrol* 21: 185-195.
1611. Maluf HM, King ME, de Luca FR, Navarro J, Talerman A, Young RH (1991). Giant multilocular prostatic cystadenoma: a distinctive lesion of the retroperitoneum in men. A report of two cases. *Am J Surg Pathol* 15: 131-135.
1612. Mancilla-Jimenez R, Stanley RJ, Blath RA (1976). Papillary renal cell carcinoma: a clinical, radiologic, and pathologic study of 34 cases. *Cancer* 38: 2469-2480.
1613. Manglani KS, Manaligod JR, Ray B (1980). Spindle cell carcinoma of the glans penis: a light and electron microscopic study. *Cancer* 46: 2266-2272.
1614. Manivel JC, Fraley EE (1988). Malignant melanoma of the penis and male urethra: 4 case reports and literature review. *J Urol* 139: 813-816.

1615. Manivel JC, Jessurun J, Wick MR, Dehner LP (1987). Placental alkaline phosphatase immunoreactivity in testicular germ-cell neoplasms. *Am J Surg Pathol* 11: 21-29.
1616. Manivel JC, Niehans G, Wick MR, Dehner LP (1987). Intermediate trophoblast in germ cell neoplasms. *Am J Surg Pathol* 11: 693-701.
1617. Manivel JC, Reinberg Y, Niehans GA, Fraley EE (1989). Intratubular germ cell neoplasia in testicular teratomas and epidermoid cysts. Correlation with prognosis and possible biologic significance. *Cancer* 64: 715-720.
1618. Manousakas T, Kyroudi A, Dimopoulos MA, Moraitis E, Mitropoulos D (2000). Plasmacytoid transitional cell carcinoma of the bladder. *BJU Int* 86: 910.
1619. Manova K, Bachvarova RF (1991). Expression of c-kit encoded at the W locus of mice in developing embryonic germ cells and presumptive melanoblasts. *Dev Biol* 146: 312-324.
1620. Manuel M, Katayama PK, Jones HWJr (1976). The age of occurrence of gonadal tumors in intersex patients with a Y chromosome. *Am J Obstet Gynecol* 124: 293-300.
1621. Manyak MJ, Hinkle GH, Olsen JO, Chiaccherini RP, Partin AW, Piantadosi S, Burgers JK, Texter JH, Neal CE, Libertino JA, Wright GLJr, Maguire RT (1999). Immunoscintigraphy with indium-111-capromab pendetide: evaluation before definitive therapy in patients with prostate cancer. *Urology* 54: 1058-1063.
1622. Maranchie JK, Bouyounes BT, Zhang PL, O'Donnell MA, Summerhayes IC, de Wolf WC (2000). Clinical and pathological characteristics of micropapillary transitional cell carcinoma: a highly aggressive variant. *J Urol* 163: 748-751.
1623. Marconis JT (1959). Primary Hodgkin's (paragranulomatous type) of the bladder lymphoma. *J Urol* 81: 275-281.
1624. Marcus PM, Vineis P, Rothman N (2000). NAT2 slow acetylation and bladder cancer risk: a meta-analysis of 22 case-control studies conducted in the general population. *Pharmacogenetics* 10: 115-122.
1625. Marks D, Crosthwaite A, Varigos G, Ellis D, Morstyn G (1988). Therapy of primary diffuse large cell lymphoma of the penis with preservation of function. *J Urol* 139: 1057-1058.
1626. Marks LB, Rutgers JL, Shipley WU, Walker TG, Stracher MS, Waltman AC, Geller SC (1990). Testicular seminoma: clinical and pathological features that may predict para-aortic lymph node metastases. *J Urol* 143: 524-527.
1627. Marley EF, Liapis H, Humphrey PA, Nadler RB, Siegel CL, Zhu X, Brandt JM, Dehner LP (1997). Primitive neuroectodermal tumor of the kidney—another enigma: a pathologic, immunohistochemical, and molecular diagnostic study. *Am J Surg Pathol* 21: 354-359.
1628. Marsden HB, Lawler W (1978). Bone-metastasizing renal tumour of childhood. *Br J Cancer* 38: 437-441.
1629. Marsden HB, Lawler W (1980). Bone metastasizing renal tumour of childhood. Histopathological and clinical review of 38 cases. *Virchows Arch A Pathol Anat Histol* 387: 341-351.
1630. Marsden HB, Lawler W, Kumar PM (1978). Bone metastasizing renal tumor of childhood: morphological and clinical features, and differences from Wilms' tumor. *Cancer* 42: 1922-1928.
1631. Marsh RJ, Ceccarelli FE (1964). Ten-year analysis of primary bladder tumors at Brooke General Hospital. *J Urol* 91: 530.
1632. Martignoni G, Bonetti F, Pea M, Tardanico R, Brunelli M, Eble JN (2002). Renal disease in adults with TSC2/PKD1 contiguous gene syndrome. *Am J Surg Pathol* 26: 198-205.
1633. Martignoni G, Pea M, Bonetti F, Brunelli M, Eble JN (2002). Oncocytoma-like angiomyolipoma. A clinicopathologic and immunohistochemical study of 2 cases. *Arch Pathol Lab Med* 126: 610-612.
1634. Martignoni G, Pea M, Bonetti F, Zamboni G, Carbonara C, Longa L, Zancanaro C, Maran M, Brisigotti M, Mariuzzi GM (1998). Carcinomalike monotypic epithelioid angiomyolipoma in patients without evidence of tuberous sclerosis: a clinicopathologic and genetic study. *Am J Surg Pathol* 22: 663-672.
1635. Martignoni G, Pea M, Chilosi M, Brunelli M, Scarpa A, Colato C, Tardanico R, Zamboni G, Bonetti F (2001). Parvalbumin is constantly expressed in chromophobe renal carcinoma. *Mod Pathol* 14: 760-767.
1636. Martignoni G, Pea M, Rigaud G, Manfrin E, Colato C, Zamboni G, Scarpa A, Tardanico R, Roncalli M, Bonetti F (2000). Renal angiomyolipoma with epithelioid sarcomatous transformation and metastases: demonstration of the same genetic defects in the primary and metastatic lesions. *Am J Surg Pathol* 24: 889-894.
1637. Martin JE, Jenkins BJ, Zuk RJ, Blandy JP, Baithun SI (1989). Clinical importance of squamous metaplasia in invasive transitional cell carcinoma of the bladder. *J Clin Pathol* 42: 250-253.
1638. Martin SA, Mynderse LA, Lager DJ, Cheville JC (2001). Juxtaglomerular cell tumor: a clinicopathologic study of four cases and review of the literature. *Am J Clin Pathol* 116: 854-863.
1639. Martin SA, Sears DL, Sebo TJ, Lohse CM, Cheville JC (2002). Smooth muscle neoplasms of the urinary bladder: a clinicopathologic comparison of leiomyoma and leiomyosarcoma. *Am J Surg Pathol* 26: 292-300.
1640. Martins AC, Faria SM, Cologna AJ, Suaid HJ, Tucci SJr (2002). Immunoexpression of p53 protein and proliferating cell nuclear antigen in penile carcinoma. *J Urol* 167: 89-92.
1641. Maru N, Ohori M, Kattan MW, Scardino PT, Wheeler TM (2001). Prognostic significance of the diameter of perineural invasion in radical prostatectomy specimens. *Hum Pathol* 32: 828-833.
1642. Masera A, Ovcak Z, Volavsek M, Bracko M (1997). Adenosquamous carcinoma of the penis. *J Urol* 157: 2261.
1643. Masih AS, Stoler MH, Farrow GM, Wooldridge TN, Johansson SL (1992). Penile verrucous carcinoma: a clinicopathologic, human papillomavirus typing and flow cytometric analysis. *Mod Pathol* 5: 48-55.
1644. Masson P (1946). Etude sur le seminoma. *Rev Can Biol* 5: 361-387.
1645. Mathew S, Murty VV, Bosl GJ, Chaganti RS (1994). Loss of heterozygosity identifies multiple sites of allelic deletions on chromosome 1 in human male germ cell tumors. *Cancer Res* 54: 6265-6269.
1646. Matoska J, Ondrus D, Hornak M (1988). Metastatic spermatocytic seminoma. A case report with light microscopic, ultrastructural, and immunohistochemical findings. *Cancer* 62: 1197-1201.
1647. Matoska J, Ondrus D, Talerman A (1992). Malignant granulosa cell tumor of the testis associated with gynecomastia and long survival. *Cancer* 69: 1769-1772.
1648. Matoska J, Talerman A (1989). Mixed germ cell-sex cord stroma tumor of the testis. A report with ultrastructural findings. *Cancer* 64: 2146-2153.
1649. Matoska J, Talerman A (1990). Spermatocytic seminoma associated with rhabdomyosarcoma. *Am J Clin Pathol* 94: 89-95.
1650. Maxwell PH, Wiesener MS, Chang GW, Clifford SC, Vaux EC, Cockman ME, Wykoff CC, Pugh CW, Maher ER, Ratcliffe PJ (1999). The tumour suppressor protein VHL targets hypoxia-inducible factors for oxygen-dependent proteolysis. *Nature* 399: 271-275.
1651. May D, Shamberger R, Newbury R, Teele RL (1992). Juvenile granulosa cell tumor of an intraabdominal testis. *Pediatr Radiol* 22: 507-508.
1652. Mayer F, Gillis AJ, Dinjens W, Oosterhuis JW, Bokemeyer C, Looijenga LH (2002). Microsatellite instability of germ cell tumors is associated with resistance to systemic treatment. *Cancer Res* 62: 2758-2760.
1653. Mayer F, Stoop H, Sen S, Bokemeyer C, Oosterhuis JW, Looijenga LH (2003). Aneuploidy of human testicular germ cell tumors is associated with amplification of centrosomes. *Oncogene* 22: 3859-3866.
1654. Maynard SE, Min JY, Merchan J, Lim KH, Li J, Mondal S, Libermann TA, Morgan JP, Sellke FW, Stillman IE, Epstein FH, Sukhatme VP, Karumanchi SA (2003). Excess placental soluble fms-like tyrosine kinase 1 (sFlt1) may contribute to endothelial dysfunction, hypertension, and proteinuria in preeclampsia. *J Clin Invest* 111: 649-658.
1655. Mazeman E (1976). Tumours of the upper urinary tract calyces, renal pelvis and ureter. *Eur Urol* 2: 120-126.
1656. Mazur MT, Myers JL, Maddox WA (1987). Cystic epithelial-stromal tumor of the seminal vesicle. *Am J Surg Pathol* 11: 210-217.
1657. Mazzu D, Jeffrey RBJr, Ralls PW (1995). Lymphoma and leukemia involving the testicles: findings on gray-scale and color Doppler sonography. *AJR Am J Roentgenol* 164: 645-647.
1658. Mazzucchelli L, Studer UE, Kraft R (1995). Small-cell undifferentiated carcinoma of the renal pelvis 26 years after subdiaphragmatic irradiation for non-Hodgkin's lymphoma. *Br J Urol* 76: 403-404.
1659. Mazzucchelli L, Studer UE, Zimmermann A (1992). Cystadenoma of the seminal vesicle: case report and literature review. *J Urol* 147: 1621-1624.
1660. Mazzucchelli R, Colanzi P, Pomante R, Muzzonigro G, Montironi R (2000). Prostate tissue and serum markers. *Adv Clin Path* 4: 111-120.
1661. Mazzucchelli R, Santinelli A, Lopez-Beltran A, Scarpelli M, Montironi R (2002). Evaluation of prognostic factors in radical prostatectomy specimens with cancer. *Urol Int* 68: 209-215.
1662. McCaffrey JA, Reuter VV, Herr HW, Macapinlac HA, Russo P, Motzer RJ (2000). Carcinoid tumor of the kidney. The use of somatostatin receptor scintigraphy in diagnosis and management. *Urol Oncol* 5: 108-111.
1663. McClaren K, Thomson D (1989). Localization of S-100 protein in a Leydig and Sertoli cell tumour of testis. *Histopathology* 15: 649-652.
1664. McCluggage WG, Ashe P, McBride H, Maxwell P, Sloan JM (1998). Localization of the cellular expression of inhibin in trophoblastic tissue. *Histopathology* 32: 252-256.
1665. McCluggage WG, Shanks JH, Arthur K, Banerjee SS (1998). Cellular proliferation and nuclear ploidy assessments augment established prognostic factors in predicting malignancy in testicular Leydig cell tumours. *Histopathology* 33: 361-368.
1666. McCluggage WG, Shanks JH, Whiteside C, Maxwell P, Banerjee SS, Biggart JD (1998). Immunohistochemical study of testicular sex cord-stromal tumors, including staining with anti-inhibin antibody. *Am J Surg Pathol* 22: 615-619.
1667. McCormack RT, Rittenhouse HG, Finlay JA, Sokoloff RL, Wang TJ, Wolfert RL, Lilja H, Oesterling JE (1995). Molecular forms of prostate-specific antigen and the human kallikrein gene family: a new era. *Urology* 45: 729-744.
1668. McCredie M, Ford JM, Taylor JS, Stewart JH (1982). Analgesics and cancer of the renal pelvis in New South Wales. *Cancer* 49: 2617-2625.
1669. McCullough DL, Lamma DL, McLaughlin AP3rd, Gittes RF (1975). Familial transitional cell carcinoma of the bladder. *J Urol* 113: 629-635.
1670. McDermott MB, O'Briain DS, Shiels OM, Daly PA (1995). Malignant lymphoma of the epididymis. A case report of bilateral involvement by a follicular large cell lymphoma. *Cancer* 75: 2174-2179.
1671. McDonald MW, O'Connell JR, Manning JT, Benjamin RS (1983). Leiomyosarcoma of the penis. *J Urol* 130: 788-789.
1672. McDougal WS (1995). Carcinoma of the penis: improved survival by early regional lymphadenectomy based on the histological grade and depth of invasion of the primary lesion. *J Urol* 154: 1364-1366.
1673. McDowell PR, Fox WM, Epstein JI (1994). Is submission of remaining tissue necessary when incidental carcinoma of the prostate is found on transurethral resection? *Hum Pathol* 25: 493-497.
1674. McGregor DH, Tanimura A, Weigel JW (1982). Basal cell carcinoma of penis. *Urology* 20: 320-323.
1675. McGregor DK, Khurana KK, Cao C, Tsao CC, Ayala G, Krishnan B, Ro JY, Lechago J, Truong LD (2001). Diagnosing primary and metastatic renal cell carcinoma: the use of the monoclonal antibody 'Renal Cell Carcinoma Marker'. *Am J Surg Pathol* 25: 1485-1492.
1676. McIntire TL, Franzini DA (1986). The presence of benign prostatic glands in perineural spaces. *J Urol* 135: 507-509.
1677. McIntosh JF, Worley G (1955). Adenocarcinoma arising in exstrophy of the bladder: report of two cases and a review of the literature. *J Urol* 73: 820-829.
1678. McKenney JK, Amin MB, Young RH (2003). Urothelial (transitional cell) papilloma of the urinary bladder: a clinicopathologic study of 26 cases. *Mod Pathol* 16: 623-629.
1679. McKusick VA (1994). *Mendelian Inheritance in Man: a Catalogue of Human Genes and Genetic Disorders. (See also http://www.ncbi.nlm.nih.gov/omim).* 11th Edition. The Johns Hopkins University Press: Baltimore.
1680. McLaughlin JK, Blot WJ, Mandel JS, Schuman LM, Mehl ES, Fraumeni JFJr (1983). Etiology of cancer of the renal pelvis. *J Natl Cancer Inst* 71: 287-291.

1681. McLaughlin JK, Silverman DT, Hsing AW, Ross RK, Schoenberg JB, Yu MC, Stemhagen A, Lynch CF, Blot WJ, Fraumeni JFJr (1992). Cigarette smoking and cancers of the renal pelvis and ureter. *Cancer Res* 52: 254-257.

1682. McNeal JE (1969). Origin and development of carcinoma in the prostate. *Cancer* 23: 24-34.

1683. McNeal JE, Bostwick DG (1986). Intraductal dysplasia: a premalignant lesion of the prostate. *Hum Pathol* 17: 64-71.

1684. McNeal JE, Haillot O (2001). Patterns of spread of adenocarcinoma in the prostate as related to cancer volume. *Prostate* 49: 48-57.

1685. McNeal JE, Price HM, Redwine EA, Freiha FS, Stamey TA (1988). Stage A versus stage B adenocarcinoma of the prostate: morphological comparison and biological significance. *J Urol* 139: 61-65.

1686. McNeal JE, Redwine EA, Freiha FS, Stamey TA (1988). Zonal distribution of prostatic adenocarcinoma. Correlation with histologic pattern and direction of spread. *Am J Surg Pathol* 12: 897-906.

1687. McNeal JE, Villers A, Redwine EA, Freiha FS, Stamey TA (1991). Microcarcinoma in the prostate: its association with duct-acinar dysplasia. *Hum Pathol* 22: 644-652.

1688. McNeal JE, Villers AA, Redwine EA, Freiha FS, Stamey TA (1990). Histologic differentiation, cancer volume, and pelvic lymph node metastasis in adenocarcinoma of the prostate. *Cancer* 66: 1225-1233.

1689. McNeal JE, Yemoto CE (1996). Spread of adenocarcinoma within prostatic ducts and acini. Morphologic and clinical correlations. *Am J Surg Pathol* 20: 802-814.

1690. McVey RJ, Banerjee SS, Eyden BP, Reeve RS, Harris M (2002). Carcinoid tumor originating in a horseshoe kidney. *In Vivo* 16: 197-199.

1691. Meacham RB, Mata JA, Espada R, Wheeler TM, Schum CW, Scardino PT (1988). Testicular metastasis as the first manifestation of colon carcinoma. *J Urol* 140: 621-622.

1692. Mearini E, Zucchi A, Costantini E, Fornetti P, Tiacci E, Mearini L (2002). Primary Burkitt's lymphoma of bladder in patient with AIDS. *J Urol* 167: 1397-1398.

1693. Medeiros LJ, Michie SA, Johnson DE, Warnke RA, Weiss LM (1988). An immunoperoxidase study of renal cell carcinomas: correlation with nuclear grade, cell type, and histologic pattern. *Hum Pathol* 19: 980-987.

1694. Medeiros LJ, Palmedo G, Krigman HR, Kovacs G, Beckwith JB (1999). Oncocytoid renal cell carcinoma after neuroblastoma: a report of four cases of a distinct clinicopathologic entity. *Am J Surg Pathol* 23: 772-780.

1695. Meduri G, Fromentin L, Vieillefond A, Fries D (1991). Donor-related non-Hodgkin's lymphoma in a renal allograft recipient. *Transplant Proc* 23: 2649.

1696. Meeker AK (2001). *Telomere Dynamics and Androgen Regulation of Telomerase Enzymatic Activity in Normal and Pathological States of the Prostate Biochemistry, Cellular and Molecular Biology.* Johns Hopkins: Baltimore.

1697. Meeker AK, Gage WR, Hicks JL, Simon I, Coffman JR, Platz EA, March GE, de Marzo AM (2002). Telomere length assessment in human archival tissues: combined telomere fluorescence in situ hybridization and immunostaining. *Am J Pathol* 160: 1259-1268.

1698. Meeker AK, Hicks JL, Platz EA, March GE, Bennet CJ, de Marzo A (2002). Telomere shortening is an early somatic DNA alteration in human prostate tumorigenesis. *Cancer Res* 62: 6405-6409.

1699. Mehlhorn J (1987). [Prostatic metastases as a differential diagnostic problem]. *Zentralbl Allg Pathol* 133: 351-353.

1700. Meis JM, Ayala AG, Johnson DE (1987). Adenocarcinoma of the urethra in women. A clinicopathologic study. *Cancer* 60: 1038-1052.

1701. Meis JM, Butler JJ, Osborne BM, Ordonez NG (1987). Solitary plasmacytomas of bone and extramedullary plasmacytomas. A clinicopathologic and immunohistochemical study. *Cancer* 59: 1475-1485.

1702. Mekori YA, Steiner ZP, Bernheim J, Manor Y, Klajman A (1984). Acute anuric bilateral ureteral obstruction in malignant lymphoma. *Am J Med Sci* 287: 70-73.

1703. Melchior SW, Brawer MK (1996). Role of transrectal ultrasound and prostate biopsy. *J Clin Ultrasound* 24: 463-471.

1704. Melen DR (1932). Multilocular cysts of the prostate. *J Urol* 27: 343-349.

1705. Melicow MM (1955). Classification of tumours of the testis: a clinical and pathological study based on 105 primary and 13 secondary cases in adults, and 3 primary and 4 secondary cases in children. *J Urol* 73: 547-574.

1706. Melicow MM, Pachter MR (1967). Endometrial carcinoma of proxtatic utricle (uterus masculinus). *Cancer* 20: 1715-1722.

1707. Melicow MM, Tannenbaum M (1971). Endometrial carcinoma of uterus masculinus (prostatic utricle). Report of 6 cases. *J Urol* 106: 892-902.

1708. Mellon JK, Lunec J, Wright C, Horne CH, Kelly P, Neal DE (1996). C-erbB-2 in bladder cancer: molecular biology, correlation with epidermal growth factor receptors and prognostic value. *J Urol* 155: 321-326.

1709. Mellon K, Wright C, Kelly P, Horne CH, Neal DE (1995). Long-term outcome related to epidermal growth factor receptor status in bladder cancer. *J Urol* 153: 919-925.

1710. Meloni AM, Dobbs RM, Pontes JE, Sandberg AA (1993). Translocation (X;1) in papillary renal cell carcinoma. A new cytogenetic subtype. *Cancer Genet Cytogenet* 65: 1-6.

1711. Mene P, Festuccia F, Polci R, Faraggiana T, Gualdi G, Cinotti GA (2001). Malignant epithelioid renal angiomyolipoma in a case of tuberous sclerosis with multiple organ involvement. *Contrib Nephrol* 136: 299-305.

1712. Meng X, de Rooij DG, Westerdahl K, Saarma M, Sariola H (2001). Promotion of seminomatous tumors by targeted overexpression of glial cell line-derived neurotrophic factor in mouse testis. *Cancer Res* 61: 3267-3271.

1713. Mentzel T, Beham A, Calonje E, Katenkamp D, Fletcher CD (1997). Epithelioid hemangioendothelioma of skin and soft tissues: clinicopathologic and immunohistochemical study of 30 cases. *Am J Surg Pathol* 21: 363-374.

1714. Mentzel T, Calonje E, Wadden C, Camplejohn RS, Beham A, Smith MA, Fletcher CD (1996). Myxofibrosarcoma. Clinicopathologic analysis of 75 cases with emphasis on the low-grade variant. *Am J Surg Pathol* 20: 391-405.

1715. Merchant SH, Mittal BV, Desai MS (1998). Haemangiopericytoma of kidney: a report of 2 cases. *J Postgrad Med* 44: 78-80.

1716. Messen S, Bonkhoff H, Bruch M, Steffens J, Ziegler M (1995). Primary renal osteosarcoma. Case report and review of the literature. *Urol Int* 55: 158-161.

1717. Messing EM (1990). Clinical implications of the expression of epidermal growth factor receptors in human transitional cell carcinoma. *Cancer Res* 50: 2530-2537.

1718. Messing EM, Vaillancourt A (1990). Hematuria screening for bladder cancer. *J Occup Med* 32: 838-845.

1719. Messing EM, Young TB, Hunt VB, Newton MA, Bram LL, Vaillancourt A, Hisgen WJ, Greenberg EB, Kuglitsch ME, Wegenke JD (1995). Hematuria home screening: repeat testing results. *J Urol* 154: 57-61.

1720. Michael H (1998). Nongerm cell tumors arising in patients with testicular germ cell tumors. *J Urol Pathol* 9: 39-60.

1721. Michael H, Hull MT, Foster RS, Sweeney CJ, Ulbright TM (1998). Nephroblastoma-like tumors in patients with testicular germ cell tumors. *Am J Surg Pathol* 22: 1107-1114.

1722. Michael H, Hull MT, Ulbright TM, Foster RS, Miller KD (1997). Primitive neuroectodermal tumors arising in testicular germ cell neoplasms. *Am J Surg Pathol* 21: 896-904.

1723. Michael H, Lucia J, Foster RS, Ulbright TM (2000). The pathology of late recurrence of testicular germ cell tumors. *Am J Surg Pathol* 24: 257-273.

1724. Michaels MM, Brown HE, Favino CJ (1974). Leiomyoma of prostate. *Urology* 3: 617-620.

1725. Michel F, Gattegno B, Roland J, Coloby P, Colbert N, Thibault P (1986). Primary nonseminomatous germ cell tumor of the prostate. *J Urol* 135: 597-599.

1726. Miettinen M, Salo J, Virtanen I (1986). Testicular stromal tumor: ultrastructural, immunohistochemical, and gel electrophoretic evidence of epithelial differentiation. *Ultrastruct Pathol* 10: 515-528.

1727. Miettinen M, Wahlstrom T, Virtanen I, Talerman A, Astengo-Osuna C (1985). Cellular differentiation in ovarian sex-cord-stromal and germ-cell tumors studied with antibodies to intermediate-filament proteins. *Am J Surg Pathol* 9: 640-651.

1728. Mihatsch MJ, Bleisch A, Six P, Heitz P (1972). Primary choriocarcinoma of the kidney in a 49-year-old woman. *J Urol* 108: 537-539.

1729. Mihatsch MJ, Knusli C (1982). Phenacetin abuse and malignant tumors. An autopsy study covering 25 years (1953-1977). *Klin Wochenschr* 60: 1339-1349.

1730. Mikuz G (1993). [Non-urothelial tumors of the urinary tract]. *Verh Dtsch Ges Pathol* 77: 180-198.

1731. Milasin J, Micic M, Micic S, Diklic V (1989). Distribution of marker chromosomes in relation to histologic grade in bladder cancer. *Cancer Genet Cytogenet* 42: 135-142.

1732. Millar DS, Ow KK, Paul CL, Russell PJ, Molloy PL, Clark SJ (1999). Detailed methylation analysis of the glutathione S-transferase pi (GSTP1) gene in prostate cancer. *Oncogene* 18: 1313-1324.

1733. Miller EC, Murray HL (1962). Congenital adrenocortical hyperplasia: case previously reported as "bilateral interstitial cell tumor of the testicle". *J Clin Endocrinol Metab* 22: 655-657.

1734. Mills SE, Bova GS, Wick MR, Young RH (1989). Leiomyosarcoma of the urinary bladder. A clinicopathologic and immunohistochemical study of 15 cases. *Am J Surg Pathol* 13: 480-489.

1735. Mills SE, Weiss MA, Swanson PE, Wick MR (1988). Small cell undifferentiated carcinoma of the renal pelvis: a light microscopic, immunohistochemical and ultrastructural study. *Surg Pathol* 1: 83-88.

1736. Milosevic MF, Warde PR, Banerjee D, Gospodarowicz MK, McLean M, Catton PA, Catton CN (2000). Urethral carcinoma in women: results of treatment with primary radiotherapy. *Radiother Oncol* 56: 29-35.

1737. Mimata H, Kasagi Y, Ohno H, Nomura Y, Iechika S (2000). Malignant neurofibroma of the urinary bladder. *Urol Int* 65: 167-168.

1738. Mineur P, de Cooman S, Hustin J, Verhoeven G, de Hertoch R (1987). Feminizing testicular Leydig cell tumor: hormonal profile before and after unilateral orchidectomy. *J Clin Endocrinol Metab* 64: 686-691.

1739. Minkowitz S, Soloway H, Soscia J (1965). Ossifying interstitial cell tumor of the testes. *J Urol* 94: 592-595.

1740. Mira JL, Fan G (2000). Leiomyoma of the male urethra: a case report and review of the literature. *Arch Pathol Lab Med* 124: 302-303.

1741. Miro AG, de Seta L, Lizza N, Kartheuser A, Detry R (1997). Malignant fibrous histiocytoma after radiation therapy for prostate cancer: case report. *J Chemother* 9: 162.

1742. Mishina M, Ogawa O, Kinoshita H, Oka H, Okumura K, Mitsumori K, Kakehi Y, Reeve AE, Yoshida O (1996). Equivalent parental distribution of frequently lost alleles and biallelic expression of the H19 gene in human testicular germ cell tumors. *Jpn J Cancer Res* 87: 816-823.

1743. Mitelman F (2000). Recurrent chromosome aberrations in cancer. *Mutat Res* 462: 247-253.

1744. Mitsudo S, Nakanishi I, Koss LG (1981). Paget's disease of the penis and adjacent skin: its association with fatal sweat gland carcinoma. *Arch Pathol Lab Med* 105: 518-520.

1745. Miyakawa M, Ueyama H, Kuze M, Matsushita T, Tachikawa Y (1971). [Renal fibrosarcoma changed from fibrolipoma: report of a case]. *Hinyokika Kiyo* 17: 517-527.

1746. Miyake H, Gleave M, Kamidono S, Hara I (2002). Overexpression of clusterin in transitional cell carcinoma of the bladder is related to disease progression and recurrence. *Urology* 59: 150-154.

1747. Miyake H, Hara I, Gohji K, Arakawa S, Kamidono S (1998). The significance of lymphadenectomy in transitional cell carcinoma of the upper urinary tract. *Br J Urol* 82: 494-498.

1748. Miyamoto H, Kubota Y, Shuin T, Torigoe S, Hosaka M, Iwasaki Y, Danenberg K, Danenberg PV (1993). Analyses of p53 gene mutations in primary human bladder cancer. *Oncol Res* 5: 245-249.

1749. Miyamoto H, Shuin T, Torigoe S, Iwasaki Y, Kubota Y (1995). Retinoblastoma gene mutations in primary human bladder cancer. *Br J Cancer* 71: 831-835.

1750. Miyao N, Masumori N, Takahashi A, Sasai M, Hisataki T, Kitamura H, Satoh M, Tsukamoto T (1998). Lymph node metastasis in patients with carcinomas of the renal pelvis and ureter. *Eur Urol* 33: 180-185.

1751. Miyao N, Tsai YC, Lerner SP, Olumi AF, Spruck CH3rd, Gonzalez-Zulueta M, Nichols PW, Skinner DG, Jones PA (1993). Role of chromosome 9 in human bladder cancer. *Cancer Res* 53: 4066-4070.

1752. Mizutani S, Okuda N, Sonoda T (1973). Granular cell myoblastoma of the bladder: report of an additional case. *J Urol* 110: 403-405.

1753. Moch H, Gasser T, Amin MB, Torhorst J, Sauter G, Mihatsch MJ (2000). Prognostic utility of the recently recommended histologic classification and revised TNM staging system of renal cell carcinoma: a Swiss experience with 588 tumors. *Cancer* 89: 604-614.

1754. Moch H, Presti JCJr, Sauter G, Buchholz N, Jordan P, Mihatsch MJ, Waldman FM (1996). Genetic aberrations detected by comparative genomic hybridization are associated with clinical outcome in renal cell carcinoma. *Cancer Res* 56: 27-30.

1755. Moch H, Sauter G, Buchholz N, Gasser TC, Bubendorf L, Waldman FM, Mihatsch MJ (1997). Epidermal growth factor receptor expression is associated with rapid tumor cell proliferation in renal cell carcinoma. *Hum Pathol* 28: 1255-1259.

1756. Moch H, Sauter G, Gasser TC, Bubendorf L, Richter J, Presti JCJr, Waldman FM, Mihatsch MJ (1998). EGF-r gene copy number changes in renal cell carcinoma detected by fluorescence in situ hybridization. *J Pathol* 184: 424-429.

1757. Moch H, Sauter G, Mihatsch MJ, Gudat F, Epper R, Waldman FM (1994). p53 but not erbB-2 expression is associated with rapid tumor proliferation in urinary bladder cancer. *Hum Pathol* 25: 1346-1351.

1758. Moch H, Sauter G, Moore D, Mihatsch MJ, Gudat F, Waldman F (1993). p53 and erbB-2 protein overexpression are associated with early invasion and metastasis in bladder cancer. *Virchows Arch A Pathol Anat Histopathol* 423: 329-334.

1759. Moch H, Schraml P, Bubendorf L, Mirlacher M, Kononen J, Gasser T, Mihatsch MJ, Kallioniemi OP, Sauter G (1999). High-throughput tissue microarray analysis to evaluate genes uncovered by cDNA microarray screening in renal cell carcinoma. *Am J Pathol* 154: 981-986.

1760. Moch H, Schraml P, Bubendorf L, Richter J, Gasser TC, Mihatsch MJ, Sauter G (1998). Intratumoral heterogeneity of von Hippel-Lindau gene deletions in renal cell carcinoma detected by fluorescence in situ hybridization. *Cancer Res* 58: 2304-2309.

1761. Moertel CL, Watterson J, McCormick SR, Simonton SC (1995). Follicular large cell lymphoma of the testis in a child. *Cancer* 75: 1182-1186.

1762. Mohammed AY, Matthew L, Harmse JL, Lang S, Townell NH (1999). Multiple leiomyoma of the renal capsule. *Scand J Urol Nephrol* 33: 138-139.

1763. Molenaar WM, Oosterhuis JW, Meiring A, Sleyfer DT, Schraffordt Koops H, Cornelisse CJ (1986). Histology and DNA contents of a secondary malignancy arising in a mature residual lesion six years after chemotherapy for a disseminated nonseminomatous testicular tumor. *Cancer* 58: 264-268.

1764. Molinie V, Liguory Brunaud MD, Chiche R (1992). [Primary carcinoid tumor of the kidney. Apropos of a case with immunohistochemical study]. *Arch Anat Cytol Pathol* 40: 289-293.

1765. Moll R, Franke WW, Schiller DL, Geiger B, Krepler R (1982). The catalog of human cytokeratins: patterns of expression in normal epithelia, tumors and cultured cells. *Cell* 31: 11-24.

1766. Moller H (1993). Clues to the aetiology of testicular germ cell tumours from descriptive epidemiology. *Eur Urol* 23: 8-13.

1767. Moller H, Evans H (2003). Epidemiology of gonadal germ cell cancer in males and females. *APMIS* 111: 43-46.

1768. Moller H, Prener A, Skakkebaek NE (1996). Testicular cancer, cryptorchidism, inguinal hernia, testicular atrophy, and genital malformations: case-control studies in Denmark. *Cancer Causes Control* 7: 264-274.

1769. Moller H, Skakkebaek NE (1997). Testicular cancer and cryptorchidism in relation to prenatal factors: case-control studies in Denmark. *Cancer Causes Control* 8: 904-912.

1770. Moller H, Skakkebaek NE (1999). Risk of testicular cancer in subfertile men: case-control study. *BMJ* 318: 559-562.

1771. Moncure CW, Prout GRJr (1970). Antigenicity of human prostatic acid phosphatase. *Cancer* 25: 463-467.

1772. Montie JE, Wood DPJr, Pontes JE, Boyett JM, Levin HS (1989). Adenocarcinoma of the prostate in cysto-prostatectomy specimens removed for bladder cancer. *Cancer* 63: 381-385.

1773. Montironi R (2001). Prognostic factors in prostate cancer. *BMJ* 322: 378-379.

1774. Montironi R (2001). Spectrum of prostatic non-epithelial tumour-like conditions and tumours. *Pathol Res Pract* 197: 653-655.

1775. Montironi R, Mazzucchelli R, Algaba F, Bostwick DG, Krongrad A (2000). Prostate-specific antigen as a marker of prostate disease. *Virchows Arch* 436: 297-304.

1776. Montironi R, Mazzucchelli R, Scarpelli M (2002). Precancerous lesions and conditions of the prostate: from morphological and biological characterization to chemoprevention. *Ann N Y Acad Sci* 963: 169-184.

1777. Montironi R, Thompson D, Bartels PH (1999). Premalignant lesions of the prostate. In: *Recent Advances in Histopathology*, DG Lowe, JCE Underwood, eds. Churchill Livingstone: Edinburgh, pp. 147-172.

1778. Mor Y, Leibovich I, Raviv G, Nass D, Medalia O, Goldwasser B, Nativ O (1995). Testicular seminoma: clinical significance of nuclear deoxyribonucleic acid ploidy pattern as studied by flow cytometry. *J Urol* 154: 1041-1043.

1779. Moran CA, Kaneko M (1990). Malignant fibrous histiocytoma of the glans penis. *Am J Dermatopathol* 12: 182-187.

1780. Moreno JG, Croce CM, Fischer R, Monne M, Vihko P, Mulholland SG, Gomella LG (1992). Detection of hematogenous micrometastasis in patients with prostate cancer. *Cancer Res* 52: 6110-6112.

1781. Morgan DR, Brame KG (1999). Granulosa cell tumour of the testis displaying immunoreactivity for inhibin. *BJU Int* 83: 731-732.

1782. Morgan DR, Dixon MF, Harnden P (1998). Villous adenoma of urethra associated with tubulovillous adenoma and adenocarcinoma of rectum. *Histopathology* 32: 87-89.

1783. Morgan E, Kidd JM (1978). Undifferentiated sarcoma of the kidney: a tumor of childhood with histopathologic and clinical characteristics distinct from Wilms' tumor. *Cancer* 42: 1916-1921.

1784. Morganti G, Gianferrari L, Cresseri A, Arrigoni G, Lovati G (1956). Recherches clinico-statistiques et génétiques sur les néoplasies de la prostate. *Acta Genet Med Gemellol (Roma)* 6: 304-305.

1785. Morin G, Houlgatte A, Camparo P, Sarrazin JL, Berlizot P, Houdelette P (1998). [Solitary fibrous tumor of the seminal vesicles: apropos of a case]. *Prog Urol* 8: 92-94.

1786. Morita R, Ishikawa J, Tsutsumi M, Hikiji K, Tsukada Y, Kamidono S, Maeda S, Nakamura Y (1991). Allelotype of renal cell carcinoma. *Cancer Res* 51: 820-823.

1787. Moriyama M, Akiyama T, Yamamoto T, Kawamoto T, Kato T, Sato K, Watanuki T, Hikage T, Katsuta N, Mori S (1991). Expression of c-erbB-2 gene product in urinary bladder cancer. *J Urol* 145: 423-427.

1788. Morrison KB, Tognon CE, Garnett MJ, Deal C, Sorensen PH (2002). ETV6-NTRK3 transformation requires insulin-like growth factor 1 receptor signaling and is associated with constitutive IRS-1 tyrosine phosphorylation. *Oncogene* 21: 5684-5695.

1789. Morrissey C, Martinez A, Zatyka M, Agathanggelou A, Honorio S, Astuti D, Morgan NV, Moch H, Richards FM, Kishida T, Yao M, Schraml P, Latif F, Maher ER (2001). Epigenetic inactivation of the RASSF1A 3p21.3 tumor suppressor gene in both clear cell and papillary renal cell carcinoma. *Cancer Res* 61: 7277-7281.

1790. Moss AH, Peterson LJ, Scott CW, Winter K, Olin DB, Garber RL (1982). Delayed diagnosis of juxtaglomerular cell tumor hypertension. *N C Med J* 43: 705-707.

1791. Mostafa MH, Helmi S, Badawi AF, Tricker AR, Spiegelhalder B, Preussmann R (1994). Nitrate, nitrite and volatile N-nitroso compounds in the urine of Schistosoma haematobium and Schistosoma mansoni infected patients. *Carcinogenesis* 15: 619-625.

1792. Mostert M, Rosenberg C, Stoop H, Schuyer M, Timmer A, Oosterhuis W, Looijenga LH (2000). Comparative genomic and in situ hybridization of germ cell tumors of the infantile testis. *Lab Invest* 80: 1055-1064.

1793. Mostert MC, Verkerk AJ, van de Pol M, Heighway J, Marynen P, Rosenberg C, van Kessel AG, van Echten J, de Jong B, Oosterhuis JW, Looijenga LH (1998). Identification of the critical region of 12p over-representation in testicular germ cell tumors of adolescents and adults. *Oncogene* 16: 2617-2627.

1794. Mostert MM, van de Pol M, Olde Weghuis D, Suijkerbuijk RF, Geurts van Kessel A, van Echten J, Oosterhuis JW, Looijenga LH (1996). Comparative genomic hybridization of germ cell tumors of the adult testis: confirmation of karyotypic findings and identification of a 12p-amplicon. *Cancer Genet Cytogenet* 89: 146-152.

1795. Mostert MM, van de Pol M, van Echten J, Olde Weghuis D, Geurts van Kessel A, Oosterhuis JW, Looijenga LH (1996). Fluorescence in situ hybridization-based approaches for detection of 12p overrepresentation, in particular i(12p), in cell lines of human testicular germ cell tumors of adults. *Cancer Genet Cytogenet* 87: 95-102.

1796. Mostofi FK (1980). Pathology of germ cell tumors of testis: a progress report. *Cancer* 45: 1735-1754.

1797. Mostofi FK (1985). Histological change ostensibly induced by therapy in the metastasis of germ cell tumors of testis. *Prog Clin Biol Res* 203: 47-60.

1798. Mostofi FK, Davis CJ, Sesterhenn IA (1999). *World Health Organization International Histological Classification of Tumours. Histological Typing of Urinary Bladder Tumours.* 2nd Edition. Springer Verlag: Berlin Heidelberg.

1799. Mostofi FK, Davis CJJr, Sesterhenn IA (1992). Carcinoma of the male and female urethra. *Urol Clin North Am* 19: 347-358.

1800. Mostofi FK, Price EB (1973). *Tumors of the Male Genital System.* 2nd Edition. AFIP: Washington, DC.

1801. Mostofi FK, Sesterhenn I, Sobin LH (1980). *International Histological Classification of Tumours. Histological Typing of Prostate Tumours.* WHO: Geneva.

1802. Mostofi FK, Sesterhenn IA (1984). Pathology of epithelial tumors and carcinoma in situ of bladder. *Prog Clin Biol Res* 162A: 55-74.

1803. Mostofi FK, Sesterhenn IA (1985). Pathology of germ cell tumors of testes. *Prog Clin Biol Res* 203: 1-34.

1804. Mostofi FK, Sesterhenn IA (1986). The diagnosis of choriocarcinoma in the male. In: *Germ Cell Tumours II*, WG Jones, A Milford-Ward, CK Anderson, eds. Pergamon Press: Oxford.

1805. Mostofi FK, Sesterhenn IA (1998). *World Health Organization International Histological Classification of Tumours. Histological Typing of Testis Tumours.* 2nd Edition. Springer-Verlag: Berlin Heidelberg.

1806. Mostofi FK, Sesterhenn IA, Davis CJ, Mesonero C (2002). Testicular teratoma in adults. *Int J Cancer Suppl* 13: 752.

1807. Mostofi FK, Sesterhenn IA, Davis CJJr (1987). Immunopathology of germ cell tumors of the testis. *Semin Diagn Pathol* 4: 320-341.

1808. Mostofi FK, Sesterhenn IA, Davis CJJr (1988). Developments in histopathology of testicular germ cell tumors. *Semin Urol* 6: 171-188.

1809. Mostofi FK, Sobin LH (1977). *World Health Organization International Histological Classification of Tumours. Histological Typing of Testicular Tumours.* WHO: Geneva.

1810. Mostofi FK, Sobin LH, Torloni H (1973). *World Health Organization International Histological Classification of Tumours. Histological Typing of Urinary Bladder Tumours.* 1st Edition. WHO: Geneva.

1811. Mostofi FK, Theiss EA, Ashley DJB (1959). Tumors of specialized gonadal stroma in human male patients. *Cancer* 12: 944-957.

1812. Mostofi FK, Theiss EA, Ashley DJB (1959). Tumors of the specialized gonadal stroma in human male patients: androblastoma, Sertoli cell tumor, granulosa Theca cell tumor of the testis, and gonadal stromal tumor. *Cancer* 12: 944-957.

1813. Mostofi FK, Thomson RV, Dean AL (1955). Mucinous adenocarcinoma of the urinary bladder. *Cancer* 8: 741-758.

1814. Mott LJ (1979). Squamous cell carcinoma of the prostate: report of 2 cases and review of the literature. *J Urol* 121: 833-835.

1815. Motzer RJ, Amsterdam A, Prieto V, Sheinfeld J, Murty VV, Mazumdar M, Bosl GJ, Chaganti RS, Reuter VE (1998). Teratoma with malignant transformation: diverse malignant histologies arising in men with germ cell tumors. *J Urol* 159: 133-138.

1816. Moudouni SM, En-Nia I, Rioux-Leclerq N, Guille F, Lobel B (2001). Leiomyosarcoma of the renal pelvis. *Scand J Urol Nephrol* 35: 425-427.

1817. Moul JW, McCarthy WF, Fernandez EB, Sesterhenn IA (1994). Percentage of embryonal carcinoma and of vascular invasion predicts pathological stage in clinical stage I nonseminomatous testicular cancer. *Cancer Res* 54: 362-364.

1818. Moul JW, Theune SM, Chang EH (1992). Detection of RAS mutations in archival testicular germ cell tumors by polymerase chain reaction and oligonucleotide hybridization. *Genes Chromosomes Cancer* 5: 109-118.

1819. Moulopoulos A, Dubrow R, David C, Dimopoulos MA (1991). Primary renal carcinoid: computed tomography, ultrasound, and angiographic findings. *J Comput Assist Tomogr* 15: 323-325.

1820. Mourad WA, Khalil S, Radwi A, Peracha A, Ezzat A (1998). Primary T-cell lymphoma of the urinary bladder. *Am J Surg Pathol* 22: 373-377.

1821. Mouradian JA, Coleman JW, McGovern JH, Gray GF (1974). Granular cell tumor (myoblastoma) of the bladder. *J Urol* 112: 343-345.

1822. Mucci NR, Akdas G, Manely S, Rubin MA (2000). Neuroendocrine expression in metastatic prostate cancer: evaluation of high throughput tissue microarrays to detect heterogeneous protein expression. *Hum Pathol* 31: 406-414.

1823. Muentener M, Hailemariam S, Dubs M, Hauri D, Sulser T (2000). Primary leiomyosarcoma of the seminal vesicle. *J Urol* 164: 2027.

1824. Muir TE, Cheville JC, Lager DJ (2001). Metanephric adenoma, nephrogenic rests, and Wilms' tumor: a histologic and immunophenotypic comparison. *Am J Surg Pathol* 25: 1290-1296.

1825. Mukai M, Torikata C, Iri H, Tamai S, Sugiura H, Tanaka Y, Sakamoto M, Hirohashi S (1992). Crystalloids in angiomyolipoma. 1. A previously unnoticed phenomenon of renal angiomyolipoma occurring at a high frequency. *Am J Surg Pathol* 16: 1-10.

1826. Mukamel E, Farrer J, Smith RB, Dekernion JB (1987). Metastatic carcinoma to penis: when is total penectomy indicated? *Urology* 29: 15-18.

1827. Mukherjee AB, Murty VV, Rodriguez E, Reuter VE, Bosl GJ, Chaganti RS (1991). Detection and analysis of origin of i(12p), a diagnostic marker of human male germ cell tumors, by fluorescence in situ hybridization. *Genes Chromosomes Cancer* 3: 300-307.

1828. Mukhopadhyay D, Knebelmann B, Cohen HT, Ananth S, Sukhatme VP (1997). The von Hippel-Lindau tumor suppressor gene product interacts with Sp1 to repress vascular endothelial growth factor promoter activity. *Mol Cell Biol* 17: 5629-5639.

1829. Mulder MP, Keijzer W, Verkerk A, Boot AJ, Prins ME, Splinter TA, Bos JL (1989). Activated ras genes in human seminoma: evidence for tumor heterogeneity. *Oncogene* 4: 1345-1351.

1830. Muller J, Skakkebaeck NE (1981). Microspectrophotometric DNA measurements of carcinoma in situ germ cells in testis. *Int J Androl* 4: 211-221.

1831. Muller J, Skakkebaek NE (1984). Testicular carcinoma in situ in children with the androgen insensitivity (testicular feminisation) syndrome. *Br Med J (Clin Res Ed)* 288: 1419-1420.

1832. Muller J, Skakkebaek NE, Parkinson MC (1987). The spermatocytic seminoma: views on pathogenesis. *Int J Androl* 10: 147-156.

1833. Muller J, Skakkebaek NE, Ritzen M, Ploen L, Petersen KE (1985). Carcinoma in situ of the testis in children with 45,X/46,XY gonadal dysgenesis. *J Pediatr* 106: 431-436.

1834. Munoz JJ, Ellison LM (2000). Upper tract urothelial neoplasms: incidence and survival during the last 2 decades. *J Urol* 164: 1523-1525.

1835. Murad T, Komaiko W, Oyasu R, Bauer K (1991). Multilocular cystic renal cell carcinoma. *Am J Clin Pathol* 95: 633-637.

1836. Murai Y (2001). Malignant mesothelioma in Japan: analysis of registered autopsy cases. *Arch Environ Health* 56: 84-88.

1837. Murphy DP, Pantuck AJ, Amenta PS, Das KM, Cummings KB, Keeney GL, Weiss RE (1999). Female urethral adenocarcinoma: immunohistochemical evidence of more than 1 tissue of origin. *J Urol* 161: 1881-1884.

1838. Murphy G, Ragde H, Kenny G, Barren R3rd, Erickson S, Tjoa B, Boynton A, Holmes E, Gilbaugh J, Douglas T (1995). Comparison of prostate specific membrane antigen, and prostate specific antigen levels in prostatic cancer patients. *Anticancer Res* 15: 1473-1479.

1839. Murphy GP, Barren RJ, Erickson SJ, Bowes VA, Wolfert RL, Bartsch G, Klocker H, Pointner J, Reissigl A, McLeod DG, Douglas T, Morgan T, Kenny GM, Ragde H, Boynton AL, Holmes EH (1996). Evaluation and comparison of two new prostate carcinoma markers. Free-prostate specific antigen and prostate specific membrane antigen. *Cancer* 78: 809-818.

1840. Murphy GP, Busch C, Abrahamsson PA, Epstein JI, McNeal JE, Miller GJ, Mostofi FK, Nagle RB, Nordling S, Parkinson C (1994). Histopathology of localized prostate cancer. Consensus Conference on Diagnosis and Prognostic Parameters in Localized Prostate Cancer. Stockholm, Sweden, May 12-13, 1993. *Scand J Urol Nephrol Suppl* 162: 7-42.

1841. Murphy GP, Holmes EH, Boynton AL, Kenny GM, Ostenson RC, Erickson SJ, Barren RJ (1995). Comparison of prostate specific antigen, prostate specific membrane antigen, and LNCaP-based enzyme-linked immunosorbent assays in prostatic cancer patients and patients with benign prostatic enlargement. *Prostate* 26: 164-168.

1842. Murphy GP, Tino WT, Holmes EH, Boynton AL, Erickson SJ, Bowes VA, Barren RJ, Tjoa BA, Misrock SL, Ragde H, Kenny GM (1996). Measurement of prostate-specific membrane antigen in the serum with a new antibody. *Prostate* 28: 266-271.

1843. Murphy WM (1989). *Urologic Pathology*. WB Saunders: Philadelphia.

1844. Murphy WM (1997). Diseases of the urinary bladder, urethra, ureters, and renal pelvis. In: *Urological Pathology*, WM Murphy, ed. 2nd Edition. WB Saunders: Philadelphia, PA, pp. 87-90.

1845. Murphy WM, Beckwith JB, Farrow GM (1994). *Atlas of Tumour Pathology. Tumours of the Kidney, Bladder, and Related Urinary Structures.* 3rd Edition. AFIP: Washington, DC.

1846. Murphy WM, Busch C, Algaba F (2000). Intraepithelial lesions of urinary bladder: morphologic considerations. *Scand J Urol Nephrol Suppl* 205: 67-81.

1847. Murphy WM, Dean PJ, Brasfield JA, Tatum L (1986). Incidental carcinoma of the prostate. How much sampling is adequate? *Am J Surg Pathol* 10: 170-174.

1848. Murphy WM, Deana DG (1992). The nested variant of transitional cell carcinoma: a neoplasm resembling proliferation of Brunn's nests. *Mod Pathol* 5: 240-243.

1849. Murphy WM, Miller AW (1984). *Bladder Cancer.* Williams & Wilkins: Baltimore, MD.

1850. Murphy WM, Nagy GK, Rao MK, Soloway MS, Parija GC, Cox CE, Friedell GH (1979). "Normal" urothelium in patients with bladder cancer: a preliminary report from the National Bladder Cancer Collaborative Group A. *Cancer* 44: 1050-1058.

1851. Murphy WM, Soloway MS (1982). Urothelial dysplasia. *J Urol* 127: 849-854.

1852. Murphy WM, Soloway MS, Barrows GH (1991). Pathologic changes associated with androgen deprivation therapy for prostate cancer. *Cancer* 68: 821-828.

1853. Murty VV, Bosl GJ, Houldsworth J, Meyers M, Mukherjee AB, Reuter V, Chaganti RS (1994). Allelic loss and somatic differentiation in human male germ cell tumors. *Oncogene* 9: 2245-2251.

1854. Murty VV, Dmitrovsky E, Bosl GJ, Chaganti RS (1990). Nonrandom chromosome abnormalities in testicular and ovarian germ cell tumor cell lines. *Cancer Genet Cytogenet* 50: 67-73.

1855. Murty VV, Houldsworth J, Baldwin S, Reuter V, Hunziker W, Besmer P, Bosl G, Chaganti RS (1992). Allelic deletions in the long arm of chromosome 12 identify sites of candidate tumor suppressor genes in male germ cell tumors. *Proc Natl Acad Sci USA* 89: 11006-11010.

1856. Murty VV, Li RG, Houldsworth J, Bronson DL, Reuter VE, Bosl GJ, Chaganti RS (1994). Frequent allelic deletions and loss of expression characterize the DCC gene in male germ cell tumors. *Oncogene* 9: 3227-3231.

1857. Murty VV, Li RG, Mathew S, Reuter VE, Bronson DL, Bosl GJ, Chaganti RS (1994). Replication error-type genetic instability at 1q42-43 in human male germ cell tumors. *Cancer Res* 54: 3983-3985.

1858. Muscheck M, Abol-Enein H, Chew K, Moore D, Bhargava V, Ghoneim MA, Carroll PR, Waldman FM (2000). Comparison of genetic changes in schistosome-related transitional and squamous bladder cancers using comparative genomic hybridization. *Carcinogenesis* 21: 1721-1726.

1859. Mustacchi P, Shimkin MS (1958). Cancer of the bladder and infestation with Schistosoma Haematobium. *J Natl Cancer Inst* 20: 825-842.

1860. Mydlo JH, Bard RH (1987). Analysis of papillary renal adenocarcinoma. *Urology* 30: 529-534.

1861. Nabi G, Ansari MS, Singh I, Sharma MC, Dogra PN (2001). Primary squamous cell carcinoma of the prostate: a rare clinicopathological entity. Report of 2 cases and review of literature. *Urol Int* 66: 216-219.

1862. Nadji M, Morales AR (1983). Immunohistochemical markers for prostatic cancer. *Ann N Y Acad Sci* 420: 134-139.

1863. Nadji M, Tabei SZ, Castro A, Chu TM, Murphy GP, Wang MC, Morales AR (1981). Prostatic-specific antigen: an immunohistologic marker for prostatic neoplasms. *Cancer* 48: 1229-1232.

1864. Nagashima Y, Miyagi Y, Udagawa K, Taki A, Misugi K, Sakai N, Kondo K, Kaneko S, Yao M, Shuin T (1996). Von Hippel-Lindau tumour suppressor gene. Localization of expression by in situ hybridization. *J Pathol* 180: 271-274.

1865. Nagashima Y, Ohaki Y, Tanaka Y, Misugi K, Horiuchi M (1988). A case of renal angiomyolipomas associated with multiple and various hamartomatous microlesions. *Virchows Arch A Pathol Anat Histopathol* 413: 177-182.

1866. Nagy GK, Frable WJ, Murphy WM (1982). Classification of premalignant urothelial abnormalities. A Delphi study of the National Bladder Cancer Collaborative Group A. *Pathol Annu* 17 (Pt 1): 219-233.

1867. Nakai Y, Namba Y, Sugao H (1999). Renal lymphangioma. *J Urol* 162: 484-485.

1868. Nakashima N, Murakami S, Fukatsu T, Nagasaka T, Fukata S, Ohiwa N, Nara Y, Sobue M, Takeuchi J (1988). Characteristics of "embryoid body" in human gonadal germ cell tumors. *Hum Pathol* 19: 1144-1154.

1869. Narducci MG, Fiorenza MT, Kang SM, Bevilacqua A, di Giacomo M, Remotti D, Picchio MC, Fidanza V, Cooper MD, Croce CM, Mangia F, Russo G (2002). TCL1 participates in early embryonic development and is overexpressed in human seminomas. *Proc Natl Acad Sci USA* 99: 11712-11717.

1870. Narla G, Heath KE, Reeves HL, Li D, Giono LE, Kimmelman AC, Glucksman MJ, Narla J, Eng FJ, Chan AM, Ferrari AC, Martignetti JA, Friedman SL (2001). KLF6, a candidate tumor suppressor gene mutated in prostate cancer. *Science* 294: 2563-2566.

1871. Nasca MR, Innocenzi D, Micali G (1999). Penile cancer among patients with genital lichen sclerosus. *J Am Acad Dermatol* 41: 911-914.

1872. Nassiri M, Ghazi C, Stivers JR, Nadji M (1994). Ganglioneuroma of the prostate. A novel finding in neurofibromatosis. *Arch Pathol Lab Med* 118: 938-939.

1873. Nativ O, Winkler HZ, Reiman HRJr, Earle JD, Lieber MM (1997). Primary testicular seminoma: prognostic significance of nuclear DNA ploidy pattern. *Eur Urol* 31: 401-404.

1874. Navon JD, Rahimzadeh M, Wong AK, Carpenter PM, Ahlering TE (1997). Angiosarcoma of the bladder after therapeutic irradiation for prostate cancer. *J Urol* 157: 1359-1360.

1875. Neal DE, Marsh C, Bennett MK, Abel PD, Hall RR, Sainsbury JR, Harris AL (1985). Epidermal-growth-factor receptors in human bladder cancer: comparison of invasive and superficial tumours. *Lancet* 1: 366-368.

1876. Neal DE, Sharples L, Smith K, Fennelly J, Hall RR, Harris AL (1990). The epidermal growth factor receptor and the prognosis of bladder cancer. *Cancer* 65: 1619-1625.

1877. Negri E, La Vecchia C (2001). Epidemiology and prevention of bladder cancer. *Eur J Cancer Prev* 10: 7-14.

1878. Nellist M, van Slegtenhorst MA, Goedbloed M, van den Ouweland AM, Halley DJ, van der Sluijs P (1999). Characterization of the cytosolic tuberin-hamartin complex. Tuberin is a cytosolic chaperone for hamartin. *J Biol Chem* 274: 35647-35652.

1879. Nelson CP, Kidd LC, Sauvageot J, Isaacs WB, de Marzo AM, Groopman JD, Nelson WG, Kensler TW (2001). Protection against 2-hydroxyamino-1-methyl-6-phenylimidazo[4,5-b]pyridine cytotoxicity and DNA adduct formation in human prostate by glutathione S-transferase P1. *Cancer Res* 61: 103-109.

1880. Nelson RS, Epstein JI (1996). Prostatic carcinoma with abundant xanthomatous cytoplasm. Foamy gland carcinoma. *Am J Surg Pathol* 20: 419-426.
1881. Neuhauser TS, Lancaster K, Haws R, Drehner D, Gulley ML, Lichy JH, Taubenberger JK (1997). Rapidly progressive T cell lymphoma presenting as acute renal failure: case report and review of the literature. *Pediatr Pathol Lab Med* 17: 449-460.
1882. Neumann HP, Bender BU (1998). Genotype-phenotype correlations in von Hippel-Lindau disease. *J Intern Med* 243: 541-545.
1883. Neumann HP, Wiestler OD (1994). Von Hippel-Lindau disease: a syndrome providing insights into growth control and tumorigenesis. *Nephrol Dial Transplant* 9: 1832-1833.
1884. Newman DM, Brown JR, Jay AC, Pontius EE (1968). Squamous cell carcinoma of the bladder. *J Urol* 100: 470-473.
1885. Newman JS, Bree RL, Rubin JM (1995). Prostate cancer: diagnosis with color Doppler sonography with histologic correlation of each biopsy site. *Radiology* 195: 86-90.
1886. Newman PL, Fletcher CD (1991). Smooth muscle tumours of the external genitalia: clinicopathological analysis of a series. *Histopathology* 18: 523-529.
1887. Newton WAJr, Soule EH, Hamoudi AB, Reiman HM, Shimada H, Beltangady M, Maurer H (1988). Histopathology of childhood sarcomas, Intergroup Rhabdomyosarcoma Studies I and II: clinicopathologic correlation. *J Clin Oncol* 6: 67-75.
1888. Ng WK, Cheung MF, Ip P, Chan KW (1999). Test and teach. Number ninety-two: Part 1. Papillary renal cell carcinoma, solid variant. *Pathology* 31: 213-214.
1889. Ng WT, Wong MK, Chan YT (1992). Re: Cavernous haemangioma of the glans penis. *Br J Urol* 70: 340.
1890. Nguyen PL, Swanson PE, Jaszcz W, Aeppli DM, Zhang G, Singleton TP, Ward S, Dykoski D, Harvey J, Niehans GA (1994). Expression of epidermal growth factor receptor in invasive transitional cell carcinoma of the urinary bladder. A multivariate survival analysis. *Am J Clin Pathol* 101: 166-176.
1891. Nickerson M, Warren M, Toro J, Matrosova V, Glenn G, Turner M, Duray P, Merino M, Choyke P, Pavlovich C, Sharma N, Walther M, Munroe D, Hill R, Maher E, Greenberg C, Lerman M, Linehan W, Zbar B, Schmidt L (2002). Mutations in a novel gene lead to kidney tumors, lung wall defects, and benign tumors of the hair follicle in patients with the Birt-Hogg-Dube syndrome. *Cancer Cell* 2: 157-164.
1892. Nicol D, Hii SI, Walsh M, Teh B, Thompson L, Kennett C, Gotley D (1997). Vascular endothelial growth factor expression is increased in renal cell carcinoma. *J Urol* 157: 1482-1486.
1893. Nicolaisen GS, Williams RD (1984). Primary transitional cell carcinoma of prostate. *Urology* 24: 544-549.
1894. Niehans GA, Manivel JC, Copland GT, Scheithauer BW, Wick MR (1988). Immunohistochemistry of germ cell and trophoblastic neoplasms. *Cancer* 62: 1113-1123.
1895. Nielsen H, Nielsen M, Skakkebaek NE (1974). The fine structure of possible carcinoma-in-situ in the seminiferous tubules in the testis of four infertile men. *Acta Pathol Microbiol Scand [A]* 82: 235-248.
1896. Nieto N, Torres-Valdivieso MJ, Aguado P, Mateos ME, Lopez-Perez J, Melero C, Vivanco JL, Gomez A (2002). Juvenile granulosa cell tumor of the testis: case report and review of literature. *Tumori* 88: 72-74.
1897. Nikzas D, Champion AE, Fox M (1990). Germ cell tumours of testis: prognostic factors and results. *Eur Urol* 18: 242-247.
1898. Nishiyama H, Gill JH, Pitt E, Kennedy W, Knowles MA (2001). Negative regulation of G(1)/S transition by the candidate bladder tumour suppressor gene DBCCR1. *Oncogene* 20: 2956-2964.
1899. Nishiyama T, Ikarashi T, Terunuma M, Ishizaki S (2001). Osteogenic sarcoma of the prostate. *Int J Urol* 8: 199-201.
1900. Nistal M, Codesal J, Paniagua R (1989). Carcinoma in situ of the testis in infertile men. A histological, immunocytochemical, and cytophotometric study of DNA content. *J Pathol* 159: 205-210.
1901. Nistal M, Lazaro R, Garcia J, Paniagua R (1992). Testicular granulosa cell tumor of the adult type. *Arch Pathol Lab Med* 116: 284-287.
1902. Nistal M, Martinez-Garcia C, Paniagua R (1992). Testicular fibroma. *J Urol* 147: 1617-1619.
1903. Nistal M, Paniagua R (1985). Primary neuroectodermal tumour of the testis. *Histopathology* 9: 1351-1359.
1904. Nistal M, Puras A, Perna C, Guarch R, Paniagua R (1996). Fusocellular gonadal stromal tumour of the testis with epithelial and myoid differentiation. *Histopathology* 29: 259-264.
1905. Nistal M, Redondo E, Paniagua R (1988). Juvenile granulosa cell tumor of the testis. *Arch Pathol Lab Med* 112: 1129-1132.
1906. Nistal M, Revestido R, Paniagua R (1992). Bilateral mucinous cystadenocarcinoma of the testis and epididymis. *Arch Pathol Lab Med* 116: 1360-1363.
1907. Nixon RG, Chang SS, Lafleur BJ, Smith JA, Cookson MS (2002). Carcinoma in situ and tumor multifocality predict the risk of prostatic urethral involvement at radical cystectomy in men with transitional cell carcinoma of the bladder. *J Urol* 167: 502-505.
1908. Nochomovitz LE, Orenstein JO (1994). Adenocarcinoma of the rete testis. Consolidation and analysis of 31 reported cases, with review of miscellaneous entities. *J Urol Pathol* 2: 1-37.
1909. Nocks BN, Dann JA (1983). Primitive neuroectodermal tumor (immature teratoma) of testis. *Urology* 22: 543-544.
1910. Nocks BN, Heney NM, Daly JJ, Perrone TA, Griffin PP, Prout GRJr (1982). Transitional cell carcinoma of renal pelvis. *Urology* 19: 472-477.
1911. Nogales FFJr, Matilla A, Ortega I, Alvarez T (1979). Mixed Brenner and adenomatoid tumor of the testis: an ultrastructural study and histogenetic considerations. *Cancer* 43: 539-543.
1912. Noguchi M, Hirabayashi Y, Kato S, Noda S (2002). Solitary fibrous tumor arising from the prostatic capsule. *J Urol* 168: 1490-1491.
1913. Noguchi M, Yahara J, Koga H, Nakashima O, Noda S (1999). Necessity of repeat biopsies in men for suspected prostate cancer. *Int J Urol* 6: 7-12.
1914. Nonomura N, Miki T, Nishimura K, Kanno N, Kojima Y, Okuyama A (1997). Altered imprinting of the H19 and insulin-like growth factor II genes in testicular tumors. *J Urol* 157: 1977-1979.
1915. Noordzij MA, van der Kwast TH, van Steenbrugge GJ, Hop WJ, Schroder FH (1995). The prognostic influence of neuroendocrine cells in prostate cancer: results of a long-term follow-up study with patients treated by radical prostatectomy. *Int J Cancer* 62: 252-258.
1916. Norden DA, Gelfand M (1972). Bilharzia and bladder cancer. An investigation of urinary -glucuronidase associated with S. haematobium infection. *Trans R Soc Trop Med Hyg* 66: 864-866.
1917. Norgaard-Pedersen B, Schultz HP, Arends J, Brincker H, Krag Jacobsen G, Lindelov B, Rorth M, Svennekjaer IL (1984). Tumour markers in testicular germ cell tumours. Five-year experience from the DATECA Study 1976-1980. *Acta Radiol Oncol* 23: 287-294.
1918. Norming U, Tribukait B, Gustafson H, Nyman CR, Wang NN, Wijkstrom H (1992). Deoxyribonucleic acid profile and tumor progression in primary carcinoma in situ of the bladder: a study of 63 patients with grade 3 lesions. *J Urol* 147: 11-15.
1919. Norton KI, Godine LB, Lempert C (1997). Leiomyosarcoma of the kidney in an HIV-infected child. *Pediatr Radiol* 27: 557-558.
1920. Nouri AM, Darakhshan F, Cannell H, Paris AM, Oliver RT (1996). The relevance of p53 mutation in urological malignancies: possible clinical implications for bladder cancer. *Br J Urol* 78: 337-344.
1921. Nouri AM, Thompson C, Cannell H, Symes M, Purkiss S, Amirghofran Z (2000). Profile of epidermal growth factor receptor (EGFr) expression in human malignancies: effects of exposure to EGF and its biological influence on established human tumour cell lines. *Int J Mol Med* 6: 495-500.
1922. Novella G, Porcaro AB, Righetti R, Cavalleri S, Beltrami P, Ficarra V, Brunelli M, Martignoni G, Malossini G, Tallarigo C (2001). Primary lymphoma of the epididymis: case report and review of the literature. *Urol Int* 67: 97-99.
1923. Novis DA, Zarbo RJ, Valenstein PA (1999). Diagnostic uncertainty expressed in prostate needle biopsies. A College of American Pathologists Q-probes Study of 15,753 prostate needle biopsies in 332 institutions. *Arch Pathol Lab Med* 123: 687-692.
1924. Nupponen NN, Kakkola L, Koivisto P, Visakorpi T (1998). Genetic alterations in hormone-refractory recurrent prostate carcinomas. *Am J Pathol* 153: 141-148.
1925. O'Brien A, Sinnott B, McLean P, Doyle GD (1992). Leiomyoma of the renal pelvis. *Br J Urol* 70: 331-332.
1926. O'dowd GJ, Miller MC, Orozco R, Veltri RW (2000). Analysis of repeated biopsy results within 1 year after a noncancer diagnosis. *Urology* 55: 553-559.
1927. O'Hara SM, Veltri RW, Skirpstunas P, Hedican SP, Partin AW, Nelson JB, Subong EN, Walsh PC (1996). Basal PSA mRNA levels detected by quantitative reverse transcriptase polymerase chain reaction (Q-RT-PCR-PSA) in blood from subjects without prostate cancer. *J Urol* 155: 418A.
1928. O'Kane HO, Megaw JM (1968). Carcinoma in the exstrophic bladder. *Br J Surg* 55: 631-635.
1929. O'Shaughnessy JA, Kelloff GJ, Gordon GB, Dannenberg AJ, Hong WK, Fabian CJ, Sigman CC, Bertagnolli MM, Stratton SP, Lam S, Nelson WG, Meyskens FL, Alberts DS, Follen M, Rustgi AK, Papadimitrakopoulou V, Scardino PT, Gazdar AF, Wattenberg LW, Sporn MB, Sakr WA, Lippman SM, Von Hoff DD (2002). Treatment and prevention of intraepithelial neoplasia: an important target for accelerated new agent development. *Clin Cancer Res* 8: 314-346.
1930. Obermann EC, Junker K, Stoehr R, Dietmaier W, Zaak D, Schubert GE, Hofstaedter F, Knuechel R, Hartmann A (2003). Frequent genetic alterations in flat urothelial hyperplasias and concomitant papillary bladder cancer as detected by CGH, LOH, and FISH analyses. *J Pathol* 199: 50-57.
1931. Oberstrass J, Reifenberger G, Reifenberger J, Wechsler W, Collins VP (1996). Mutation of the Von Hippel-Lindau tumour suppressor gene in capillary haemangioblastomas of the central nervous system. *J Pathol* 179: 151-156.
1932. Oda H, Nakatsuru Y, Ishikawa T (1995). Mutations of the p53 gene and p53 protein overexpression are associated with sarcomatoid transformation in renal cell carcinomas. *Cancer Res* 55: 658-662.
1933. Oertel J, Duarte S, Ayala J, Vaux A, Velazquez EF, Cubilla AL (2002). Squamous cell carcinoma exclusive of the foreskin: distinctive association with low grade variants, multicentricity and lichen sclerosus. *Mod Pathol* 15: 175A.
1934. Oesterling JE, Brendler CB, Burgers JK, Marshall FF, Epstein JI (1990). Advanced small cell carcinoma of the bladder. Successful treatment with combined radical cystoprostatectomy and adjuvant methotrexate, vinblastine, doxorubicin, and cisplatin chemotherapy. *Cancer* 65: 1928-1936.
1935. Oesterling JE, Epstein JI, Brendler CB (1990). Myxoid malignant fibrous histiocytoma of the bladder. *Cancer* 66: 1836-1842.
1936. Oesterling JE, Fishman EK, Goldman SM, Marshall FF (1986). The management of renal angiomyolipoma. *J Urol* 135: 1121-1124.
1937. Oesterling JE, Jacobsen SJ, Chute CG, Guess HA, Girman CJ, Panser LA, Lieber MM (1993). Serum prostate-specific antigen in a community-based population of healthy men. Establishment of age-specific reference ranges. *JAMA* 270: 860-864.
1938. Ogawa A, Sugihara S, Nakazawa Y, Kumasaka F, Sato J, Nakanishi Y, Nakazato Y, Honma M (1988). [A case of primary carcinoid tumor of the testis]. *Gan No Rinsho* 34: 1629-1634.
1939. Ogawa O, Habuchi T, Kakehi Y, Koshiba M, Sugiyama T, Yoshida O (1992). Allelic losses at chromosome 17p in human renal cell carcinoma are inversely related to allelic losses at chromosome 3p. *Cancer Res* 52: 1881-1885.
1940. Oguchi K, Takeuchi T, Kuriyama M, Tanaka T (1988). Primary carcinoma of the seminal vesicle (cross-imaging diagnosis). *Br J Urol* 62: 383-384.
1941. Oh YL, Kim KR (2000). Micropapillary variant of transitional cell carcinoma of the ureter. *Pathol Int* 50: 52-56.
1942. Ohh M, Kaelin WGJr (1999). The von Hippel-Lindau tumour suppressor protein: new perspectives. *Mol Med Today* 5: 257-263.
1943. Ohh M, Yauch RL, Lonergan KM, Whaley JM, Stemmer-Rachamimov AO, Louis DN, Gavin BJ, Kley N, Kaelin WGJr, Iliopoulos O (1998). The von Hippel-Lindau tumor suppressor protein is required for proper assembly of an extracellular fibronectin matrix. *Mol Cell* 1: 959-968.
1944. Ohori M, Scardino PT, Lapin SL, Seale-Hawkins C, Link J, Wheeler TM (1993). The mechanisms and prognostic significance of seminal vesicle involvement by prostate cancer. *Am J Surg Pathol* 17: 1252-1261.

1945. Ohori M, Wheeler TM, Kattan MW, Goto Y, Scardino PT (1995). Prognostic significance of positive surgical margins in radical prostatectomy specimens. *J Urol* 154: 1818-1824.
1946. Ohsawa M, Aozasa K, Horiuchi K, Kanamaru A (1993). Malignant lymphoma of bladder. Report of three cases and review of the literature. *Cancer* 72: 1969-1974.
1947. Ohsawa M, Mishima K, Suzuki A, Hagino K, Doi J, Aozasa K (1994). Malignant lymphoma of the urethra: report of a case with detection of Epstein-Barr virus genome in the tumour cells. *Histopathology* 24: 525-529.
1948. Okegawa T, Nutahara K, Higashihara E (2000). Detection of micrometastatic prostate cancer cells in the lymph nodes by reverse transcriptase polymerase chain reaction is predictive of biochemical recurrence in pathological stage T2 prostate cancer. *J Urol* 163: 1183-1188.
1949. Okuda N, Okawa T, Nakamura T, Ishida O, Uchida H (1969). [Granular cell myoblastoma of the urinary bladder: report of a case]. *Hinyokika Kiyo* 15: 505-513.
1950. Oldbring J, Mikulowski P (1987). Malignant melanoma of the penis and male urethra. Report of nine cases and review of the literature. *Cancer* 59: 581-587.
1951. Oliai BR, Kahane H, Epstein JI (2001). A clinicopathologic analysis of urothelial carcinomas diagnosed on prostate needle biopsy. *Am J Surg Pathol* 25: 794-801.
1952. Oliai BR, Kahane H, Epstein JI (2002). Can basal cells be seen in adenocarcinoma of the prostate?: an immunohistochemical study using high molecular weight cytokeratin (clone 34betaE12) antibody. *Am J Surg Pathol* 26: 1151-1160.
1953. Olie RA, Looijenga LH, Boerrigter L, Top B, Rodenhuis S, Langeveld A, Mulder MP, Oosterhuis JW (1995). N- and KRAS mutations in primary testicular germ cell tumors: incidence and possible biological implications. *Genes Chromosomes Cancer* 12: 110-116.
1954. Oliva E, Amin MB, Jimenez R, Young RH (2002). Clear cell carcinoma of the urinary bladder: a report and comparison of four tumors of mullerian origin and nine of probable urothelial origin with discussion of histogenesis and diagnostic problems. *Am J Surg Pathol* 26: 190-197.
1955. Oliva E, Young RH (1996). Clear cell adenocarcinoma of the urethra: a clinicopathologic analysis of 19 cases. *Mod Pathol* 9: 513-520.
1956. Oliver SE, May MT, Gunnell D (2001). International trends in prostate-cancer mortality in the "PSA ERA". *Int J Cancer* 92: 893-898.
1957. Olivier M, Eeles R, Hollstein M, Khan MA, Harris CC, Hainaut P (2002). The IARC TP53 database: new online mutation analysis and recommendations to users. *Hum Mutat* 19: 607-614.
1958. Olschwang S, Richard S, Boisson C, Giraud S, Laurent-Puig P, Resche F, Thomas G (1998). Germline mutation profile of the VHL gene in von Hippel-Lindau disease and in sporadic hemangioblastoma. *Hum Mutat* 12: 424-430.
1959. Olsen TG, Helwig EB (1985). Angiolymphoid hyperplasia with eosinophilia. A clinicopathologic study of 116 patients. *J Am Acad Dermatol* 12: 781-796.
1960. Omeroglu A, Paner GP, Wojcik EM, Siziopikou K (2002). A carcinosarcoma/sarcomatoid carcinoma arising in a urinary bladder diverticulum. *Arch Pathol Lab Med* 126: 853-855.
1961. Ono Y, Ozawa M, Tamura Y, Suzuki T, Suzuki K, Kurokawa K, Fukabori Y, Yamanaka H (2002). Tumor-associated tissue eosinophilia of penile cancer. *Int J Urol* 9: 82-87.
1962. Oosterhuis JW, Castedo SM, de Jong B, Cornelisse CJ, Dam A, Sleijfer DT, Schraffordt Koops H (1989). Ploidy of primary germ cell tumors of the testis. Pathogenetic and clinical relevance. *Lab Invest* 60: 14-21.
1963. Oosterhuis JW, de Jong B, Cornelisse CJ, Molenaar IM, Meiring A, Idenburg V, Koops HS, Sleijfer DT (1986). Karyotyping and DNA flow cytometry of mature residual teratoma after intensive chemotherapy of disseminated nonseminomatous germ cell tumor of the testis: a report of two cases. *Cancer Genet Cytogenet* 22: 149-157.
1964. Oosterhuis JW, Looijenga LH (1993). The biology of human germ cell tumours: retrospective speculations and new prospectives. *Eur Urol* 23: 245-250.
1965. Oosterhuis JW, Looijenga LH, van Echten J, de Jong B (1997). Chromosomal constitution and developmental potential of human germ cell tumors and teratomas. *Cancer Genet Cytogenet* 95: 96-102.
1966. Oosterhuis JW, Suurmeyer AJ, Sleyfer DT, Koops HS, Oldhoff J, Fleuren G (1983). Effects of multiple-drug chemotherapy (cis-diammine-dichloroplatinum, bleomycin, and vinblastine) on the maturation of retroperitoneal lymph node metastases of nonseminomatous germ cell tumors of the testis. No evidence for De Novo induction of differentiation. *Cancer* 51: 408-416.
1967. Oppenheim AR (1981). Sebaceous carcinoma of the penis. *Arch Dermatol* 117: 306-307.
1968. Oppenheim PI, Cohen S, Anders KH (1991). Testicular plasmacytoma. A case report with immunohistochemical studies and literature review. *Arch Pathol Lab Med* 115: 629-632.
1969. Ordonez NG (2000). Value of thyroid transcription factor-1 immunostaining in distinguishing small cell lung carcinomas from other small cell carcinomas. *Am J Surg Pathol* 24: 1217-1223.
1970. Ordonez NG, Ayala AG, Sneige N, Mackay B (1982). Immunohistochemical demonstration of multiple neurohormonal polypeptides in a case of pure testicular carcinoid. *Am J Clin Pathol* 78: 860-864.
1971. Ordonez NG, el-Naggar AK, Ro JY, Silva EG, Mackay B (1993). Intra-abdominal desmoplastic small cell tumor: a light microscopic, immunocytochemical, ultrastructural, and flow cytometric study. *Hum Pathol* 24: 850-865.
1972. Ordonez NG, Ro JY, Ayala AG (1992). Metastatic prostatic carcinoma presenting as an oncocytic tumor. *Am J Surg Pathol* 16: 1007-1012.
1973. Ordonez NG, Ro JY, Ayala AG (1998). Lesions described as nodular mesothelial hyperplasia are primarily composed of histiocytes. *Am J Surg Pathol* 22: 285-292.
1974. Orlando C, Sestini R, Vona G, Pinzani P, Bianchi S, Giacca M, Pazzagli M, Selli C (1996). Detection of c-erbB-2 amplification in transitional cell bladder carcinoma using competitive PCR technique. *J Urol* 156: 2089-2093.
1975. Orlow I, Lacombe L, Hannon GJ, Serrano M, Pellicer I, Dalbagni G, Reuter VE, Zhang ZF, Beach D, Cordon-Cardo C (1995). Deletion of the p16 and p15 genes in human bladder tumors. *J Natl Cancer Inst* 87: 1524-1529.
1976. Orlowski JP, Levin HS, Dyment PG (1980). Intrascrotal Wilms' tumor developing in a heterotopic renal anlage of probable mesonephric origin. *J Pediatr Surg* 15: 679-682.
1977. Ormsby AH, Haskell R, Ruthven SE, Mylne GE (1996). Bilateral primary seminal vesicle carcinoma. *Pathology* 28: 196-200.
1978. Ormsby AH, Liou LS, Oriba HA, Angermeier KW, Goldblum JR (2000). Epithelioid sarcoma of the penis: report of an unusual case and review of the literature. *Ann Diagn Pathol* 4: 88-94.
1979. Ornstein DK, Lubensky IA, Venzon D, Zbar B, Linehan WM, Walther MM (2000). Prevalence of microscopic tumors in normal appearing renal parenchyma of patients with hereditary papillary renal cancer. *J Urol* 163: 431-433.
1980. Orntoft TF, Wolf H (1998). Molecular alterations in bladder cancer. *Urol Res* 26: 223-233.
1981. Orozco RE, Martin AA, Murphy WM (1994). Carcinoma in situ of the urinary bladder. Clues to host involvement in human carcinogenesis. *Cancer* 74: 115-122.
1982. Orozco RE, vander Zwaag R, Murphy WM (1993). The pagetoid variant of urothelial carcinoma in situ. *Hum Pathol* 24: 1199-1202.
1983. Osborne GE, Chinn RJ, Francis ND, Bunker CB (2000). Magnetic Resonance Imaging in the investigation of penile lymphangioma circumscriptum. *Br J Dermatol* 143: 467-468.
1984. Osman I, Scher H, Zhang ZF, Soos TJ, Hamza R, Eissa S, Khaled H, Koff A, Cordon-Cardo C (1997). Expression of cyclin D1, but not cyclins E and A, is related to progression in bilharzial bladder cancer. *Clin Cancer Res* 3: 2247-2251.
1985. Osterlind A, Berthelsen JG, Abildgaard N, Hansen SO, Hjalgrim H, Johansen B, Munck-Hansen J, Rasmussen LH (1991). Risk of bilateral testicular germ cell cancer in Denmark: 1960-1984. *J Natl Cancer Inst* 83: 1391-1395.
1986. Otani M, Tsujimoto S, Miura M, Nagashima Y (2001). Intrarenal mature cystic teratoma associated with renal dysplasia: case report and literature review. *Pathol Int* 51: 560-564.
1987. Oto A, Meyer J (1999). MR appearance of penile epithelioid sarcoma. *AJR Am J Roentgenol* 172: 555-556.
1988. Ottesen AM, Kirchhoff M, de Meyts ER, Maahr J, Gerdes T, Rose H, Lundsteen C, Petersen PM, Philip J, Skakkebaek NE (1997). Detection of chromosomal aberrations in seminomatous germ cell tumours using comparative genomic hybridization. *Genes Chromosomes Cancer* 20: 412-418.
1989. Otto T, Rembrink K, Goepel M, Meyer-Schwickerath M, Rubben H (1993). E-cadherin: a marker for differentiation and invasiveness in prostatic carcinoma. *Urol Res* 21: 359-362.
1990. Oxley JD, Abbott CD, Gillatt DA, MacIver AG (1998). Ductal carcinomas of the prostate: a clinicopathological and immunohistochemical study. *Br J Urol* 81: 109-115.
1991. Oya M, Schmidt B, Schmitz-Drager BJ, Schulz WA (1998). Expression of G1—>S transition regulatory molecules in human urothelial cancer. *Jpn J Cancer Res* 89: 719-726.
1992. Oyama H, Fukui I, Maeda Y, Yoshimura K, Maeda H, Izutani T, Yamauchi T, Kawai T, Ishikawa Y, Yamamoto N (1998). [Renal hemangiopericytoma: report of a case]. *Nippon Hinyokika Gakkai Zasshi* 89: 50-53.
1993. Oyasu R, Bahnson RR, Nowels K, Garnett JE (1986). Cytological atypia in the prostate gland: frequency, distribution and possible relevance to carcinoma. *J Urol* 135: 959-962.
1994. Ozdemir BH, Ozdemir OG, Sertcelik A (2001). The prognostic importance of the nucleolar organizer region (AgNOR), Ki-67 and proliferating cell nuclear antigen (PCNA) in primary nonurachal bladder adenocarcinoma. *APMIS* 109: 428-434.
1995. Ozsahin M, Zouhair A, Villa S, Storme G, Chauvet B, Taussky D, Gouders D, Ries G, Bontemps P, Coucke PA, Mirimanoff RO (1999). Prognostic factors in urothelial renal pelvis and ureter tumours: a multicentre Rare Cancer Network study. *Eur J Cancer* 35: 738-743.
1996. Pacelli A, Bostwick DG (1997). Clinical significance of high-grade prostatic intraepithelial neoplasia in transurethral resection specimens. *Urology* 50: 355-359.
1997. Paik ML, Scolieri MJ, Brown SL, Spirnak JP, Resnick MI (2000). Limitations of computerized tomography in staging invasive bladder cancer before radical cystectomy. *J Urol* 163: 1693-1696.
1998. Pak K, Sakaguchi N, Takayama H, Tomoyoshi T (1986). Rhabdomyosarcoma of the penis. *J Urol* 136: 438-439.
1999. Pakzad K, MacLennan GT, Elder JS, Flom LS, Trujillo YP, Sutherland SE, Meyerson HJ (2002). Follicular large cell lymphoma localized to the testis in children. *J Urol* 168: 225-228.
2000. Pal N, Wadey RB, Buckle B, Yeomans E, Pritchard J, Cowell JK (1990). Preferential loss of maternal alleles in sporadic Wilms' tumour. *Oncogene* 5: 1665-1668.
2001. Paladugu RR, Bearman RM, Rappaport H (1980). Malignant lymphoma with primary manifestation in the gonad: a clinicopathologic study of 38 patients. *Cancer* 45: 561-571.
2002. Pallesen G, Hamilton-Dutoit SJ (1988). Ki-1 (CD30) antigen is regularly expressed by tumor cells of embryonal carcinoma. *Am J Pathol* 133: 446-450.
2003. Palumbo C, van Roozendaal K, Gillis AJ, van Gurp RH, de Munnik H, Oosterhuis JW, van Zoelen EJ, Looijenga LH (2002). Expression of the PDGF alpha-receptor 1.5 kb transcript, OCT-4, and c-KIT in human normal and malignant tissues. Implications for the early diagnosis of testicular germ cell tumours and for our understanding of regulatory mechanisms. *J Pathol* 196: 467-477.
2004. Pan CC, Chiang H, Chang YH, Epstein JI (2000). Tubulocystic clear cell adenocarcinoma arising within the prostate. *Am J Surg Pathol* 24: 1433-1436.
2005. Pan CC, Potter SR, Partin AW, Epstein JI (2000). The prognostic significance of tertiary Gleason patterns of higher grade in radical prostatectomy specimens: a proposal to modify the Gleason grading system. *Am J Surg Pathol* 24: 563-569.
2006. Panageas E, Kuligowska E, Dunlop R, Babayan R (1990). Angiosarcoma of the seminal vesicle: early detection using transrectal ultrasound-guided biopsy. *J Clin Ultrasound* 18: 666-670.
2007. Paradis V, Dargere D, Laurendeau I, Benoit G, Vidaud M, Jardin A, Bedossa P (1999). Expression of the RNA component of human telomerase (hTR) in prostate cancer, prostatic intraepithelial neoplasia, and normal prostate tissue. *J Pathol* 189: 213-218.

2008. Paradis V, Laurendeau I, Vieillefond A, Blanchet P, Eschwege P, Benoit G, Vidaud M, Jardin A, Bedossa P (1998). Clonal analysis of renal sporadic angiomyolipomas. *Hum Pathol* 29: 1063-1067.
2009. Parham DM, Roloson GJ, Feely M, Green DM, Bridge JA, Beckwith JB (2001). Primary malignant neuroepithelial tumors of the kidney: a clinicopathologic analysis of 146 adult and pediatric cases from the National Wilms' Tumor Study Group Pathology Center. *Am J Surg Pathol* 25: 133-146.
2010. Park S, Shinohara K, Grossfeld GD, Carroll PR (2001). Prostate cancer detection in men with prior high grade prostatic intraepithelial neoplasia or atypical prostate biopsy. *J Urol* 165: 1409-1414.
2011. Park SH, Kim TJ, Chi JG (1991). Congenital granular cell tumor with systemic involvement. Immunohistochemical and ultrastructural study. *Arch Pathol Lab Med* 115: 934-938.
2012. Parkin DM (2001). Global cancer statistics in the year 2000. *Lancet Oncol* 2: 533-543.
2013. Parkin DM, Ferlay J, Hamdi-Cherif M, Sitas F, Thomas JO, Wabinga H, Whelan SL (2003). *Cancer in Africa: Epidemiology and Prevention. IARC Scientific Publication No 153.* IARC Press: Lyon.
2014. Parkin DM, Pisani P, Ferlay J (1999). Estimates of the worldwide incidence of 25 major cancers in 1990. *Int J Cancer* 80: 827-841.
2015. Parkin DM, Pisani P, Lopez AD, Masuyer E (1994). At least one in seven cases of cancer is caused by smoking. Global estimates for 1985. *Int J Cancer* 59: 494-504.
2016. Parkin DM, Whelan SL, Ferlay J, Teppo L, Thomas DB (2003). *Cancer Incidence in Five Continents. IARC Scientific Publications No155.* IARC Press: Lyon.
2017. Parkinson C, Harland SJ (1999). Testis cancer. In: *The Scientific Basis of Urology*, AR Mundy, JM Fitzpatrick, DE Neal, NJR George, eds. ISIS Medical Media: Oxford.
2018. Parkinson MC, Swerdlow AJ, Pike MC (1994). Carcinoma in situ in boys with cryptorchidism: when can it be detected? *Br J Urol* 73: 431-435.
2019. Parmar MK, Freedman LS, Hargreave TB, Tolley DA (1989). Prognostic factors for recurrence and followup policies in the treatment of superficial bladder cancer: report from the British Medical Research Council Subgroup on Superficial Bladder Cancer (Urological Cancer Working Party). *J Urol* 142: 284-288.
2020. Parshad S, Yadav SP, Arora B (2001). Urethral hemangioma. An unusual cause of hematuria. *Urol Int* 66: 43-45.
2021. Partanen S, Asikainen U (1985). Oat cell carcinoma of the urinary bladder with ectopic adrenocorticotropic hormone production. *Hum Pathol* 16: 313-315.
2022. Partin AW, Criley SR, Subong EN, Zincke H, Walsh PC, Oesterling JE (1996). Standard versus age-specific prostate specific antigen reference ranges among men with clinically localized prostate cancer: A pathological analysis. *J Urol* 155: 1336-1339.
2023. Partin AW, Mangold LA, Lamm DM, Walsh PC, Epstein JI, Pearson JD (2001). Contemporary update of prostate cancer staging nomograms (Partin Tables) for the new millennium. *Urology* 58: 843-848.
2024. Parwani AV, Husain AN, Epstein JI, Beckwith JB, Argani P (2001). Low-grade myxoid renal epithelial neoplasms with distal nephron differentiation. *Hum Pathol* 32: 506-512.
2025. Pashos CL, Botteman MF, Laskin BL, Redaelli A (2002). Bladder cancer: epidemiology, diagnosis, and management. *Cancer Pract* 10: 311-322.
2026. Patsalis PC, Sismani C, Hadjimarcou MI, Kitsiou-Tzeli S, Tzezou A, Hadjiathanasiou CG, Velissariou V, Lymberatou E, Moschonas NK, Skordis N (1998). Detection and incidence of cryptic Y chromosome sequences in Turner syndrome patients. *Clin Genet* 53: 249-257.
2027. Pause A, Lee S, Lonergan KM, Klausner RD (1998). The von Hippel-Lindau tumor suppressor gene is required for cell cycle exit upon serum withdrawal. *Proc Natl Acad Sci USA* 95: 993-998.
2028. Pause A, Lee S, Worrell RA, Chen DY, Burgess WH, Linehan WM, Klausner RD (1997). The von Hippel-Lindau tumor-suppressor gene product forms a stable complex with human CUL-2, a member of the Cdc53 family of proteins. *Proc Natl Acad Sci USA* 94: 2156-2161.
2029. Pauwels RP, Smeets AW, Schapers RF, Geraedts JP, Debruyne FM (1988). Grading in superficial bladder cancer. (2). Cytogenetic classification. *Br J Urol* 61: 135-139.
2030. Pauwels RP, Smeets WW, Geraedts JP, Debruyne FM (1987). Cytogenetic analysis in urothelial cell carcinoma. *J Urol* 137: 210-215.
2031. Pavlovich CP, Glenn GM, Hewitt S (2001). Renal tumours in the Birt-Hogg-Dube syndrome: Disease spectrum and clinical management. *Am Urol Assoc Program Abstracts* 165: 159.
2032. Pavlovich CP, Schmidt LS, Phillips JL (2003). The genetic basis of renal cell carcinoma. *Urol Clin North Am* 30: 437-454.
2033. Pavlovich CP, Walther MM, Eyler RA, Hewitt SM, Zbar B, Linehan WM, Merino MJ (2002). Renal tumors in the Birt-Hogg-Dube' syndrome. *Am J Surg Pathol* 26: 1542-1552.
2034. Pawade J, Banerjee SS, Harris M, Isaacson P, Wright D (1993). Lymphomas of mucosa-associated lymphoid tissue arising in the urinary bladder. *Histopathology* 23: 147-151.
2035. Pawade J, Soosay GN, Delprado W, Parkinson MC, Rode J (1993). Cystic hamartoma of the renal pelvis. *Am J Surg Pathol* 17: 1169-1175.
2036. Pea M, Bonetti F, Martignoni G, Henske EP, Manfrin E, Colato C, Bernstein J (1998). Apparent renal cell carcinomas in tuberous sclerosis are heterogeneous: the identification of malignant epithelioid angiomyolipoma. *Am J Surg Pathol* 22: 180-187.
2037. Pea M, Bonetti F, Zamboni G, Martignoni G, Riva M, Colombari R, Mombello A, Bonzanini M, Scarpa A, Ghimenton C, Donati LF (1991). Melanocyte-marker-HMB-45 is regularly expressed in angiomyolipoma of the kidney. *Pathology* 23: 185-188.
2038. Pearson JM, Banerjee SS, Haboubi NY (1989). Two cases of pseudosarcomatous invasive transitional cell carcinoma of the urinary bladder mimicking malignant fibrous histiocytoma. *Histopathology* 15: 93-96.
2039. Pedersen-Bjergaard J, Jonsson V, Pedersen M, Hou-Jensen K (1995). Leiomyosarcoma of the urinary bladder after cyclophosphamide. *J Clin Oncol* 13: 532-533.
2040. Pedersen KV, Boiesen P, Zetterlund CG (1987). Experience of screening for carcinoma-in-situ of the testis among young men with surgically corrected maldescended testes. *Int J Androl* 10: 181-185.
2041. Peison B, Benisch B, Nicora B (1985). Multicentric basal cell carcinoma of penile skin. *Urology* 25: 322-323.
2042. Pelkey TJ, Frierson HFJr, Mills SE, Stoler MH (1999). Detection of the alpha-subunit of inhibin in trophoblastic neoplasia. *Hum Pathol* 30: 26-31.
2043. Pelletier J, Bruening W, Kashtan CE, Mauer SM, Manivel JC, Striegel JE, Houghton DC, Junien C, Habib R, Fouser L, Fine RN, Silverman BL, Haber DA, Housman DE (1991). Germline mutations in the Wilms' tumor suppressor gene are associated with abnormal urogenital development in Denys-Drash syndrome. *Cell* 67: 437-447.
2044. Peltomaki P, Lothe RA, Aaltonen LA, Pylkkanen L, Nystrom-Lahti M, Seruca R, David L, Holm R, Ryberg D, Haugen A, Brogger A, Borresen AL, de la Chapelle A (1993). Microsatellite instability is associated with tumors that characterize the hereditary non-polyposis colorectal carcinoma syndrome. *Cancer Res* 53: 5853-5855.
2045. Peng HQ, Liu L, Goss PE, Bailey D, Hogg D (1999). Chromosomal deletions occur in restricted regions of 5q in testicular germ cell cancer. *Oncogene* 18: 3277-3283.
2046. Perachino M, di Ciolo L, Barbetti V, Ardoino S, Vitali A, Introini C, Vigliercio G, Puppo P (1997). Results of rebiopsy for suspected prostate cancer in symptomatic men with elevated PSA levels. *Eur Urol* 32: 155-159.
2047. Peralta-Venturina M, Moch H, Amin M, Tamboli P, Hailemariam S, Mihatsch M, Javidan J, Stricker H, Ro JY, Amin MB (2001). Sarcomatoid differentiation in renal cell carcinoma: a study of 101 cases. *Am J Surg Pathol* 25: 275-284.
2048. Perez-Atayde AR, Joste N, Mulhern H (1996). Juvenile granulosa cell tumor of the infantile testis. Evidence of a dual epithelial-smooth muscle differentiation. *Am J Surg Pathol* 20: 72-79.
2049. Perez-Mesa C, Oxenhandler R (1989). Metastatic tumors of the penis. *J Surg Oncol* 42: 11-15.
2050. Perez-Ordonez B, Hamed G, Campbell S, Erlandson RA, Russo P, Gaudin PB, Reuter VE (1997). Renal oncocytoma: a clinicopathologic study of 70 cases. *Am J Surg Pathol* 21: 871-883.
2051. Perez-Ordonez B, Srigley JR (2000). Mesothelial lesions of the paratesticular region. *Semin Diagn Pathol* 17: 294-306.
2052. Perez C, Novoa J, Alcaniz J, Salto L, Barcelo B (1980). Leydig cell tumour of the testis with gynaecomastia and elevated oestrogen, progesterone and prolactin levels: case report. *Clin Endocrinol (Oxf)* 13: 409-412.
2053. Perito PE, Ciancio G, Civantos F, Politano VA (1992). Sertoli-Leydig cell testicular tumor: case report and review of sex cord/gonadal stromal tumor histogenesis. *J Urol* 148: 883-885.
2054. Perlman EJ, Hu J, Ho D, Cushing B, Lauer S, Castleberry RP (2000). Genetic analysis of childhood endodermal sinus tumors by comparative genomic hybridization. *J Pediatr Hematol Oncol* 22: 100-105.
2055. Pero R, Lembo F, di Vizio D, Boccia A, Chieffi P, Fedele M, Pierantoni GM, Rossi P, Iuliano R, Santoro M, Viglietto G, Bruni CB, Fusco A, Chiariotti L (2001). RNF4 is a growth inhibitor expressed in germ cells but not in human testicular tumors. *Am J Pathol* 159: 1225-1230.
2056. Perou CM, Sorlie T, Eisen MB, van de Rijn M, Jeffrey SS, Rees CA, Pollack JR, Ross DT, Johnsen H, Akslen LA, Fluge O, Pergamenschikov A, Williams C, Zhu SX, Lonning PE, Borresen-Dale AL, Brown PO, Botstein D (2000). Molecular portraits of human breast tumours. *Nature* 406: 747-752.
2057. Perret L, Chaubert P, Hessler D, Guillou L (1998). Primary heterologous carcinosarcoma (metaplastic carcinoma) of the urinary bladder: a clinicopathologic, immunohistochemical, and ultrastructural analysis of eight cases and a review of the literature. *Cancer* 82: 1535-1549.
2058. Pesti T, Sukosd F, Jones EC, Kovacs G (2001). Mapping a tumor suppressor gene to chromosome 2p13 in metanephric adenoma by microsatellite allelotyping. *Hum Pathol* 32: 101-104.
2059. Petersen I, Ohgaki H, Ludeke BI, Kleihues P (1993). p53 mutations in phenacetin-associated human urothelial carcinomas. *Carcinogenesis* 14: 2119-2122.
2060. Petersen SE, Harving N, Orntoft T, Wolf H (1988). Clonal heterogeneity of aneuploid cell populations in carcinoma in situ of the bladder: a flow cytometric study. *Scand J Urol Nephrol Suppl* 110: 213-217.
2061. Pettijohn DE, Stranahan PL, Due C, Ronne E, Sorensen HR, Olsson L (1987). Glycoproteins distinguishing non-small cell from small cell human lung carcinoma recognized by monoclonal antibody 43-9F. *Cancer Res* 47: 1161-1169.
2062. Pettinato G, Manivel JC, d'Amore ES, Jaszcz W, Gorlin RJ (1991). Melanotic neuroectodermal tumor of infancy. A reexamination of a histogenetic problem based on immunohistochemical, flow cytometric, and ultrastructural study of 10 cases. *Am J Surg Pathol* 15: 233-245.
2063. Pettinato G, Manivel JC, Wick MR, Dehner LP (1989). Classical and cellular (atypical) congenital mesoblastic nephroma: a clinicopathologic, ultrastructural, immunohistochemical, and flow cytometric study. *Hum Pathol* 20: 682-690.
2064. Peyromaure M, Weibing S, Sebe P, Verpillat P, Toublanc M, Dauge MC, Boccon-Gibod L, Ravery V (2002). Prognostic value of p53 overexpression in T1G3 bladder tumors treated with bacillus Calmette-Guerin therapy. *Urology* 59: 409-413.
2065. Pfister C, Buzelin F, Casse C, Bochereau G, Buzelin JM, Bouchot O (1998). Comparative analysis of MiB1 and p53 expression in human bladder tumors and their correlation with cancer progression. *Eur Urol* 33: 278-284.
2066. Pfister C, Flaman JM, Martin C, Grise P, Frebourg T (1999). Selective detection of inactivating mutations of the tumor suppressor gene p53 in bladder tumors. *J Urol* 161: 1973-1975.
2067. Pfister C, Larue H, Moore L, Lacombe L, Veilleux C, Tetu B, Meyer F, Fradet Y (2000). Tumorigenic pathways in low-stage bladder cancer based on p53, MDM2 and p21 phenotypes. *Int J Cancer* 89: 100-104.
2068. Pfister C, Moore L, Allard P, Larue H, Lacombe L, Tetu B, Meyer F, Fradet Y (1999). Predictive value of cell cycle markers p53, MDM2, p21, and Ki-67 in superficial bladder tumor recurrence. *Clin Cancer Res* 5: 4079-4084.
2069. Philip AT, Amin MB, Tamboli P, Lee TJ, Hill CE, Ro JY (2000). Intravesical adipose tissue: a quantitative study of its presence and location with implications for therapy and prognosis. *Am J Surg Pathol* 24: 1286-1290.

2070. Phillips G, Kumari-Subaiya S, Sawitsky A (1987). Ultrasonic evaluation of the scrotum in lymphoproliferative disease. *J Ultrasound Med* 6: 169-175.
2071. Pich A, Chiusa L, Formiconi A, Galliano D, Bortolin P, Navone R (2001). Biologic differences between noninvasive papillary urothelial neoplasms of low malignant potential and low-grade (grade 1) papillary carcinomas of the bladder. *Am J Surg Pathol* 25: 1528-1533.
2072. Picken MM, Curry JL, Lindgren V, Clark JI, Eble JN (2001). Metanephric adenosarcoma in a young adult: morphologic, immunophenotypic, ultrastructural, and fluorescence in situ hybridization analyses: a case report and review of the literature. *Am J Surg Pathol* 25: 1451-1457.
2073. Pierson CR, Schober MS, Wallis T, Sarkar FH, Sorensen PH, Eble JN, Srigley JR, Jones EC, Grignon DJ, Adsay V (2001). Mixed epithelial and stromal tumor of the kidney lacks the genetic alterations of cellular congenital mesoblastic nephroma. *Hum Pathol* 32: 513-520.
2074. Piironen T, Lovgren J, Karp M, Eerola R, Lundwall A, Dowell B, Lovgren T, Lilja H, Pettersson K (1996). Immunofluorometric assay for sensitive and specific measurement of human prostatic glandular kallikrein (hK2) in serum. *Clin Chem* 42: 1034-1041.
2075. Pila Perez R, Pila Pelaez R, Boladeres Iniquez C, Caceres Diaz C (1994). [Hodgkin's disease of the penis. Report of a new case]. *Arch Esp Urol* 47: 283-285.
2076. Pileri SA, Sabattini E, Rosito P, Zinzani PL, Ascani S, Fraternali-Orcioni G, Gamberi B, Piccioli M, Vivenza D, Falini B, Gaidano G (2002). Primary follicular lymphoma of the testis in childhood: an entity with peculiar clinical and molecular characteristics. *J Clin Pathol* 55: 684-688.
2077. Ping AJ, Reeve AE, Law DJ, Young MR, Boehnke M, Feinberg AP (1989). Genetic linkage of Beckwith-Wiedemann syndrome to 11p15. *Am J Hum Genet* 44: 720-723.
2078. Pinkerton CR (1997). Malignant germ cell tumours in childhood. *Eur J Cancer* 33: 895-901.
2079. Pins MR, Campbell SC, Laskin WB, Steinbronn K, Dalton DP (2001). Solitary fibrous tumor of the prostate a report of 2 cases and review of the literature. *Arch Pathol Lab Med* 125: 274-277.
2080. Pinto JA, Gonzalez JE, Granadillo MA (1994). Primary carcinoma of the prostate with diffuse oncocytic changes. *Histopathology* 25: 286-288.
2081. Pinto KJ, Jerkins GR (1997). Bladder pheochromocytoma in a 10-year-old girl. *J Urol* 158: 583-584.
2082. Pinto MM (1985). Juvenile granulosa cell tumor of the infant testis: case report with ultrastructural observations. *Pediatr Pathol* 4: 277-289.
2083. Pirich LM, Chou P, Walterhouse DO (1999). Prolonged survival of a patient with sickle cell trait and metastatic renal medullary carcinoma. *J Pediatr Hematol Oncol* 21: 67-69.
2084. Pisani P, Bray F, Parkin DM (2002). Estimates of the world-wide prevalence of cancer for 25 sites in the adult population. *Int J Cancer* 97: 72-81.
2085. Pitt MA, Morphopoulos G, Wells S, Bisset DL (1995). Pseudoangiosarcomatous carcinoma of the genitourinary tract. *J Clin Pathol* 48: 1059-1061.
2086. Pitz S, Moll R, Storkel S, Thoenes W (1987). Expression of intermediate filament proteins in subtypes of renal cell carcinomas and in renal oncocytomas. Distinction of two classes of renal cell tumors. *Lab Invest* 56: 642-653.
2087. Pizzo PA, Cassady JR, Miser JS (1989). Solid tumors of childhood. In: *Cancer: Principles and Practice of Oncology*, VTJr de Vita, S Hellman, SA Rosenberg, eds. 3rd Edition. J.B. Lippincott: Philadelphia, pp. 1511-1589.
2088. Plank TL, Yeung RS, Henske EP (1998). Hamartin, the product of the tuberous sclerosis 1 (TSC1) gene, interacts with tuberin and appears to be localized to cytoplasmic vesicles. *Cancer Res* 58: 4766-4770.
2089. Planz B, George R, Adam G, Jakse G, Planz K (1995). Computed tomography for detection and staging of transitional cell carcinoma of the upper urinary tract. *Eur Urol* 27: 146-150.
2090. Plas E, Riedl CR, Pfluger H (1998). Malignant mesothelioma of the tunica vaginalis testis: review of the literature and assessment of prognostic parameters. *Cancer* 83: 2437-2446.
2091. Platz EA, Rimm EB, Willett WC, Kantoff PW, Giovannucci E (2000). Racial variation in prostate cancer incidence and in hormonal system markers among male health professionals. *J Natl Cancer Inst* 92: 2009-2017.
2092. Plesner KB, Jacobsen BB, Kock KE, Rix M, Rosthoj S (2000). [Granulosa cell tumors in children]. *Ugeskr Laeger* 162: 3731-3733.
2093. Poblet E, Gomez-Tierno A, Alfaro L (2000). Prostatic carcinosarcoma: a case originating in a previous ductal adenocarcinoma of the prostate. *Pathol Res Pract* 196: 569-572.
2094. Polascik TJ, Cairns P, Epstein JI, Fuzesi L, Ro JY, Marshall FF, Sidransky D, Schoenberg M (1996). Distal nephron renal tumors: microsatellite allelotype. *Cancer Res* 56: 1892-1895.
2095. Pollack A, Czerniak B, Zagars GK, Hu SX, Wu CS, Dinney CP, Chyle V, Benedict WF (1997). Retinoblastoma protein expression and radiation response in muscle-invasive bladder cancer. *Int J Radiat Oncol Biol Phys* 39: 687-695.
2096. Popek EJ, Montgomery EA, Fourcroy JL (1994). Fibrous hamartoma of infancy in the genital region: findings in 15 cases. *J Urol* 152: 990-993.
2097. Porcaro AB, D'Amico A, Novella G, Curti P, Ficarra V, Antoniolli SZ, Martignoni G, Matteo B, Malossini G (2002). Primary lymphoma of the kidney. Report of a case and update of the literature. *Arch Ital Urol Androl* 74: 44-47.
2098. Porter JR, Brawer MK (1993). Prostatic intraepithelial neoplasia and prostate-specific antigen. *World J Urol* 11: 196-200.
2099. Potosky AL, Kessler L, Gridley G, Brown CC, Horm JW (1990). Rise in prostatic cancer incidence associated with increased use of transurethral resection. *J Natl Cancer Inst* 82: 1624-1628.
2100. Potosky AL, Miller BA, Albertsen PC, Kramer BS (1995). The role of increasing detection in the rising incidence of prostate cancer. *JAMA* 273: 548-552.
2101. Potts IF, Hirst E (1963). Inverted papilloma of the bladder. *J Urol* 90: 175.
2102. Poulsen AL, Horn T, Steven K (1998). Radical cystectomy: extending the limits of pelvic lymph node dissection improves survival for patients with bladder cancer confined to the bladder wall. *J Urol* 160: 2015-2019.
2103. Pow-Sang MR, Orihuela E (1994). Leiomyosarcoma of the penis. *J Urol* 151: 1643-1645.
2104. Pozza D, Masci P, Amodeo S, Marchionni L (1994). Papillary cystadenoma of the epididymis as a cause of obstructive azoospermia. *Urol Int* 53: 222-224.
2105. Prener A, Engholm G, Jensen OM (1996). Genital anomalies and risk for testicular cancer in Danish men. *Epidemiology* 7: 14-19.
2106. Prescott RJ, Mainwaring AR (1990). Irradiation-induced penile angiosarcoma. *Postgrad Med J* 66: 576-579.
2107. Presti JCJr, Moch H, Gelb AB, Huynh D, Waldman FM (1998). Initiating genetic events in small renal neoplasms detected by comparative genomic hybridization. *J Urol* 160: 1557-1561.
2108. Presti JCJr, Moch H, Reuter VE, Huynh D, Waldman FM (1996). Comparative genomic hybridization for genetic analysis of renal oncocytomas. *Genes Chromosomes Cancer* 17: 199-204.
2109. Presti JCJr, Rao PH, Chen Q, Reuter VE, Li FP, Fair WR, Jhanwar SC (1991). Histopathological, cytogenetic, and molecular characterization of renal cortical tumors. *Cancer Res* 51: 1544-1552.
2110. Presti JCJr, Reuter VE, Galan T, Fair WR, Cordon-Cardo C (1991). Molecular genetic alterations in superficial and locally advanced human bladder cancer. *Cancer Res* 51: 5405-5409.
2111. Price EBJr (1971). Papillary cystadenoma of the epididymis. A clinicopathologic analysis of 20 cases. *Arch Pathol* 91: 456-470.
2112. Primdahl H, von der Maase H, Christensen M, Wolf H, Orntoft TF (2000). Allelic deletions of cell growth regulators during progression of bladder cancer. *Cancer Res* 60: 6623-6629.
2113. Pritchard-Jones K, Fleming S (1991). Cell types expressing the Wilms' tumour gene (WT1) in Wilms' tumours: implications for tumour histogenesis. *Oncogene* 6: 2211-2220.
2114. Proctor AJ, Coombs LM, Cairns JP, Knowles MA (1991). Amplification at chromosome 11q13 in transitional cell tumours of the bladder. *Oncogene* 6: 789-795.
2115. Prout GRJr, Griffin PP, Daly JJ, Heney NM (1983). Carcinoma in situ of the urinary bladder with and without associated vesical neoplasms. *Cancer* 52: 524-532.
2116. Pryor JP, Cameron KM, Chilton CP, Ford TF, Parkinson MC, Sinokrot J, Westwood CA (1983). Carcinoma in situ in testicular biopsies from men presenting with infertility. *Br J Urol* 55: 780-784.
2117. Przybojewska B, Jagiello A, Jalmuzna P (2000). H-RAS, K-RAS, and N-RAS gene activation in human bladder cancers. *Cancer Genet Cytogenet* 121: 73-77.
2118. Pycha A, Mian C, Posch B, Haitel A, Mokhtar AA, el Baz M, Ghoneim MA, Marberger M (1999). Numerical chromosomal aberrations in muscle invasive squamous cell and transitional cell cancer of the urinary bladder: an alternative to classic prognostic indicators? *Urology* 53: 1005-1010.
2119. Qi J, Shen PU, Rezuke WN, Currier AA, Westfall PK, Mandavilli SR (2001). Fine needle aspiration cytology diagnosis of renal medullary carcinoma: a case report. *Acta Cytol* 45: 735-739.
2120. Qian J, Bostwick DG, Takahashi S, Borell TJ, Herath JF, Lieber MM, Jenkins RB (1995). Chromosomal anomalies in prostatic intraepithelial neoplasia and carcinoma detected by fluorescence in situ hybridization. *Cancer Res* 55: 5408-5414.
2121. Qian J, Jenkins RB, Bostwick DG (1997). Detection of chromosomal anomalies and c-myc gene amplification in the cribriform pattern of prostatic intraepithelial neoplasia and carcinoma by fluorescence in situ hybridization. *Mod Pathol* 10: 1113-1119.
2122. Qian J, Wollan P, Bostwick DG (1997). The extent and multicentricity of high-grade prostatic intraepithelial neoplasia in clinically localized prostatic adenocarcinoma. *Hum Pathol* 28: 143-148.
2123. Qiao D, Zeeman AM, Deng W, Looijenga LH, Lin H (2002). Molecular characterization of hiwi, a human member of the piwi gene family whose overexpression is correlated to seminomas. *Oncogene* 21: 3988-3999.
2124. Quezado M, Benjamin DR, Tsokos M (1997). EWS/FLI-1 fusion transcripts in three peripheral primitive neuroectodermal tumors of the kidney. *Hum Pathol* 28: 767-771.
2125. Quinn BD, Cho KR, Epstein JI (1990). Relationship of severe dysplasia to stage B adenocarcinoma of the prostate. *Cancer* 65: 2328-2337.
2126. Qureshi KN, Griffiths TR, Robinson MC, Marsh C, Roberts JT, Lunec J, Neal DE, Mellon JK (2001). Combined p21WAF1/CIP1 and p53 overexpression predict improved survival in muscle-invasive bladder cancer treated by radical radiotherapy. *Int J Radiat Oncol Biol Phys* 51: 1234-1240.
2127. Rabbani F, Cordon-Cardo C (2000). Mutation of cell cycle regulators and their impact on superficial bladder cancer. *Urol Clin North Am* 27: 83-102.
2128. Rabbani F, Gleave ME, Coppin CM, Murray N, Sullivan LD (1996). Teratoma in primary testis tumor reduces complete response rates in the retroperitoneum after primary chemotherapy. The case for primary retroperitoneal lymph node dissection of stage IIb germ cell tumors with teratomatous elements. *Cancer* 78: 480-486.
2129. Rachmilewitz J, Elkin M, Looijenga LH, Verkerk AJ, Gonik B, Lustig O, Werner D, de Groot N, Hochberg A (1996). Characterization of the imprinted IPW gene: allelic expression in normal and tumorigenic human tissues. *Oncogene* 13: 1687-1692.
2130. Radhi JM (1997). Urethral malignant melanoma closely mimicking urothelial carcinoma. *J Clin Pathol* 50: 250-252.
2131. Radojkovic M, Ilic S (1992). [Carcinoma in situ in cryptorchid testes in post-pubertal patients]. *Vojnosanit Pregl* 49: 493-497.
2132. Raghavan D, Scher HI, Leibel SA, Lange PH (1997). *Principle and Practice of Genitourinary Oncology.* Lippincott-Raven: Philadelphia.
2133. Raghavan D, Shipley WU, Garnick MB, Russell PJ, Richie JP (1990). Biology and management of bladder cancer. *N Engl J Med* 322: 1129-1138.
2134. Rahman N, Abidi F, Ford D, Arbour L, Rapley E, Tonin P, Barton D, Batcup G, Berry J, Cotter F, Davison V, Gerrard M, Gray E, Grundy R, Hanafy M, King D, Lewis I, Ridolfi Luethy A, Madlensky L, Mann J, O'Meara A, Oakhill T, Skolnick M, Strong L, Variend D, Narod S, Schwartz C, Pritchard-Jones K, Stratton MR (1998). Confirmation of FWT1 as a Wilms' tumour susceptibility gene and phenotypic characteristics of Wilms' tumour attributable to FWT1. *Hum Genet* 103: 547-556.

2135. Rajpert-de Meyts E, Skakkebaek NE (1994). Expression of the c-kit protein product in carcinoma-in-situ and invasive testicular germ cell tumours. *Int J Androl* 17: 85-92.
2136. Raju U, Fine G, Warrier R, Kini R, Weiss L (1986). Congenital testicular juvenile granulosa cell tumor in a neonate with X/XY mosaicism. *Am J Surg Pathol* 10: 577-583.
2137. Rakozy C, Schmahl GE, Bogner S, Stoerkel S (2002). Low-grade tubular-mucinous renal neoplasms: morphologic, immunohistochemical, and genetic features. *Mod Pathol* 15: 1162-1171.
2138. Ramadan A, Naab T, Frederick W, Green W (2000). Testicular plasmacytoma in a patient with the acquired immunodeficiency syndrome. *Tumori* 86: 480-482.
2139. Ramani P, Cowell JK (1996). The expression pattern of Wilms' tumour gene (WT1) product in normal tissues and paediatric renal tumours. *J Pathol* 179: 162-168.
2140. Ramani P, Yeung CK, Habeebu SS (1993). Testicular intratubular germ cell neoplasia in children and adolescents with intersex. *Am J Surg Pathol* 17: 1124-1133.
2141. Ramchurren N, Cooper K, Summerhayes IC (1995). Molecular events underlying schistosomiasis-related bladder cancer. *Int J Cancer* 62: 237-244.
2142. Rames RA, Richardson M, Swiger F, Kaczmarek A (1995). Mixed germ cell-sex cord stromal tumor of the testis: the incidental finding of a rare testicular neoplasm. *J Urol* 154: 1479.
2143. Rames RA, Smith MT (1999). Malignant peripheral nerve sheath tumor of the prostate: a rare manifestion of neurofibromatosis type 1. *J Urol* 162: 165-166.
2144. Ramos CG, Carvahal GF, Mager DE, Haberer B, Catalona WJ (1999). The effect of high grade prostatic intraepithelial neoplasia on serum total and percentage of free prostate specific antigen levels. *J Urol* 162: 1587-1590.
2145. Randolph TL, Amin MB, Ro JY, Ayala AG (1997). Histologic variants of adenocarcinoma and other carcinomas of prostate: pathologic criteria and clinical significance. *Mod Pathol* 10: 612-629.
2146. Raney RBJr, Tefft M, Lawrence WJr, Ragab AH, Soule EH, Beltangady M, Gehan EA (1987). Paratesticular sarcoma in childhood and adolescence. A report from the Intergroup Rhabdomyosarcoma Studies I and II, 1973-1983. *Cancer* 60: 2337-2343.
2147. Rao PH, Houldsworth J, Palanisamy N, Murty VV, Reuter VE, Motzer RJ, Bosl GJ, Chaganti RS (1998). Chromosomal amplification is associated with cisplatin resistance of human male germ cell tumors. *Cancer Res* 58: 4260-4263.
2148. Rapley EA, Crockford GP, Teare D, Biggs P, Seal S, Barfoot R, Edwards S, Hamoudi R, Heimdal K, Fossa SD, Tucker K, Donald J, Collins F, Friedlander M, Hogg D, Goss P, Heidenreich A, Ormiston W, Daly PA, Forman D, Oliver TD, Leahy M, Huddart R, Cooper CS, Bodmer JG, Easton DF, Stratton MR, Bishop DT (2000). Localization to Xq27 of a susceptibility gene for testicular germ-cell tumours. *Nat Genet* 24: 197-200.
2149. Rasch C, Barillot I, Remeijer P, Touw A, van Herk M, Lebesque JV (1999). Definition of the prostate in CT and MRI: a multi-observer study. *Int J Radiat Oncol Biol Phys* 43: 57-66.
2150. Raslan WF, Ro JY, Ordonez NG, Amin MB, Troncoso P, Sella A, Ayala AG (1993). Primary carcinoid of the kidney. Immunohistochemical and ultrastructural studies of five patients. *Cancer* 72: 2660-2666.
2151. Ravery V, Goldblatt L, Royer B, Blanc E, Toublanc M, Boccon-Gibod L (2000). Extensive biopsy protocol improves the detection rate of prostate cancer. *J Urol* 164: 393-396.
2152. Ravery V, Grignon DJ, Angulo J, Pontes E, Montie J, Crissman J, Chopin D (1997). Evaluation of epidermal growth factor receptor, transforming growth factor alpha, epidermal growth factor and c-erbB2 in the progression of invasive bladder cancer. *Urol Res* 25: 9-17.
2153. Ravich A, Stout AP, Ravich RA (1945). Malignant granular cell myoblastoma involving the urinary bladder. *Ann Surg* 121: 361-372.
2154. Ray B, Canto AR, Whitmore WFJr (1977). Experience with primary carcinoma of the male urethra. *J Urol* 117: 591-594.
2155. Ray B, Guinan PD (1979). Primary carcinoma of the urethra. In: *Principles and Management of Urologic Cancer*, N Javadpour, ed. Williams and Wilkins: Baltimore, MD, pp. 445-473.
2156. Raziuddin S, Masihuzzaman M, Shetty S, Ibrahim A (1993). Tumor necrosis factor alpha production in schistosomiasis with carcinoma of urinary bladder. *J Clin Immunol* 13: 23-29.
2157. Raziuddin S, Shetty S, Ibrahim A (1991). T-cell abnormality and defective interleukin-2 production in patients with carcinoma of the urinary bladder with schistosomiasis. *J Clin Immunol* 11: 103-113.
2158. Raziuddin S, Shetty S, Ibrahim A (1992). Soluble interleukin-2 receptor levels and immune activation in patients with schistosomiasis and carcinoma of the urinary bladder. *Scand J Immunol* 35: 637-641.
2159. Razvi M, Fifer R, Berkson B (1975). Occult transitional cell carcinoma of the prostate presenting as skin metastasis. *J Urol* 113: 734-735.
2160. Reek C, Graefen M, Noldus J, Fernandez S (2000). [Mixed squamous epithelial and adenocarcinoma of the female urethra. A case report]. *Urologe A* 39: 174-177.
2161. Reese AJM, Winstanley DP (1958). The small tumor-like lesions of the kidney. *Br J Cancer* 12: 507-516.
2162. Regan JB, Barrett DM, Wold LE (1987). Giant leiomyoma of the prostate. *Arch Pathol Lab Med* 111: 381-382.
2163. Reis M, Faria V, Lindoro J, Adolfo A (1988). The small cystic and noncystic noninflammatory renal nodules: a postmortem study. *J Urol* 140: 721-724.
2164. Reiter RE, Anglard P, Liu S, Gnarra JR, Linehan WM (1993). Chromosome 17p deletions and p53 mutations in renal cell carcinoma. *Cancer Res* 53: 3092-3097.
2165. Reiter RE, Gu Z, Watabe T, Thomas G, Szigeti K, Davis E, Wahl M, Nisitani S, Yamashiro J, Le Beau MM, Loda M, Witte ON (1998). Prostate stem cell antigen: a cell surface marker overexpressed in prostate cancer. *Proc Natl Acad Sci USA* 95: 1735-1740.
2166. Remmele W, Kaiserling E, Zerban U, Hildebrand U, Bennek M, Jacobi-Nolde P, Pinkenburg FA (1992). Serous papillary cystic tumor of borderline malignancy with focal carcinoma arising in testis: case report with immunohistochemical and ultrastructural observations. *Hum Pathol* 23: 75-79.
2167. Renedo DE, Trainer TD (1994). Intratubular germ cell neoplasia (ITGCN) with p53 and PCNA expression and adjacent mature teratoma in an infant testis. An immunohistochemical and morphologic study with a review of the literature. *Am J Surg Pathol* 18: 947-952.
2168. Renshaw AA (1998). Correlation of gross morphologic features with histologic features in radical prostatectomy specimens. *Am J Clin Pathol* 110: 38-42.
2169. Renshaw AA, Corless CL (1995). Papillary renal cell carcinoma. Histology and immunohistochemistry. *Am J Surg Pathol* 19: 842-849.
2170. Renshaw AA, Gordon M, Corless CL (1997). Immunohistochemistry of unclassified sex cord-stromal tumors of the testis with a predominance of spindle cells. *Mod Pathol* 10: 693-700.
2171. Renshaw AA, Maurici D, Fletcher JA (1997). Cytologic and fluorescence in situ hybridization (FISH) examination of metanephric adenoma. *Diagn Cytopathol* 16: 107-111.
2172. Renshaw AA, Richie JP (1999). Subtypes of renal cell carcinoma. Different onset and sites of metastatic disease. *Am J Clin Pathol* 111: 539-543.
2173. Renshaw AA, Zhang H, Corless CL, Fletcher JA, Pins MR (1997). Solid variants of papillary (chromophil) renal cell carcinoma: clinicopathologic and genetic features. *Am J Surg Pathol* 21: 1203-1209.
2174. Resnick ME, Unterberger H, McLoughlin PT (1966). Renal carcinoid producing the carcinoid syndrome. *Med Times* 94: 895-896.
2175. Reuter VE (1993). Sarcomatoid lesions of the urogenital tract. *Semin Diagn Pathol* 10: 188-201.
2176. Reuter VE (1997). Pathological changes in benign and malignant prostatic tissue following androgen deprivation therapy. *Urology* 49: 16-22.
2177. Reuter VE (1999). Bladder. Risk and prognostic factors—a pathologist's perspective. *Urol Clin North Am* 26: 481-492.
2178. Reuter VE, Gaudin PG (1999). Adult renal tumors. In: *Diagnostic Surgical Pathology*, SS Sternberg, ed. 3rd Edition. Lippincott Williams and Wilkins: New York, pp. 1785-1824.
2179. Reutzel D, Mende M, Naumann S, Storkel S, Brenner W, Zabel B, Decker J (2001). Genomic imbalances in 61 renal cancers from the proximal tubulus detected by comparative genomic hybridization. *Cytogenet Cell Genet* 93: 221-227.
2180. Rey R, Sabourin JC, Venara M, Long WQ, Jaubert F, Zeller WP, Duvillard P, Chemes H, Bidart JM (2000). Anti-Mullerian hormone is a specific marker of Sertoli- and granulosa-cell origin in gonadal tumors. *Hum Pathol* 31: 1202-1208.
2181. Reyes AO, Swanson PE, Carbone JM, Humphrey PA (1997). Unusual histologic types of high-grade prostatic intraepithelial neoplasia. *Am J Surg Pathol* 21: 1215-1222.
2182. Reyes CV, Soneru I (1985). Small cell carcinoma of the urinary bladder with hypercalcemia. *Cancer* 56: 2530-2533.
2183. Rha SE, Byun JY, Kim HH, Baek JH, Hwang TK, Kang SJ (2000). Kaposi's sarcoma involving a transplanted kidney, ureter and urinary bladder: ultrasound and CT findings. *Br J Radiol* 73: 1221-1223.
2183a. Rhodes DR, Barrette TR, Rubin MA, Ghosh D, Chinnaiyan AM (2002). Meta-analysis of microarrays: interstudy validation of gene expression profiles reveals pathway dysregulation in prostate cancer. *Cancer Res*, 62: 4427-4433.
2184. Ribalta T, Lloreta J, Munne A, Serrano S, Cardesa A (2000). Malignant pigmented clear cell epithelioid tumor of the kidney: clear cell ("sugar") tumor versus malignant melanoma. *Hum Pathol* 31: 516-519.
2185. Richardson TD, Oesterling JE (1997). Age-specific reference ranges for serum prostate-specific antigen. *Urol Clin North Am* 24: 339-351.
2186. Richiardi L, Akre O, Bellocco R, Ekbom A (2002). Perinatal determinants of germ-cell testicular cancer in relation to histological subtypes. *Br J Cancer* 87: 545-550.
2187. Richie JP, Skinner DG (1978). Carcinoma in situ of the urethra associated with bladder carcinoma: the role of urethrectomy. *J Urol* 119: 80-81.
2188. Richter J, Beffa L, Wagner U, Schraml P, Gasser TC, Moch H, Mihatsch MJ, Sauter G (1998). Patterns of chromosomal imbalances in advanced urinary bladder cancer detected by comparative genomic hybridization. *Am J Pathol* 153: 1615-1621.
2189. Richter J, Jiang F, Gorog JP, Sartorius G, Egenter C, Gasser TC, Moch H, Mihatsch MJ, Sauter G (1997). Marked genetic differences between stage pTa and stage pT1 papillary bladder cancer detected by comparative genomic hybridization. *Cancer Res* 57: 2860-2864.
2190. Richter J, Wagner U, Kononen J, Fijan A, Bruderer J, Schmid U, Ackermann D, Maurer R, Alund G, Knonagel H, Rist M, Wilber K, Anabitarte M, Hering F, Hardmeier T, Schonenberger A, Flury R, Jager P, Fehr JL, Schraml P, Moch H, Mihatsch MJ, Gasser T, Kallioniemi OP, Sauter G (2000). High-throughput tissue microarray analysis of cyclin E gene amplification and overexpression in urinary bladder cancer. *Am J Pathol* 157: 787-794.
2191. Richter J, Wagner U, Schraml P, Maurer R, Alund G, Knonagel H, Moch H, Mihatsch MJ, Gasser TC, Sauter G (1999). Chromosomal imbalances are associated with a high risk of progression in early invasive (pT1) urinary bladder cancer. *Cancer Res* 59: 5687-5691.
2192. Ridanpaa M, Lothe RA, Onfelt A, Fossa S, Borresen AL, Husgafvel-Pursiainen K (1993). K-ras oncogene codon 12 point mutations in testicular cancer. *Environ Health Perspect* 101 Suppl 3: 185-187.
2193. Rifkin MD, Choi H (1988). Implications of small, peripheral hypoechoic lesions in endorectal US of the prostate. *Radiology* 166: 619-622.
2194. Rifkin MD, Kurtz AB, Pasto ME, Goldberg BB (1985). Diagnostic capabilities of high-resolution scrotal ultrasonography: prospective evaluation. *J Ultrasound Med* 4: 13-19.
2195. Rifkin MD, Sudakoff GS, Alexander AA (1993). Prostate: techniques, results, and potential applications of color Doppler US scanning. *Radiology* 186: 509-513.
2196. Rifkin MD, Zerhouni EA, Gatsonis CA, Quint LE, Paushter DM, Epstein JI, Hamper U, Walsh PC, McNeil BJ (1990). Comparison of magnetic resonance imaging and ultrasonography in staging early prostate cancer. Results of a multi-institutional cooperative trial. *N Engl J Med* 323: 621-626.
2197. Rigola MA, Fuster C, Casadevall C, Bernues M, Caballin MR, Gelabert A, Egozcue J, Miro R (2001). Comparative genomic hybridization analysis of transitional cell carcinomas of the renal pelvis. *Cancer Genet Cytogenet* 127: 59-63.
2198. Riopel MA, Spellerberg A, Griffin CA, Perlman EJ (1998). Genetic analysis of ovarian germ cell tumors by comparative genomic hybridization. *Cancer Res* 58: 3105-3110.

2199. Riou G, Barrois M, Prost S, Terrier MJ, Theodore C, Levine AJ (1995). The p53 and mdm-2 genes in human testicular germ-cell tumors. *Mol Carcinog* 12: 124-131.

2200. Ritchey ML, Bagnall JW, McDonald EC, Sago AL (1985). Development of nongerm cell malignancies in nonseminomatous germ cell tumors. *J Urol* 134: 146-149.

2201. Ritter MM, Frilling A, Crossey PA, Hoppner W, Maher ER, Mulligan L, Ponder BA, Engelhardt D (1996). Isolated familial pheochromocytoma as a variant of von Hippel-Lindau disease. *J Clin Endocrinol Metab* 81: 1035-1037.

2202. Ro JY, Amin MB, Ayala AG (1997). Penis and scrotum. In: *Urologic Surgical Pathology*, DG Bostwick, JN Eble, eds. Mosby: St Louis.

2203. Ro JY, Ayala AG, el-Naggar A (1987). Muscularis mucosae of urinary bladder. Importance for staging and treatment. *Am J Surg Pathol* 11: 668-673.

2204. Ro JY, Ayala AG, Ordonez NG, Cartwright JJr, Mackay B (1986). Intraluminal crystalloids in prostatic adenocarcinoma. Immunohistochemical, electron microscopic, and x-ray microanalytic studies. *Cancer* 57: 2397-2407.

2205. Ro JY, Ayala AG, Wishnow KI, Ordonez NG (1988). Prostatic duct adenocarcinoma with endometrioid features: immunohistochemical and electron microscopic study. *Semin Diagn Pathol* 5: 301-311.

2206. Ro JY, el-Naggar A, Ayala AG, Mody DR, Ordonez NG (1988). Signet-ring-cell carcinoma of the prostate. Electron-microscopic and immunohistochemical studies of eight cases. *Am J Surg Pathol* 12: 453-460.

2207. Ro JY, Grignon DJ, Ayala AG, Fernandez PL, Ordonez NG, Wishnow KI (1990). Mucinous adenocarcinoma of the prostate: histochemical and immunohistochemical studies. *Hum Pathol* 21: 593-600.

2208. Ro JY, Grignon DJ, Ayala AG, Hogan SF, Tetu B, Ordonez NG (1988). Blue nevus and melanosis of the prostate. Electron-microscopic and immunohistochemical studies. *Am J Clin Pathol* 90: 530-535.

2209. Ro JY, Sella A, el-Naggar A, Ayala AG (1990). Mature growing teratoma: clinicopathologic and DNA flow cytometric analysis. *Lab Invest* 62: 83A.

2210. Ro JY, Tetu B, Ayala AG, Ordonez NG (1987). Small cell carcinoma of the prostate. II. Immunohistochemical and electron microscopic studies of 18 cases. *Cancer* 59: 977-982.

2211. Robel P (1994). Prostate-specific antigen: present and future. In: *Local Prostatic Carcinoma*, M Bolla, JJ Rambeaud, F Vincent, eds. Karger: Basel, pp. 46-56.

2212. Robertson KA, Bullock HA, Xu Y, Tritt R, Zimmerman E, Ulbright TM, Foster RS, Einhorn LH, Kelley MR (2001). Altered expression of Ape1/ref-1 in germ cell tumors and overexpression in NT2 cells confers resistance to bleomycin and radiation. *Cancer Res* 61: 2220-2225.

2213. Robertson PW, Klidjian A, Harding LK, Walters G, Lee MR, Robb-Smith AH (1967). Hypertension due to a renin-secreting renal tumour. *Am J Med* 43: 963-976.

2214. Rochon YP, Horoszewicz JS, Boynton AL, Holmes EH, Barren RJ3rd, Erickson SJ, Kenny GM, Murphy GP (1994). Western blot assay for prostate-specific membrane antigen in serum of prostate cancer patients. *Prostate* 25: 219-223.

2215. Rodriguez-Alonso A, Pita-Fernandez S, Gonzalez-Carrero J, Nogueira-March JL (2002). Multivariate analysis of survival, recurrence, progression and development of mestastasis in T1 and T2a transitional cell bladder carcinoma. *Cancer* 94: 1677-1684.

2216. Rodriguez E, Houldsworth J, Reuter VE, Meltzer P, Zhang J, Trent JM, Bosl GJ, Chaganti RS (1993). Molecular cytogenetic analysis of i(12p)-negative human male germ cell tumors. *Genes Chromosomes Cancer* 8: 230-236.

2217. Rodriguez E, Mathew S, Reuter V, Ilson DH, Bosl GJ, Chaganti RS (1992). Cytogenetic analysis of 124 prospectively ascertained male germ cell tumors. *Cancer Res* 52: 2285-2291.

2218. Rodriguez E, Sreekantaiah C, Gerald W, Reuter VE, Motzer RJ, Chaganti RS (1993). A recurring translocation, t(11;22) (p13;q11.2), characterizes intra-abdominal desmoplastic small round-cell tumors. *Cancer Genet Cytogenet* 69: 17-21.

2219. Rodriguez S, Jafer O, Goker H, Summersgill BM, Zafarana G, Gillis AJ, van Gurp RJ, Oosterhuis JW, Lu YJ, Huddart R, Cooper CS, Clark J, Looijenga LH, Shipley JM (2003). Expression profile of genes from 12p in testicular germ cell tumors of adolescents and adults associated with i(12p) and amplification at 12p11.2-p12.1. *Oncogene* 22: 1880-1891.

2220. Rodriquez-Jurado R, Gonzalez-Crussi F (1996). Renal medullary carcinoma. Immunohistochemical and ultrastructural observations. *J Urol Pathol* 4: 191-203.

2221. Roelofs H, Mostert MC, Pompe K, Zafarana G, van Oorschot M, van Gurp RJ, Gillis AJ, Stoop H, Beverloo B, Oosterhuis JW, Bokemeyer C, Looijenga LH (2000). Restricted 12p amplification and RAS mutation in human germ cell tumors of the adult testis. *Am J Pathol* 157: 1155-1166.

2222. Rogers E, Teahan S, Gallagher H, Butler MR, Grainger R, McDermott TE, Thornhill JA (1998). The role of orchiectomy in the management of postpubertal cryptorchidism. *J Urol* 159: 851-854.

2223. Rohr LR (1987). Incidental adenocarcinoma in transurethral resections of the prostate. Partial versus complete microscopic examination. *Am J Surg Pathol* 11: 53-58.

2224. Roig JM, Amerigo J, Velasco FJ, Gimenez A, Guerrero E, Soler JL, Gonzalez-Campora R (2001). Lymphoepithelioma-like carcinoma of ureter. *Histopathology* 39: 106-107.

2225. Rolonson GJ, Beckwith JB (1993). Primary neuroepithelial tumors of the kidney in children and adults. A report from the NTWS pathology center. *Mod Pathol* 6: 67A.

2226. Romanenko AM, Persidsky YV, Mostofi FK (1993). Ultrastructure and histogenesis of spermatocytic seminoma. *J Urol Pathol* 1: 387-395.

2227. Ronnett BM, Carmichael MJ, Carter HB, Epstein JI (1993). Does high grade prostatic intraepithelial neoplasia result in elevated serum prostate specific antigen levels? *J Urol* 150: 386-389.

2228. Rosai J, Dehner LP (1975). Nodular mesothelial hyperplasia in hernia sacs: a benign reactive condition simulating a neoplastic process. *Cancer* 35: 165-175.

2229. Rosai J, Silber I, Khodadoust K (1969). Spermatocytic seminoma. I. Clinicopathologic study of six cases and review of the literature. *Cancer* 24: 92-102.

2230. Rose EK, Enterline HT, Rhoads JE, Rose E (1952). Adrenal cortical hyperfunction in childhood. Report of a case with adrenocortical hyperplasia and testicular adrenal rests. *Pediatrics* 9: 475-484.

2231. Rosen MA, Goldstone L, Lapin S, Wheeler T, Scardino PT (1992). Frequency and location of extracapsular extension and positive surgical margins in radical prostatectomy specimens. *J Urol* 148: 331-337.

2232. Rosen T, Hoffman J, Jones A (1999). Penile Kaposi's sarcoma. *J Eur Acad Dermatol Venereol* 13: 71-73.

2233. Rosen Y, Ambiavagar PC, Vuletin JC, Macchia RJ (1980). Atypical leiomyoma of prostate. *Urology* 15: 183-185.

2234. Rosenberg C, Mostert MC, Schut TB, van de Pol M, van Echten J, de Jong B, Raap AK, Tanke H, Oosterhuis JW, Looijenga LH (1998). Chromosomal constitution of human spermatocytic seminomas: comparative genomic hybridization supported by conventional and interphase cytogenetics. *Genes Chromosomes Cancer* 23: 286-291.

2235. Rosenberg C, Schut TB, Mostert M, Tanke H, Raap A, Oosterhuis JW, Looijenga LH (1999). Chromosomal gains and losses in testicular germ cell tumors of adolescents and adults investigated by a modified comparative genomic hybridization approach. *Lab Invest* 79: 1447-1451.

2236. Rosenberg C, van Gurp RJ, Geelen E, Oosterhuis JW, Looijenga LH (2000). Overrepresentation of the short arm of chromosome 12 is related to invasive growth of human testicular seminomas and nonseminomas. *Oncogene* 19: 5858-5862.

2237. Rosenkilde-Olsen P, Wolf H, Schroeder T, Fisher A, Hojgaard K (1988). Urothelial atypia and survival rate of 500 unselected patients with primary transitional cell tumour of the urinary bladder. *Scand J Urol Nephrol* 22: 257-263.

2238. Rosenwald A, Wright G, Chan WC, Connors JM, Campo E, Fisher RI, Gascoyne RD, Muller-Hermelink HK, Smeland EB, Giltnane JM, Hurt EM, Zhao H, Averett L, Yang L, Wilson WH, Jaffe ES, Simon R, Klausner RD, Powell J, Duffey PL, Longo DL, Greiner TC, Weisenburger DD, Sanger WG, Dave BJ, Lynch JC, Vose J, Armitage JO, Montserrat E, Lopez-Guillermo A, Grogan TM, Miller TP, LeBlanc M, Ott G, Kvaloy S, Delabie J, Holte H, Krajci P, Stokke T, Staudt LM (2002). The use of molecular profiling to predict survival after chemotherapy for diffuse large-B-cell lymphoma. *N Engl J Med* 346: 1937-1947.

2239. Rosin MP, Anwar W (1992). Chromosomal damage in urothelial cells from Egyptians with chronic Schistosoma haematobium infections. *Int J Cancer* 50: 539-543.

2240. Rosin MP, Anwar WA, Ward AJ (1994). Inflammation, chromosomal instability, and cancer: the schistosomiasis model. *Cancer Res* 54: 1929s-1933s.

2241. Rosin MP, Cairns P, Epstein JI, Schoenberg MP, Sidransky D (1995). Partial allelotype of carcinoma in situ of the human bladder. *Cancer Res* 55: 5213-5216.

2242. Rosin MP, Saad el Din Zaki S, Ward AJ, Anwar WA (1994). Involvement of inflammatory reactions and elevated cell proliferation in the development of bladder cancer in schistosomiasis patients. *Mutat Res* 305: 283-292.

2243. Ross JA, Schmidt PT, Perentesis JP, Davies SM (1999). Genomic imprinting of H19 and insulin-like growth factor-2 in pediatric germ cell tumors. *Cancer* 85: 1389-1394.

2244. Ross JH, Rybicki L, Kay R (2002). Clinical behavior and a contemporary management algorithm for prepubertal testis tumors: a summary of the prepubertal testis tumor registry. *J Urol* 168: 1675-1678.

2245. Ross RK, Paganini-Hill A, Landolph J, Gerkins V, Henderson BE (1989). Analgesics, cigarette smoking, and other risk factors for cancer of the renal pelvis and ureter. *Cancer Res* 49: 1045-1048.

2246. Ross RK, Pike MC, Coetzee GA, Reichardt JK, Yu MC, Feigelson H, Stanczyk FZ, Kolonel LN, Henderson BE (1998). Androgen metabolism and prostate cancer: establishing a model of genetic susceptibility. *Cancer Res* 58: 4497-4504.

2247. Rossi G, Ferrari G, Longo L, Trentini GP (2000). Epithelioid sarcoma of the penis: a case report and review of the literature. *Pathol Int* 50: 579-585.

2248. Roszkiewicz A, Roszkiewicz J, Lange M, Tukaj C (1998). Kaposi's sarcoma following long-term immunosuppressive therapy: clinical, histologic, and ultrastructural study. *Cutis* 61: 137-141.

2249. Roth BJ, Greist A, Kubilis PS, Williams SD, Einhorn LH (1988). Cisplatin-based combination chemotherapy for disseminated germ cell tumors: long-term follow-up. *J Clin Oncol* 6: 1239-1247.

2250. Rothe M, Albers P, Wernert N (1999). Loss of heterozygosity, differentiation, and clonality in microdissected male germ cell tumours. *J Pathol* 188: 389-394.

2251. Rothe M, Ko Y, Albers P, Wernert N (2000). Eukaryotic initiation factor 3 p110 mRNA is overexpressed in testicular seminomas. *Am J Pathol* 157: 1597-1604.

2252. Rottinto A, Debellis H (1944). Extragenital chorioma: its relation to teratoid vestiges in the testicles. *Arch Pathol* 37: 78-80.

2253. Rowland RG, Eble JN (1983). Bladder leiomyosarcoma and pelvic fibroblastic tumor following cyclophosphamide therapy. *J Urol* 130: 344-346.

2254. Rubenstein JH, Katin MJ, Mangano MM, Dauphin J, Salenius SA, Dosoretz DE, Blitzer PH (1997). Small cell anaplastic carcinoma of the prostate: seven new cases, review of the literature, and discussion of a therapeutic strategy. *Am J Clin Oncol* 20: 376-380.

2255. Rubin BP, Chen CJ, Morgan TW, Xiao S, Grier HE, Kozakewich HP, Perez-Atayde AR, Fletcher JA (1998). Congenital mesoblastic nephroma t(12;15) is associated with ETV6-NTRK3 gene fusion: cytogenetic and molecular relationship to congenital (infantile) fibrosarcoma. *Am J Pathol* 153: 1451-1458.

2256. Rubin MA, de La Taille A, Bagiella E, Olsson CA, O'Toole KM (1998). Cribriform carcinoma of the prostate and cribriform prostatic intraepithelial neoplasia: incidence and clinical implications. *Am J Surg Pathol* 22: 840-848.

2257. Rubin MA, Dunn R, Kambham N, Misick CP, O'Toole KM (2000). Should a Gleason score be assigned to a minute focus of carcinoma on prostate biopsy? *Am J Surg Pathol* 24: 1634-1640.

2258. Rubin MA, Kleter B, Zhou M, Ayala G, Cubilla AL, Quint WG, Pirog EC (2001). Detection and typing of human papillomavirus DNA in penile carcinoma: evidence for multiple independent pathways of penile carcinogenesis. *Am J Pathol* 159: 1211-1218.

2259. Rubin MA, Zhou M, Dhanasekaran SM, Varambally S, Barrette TR, Sanda MG, Pienta KJ, Ghosh D, Chinnaiyan AM (2002). alpha-Methylacyl coenzyme A racemase as a tissue biomarker for prostate cancer. *JAMA* 287: 1662-1670.
2260. Rudrick B, Nguyen GK, Lakey WH (1995). Carcinoid tumor of the renal pelvis: report of a case with positive urine cytology. *Diagn Cytopathol* 12: 360-363.
2261. Ruijter ET, van de Kaa CA, Schalken JA, Debruyne FM, Ruiter DJ (1996). Histological grade heterogeneity in multifocal prostate cancer. Biological and clinical implications. *J Pathol* 180: 295-299.
2262. Rumpelt HJ, Storkel S, Moll R, Scharfe T, Thoenes W (1991). Bellini duct carcinoma: further evidence for this rare variant of renal cell carcinoma. *Histopathology* 18: 115-122.
2263. Rundle JS, Hart AJ, McGeorge A, Smith JS, Malcolm AJ, Smith PM (1982). Squamous cell carcinoma of bladder. A review of 114 patients. *Br J Urol* 54: 522-526.
2264. Rushton HG, Belman AB, Sesterhenn I, Patterson K, Mostofi FK (1990). Testicular sparing surgery for prepubertal teratoma of the testis: a clinical and pathological study. *J Urol* 144: 726-730.
2265. Rustin GJ, Vogelzang NJ, Sleijfer DT, Nisselbaum JN (1990). Consensus statement on circulating tumour markers and staging patients with germ cell tumours. *Prog Clin Biol Res* 357: 277-284.
2266. Rutgers JL (1991). Adenomas in the pathology of intersex syndrome. *Hum Pathol* 22: 384-394.
2267. Rutgers JL, Scully RE (1987). Pathology of the testis in intersex syndromes. *Semin Diagn Pathol* 4: 275-291.
2268. Rutgers JL, Scully RE (1991). The androgen insensitivity syndrome (testicular feminization): a clinicopathologic study of 43 cases. *Int J Gynecol Pathol* 10: 126-144.
2269. Rutgers JL, Young RH, Scully RE (1988). The testicular "tumor" of the adrenogenital syndrome. A report of six cases and review of the literature on testicular masses in patients with adrenocortical disorders. *Am J Surg Pathol* 12: 503-513.
2270. Sabroe S, Olsen J (1998). Perinatal correlates of specific histological types of testicular cancer in patients below 35 years of age: a case-cohort study based on midwives' records in Denmark. *Int J Cancer* 78: 140-143.
2271. Sacker AR, Oyama KK, Kessler S (1994). Primary osteosarcoma of the penis. *Am J Dermatopathol* 16: 285-287.
2272. Sahin AA, Myhre M, Ro JY, Sneige N, Dekmezian RH, Ayala AG (1991). Plasmacytoid transitional cell carcinoma. Report of a case with initial presentation mimicking multiple myeloma. *Acta Cytol* 35: 277-280.
2273. Saint-Andre JP, Chapeau MC, Pein F (1988). [Nephroblastoma with symptomatic neuronal differentiation]. *Ann Pathol* 8: 144-148.
2274. Saito S, Iwaki H (1999). Mucin-producing carcinoma of the prostate: review of 88 cases. *Urology* 54: 141-144.
2275. Saito T (2000). Glomus tumor of the penis. *Int J Urol* 7: 115-117.
2276. Sakamoto N, Tsuneyoshi M, Enjoji M (1992). Urinary bladder carcinoma with a neoplastic squamous component: a mapping study of 31 cases. *Histopathology* 21: 135-141.
2277. Sakashita N, Takeya M, Kishida T, Stackhouse TM, Zbar B, Takahashi K (1999). Expression of von Hippel-Lindau protein in normal and pathological human tissues. *Histochem J* 31: 133-144.
2278. Sakr WA (1999). Prostatic intraepithelial neoplasia: A marker for high-risk groups and a potential target for chemoprevention. *Eur Urol* 35: 474-478.
2279. Sakr WA, Grignon DJ, Haas GP (1998). Pathology of premalignant lesions and carcinoma of the prostate in African-American men. *Semin Urol Oncol* 16: 214-220.
2280. Sakr WA, Haas GP, Cassin BF, Pontes JE, Crissman JD (1993). The frequency of carcinoma and intraepithelial neoplasia of the prostate in young male patients. *J Urol* 150: 379-385.
2281. Sakr WA, Macoska JA, Benson P, Grignon DJ, Wolman SR, Pontes JE, Crissman JD (1994). Allelic loss in locally metastatic, multisampled prostate cancer. *Cancer Res* 54: 3273-3277.
2282. Sakr WA, Tefilli MV, Grignon DJ, Banerjee M, Dey J, Gheiler EL, Tiguert R, Powell IJ, Wood DP (2000). Gleason score 7 prostate cancer: a heterogeneous entity? Correlation with pathologic parameters and disease-free survival. *Urology* 56: 730-734.
2283. Sakr WA, Wheeler TM, Blute M, Bodo M, Calle-Rodrigue R, Henson DE, Mostofi FK, Seiffert J, Wojno K, Zincke H (1996). Staging and reporting of prostate cancer—sampling of the radical prostatectomy specimen. *Cancer* 78: 366-368.
2284. Salem Y, Pagliaro LC, Manyak MJ (1993). Primary small noncleaved cell lymphoma of kidney. *Urology* 42: 331-335.
2285. Salo JO, Rannikko S, Makinen J, Lehtonen T (1987). Echogenic structure of prostatic cancer imaged on radical prostatectomy specimens. *Prostate* 10: 1-9.
2286. Salo P, Kaariainen H, Petrovic V, Peltomaki P, Page DC, de la Chapelle A (1995). Molecular mapping of the putative gonadoblastoma locus on the Y chromosome. *Genes Chromosomes Cancer* 14: 210-214.
2287. Salomao DR, Graham SD, Bostwick DG (1995). Microvascular invasion in prostate cancer correlates with pathologic stage. *Arch Pathol Lab Med* 119: 1050-1054.
2288. Sanchez-Chapado M, Angulo JC, Haas GP (1995). Adenocarcinoma of the rete testis. *Urology* 46: 468-475.
2289. Sandberg AA (1986). Chromosome changes in bladder cancer: clinical and other correlations. *Cancer Genet Cytogenet* 19: 163-175.
2290. Sandberg AA, Meloni AM, Suijkerbuijk RF (1996). Reviews of chromosome studies in urological tumors. III. Cytogenetics and genes in testicular tumors. *J Urol* 155: 1531-1556.
2291. Sanders ME, Mick R, Tomaszewski JE, Barr FG (2002). Unique patterns of allelic imbalance distinguish type 1 from type 2 sporadic papillary renal cell carcinoma. *Am J Pathol* 161: 997-1005.
2292. Santos LD, Wong CS, Killingsworth M (2001). Cystadenoma of the seminal vesicle: report of a case with ultrastructural findings. *Pathology* 33: 399-402.
2293. Sarkis AS, Bajorin DF, Reuter VE, Herr HW, Netto G, Zhang ZF, Schultz PK, Cordon-Cardo C, Scher HI (1995). Prognostic value of p53 nuclear overexpression in patients with invasive bladder cancer treated with neoadjuvant MVAC. *J Clin Oncol* 13: 1384-1390.
2294. Sarkis AS, Dalbagni G, Cordon-Cardo C, Melamed J, Zhang ZF, Sheinfeld J, Fair WR, Herr HW, Reuter VE (1994). Association of P53 nuclear overexpression and tumor progression in carcinoma in situ of the bladder. *J Urol* 152: 388-392.
2295. Sarkis AS, Dalbagni G, Cordon-Cardo C, Zhang ZF, Sheinfeld J, Fair WR, Herr HW, Reuter VE (1993). Nuclear overexpression of p53 protein in transitional cell bladder carcinoma: a marker for disease progression. *J Natl Cancer Inst* 85: 53-59.
2296. Sarkis AS, Zhang ZF, Cordon CC, Melamed J, Dalbagni G, Sheinfeld J, Fair WR, Herr HW, Reuter VE (1993). p53 Nuclear overexpression and disease progression in Ta bladder carcinoma. *Int J Oncol* 3: 355-360.
2297. Sarma KP (1970). Squamous cell carcinoma of the bladder. *Int Surg* 53: 313-319.
2298. Sarosdy MF, Schellhammer P, Bokinsky G, Kahn P, Chao R, Yore L, Zadra J, Burzon D, Osher G, Bridge JA, Anderson S, Johansson SL, Lieber M, Soloway M, Flom K (2002). Clinical evaluation of a multi-target fluorescent in situ hybridization assay for detection of bladder cancer. *J Urol* 168: 1950-1954.
2299. Satie AP, Rajpert-de Meyts E, Spagnoli GC, Henno S, Olivo L, Jacobsen GK, Rioux-Leclercq N, Jegou B, Samson M (2002). The cancer-testis gene, NY-ESO-1, is expressed in normal fetal and adult testes and in spermatocytic seminomas and testicular carcinoma in situ. *Lab Invest* 82: 775-780.
2300. Sato D, Kase T, Tajima M, Sawamura Y, Matsushima M, Wakayama M, Kuwajima A (2001). Penile schwannoma. *Int J Urol* 8: 87-89.
2301. Sato K, Moriyama M, Mori S, Saito M, Watanuki T, Terada K, Okuhara E, Akiyama T, Toyoshima K, Yamamoto T, Kato T (1992). An immunohistologic evaluation of C-erbB-2 gene product in patients with urinary bladder carcinoma. *Cancer* 70: 2493-2498.
2302. Satoh E, Miyao N, Tachiki H, Fujisawa Y (2002). Prediction of muscle invasion of bladder cancer by cystoscopy. *Eur Urol* 41: 178-181.
2303. Sauter ER, Schorin MA, Farr GHJr, Falterman KW, Arensman RM (1990). Wilms' tumor with metastasis to the left testis. *Am Surg* 56: 260-262.
2304. Sauter G, Gasser TC, Moch H, Richter J, Jiang F, Albrecht R, Novotny H, Wagner U, Bubendorf L, Mihatsch MJ (1997). DNA aberrations in urinary bladder cancer detected by flow cytometry and FISH. *Urol Res* 25 Suppl 1: 37-43.
2305. Sauter G, Haley J, Chew K, Kerschmann R, Moore D, Carroll P, Moch H, Gudat F, Mihatsch MJ, Waldman F (1994). Epidermal-growth-factor-receptor expression is associated with rapid tumor proliferation in bladder cancer. *Int J Cancer* 57: 508-514.
2306. Sauter G, Mihatsch MJ (1998). Pussycats and baby tigers: non-invasive (pTa) and minimally invasive (pT1) bladder carcinomas are not the same! *J Pathol* 185: 339-341.
2307. Sauter G, Moch H, Carroll P, Kerschmann R, Mihatsch MJ, Waldman FM (1995). Chromosome-9 loss detected by fluorescence in situ hybridization in bladder cancer. *Int J Cancer* 64: 99-103.
2308. Sauter G, Moch H, Gudat F, Mihatsch MJ, Haley J, Meecker T, Waldman F (1993). [Demonstration of gene amplification in urinary bladder cancer by fluorescent in situ hybridization (FISH)]. *Verh Dtsch Ges Pathol* 77: 247-251.
2309. Sauter G, Moch H, Moore D, Carroll P, Kerschmann R, Chew K, Mihatsch MJ, Gudat F, Waldman F (1993). Heterogeneity of erbB-2 gene amplification in bladder cancer. *Cancer Res* 53: 2199-2203.
2310. Sauter G, Moch H, Wagner U, Novotna H, Gasser TC, Mattarelli G, Mihatsch MJ, Waldman FM (1995). Y chromosome loss detected by FISH in bladder cancer. *Cancer Genet Cytogenet* 82: 163-169.
2311. Savla J, Chen TT, Schneider NR, Timmons CF, Delattre O, Tomlinson GE (2000). Mutations of the hSNF5/INI1 gene in renal rhabdoid tumors with second primary brain tumors. *J Natl Cancer Inst* 92: 648-650.
2312. Saw D, Tse CH, Chan J, Watt CY, Ng CS, Poon YF (1986). Clear cell sarcoma of the penis. *Hum Pathol* 17: 423-425.
2313. Sawczuk I, Tannenbaum M, Olsson CA, de Vere White R (1985). Primary transitional cell carcinoma of prostatic periurethral ducts. *Urology* 25: 339-343.
2314. Sawyer JR, Tryka AF, Lewis JM (1992). A novel reciprocal chromosome translocation t(11;22)(p13;q12) in an intraabdominal desmoplastic small round-cell tumor. *Am J Surg Pathol* 16: 411-416.
2315. Schade RO, Swinney J (1968). Pre-cancerous changes in bladder epithelium. *Lancet* 2: 943-946.
2316. Schaffer AA, Simon R, Desper R, Richter J, Sauter G (2001). Tree models for dependent copy number changes in bladder cancer. *Int J Oncol* 18: 349-354.
2317. Schally AV, Comaru-Schally AM, Plonowski A, Nagy A, Halmos G, Rekasi Z (2000). Peptide analogs in the therapy of prostate cancer. *Prostate* 45: 158-166.
2318. Schellhammer PF (1983). Urethral carcinoma. *Semin Urol* 1: 82-89.
2319. Schellhammer PF, Whitmore WFJr (1976). Transitional cell carcinoma of the urethra in men having cystectomy for bladder cancer. *J Urol* 115: 56-60.
2320. Schenkman NS, Moul JW, Nicely ER, Maggio MI, Ho CK (1993). Synchronous bilateral testis tumor: mixed germ cell and theca cell tumors. *Urology* 42: 593-595.
2321. Schillinger F, Montagnac R (1996). Chronic renal failure and its treatment in tuberous sclerosis. *Nephrol Dial Transplant* 11: 481-485.
2322. Schindler S, de Frias DV, Yu GH (1999). Primary angiosarcoma of the bladder: cytomorphology and differential diagnosis. *Cytopathology* 10: 137-143.
2323. Schips L, Augustin H, Zigeuner RE, Galle G, Habermann H, Trummer H, Pummer K, Hubmer G (2002). Is repeated transurethral resection justified in patients with newly diagnosed superficial bladder cancer? *Urology* 59: 220-223.
2324. Schmauz R, Cole P (1974). Epidemiology of cancer of the renal pelvis and ureter. *J Natl Cancer Inst* 52: 1431-1434.
2325. Schmidt BA, Rose A, Steinhoff C, Strohmeyer T, Hartmann M, Ackermann R (2001). Up-regulation of cyclin-dependent kinase 4/cyclin D2 expression but down-regulation of cyclin-dependent kinase 2/cyclin E in testicular germ cell tumors. *Cancer Res* 61: 4214-4221.
2326. Schmidt L, Duh FM, Chen F, Kishida T, Glenn G, Choyke P, Scherer SW, Zhuang Z, Lubensky I, Dean M, Allikmets R, Chidambaram A, Bergerheim UR, Feltis JT, Casadevall C, Zamarron A, Bernues M, Richard S, Lips CJ, Walther MM, Tsui LC, Geil L, Orcutt ML, Stackhouse T, Lipan J, Slife L, Brauch H, Decker J, Niehans G, Hughson MD, Moch H, Storkel S, Lerman MI, Linehan WM, Zbar B (1997). Germline and somatic mutations in the tyrosine kinase domain of the MET proto-oncogene in papillary renal carcinomas. *Nat Genet* 16: 68-73.

2327. Schmidt L, Junker K, Weirich G, Glenn G, Choyke P, Lubensky I, Zhuang Z, Jeffers M, Vande Woude G, Neumann H, Walther M, Linehan WM, Zbar B (1998). Two North American families with hereditary papillary renal carcinoma and identical novel mutations in the MET proto-oncogene. *Cancer Res* 58: 1719-1722.
2328. Schmidt LS, Warren MB, Nickerson ML, Weirich G, Matrosova V, Toro JR, Turner ML, Duray P, Merino M, Hewitt S, Pavlovich CP, Glenn G, Greenberg CR, Linehan WM, Zbar B (2001). Birt-Hogg-Dube syndrome, a genodermatosis associated with spontaneous pneumothorax and kidney neoplasia, maps to chromosome 17p11.2. *Am J Hum Genet* 69: 876-882.
2329. Schmitz-Drager BJ, Goebell PJ, Ebert T, Fradet Y (2000). p53 immunohistochemistry as a prognostic marker in bladder cancer. Playground for urology scientists? *Eur Urol* 38: 691-699.
2330. Schmitz-Drager BJ, Kushima M, Goebell P, Jax TW, Gerharz CD, Bultel H, Schulz WA, Ebert T, Ackermann R (1997). p53 and MDM2 in the development and progression of bladder cancer. *Eur Urol* 32: 487-493.
2331. Schmitz-Drager BJ, van Roeyen CR, Grimm MO, Gerharz CD, Decken K, Schulz WA, Bultel H, Makri D, Ebert T, Ackermann R (1994). P53 accumulation in precursor lesions and early stages of bladder cancer. *World J Urol* 12: 79-83.
2332. Schned AR, Ledbetter JS, Selikowitz SM (1986). Primary leiomyosarcoma of the seminal vesicle. *Cancer* 57: 2202-2206.
2333. Schneider A, Brand T, Zweigerdt R, Arnold H (2000). Targeted disruption of the Nkx3.1 gene in mice results in morphogenetic defects of minor salivary glands: parallels to glandular duct morphogenesis in prostate. *Mech Dev* 95: 163-174.
2334. Schneider DT, Schuster AE, Fritsch MK, Hu J, Olson T, Lauer S, Gobel U, Perlman EJ (2001). Multipoint imprinting analysis indicates a common precursor cell for gonadal and nongonadal pediatric germ cell tumors. *Cancer Res* 61: 7268-7276.
2335. Schoenberg M, Cairns P, Brooks JD, Marshall FF, Epstein JI, Isaacs WB, Sidransky D (1995). Frequent loss of chromosome arms 8p and 13q in collecting duct carcinoma (CDC) of the kidney. *Genes Chromosomes Cancer* 12: 76-80.
2336. Schoenberg M, Kiemeney L, Walsh PC, Griffin CA, Sidransky D (1996). Germline translocation t(5;20)(p15;q11) and familial transitional cell carcinoma. *J Urol* 155: 1035-1036.
2337. Schoenberg MP, Hakimi JM, Wang S, Bova GS, Epstein JI, Fischbeck KH, Isaacs WB, Walsh PC, Barrack ER (1994). Microsatellite mutation (CAG24—>18) in the androgen receptor gene in human prostate cancer. *Biochem Biophys Res Commun* 198: 74-80.
2338. Schofield DE, Yunis EJ, Fletcher JA (1993). Chromosome aberrations in mesoblastic nephroma. *Am J Pathol* 143: 714-724.
2339. Schraml P, Kononen J, Bubendorf L, Moch H, Bissig H, Nocito A, Mihatsch MJ, Kallioniemi OP, Sauter G (1999). Tissue microarrays for gene amplification surveys in many different tumor types. *Clin Cancer Res* 5: 1966-1975.
2340. Schraml P, Muller D, Bednar R, Gasser T, Sauter G, Mihatsch MJ, Moch H (2000). Allelic loss at the D9S171 locus on chromosome 9p13 is associated with progression of papillary renal cell carcinoma. *J Pathol* 190: 457-461.
2341. Schraml P, Struckmann K, Bednar R, Fu W, Gasser T, Wilber K, Kononen J, Sauter G, Mihatsch MJ, Moch H (2001). CDKNA2A mutation analysis, protein expression, and deletion mapping of chromosome 9p in conventional clear-cell renal carcinomas: evidence for a second tumor suppressor gene proximal to CDKN2A. *Am J Pathol* 158: 593-601.
2342. Schraml P, Struckmann K, Hatz F, Sonnet S, Kully C, Gasser T, Sauter G, Mihatsch MJ, Moch H (2002). VHL mutations and their correlation with tumour cell proliferation, microvessel density, and patient prognosis in clear cell renal cell carcinoma. *J Pathol* 196: 186-193.
2343. Schubert GE, Pavkovic MB, Bethke-Bedurftig BA (1982). Tubular urachal remnants in adult bladders. *J Urol* 127: 40-42.
2344. Schullerus D, Herbers J, Chudek J, Kanamaru H, Kovacs G (1997). Loss of heterozygosity at chromosomes 8p, 9p, and 14q is associated with stage and grade of non-papillary renal cell carcinomas. *J Pathol* 183: 151-155.
2345. Schullerus D, von Knobloch R, Chudek J, Herbers J, Kovacs G (1999). Microsatellite analysis reveals deletion of a large region at chromosome 8p in conventional renal cell carcinoma. *Int J Cancer* 80: 22-24.
2346. Schutte B (1988). Early testicular cancer in severe oligozoospermia. In: *Carl Schirren Symposium: Advances in Andrology*, AF Holstein, F Leidenberger, HK Holzer, G Bettendorf, eds. Diesbach Verlag: Berlin, pp. 188-190.
2347. Schwerk WB, Schwerk WN, Rodeck G (1987). Testicular tumors: prospective analysis of real-time US patterns and abdominal staging. *Radiology* 164: 369-374.
2348. Scott RJr, Mutchnik DL, Laskowski TZ, Schmalhorst WR (1969). Carcinoma of the prostate in elderly men: incidence, growth characteristics and clinical significance. *J Urol* 101: 602-607.
2349. Scully RE (1950). Spermatocytic seminoma of the testis. A report of 3 cases and review of the literature. *Cancer* 14: 788-794.
2350. Scully RE (1970). Gonadoblastoma. A review of 74 cases. *Cancer* 25: 1340-1356.
2351. Seery WH (1968). Granular cell myoblastoma of the bladder: report of a case. *J Urol* 100: 735-737.
2352. Segawa N, Mori I, Utsunomiya H, Nakamura M, Nakamura Y, Shan L, Kakudo K, Katsuoka Y (2001). Prognostic significance of neuroendocrine differentiation, proliferation activity and androgen receptor expression in prostate cancer. *Pathol Int* 51: 452-459.
2353. Segelov E, Cox KM, Raghavan D, McNeil E, Lancaster L, Rogers J (1993). The impact of histological review on clinical management of testicular cancer. *Br J Urol* 71: 736-738.
2354. Sehdev AE, Pan CC, Epstein JI (2001). Comparative analysis of sampling methods for grossing radical prostatectomy specimens performed for nonpalpable (stage T1c) prostatic adenocarcinoma. *Hum Pathol* 32: 494-499.
2355. Sehested M, Jacobsen GK (1987). Ultrastructure of syncytiotrophoblast-like cells in seminomas of the testis. *Int J Androl* 10: 121-126.
2356. Seibel JL, Prasad S, Weiss RE, Bancila E, Epstein JI (2002). Villous adenoma of the urinary tract: a lesion frequently associated with malignancy. *Hum Pathol* 33: 236-241.
2357. Selli C, Amorosi A, Vona G, Sestini R, Travaglini F, Bartoletti R, Orlando C (1997). Retrospective evaluation of c-erbB-2 oncogene amplification using competitive PCR in collecting duct carcinoma of the kidney. *J Urol* 158: 245-247.
2358. Selli C, Montironi R, Bono A, Pagano F, Zattoni F, Manganelli A, Selvaggi FP, Comeri G, Fiaccavento G, Guazzieri S, Lembo A, Cosciani-Cunico S, Potenzoni D, Muto G, Mazzucchelli R, Santinelli A (2002). Effects of complete androgen blockade for 12 and 24 weeks on the pathological stage and resection margin status of prostate cancer. *J Clin Pathol* 55: 508-513.
2359. Semenza JC, Ziogas A, Largent J, Peel D, Anton-Culver H (2001). Gene-environment interactions in renal cell carcinoma. *Am J Epidemiol* 153: 851-859.
2360. Senel MF, van Buren CT, Riggs S, Clark J3rd, Etheridge WB, Kahan BD (1996). Post-transplantation lymphoproliferative disorder in the renal transplant ureter. *J Urol* 155: 2025.
2361. Senoh H, Ichikawa Y, Okuyama A, Takaha M, Sonoda T (1986). Cavernous hemangioma of scrotum and penile shaft. *Urol Int* 41: 309-311.
2362. Serra AD, Hricak H, Coakley FV, Kim B, Dudley A, Morey A, Tschumper B, Carroll PR (1998). Inconclusive clinical and ultrasound evaluation of the scrotum: impact of magnetic resonance imaging on patient management and cost. *Urology* 51: 1018-1021.
2363. Serrano-Olmo J, Tang CK, Seidmon EJ, Ellison NE, Elfenbein IB, Ming PM (1993). Neuroblastoma as a prominent component of a mixed germ cell tumor of testis. *Cancer* 72: 3271-3276.
2364. Serth J, Kuczyk MA, Bokemeyer C, Hervatin C, Nafe R, Tan HK, Jonas U (1995). p53 immunohistochemistry as an independent prognostic factor for superficial transitional cell carcinoma of the bladder. *Br J Cancer* 71: 201-205.
2365. Sesterhenn I, Davis CJJr, Mostofi FK (1987). Undifferentiated malignant epithelial tumors involving serosal surfaces of scrotum and abdomen in young males. *J Urol* 137: 214.
2366. Sesterhenn IA, Mostofi FK, Davis CJ (1986). Testicular tumours in infants and children. In: *Advances in the Biosciences Germ Cell Tumours II*, WG Jones, ed. Pergamon Press: Oxford, pp. 173-184.
2367. Sesterhenn IA, Weiss RB, Mostofi FK, Stablein DM, Rowland RG, Falkson G, Rivkind SE, Vogelzang NJ (1992). Prognosis and other clinical correlates of pathologic review in stage I and II testicular carcinoma: a report from the Testicular Cancer Intergroup Study. *J Clin Oncol* 10: 69-78.
2368. Sevenet N, Sheridan E, Amram D, Schneider P, Handgretinger R, Delattre O (1999). Constitutional mutations of the hSNF5/INI1 gene predispose to a variety of cancers. *Am J Hum Genet* 65: 1342-1348.
2369. Sexton WJ, Lance RE, Reyes AO, Pisters PW, Tu SM, Pisters LL (2001). Adult prostate sarcoma: the M.D. Anderson Cancer Center Experience. *J Urol* 166: 521-525.
2370. Seymour JF, Solomon B, Wolf MM, Janusczewicz EH, Wirth A, Prince HM (2001). Primary large-cell non-Hodgkin's lymphoma of the testis: a retrospective analysis of patterns of failure and prognostic factors. *Clin Lymphoma* 2: 109-115.
2371. Sgambato A, Migaldi M, Faraglia B, de Aloysio G, Ferrari P, Ardito R, de Gaetani C, Capelli G, Cittadini A, Trentini GP (2002). Cyclin D1 expression in papillary superficial bladder cancer: its association with other cell cycle-associated proteins, cell proliferation and clinical outcome. *Int J Cancer* 97: 671-678.
2372. Sgrignoli AR, Walsh PC, Steinberg GD, Steiner MS, Epstein JI (1994). Prognostic factors in men with stage D1 prostate cancer: identification of patients less likely to have prolonged survival after radical prostatectomy. *J Urol* 152: 1077-1081.
2373. Shaaban AA, Javadpour N, Tribukait B, Ghoneim MA (1992). Prognostic significance of flow-DNA analysis and cell surface isoantigens in carcinoma of bilharzial bladder. *Urology* 39: 207-210.
2374. Shah RB, Zhou M, LeBlanc M, Snyder M, Rubin MA (2002). Comparison of the basal cell-specific markers, 34betaE12 and p63, in the diagnosis of prostate cancer. *Am J Surg Pathol* 26: 1161-1168.
2375. Shamberger RC, Smith EI, Joshi VV, Rao PV, Hayes FA, Bowman LC, Castleberry RP (1998). The risk of nephrectomy during local control in abdominal neuroblastoma. *J Pediatr Surg* 33: 161-164.
2376. Shannon RL, Ro JY, Grignon DJ, Ordonez NG, Johnson DE, Mackay B, Tetu B, Ayala AG (1992). Sarcomatoid carcinoma of the prostate. A clinicopathologic study of 12 patients. *Cancer* 69: 2676-2682.
2377. Shapeero LG, Vordermark JS (1993). Epidermoid cysts of testes and role of sonography. *Urology* 41: 75-79.
2378. Sharpe RM, Skakkebaek NE (1993). Are oestrogens involved in falling sperm counts and disorders of the male reproductive tract? *Lancet* 341: 1392-1395.
2379. Shaw JL, Gislason GJ, Imbriglia JE (1958). Transition of cystitis glandularis to primary adenocarcinoma of the bladder. *J Urol* 79: 815-822.
2380. Shaw ME, Elder PA, Abbas A, Knowles MA (1999). Partial allelotype of schistosomiasis-associated bladder cancer. *Int J Cancer* 80: 656-661.
2381. Shearer P, Parham DM, Fontanesi J, Kumar M, Lobe TE, Fairclough D, Douglass EC, Wilimas J (1993). Bilateral Wilms tumor. Review of outcome, associated abnormalities, and late effects in 36 pediatric patients treated at a single institution. *Cancer* 72: 1422-1426.
2382. Sheil O, Redman CW, Pugh C (1991). Renal failure in pregnancy due to primary renal lymphoma. Case report. *Br J Obstet Gynaecol* 98: 216-217.
2383. Sheldon CA, Clayman RV, Gonzalez R, Williams RD, Fraley EE (1984). Malignant urachal lesions. *J Urol* 131: 1-8.
2384. Shen T, Zhuang Z, Gersell DJ, Tavassoli FA (2000). Allelic deletion of VHL gene detected in papillary tumors of the broad ligament, epididymis, and retroperitoneum in von Hippel-Lindau disease patients. *Int J Surg Pathol* 8: 207-212.
2385. Shende A, Wind ES, Lanzkowsky P (1979). Intrarenal neuroblastoma mimicking Wilms' tumor. *N Y State J Med* 79: 93.
2386. Shepherd D, Keetch DW, Humphrey PA, Smith DS, Stahl D (1996). Repeat biopsy strategy in men with isolated prostatic intraepithelial neoplasia on prostate needle biopsy. *J Urol* 156: 460-462.
2387. Sherif A, de la Torre M, Malmstrom PU, Thorn M (2001). Lymphatic mapping and detection of sentinel nodes in patients with bladder cancer. *J Urol* 166: 812-815.

2388. Sherman JL, Hartman DS, Friedman AC, Madewell JE, Davis CJ, Goldman SM (1981). Angiomyolipoma: computed tomographic-pathologic correlation of 17 cases. *AJR Am J Roentgenol* 137: 1221-1226.

2389. Shibata A, Whittemore AS (1997). Genetic predisposition to prostate cancer: possible explanations for ethnic differences in risk. *Prostate* 32: 65-72.

2390. Shiina H, Igawa M, Shigeno K, Yamasaki Y, Urakami S, Yoneda T, Wada Y, Honda S, Nagasaki M (1999). Clinical significance of mdm2 and p53 expression in bladder cancer. A comparison with cell proliferation and apoptosis. *Oncology* 56: 239-247.

2391. Shimazui T, Giroldi LA, Bringuier PP, Oosterwijk E, Schalken JA (1996). Complex cadherin expression in renal cell carcinoma. *Cancer Res* 56: 3234-3237.

2392. Shimizu H, Ross RK, Bernstein L (1991). Possible underestimation of the incidence rate of prostate cancer in Japan. *Jpn J Cancer Res* 82: 483-485.

2393. Shimura S, Uchida T, Shitara T, Nishimura K, Murayama M, Honda N, Koshiba K (1991). [Primary carcinoid tumor of the testis with metastasis to the upper vertebrae. Report of a case]. *Nippon Hinyokika Gakkai Zasshi* 82: 1157-1160.

2394. Shin KY, Kong G, Kim WS, Lee TY, Woo YN, Lee JD (1997). Overexpression of cyclin D1 correlates with early recurrence in superficial bladder cancers. *Br J Cancer* 75: 1788-1792.

2395. Shinohara N, Koyanagi T (2002). Ras signal transduction in carcinogenesis and progression of bladder cancer: molecular target for treatment? *Urol Res* 30: 273-281.

2396. Shipman R, Schraml P, Colombi M, Raefle G, Ludwig CU (1993). Loss of heterozygosity on chromosome 11p13 in primary bladder carcinoma. *Hum Genet* 91: 455-458.

2397. Shirahama T (2000). Cyclooxygenase-2 expression is up-regulated in transitional cell carcinoma and its preneoplastic lesions in the human urinary bladder. *Clin Cancer Res* 6: 2424-2430.

2398. Shmookler BM, Enzinger FM, Weiss SW (1989). Giant cell fibroblastoma. A juvenile form of dermatofibrosarcoma protuberans. *Cancer* 64: 2154-2161.

2399. Shubber EK (1987). Sister-chromatid exchanges in lymphocytes from patients with Schistosoma hematobium. *Mutat Res* 180: 93-99.

2400. Shuin T, Kondo K, Torigoe S, Kishida T, Kubota Y, Hosaka M, Nagashima Y, Kitamura H, Latif F, Zbar B, Lerman MI, Yao M (1994). Frequent somatic mutations and loss of heterozygosity of the von Hippel-Lindau tumor suppressor gene in primary human renal cell carcinomas. *Cancer Res* 54: 2852-2855.

2401. Shurbaji MS, Kuhajda FP, Pasternack GR, Thurmond TS (1992). Expression of oncogenic antigen 519 (OA-519) in prostate cancer is a potential prognostic indicator. *Am J Clin Pathol* 97: 686-691.

2402. Shvarts O, Han KR, Seltzer M, Pantuck AJ, Belldegrun AS (2002). Positron emission tomography in urologic oncology. *Cancer Control* 9: 335-342.

2403. Sibley K, Cuthbert-Heavens D, Knowles MA (2001). Loss of heterozygosity at 4p16.3 and mutation of FGFR3 in transitional cell carcinoma. *Oncogene* 20: 686-691.

2404. Sicinski P, Donaher JL, Geng Y, Parker SB, Gardner H, Park MY, Robker RL, Richards JS, McGinnis LK, Biggers JD, Eppig JJ, Bronson RT, Elledge SJ, Weinberg RA (1996). Cyclin D2 is an FSH-responsive gene involved in gonadal cell proliferation and oncogenesis. *Nature* 384: 470-474.

2405. Sidransky D, Frost P, von Eschenbach A, Oyasu R, Preisinger AC, Vogelstein B (1992). Clonal origin bladder cancer. *N Engl J Med* 326: 737-740.

2406. Siegal GP, Gaffey TA (1976). Solitary leiomyomas arising from the tunica dartos scroti. *J Urol* 116: 69-71.

2407. Siegrist S, Feral C, Chami M, Solhonne B, Mattei MG, Rajpert-de Meyts E, Guellaen G, Bulle F (2001). hH-Rev107, a class II tumor suppressor gene, is expressed by post-meiotic testicular germ cells and CIS cells but not by human testicular germ cell tumors. *Oncogene* 20: 5155-5163.

2408. Sieniawska M, Bialasik D, Jedrzejowski A, Sopylo B, Maldyk J (1997). Bilateral primary renal Burkitt lymphoma in a child presenting with acute renal failure. *Nephrol Dial Transplant* 12: 1490-1492.

2409. Sigg C, Hedinger C (1984). Atypical germ cells of the testis. Comparative ultrastructural and immunohistochemical investigations. *Virchows Arch A Pathol Anat Histopathol* 402: 439-450.

2410. Signoretti S, Waltregny D, Dilks J, Isaac B, Lin D, Garraway L, Yang A, Montironi R, McKeon F, Loda M (2000). p63 is a prostate basal cell marker and is required for prostate development. *Am J Pathol* 157: 1769-1775.

2411. Sijmons RH, Kiemeney LA, Witjes JA, Vasen HF (1998). Urinary tract cancer and hereditary nonpolyposis colorectal cancer: risks and screening options. *J Urol* 160: 466-470.

2412. Silver DA, Pellicer I, Fair WR, Heston WD, Cordon-Cardo C (1997). Prostate-specific membrane antigen expression in normal and malignant human tissues. *Clin Cancer Res* 3: 81-85.

2413. Silver SA, Wiley JM, Perlman EJ (1994). DNA ploidy analysis of pediatric germ cell tumors. *Mod Pathol* 7: 951-956.

2414. Silverman ML, Eyre RC, Zinman LA, Corsson AW (1981). Mixed mucinous and papillary adenocarcinoma involving male urethra, probably originating in periurethral glands. *Cancer* 47: 1398-1402.

2415. Sim SJ, Ro JY, Ordonez NG, Park YW, Kee KH, Ayala AG (1999). Metastatic renal cell carcinoma to the bladder: a clinicopathologic and immunohistochemical study. *Mod Pathol* 12: 351-355.

2416. Simard C, Tayot J, Francois H, Bertrand G, Soret JY, Pantin J (1975). [Potts-Hirst "inverted" urothelial papilloma. Apropos of 2 vesical cases]. *Arch Anat Pathol (Paris)* 23: 139-144.

2417. Simon R, Atefy R, Wagner U, Forster T, Fijan A, Bruderer J, Wilber K, Mihatsch MJ, Gasser T, Sauter G (2003). HER-2 and TOP2A coamplification in urinary bladder cancer. *Int J Cancer* 107: 764-772.

2418. Simon R, Burger H, Brinkschmidt C, Bocker W, Hertle L, Terpe HJ (1998). Chromosomal aberrations associated with invasion in papillary superficial bladder cancer. *J Pathol* 185: 345-351.

2419. Simon R, Burger H, Semjonow A, Hertle L, Terpe HJ, Bocker W (2000). Patterns of chromosomal imbalances in muscle invasive bladder cancer. *Int J Oncol* 17: 1025-1029.

2420. Simon R, Eltze E, Schafer KL, Burger H, Semjonow A, Hertle L, Dockhorn-Dworniczak B, Terpe HJ, Bocker W (2001). Cytogenetic analysis of multifocal bladder cancer supports a monoclonal origin and intraepithelial spread of tumor cells. *Cancer Res* 61: 355-362.

2421. Simon R, Richter J, Wagner U, Fijan A, Bruderer J, Schmid U, Ackermann D, Maurer R, Alund G, Knonagel H, Rist M, Wilber K, Anabitarte M, Hering F, Hardmeier T, Schonenberger A, Flury R, Jager P, Fehr JL, Schraml P, Moch H, Mihatsch MJ, Gasser T, Sauter G (2001). High-throughput tissue microarray analysis of 3p25 (RAF1) and 8p12 (FGFR1) copy number alterations in urinary bladder cancer. *Cancer Res* 61: 4514-4519.

2422. Simon R, Struckmann K, Schraml P, Wagner U, Forster T, Moch H, Fijan A, Bruderer J, Wilber K, Mihatsch MJ, Gasser T, Sauter G (2002). Amplification pattern of 12q13-q15 genes (MDM2, CDK4, GLI) in urinary bladder cancer. *Oncogene* 21: 2476-2483.

2423. Simoneau AR, Spruck CH3rd, Gonzalez-Zulueta M, Gonzalgo ML, Chan MF, Tsai YC, Dean M, Steven K, Horn T, Jones PA (1996). Evidence for two tumor suppressor loci associated with proximal chromosome 9p to q and distal chromosome 9q in bladder cancer and the initial screening for GAS1 and PTC mutations. *Cancer Res* 56: 5039-5043.

2424. Singer AJ, Anders KH (1996). Neurilemoma of the kidney. *Urology* 47: 575-581.

2425. Singer G, Kurman RJ, McMaster MT, Shih IeM (2002). HLA-G immunoreactivity is specific for intermediate trophoblast in gestational trophoblastic disease and can serve as a useful marker in differential diagnosis. *Am J Surg Pathol* 26: 914-920.

2426. Singh D, Febbo PG, Ross K, Jackson DG, Manola J, Ladd C, Tamayo P, Renshaw AA, D'Amico AV, Richie JP, Lander ES, Loda M, Kantoff PW, Golub TR, Sellers WR (2002). Gene expression correlates of clinical prostate cancer behavior. *Cancer Cell* 1: 203-209.

2427. Singh N, Cumming J, Theaker JM (1997). Pure cartilaginous teratoma differentiated of the testis. *Histopathology* 30: 373-374.

2428. Sinke RJ, Suijkerbuijk RF, de Jong B, Oosterhuis JW, Geurts van Kessel A (1993). Uniparental origin of i(12p) in human germ cell tumors. *Genes Chromosomes Cancer* 6: 161-165.

2429. Skailes GE, Menasce L, Banerjee SS, Shanks JH, Logue JP (1998). Adenocarcinoma of the rete testis. *Clin Oncol (R Coll Radiol)* 10: 401-403.

2430. Skakkebaek NE (2002). Carcinoma in situ of the testis: frequency and relationship to invasive germ cell tumours in infertile men. N.E. Skakkebaek. *Histopathology* (1978) 2: 157-170. *Histopathology* 41: 2.

2431. Skakkebaek NE, Berthelsen JG, Muller J (1982). Carcinoma-in-situ of the undescended testis. *Urol Clin North Am* 9: 377-385.

2432. Skalsky YM, Ajuh PM, Parker C, Lamond AI, Goodwin G, Cooper CS (2001). PRCC, the commonest TFE3 fusion partner in papillary renal carcinoma is associated with pre-mRNA splicing factors. *Oncogene* 20: 178-187.

2433. Skinner DG, Colvin RB, Vermillion CD, Pfister RC, Leadbetter WF (1971). Diagnosis and management of renal cell carcinoma. A clinical and pathologic study of 309 cases. *Cancer* 28: 1165-1177.

2434. Skjorten FJ, Berner A, Harvei S, Robsahm TE, Tretli S (1997). Prostatic intraepithelial neoplasia in surgical resections: relationship to coexistent adenocarcinoma and atypical adenomatous hyperplasia of the prostate. *Cancer* 79: 1172-1179.

2435. Skotheim RI, Kraggerud SM, Fossa SD, Stenwig AE, Gedde-Dahl TJr, Danielsen HE, Jakobsen KS, Lothe RA (2001). Familial/bilateral and sporadic testicular germ cell tumors show frequent genetic changes at loci with suggestive linkage evidence. *Neoplasia* 3: 196-203.

2436. Skotheim RI, Monni O, Mousses S, Fossa SD, Kallioniemi OP, Lothe RA, Kallioniemi A (2002). New insights into testicular germ cell tumorigenesis from gene expression profiling. *Cancer Res* 62: 2359-2364.

2437. Slaton JW, Inoue K, Perrotte P, el-Naggar AK, Swanson DA, Fidler IJ, Dinney CP (2001). Expression levels of genes that regulate metastasis and angiogenesis correlate with advanced pathological stage of renal cell carcinoma. *Am J Pathol* 158: 735-743.

2438. Slaton JW, Morgenstern N, Levy DA, Santos MWJr, Tamboli P, Ro JY, Ayala AG, Pettaway CA (2001). Tumor stage, vascular invasion and the percentage of poorly differentiated cancer: independent prognosticators for inguinal lymph node metastasis in penile squamous cancer. *J Urol* 165: 1138-1142.

2439. Sloan SE, Rapoport JM (1985). Prostatic chondroma. *Urology* 25: 319-321.

2440. Small JD, Albertsen PC, Graydon RJ, Ricci AJr, Sardella WV (1992). Adenoid cystic carcinoma of Cowper's gland. *J Urol* 147: 699-701.

2441. Smeets W, Pauwels R, Geraedts J (1985). Chromosomal analysis of bladder cancer: technical aspects. *Cancer Genet Cytogenet* 16: 259-268.

2442. Smeets W, Pauwels R, Laarakkers L, Debruyne F, Geraedts J (1987). Chromosomal analysis of bladder cancer. III. Nonrandom alterations. *Cancer Genet Cytogenet* 29: 29-41.

2443. Smiraglia DJ, Szymanska J, Kraggerud SM, Lothe RA, Peltomaki P, Plass C (2002). Distinct epigenetic phenotypes in seminomatous and nonseminomatous testicular germ cell tumors. *Oncogene* 21: 3909-3916.

2444. Smith AH, Goycolea M, Haque R, Biggs ML (1998). Marked increase in bladder and lung cancer mortality in a region of Northern Chile due to arsenic in drinking water. *Am J Epidemiol* 147: 660-669.

2445. Smith BD, Flegel G (1983). Primary transitional cell carcinoma of the prostate: report of two cases. *J Am Osteopath Assoc* 82: 547-548.

2446. Smith DM, Manivel C, Kapps D, Uecker J (1986). Angiosarcoma of the prostate: report of 2 cases and review of the literature. *J Urol* 135: 382-384.

2447. Smith DM, Murphy WM (1994). Histologic changes in prostate carcinomas treated with leuprolide (luteinizing hormone-releasing hormone effect). Distinction from poor tumor differentiation. *Cancer* 73: 1472-1477.

2448. Smith DS, Catalona WJ (1994). The nature of prostate cancer detected through prostate specific antigen based screening. *J Urol* 152: 1732-1736.

2449. Smith EM, Resnick MI (1994). Ureteropelvic junction obstruction secondary to periureteral lipoma. *J Urol* 151: 150-151.

2450. Smith G, Elton RA, Beynon LL, Newsam JE, Chisholm GD, Hargreave TB (1983). Prognostic significance of biopsy results of normal-looking mucosa in cases of superficial bladder cancer. *Br J Urol* 55: 665-669.

2451. Smith JR, Freije D, Carpten JD, Gronberg H, Xu J, Isaacs SD, Brownstein MJ, Bova GS, Guo H, Bujnovszky P, Nusskern DR, Damber JE, Bergh A, Emanuelsson M, Kallioniemi OP, Walker-Daniels J, Bailey-Wilson JE, Beaty TH, Meyers DA, Walsh PC, Collins FS, Trent JM, Isaacs WB (1996). Major susceptibility locus for prostate cancer on chromosome 1 suggested by a genome-wide search. *Science* 274: 1371-1374.

2452. Soejima H, Ogawa O, Nomura Y, Ogata J (1977). Pheochromocytoma of the spermatic cord: a case report. *J Urol* 118: 495-496.

2453. Sogbein SK, Steele AA (1989). Papillary prostatic epithelial hyperplasia of the urethra: a cause of hematuria in young men. *J Urol* 142: 1218-1220.

2454. Sohn M, Neuerburg J, Teufl F, Bohndorf K (1990). Gadolinium-enhanced magnetic resonance imaging in the staging of urinary bladder neoplasms. *Urol Int* 45: 142-147.

2455. Sohval AR, Churg J, Gabrilove JL, Freiberg EK, Katz N (1982). Ultrastructure of feminizing testicular Leydig cell tumors. *Ultrastruct Pathol* 3: 335-345.

2456. Sohval AR, Churg J, Suzuki Y, Katz N, Gabrilove JL (1977). Electron microscopy of a feminizing Leydig cell tumor of the testis. *Hum Pathol* 8: 621-634.

2457. Soini Y, Turpeenniemi-Hujanen T, Kamel D, Autio-Harmainen H, Risteli J, Risteli L, Nuorva K, Paakko P, Vahakangas K (1993). p53 immunohistochemistry in transitional cell carcinoma and dysplasia of the urinary bladder correlates with disease progression. *Br J Cancer* 68: 1029-1035.

2458. Solsona E, Iborra I, Rubio J, Casanova JL, Ricos JV, Calabuig C (2001). Prospective validation of the association of local tumor stage and grade as a predictive factor for occult lymph node micrometastasis in patients with penile carcinoma and clinically negative inguinal lymph nodes. *J Urol* 165: 1506-1509.

2459. Solter D (1988). Differential imprinting and expression of maternal and paternal genomes. *Annu Rev Genet* 22: 127-146.

2460. Somers WJ, Terpenning B, Lowe FC, Romas NA (1988). Renal parenchymal neurilemoma: a rare and unusual kidney tumor. *J Urol* 139: 109-110.

2461. Sommerfeld HJ, Meeker AK, Piatyszek MA, Bova GS, Shay JW, Coffey DS (1996). Telomerase activity: a prevalent marker of malignant human prostate tissue. *Cancer Res* 56: 218-222.

2462. Sotelo-Avila C, Beckwith JB, Johnson JE (1995). Ossifying renal tumor of infancy: a clinicopathologic study of nine cases. *Pediatr Pathol Lab Med* 15: 745-762.

2463. Soulie M, Escourrou G, Vazzoler N, Seguin P, Suc B, Pontonnier F, Plante P (2001). [Primary carcinoid tumor and horseshoe kidney: potential association]. *Prog Urol* 11: 301-303.

2464. Speicher MR, Schoell B, du Manoir S, Schrock E, Ried T, Cremer T, Storkel S, Kovacs A, Kovacs G (1994). Specific loss of chromosomes 1, 2, 6, 10, 13, 17, and 21 in chromophobe renal cell carcinomas revealed by comparative genomic hybridization. *Am J Pathol* 145: 356-364.

2465. Speights VOJr, Cohen MK, Riggs MW, Coffield KS, Keegan G, Arber DA (1997). Neuroendocrine stains and proliferative indices of prostatic adenocarcinomas in transurethral resection samples. *Br J Urol* 80: 281-286.

2466. Spencer JR, Brodin AG, Ignatoff JM (1990). Clear cell adenocarcinoma of the urethra: evidence for origin within paraurethral ducts. *J Urol* 143: 122-125.

2467. Spruck CH3rd, Ohneseit PF, Gonzalez-Zulueta M, Esrig D, Miyao N, Tsai YC, Lerner SP, Schmutte C, Yang AS, Cote R, Dubeau L, Nichols PW, Hermann GG, Steven K, Horn T, Skinner DG, Jones PA (1994). Two molecular pathways to transitional cell carcinoma of the bladder. *Cancer Res* 54: 784-788.

2468. Spruck CH3rd, Rideout WM3rd, Olumi AF, Ohneseit PF, Yang AS, Tsai YC, Nichols PW, Horn T, Hermann GG, Steven K, Ross RK, Yu MC, Jones PA (1993). Distinct pattern of p53 mutations in bladder cancer: relationship to tobacco usage. *Cancer Res* 53: 1162-1166.

2469. Srigley J, Kapusta L, Reuter V, Amin M, Grignon DJ, Eble JN, Weber A, Moch H (2002). Phenotypic, molecular and ultrastructural studies of a novel low-grade renal epithelial neoplasm possible related to the loop of Henle. *Mod Pathol* 15: 182.

2470. Srigley JR, Eble JN (1998). Collecting duct carcinoma of kidney. *Semin Diagn Pathol* 15: 54-67.

2471. Srigley JR, Eble JN, Grignon DJ, Hartwick RWJ (1999). Unusual renal cell carcinoma (RCC) with prominent spindle cell change possibly related to the loop of Henle. *Mod Pathol* 12: 107.

2472. Srigley JR, Grignon DJ, Young RH (2002). The distinction between pure carcinoid tumor and carcinoid-like adenocarcinoma of the prostate. *Mod Pathol* 15: 182A-183A.

2473. Srigley JR, Hutter RV, Gelb AB, Henson DE, Kenney G, King BF, Raziuddin S, Pisansky TM (1997). Current prognostic factors—renal cell carcinoma: Workgroup No. 4. Union Internationale Contre le Cancer (UICC) and the American Joint Committee on Cancer (AJCC). *Cancer* 80: 994-996.

2474. Srinivas V, Herr HW, Hajdu EO (1985). Partial nephrectomy for a renal oncocytoma associated with tuberous sclerosis. *J Urol* 133: 263-265.

2475. Sriplakich S, Jahnson S, Karlsson MG (1999). Epidermal growth factor receptor expression: predictive value for the outcome after cystectomy for bladder cancer? *BJU Int* 83: 498-503.

2476. Stadler WM, Steinberg G, Yang X, Hagos F, Turner C, Olopade OI (2001). Alterations of the 9p21 and 9q33 chromosomal bands in clinical bladder cancer specimens by fluorescence in situ hybridization. *Clin Cancer Res* 7: 1676-1682.

2477. Stallone G, Infante B, Manno C, Campobasso N, Pannarale G, Schena FP (2000). Primary renal lymphoma does exist: case report and review of the literature. *J Nephrol* 13: 367-372.

2478. Stamey TA, Johnstone IM, McNeal JE, Lu AY, Yemoto CM (2002). Preoperative serum prostate specific antigen levels between 2 and 22 ng/ml correlate poorly with post-radical prostatectomy cancer morphology: prostate specific antigen cure rates appear constant between 2 and 9 ng/ml. *J Urol* 167: 103-111.

2479. Stamey TA, McNeal JE, Yemoto CM, Sigal BM, Johnstone IM (1999). Biological determinants of cancer progression in men with prostate cancer. *JAMA* 281: 1395-1400.

2480. Stamey TA, Villers AA, McNeal JE, Link PC, Freiha FS (1990). Positive surgical margins at radical prostatectomy: importance of the apical dissection. *J Urol* 143: 1166-1172.

2481. Stamey TA, Warrington JA, Caldwell MC, Chen Z, Fan Z, Mahadevappa M, McNeal JE, Nolley R, Zhang Z (2001). Molecular genetic profiling of Gleason grade 4/5 prostate cancers compared to benign prostatic hyperplasia. *J Urol* 166: 2171-2177.

2482. Stamp IM, Barlebo H, Rix M, Jacobsen GK (1993). Intratubular germ cell neoplasia in an infantile testis with immature teratoma. *Histopathology* 22: 69-72.

2483. Stamp IM, Jacobsen GK (1995). Infant intratubular germ cell neoplasia. *Am J Surg Pathol* 19: 489.

2484. Stampfer DS, Carpinito GA, Rodriguez-Villanueva J, Willsey LW, Dinney CP, Grossman HB, Fritsche HA, McDougal WS (1998). Evaluation of NMP22 in the detection of transitional cell carcinoma of the bladder. *J Urol* 159: 394-398.

2485. Stanfield BL, Grimes MM, Kay S (1994). Primary carcinoid tumor of the bladder arising beneath an inverted papilloma. *Arch Pathol Lab Med* 118: 666-667.

2486. Stanisic TH, Donovan J (1986). Prolactin secreting renal cell carcinoma. *J Urol* 136: 85-86.

2487. Stattin P, Bergh A, Karlberg L, Tavelin B, Damber JE (1997). Long-term outcome of conservative therapy in men presenting with voiding symptoms and prostate cancer. *Eur Urol* 32: 404-409.

2488. Stebbins CE, Kaelin WGJr, Pavletich NP (1999). Structure of the VHL-ElonginC-ElonginB complex: implications for VHL tumor suppressor function. *Science* 284: 455-461.

2489. Steck PA, Pershouse MA, Jasser SA, Yung WK, Lin H, Ligon AH, Langford LA, Baumgard ML, Hattier T, Davis T, Frye C, Hu R, Swedlund B, Teng DH, Tavtigian SV (1997). Identification of a candidate tumour suppressor gene, MMAC1, at chromosome 10q23.3 that is mutated in multiple advanced cancers. *Nat Genet* 15: 356-362.

2490. Stefansson K, Wollmann RL (1982). S-100 protein in granular cell tumors (granular cell myoblastomas). *Cancer* 49: 1834-1838.

2491. Steffens J, Girardot P, Bock R, Braedel HU, Alloussi S, Ziegler M (1992). [Carcinoma of the kidney with production of renin. A special form of hypertension]. *Ann Urol (Paris)* 26: 5-9.

2492. Steidl C, Simon R, Burger H, Brinkschmidt C, Hertle L, Bocker W, Terpe HJ (2002). Patterns of chromosomal aberrations in urinary bladder tumours and adjacent urothelium. *J Pathol* 198: 115-120.

2493. Stein BS, Kendall AR (1984). Malignant melanoma of the genitourinary tract. *J Urol* 132: 859-868.

2494. Stein BS, Rosen S, Kendall AR (1984). The association of inverted papilloma and transitional cell carcinoma of the urothelium. *J Urol* 131: 751-752.

2495. Stein JP, Ginsberg DA, Grossfeld GD, Chatterjee SJ, Esrig D, Dickinson MG, Groshen S, Taylor CR, Jones PA, Skinner DG, Cote RJ (1998). Effect of p21WAF1/CIP1 expression on tumor progression in bladder cancer. *J Natl Cancer Inst* 90: 1072-1079.

2496. Stein JP, Grossfeld GD, Ginsberg DA, Esrig D, Freeman JA, Figueroa AJ, Skinner DG, Cote RJ (1998). Prognostic markers in bladder cancer: a contemporary review of the literature. *J Urol* 160: 645-659.

2497. Steinberg D (1975). Plasmacytoma of the testis. Report of a case. *Cancer* 36: 1470-1472.

2498. Steinberg DM, Sauvageot J, Piantadosi S, Epstein JI (1997). Correlation of prostate needle biopsy and radical prostatectomy Gleason grade in academic and community settings. *Am J Surg Pathol* 21: 566-576.

2499. Steinberg GD, Carter BS, Beaty TH, Childs B, Walsh PC (1990). Family history and the risk of prostate cancer. *Prostate* 17: 337-347.

2500. Steinberg GD, Epstein JI, Piantadosi S, Walsh PC (1990). Management of stage D1 adenocarcinoma of the prostate: the Johns Hopkins experience 1974 to 1987. *J Urol* 144: 1425-1432.

2501. Steiner G, Cairns P, Polascik TJ, Marshall FF, Epstein JI, Sidransky D, Schoenberg M (1996). High-density mapping of chromosomal arm 1q in renal collecting duct carcinoma: region of minimal deletion at 1q32.1-32.2. *Cancer Res* 56: 5044-5046.

2502. Steiner M, Quinlan D, Goldman SM, Millmond S, Hallowell MJ, Stutzman RE, Korobkin M (1990). Leiomyoma of the kidney: presentation of 4 new cases and the role of computerized tomography. *J Urol* 143: 994-998.

2503. Steiner MS, Goldman SM, Fishman EK, Marshall FF (1993). The natural history of renal angiomyolipoma. *J Urol* 150: 1782-1786.

2504. Stenman UH, Leinonen J, Alfthan H, Rannikko S, Tuhkanen K, Alfthan O (1991). A complex between prostate-specific antigen and alpha 1-antichymotrypsin is the major form of prostate-specific antigen in serum of patients with prostatic cancer: assay of the complex improves clinical sensitivity for cancer. *Cancer Res* 51: 222-226.

2505. Stenram U, Holby LE (1969). A case of circumscribed myosarcoma of the prostate. *Cancer* 24: 803-806.

2506. Stephan C, Lein M, Jung K, Schnorr D, Loening SA (1997). The influence of prostate volume on the ratio of free to total prostate specific antigen in serum of patients with prostate carcinoma and benign prostate hyperplasia. *Cancer* 79: 104-109.

2507. Stern RS (1990). Genital tumors among men with psoriasis exposed to psoralens and ultraviolet A radiation (PUVA) and ultraviolet B radiation. The Photochemotherapy Follow-up Study. *N Engl J Med* 322: 1093-1097.

2508. Stewart AL, Grieve RJ, Banerjee SS (1985). Primary lymphoma of the penis. *Eur J Surg Oncol* 11: 179-181.

2509. Steyerberg EW, Keizer HJ, Stoter G, Habbema JD (1994). Predictors of residual mass histology following chemotherapy for metastatic non-seminomatous testicular cancer: a quantitative overview of 996 resections. *Eur J Cancer* 30A: 1231-1239.

2510. Stolle C, Glenn G, Zbar B, Humphrey JS, Choyke P, Walther M, Pack S, Hurley K, Andrey C, Klausner R, Linehan WM (1998). Improved detection of germline mutations in the von Hippel-Lindau disease tumor suppressor gene. *Hum Mutat* 12: 417-423.

2511. Stone CH, Lee MW, Amin MB, Yaziji H, Gown AM, Ro JY, Tetu B, Paraf F, Zarbo RJ (2001). Renal angiomyolipoma: further immunophenotypic characterization of an expanding morphologic spectrum. *Arch Pathol Lab Med* 125: 751-758.
2512. Stoop H, van Gurp R, de Krijger R, Geurts van Kessel A, Koberle B, Oosterhuis W, Looijenga LH (2001). Reactivity of germ cell maturation stage-specific markers in spermatocytic seminoma: diagnostic and etiological implications. *Lab Invest* 81: 919-928.
2513. Storkel S (1993). *Karzinome und Onkozytome der Niere. Phänotypische Charakterisierung und prognostische Merkmale.* Gustav Fischer Verlag: Stuttgart.
2514. Storkel S, Eble JN, Adlakha K, Amin M, Blute ML, Bostwick DG, Darson M, Delahunt B, Iczkowski K (1997). Classification of renal cell carcinoma: Workgroup No. 1. Union Internationale Contre le Cancer (UICC) and the American Joint Committee on Cancer (AJCC). *Cancer* 80: 987-989.
2515. Storkel S, Steart PV, Drenckhahn D, Thoenes W (1989). The human chromophobe cell renal carcinoma: its probable relation to intercalated cells of the collecting duct. *Virchows Arch B Cell Pathol Incl Mol Pathol* 56: 237-245.
2516. Strohmeyer D, Langenhof S, Ackermann R, Hartmann M, Strohmeyer T, Schmidt B (1997). Analysis of the DCC tumor suppressor gene in testicular germ cell tumors: mutations and loss of expression. *J Urol* 157: 1973-1976.
2517. Strohmeyer T, Peter S, Hartmann M, Munemitsu S, Ackermann R, Ullrich A, Slamon DJ (1991). Expression of the hst-1 and c-kit protooncogenes in human testicular germ cell tumors. *Cancer Res* 51: 1811-1816.
2518. Strohmeyer T, Reese D, Press M, Ackermann R, Hartmann M, Slamon D (1995). Expression of the c-kit proto-oncogene and its ligand stem cell factor (SCF) in normal and malignant human testicular tissue. *J Urol* 153: 511-515.
2519. Strohmeyer T, Reissmann P, Cordon-Cardo C, Hartmann M, Ackermann R, Slamon D (1991). Correlation between retinoblastoma gene expression and differentiation in human testicular tumors. *Proc Natl Acad Sci USA* 88: 6662-6666.
2520. Strohsnitter WC, Noller KL, Hoover RN, Robboy SJ, Palmer JR, Titus-Ernstoff L, Kaufman RH, Adam E, Herbst AL, Hatch EE (2001). Cancer risk in men exposed in utero to diethylstilbestrol. *J Natl Cancer Inst* 93: 545-551.
2521. Stuart WT (1962). Carcinoma of the bladder associated with exstrophy: report of a case and review of the literature. *Va Med Mon* 89: 39-42.
2522. Stumm M, Koch A, Wieacker PF, Phillip C, Steinbach F, Allhoff EP, Buhtz P, Walter H, Tonnies H, Wirth J (1999). Partial monosomy 2p as the single chromosomal anomaly in a case of renal metanephric adenoma. *Cancer Genet Cytogenet* 115: 82-85.
2523. Suarez GM, Lewis RW (1986). Granular cell tumor of the glans penis. *J Urol* 135: 1252-1253.
2524. Subramaniam K, Seydoux G (2003). Dedifferentiation of primary spermatocytes into germ cell tumors in C. elegans lacking the Pumilio-like protein PUF-8. *Curr Biol* 13: 134-139.
2525. Sufrin G, Chasan S, Golio A, Murphy GP (1989). Paraneoplastic and serologic syndromes of renal adenocarcinoma. *Semin Urol* 7: 158-171.
2526. Sufrin G, Mirand EA, Moore RH, Chu TM, Murphy GP (1977). Hormones in renal cancer. *J Urol* 117: 433-438.
2527. Sugihara A, Kajio K, Yoshimoto T, Tsujimura T, Iwasaki T, Yamada N, Terada N, Tsuji M, Nojima M, Yabumoto H, Mori Y, Shima H (2002). Primary carcinoid tumor of the urinary bladder. *Int Urol Nephrol* 33: 53-57.
2528. Sugita Y, Clarnette TD, Cooke-Yarborough C, Chow CW, Waters K, Hutson JM (1999). Testicular and paratesticular tumours in children: 30 years' experience. *Aust N Z J Surg* 69: 505-508.
2529. Suijkerbuijk RF, Sinke RJ, Meloni AM, Parrington JM, van Echten J, de Jong B, Oosterhuis JW, Sandberg AA, Geurts van Kessel A (1993). Overrepresentation of chromosome 12p sequences and karyotypic evolution in i(12p)-negative testicular germ-cell tumors revealed by fluorescence in situ hybridization. *Cancer Genet Cytogenet* 70: 85-93.
2530. Suijkerbuijk RF, Sinke RJ, Weghuis DE, Roque L, Forus A, Stellink F, Siepman A, van de Kaa C, Soares J, Geurts van Kessel A (1994). Amplification of chromosome subregion 12p11.2-p12.1 in a metastasis of an i(12p)-negative seminoma: relationship to tumor progression? *Cancer Genet Cytogenet* 78: 145-152.
2531. Sukosd F, Digon B, Fischer J, Pietsch T, Kovacs G (2001). Allelic loss at 10q23.3 but lack of mutation of PTEN/MMAC1 in chromophobe renal cell carcinoma. *Cancer Genet Cytogenet* 128: 161-163.
2532. Sullivan J, Grabstald H (1978). Management of carcinoma of the urethra. In: *Genitourinary Cancer*, DG Skinner, JB Dekernion, eds. WB Saunders: Philadelphia, PA, pp. 419-429.
2533. Sullivan JL, Packer JT, Bryant M (1981). Primary malignant carcinoid of the testis. *Arch Pathol Lab Med* 105: 515-517.
2534. Summers DE, Rushin JM, Frazier HA, Cotelingam JD (1991). Inverted papilloma of the urinary bladder with granular eosinophilic cells. An unusual neuroendocrine variant. *Arch Pathol Lab Med* 115: 802-806.
2535. Summersgill B, Goker H, Weber-Hall S, Huddart R, Horwich A, Shipley J (1998). Molecular cytogenetic analysis of adult testicular germ cell tumours and identification of regions of consensus copy number change. *Br J Cancer* 77: 305-313.
2536. Summersgill B, Osin P, Lu YJ, Huddart R, Shipley J (2001). Chromosomal imbalances associated with carcinoma in situ and associated testicular germ cell tumours of adolescents and adults. *Br J Cancer* 85: 213-220.
2537. Sun B, Halmos G, Schally AV, Wang X, Martinez M (2000). Presence of receptors for bombesin/gastrin-releasing peptide and mRNA for three receptor subtypes in human prostate cancers. *Prostate* 42: 295-303.
2538. Susmano D, Rubenstein AB, Dakin AR, Lloyd FA (1971). Cystitis glandularis and adenocarcinoma of the bladder. *J Urol* 105: 671-674.
2539. Suster S, Wong TY, Moran CA (1993). Sarcomas with combined features of liposarcoma and leiomyosarcoma. Study of two cases of an unusual soft-tissue tumor showing dual lineage differentiation. *Am J Surg Pathol* 17: 905-911.
2540. Suwa Y, Takano Y, Iki M, Takeda M, Asakura T, Noguchi S, Masuda M (1998). Cyclin D1 protein overexpression is related to tumor differentiation, but not to tumor progression or proliferative activity, in transitional cell carcinoma of the bladder. *J Urol* 160: 897-900.
2541. Suzuki K, Shioji Y, Morita T, Tokue A (2001). Primary testicular plasmacytoma with hydrocele of the testis. *Int J Urol* 8: 139-140.
2542. Suzuki T, Sasano H, Aoki H, Nagura H, Sasano N, Sano T, Saito M, Watanuki T, Kato H, Aizawa S (1993). Immunohistochemical comparison between anaplastic seminoma and typical seminoma. *Acta Pathol Jpn* 43: 751-757.
2543. Swartz DA, Johnson DE, Ayala AG, Watkins DL (1985). Bladder leiomyosarcoma: a review of 10 cases with 5-year followup. *J Urol* 133: 200-202.
2544. Sweeney C, Farrow DC, Schwartz SM, Eaton DL, Checkoway H, Vaughan TL (2000). Glutathione S-transferase M1, T1, and P1 polymorphisms as risk factors for renal cell carcinoma: a case-control study. *Cancer Epidemiol Biomarkers Prev* 9: 449-454.
2545. Swierczynski SL, Epstein JI (2002). Prognostic significance of atypical papillary urothelial hyperplasia. *Hum Pathol* 33: 512-517.
2546. Swinnen JV, Roskams T, Joniau S, van Poppel H, Oyen R, Baert L, Heyns W, Verhoeven G (2002). Overexpression of fatty acid synthase is an early and common event in the development of prostate cancer. *Int J Cancer* 98: 19-22.
2547. Symington T, Cameron KM (1976). Testicular tumours — Sertoli-cell/mesenchymal tumours. In: *Pathology of the Testis*, RCG Pugh, ed. Blackwell: Oxford, pp. 281-290.
2548. Szabo PE, Mann JR (1995). Biallelic expression of imprinted genes in the mouse germ line: implications for erasure, establishment, and mechanisms of genomic imprinting. *Genes Dev* 9: 1857-1868.
2549. Ta S, Klausner AP, Savage SJ, Unger P, Bar-Chama N (2000). Male infertility due to a benign prostatic polyp. *J Urol* 164: 1659-1660.
2550. Tainio HM, Kylmala TM, Haapasalo HK (1999). Primary malignant melanoma of the urinary bladder associated with widespread metastases. *Scand J Urol Nephrol* 33: 406-407.
2551. Takahashi M, Rhodes DR, Furge KA, Kanayama H, Kagawa S, Haab BB, Teh BT (2001). Gene expression profiling of clear cell renal cell carcinoma: gene identification and prognostic classification. *Proc Natl Acad Sci USA* 98: 9754-9759.
2552. Takahashi T, Habuchi T, Kakehi Y, Mitsumori K, Akao T, Terachi T, Yoshida O (1998). Clonal and chronological genetic analysis of multifocal cancers of the bladder and upper urinary tract. *Cancer Res* 58: 5835-5841.
2553. Takahashi T, Habuchi T, Kakehi Y, Okuno H, Terachi T, Kato T, Ogawa O (2000). Molecular diagnosis of metastatic origin in a patient with metachronous multiple cancers of the renal pelvis and bladder. *Urology* 56: 331.
2554. Takahashi T, Kakehi Y, Mitsumori K, Akao T, Terachi T, Kato T, Ogawa O, Habuchi T (2001). Distinct microsatellite alterations in upper urinary tract tumors and subsequent bladder tumors. *J Urol* 165: 672-677.
2555. Takashashi H (1993). Cytometric analysis of testicular seminoma and spermatocytic seminoma. *Acta Pathol Jap* 43: 121-129.
2556. Takashi M, Sakata T, Nagai T, Kato T, Sahashi M, Koshikawa T, Miyake K (1990). Primary transitional cell carcinoma of prostate: case with lymph node metastasis eradicated by neoadjuvant methotrexate, vinblastine, doxorubicin, and cisplatin (M-VAC) therapy. *Urology* 36: 96-98.
2557. Takayama H, Takakuwa T, Tsujimoto Y, Tani Y, Nonomura N, Okuyama A, Nagata S, Aozasa K (2002). Frequent Fas gene mutations in testicular germ cell tumors. *Am J Pathol* 161: 635-641.
2558. Takayama TK, Vessella RL, Lange PH (1994). Newer applications of serum prostate-specific antigen in the management of prostate cancer. *Semin Oncol* 21: 542-553.
2559. Takeda H, Akakura K, Masai M, Akimoto S, Yatani R, Shimazaki J (1996). Androgen receptor content of prostate carcinoma cells estimated by immunohistochemistry is related to prognosis of patients with stage D2 prostate carcinoma. *Cancer* 77: 934-940.
2560. Takeshima Y, Inai K, Yoneda K (1996). Primary carcinoid tumor of the kidney with special reference to its histogenesis. *Pathol Int* 46: 894-900.
2561. Takeuchi T, Tanaka T, Tokuyama H, Kuriyama M, Nishiura T (1984). Multilocular cystic renal adenocarcinoma: a case report and review of the literature. *J Surg Oncol* 25: 136-140.
2562. Talbert ML, Young RH (1989). Carcinomas of the urinary bladder with deceptively benign-appearing foci. A report of three cases. *Am J Surg Pathol* 13: 374-381.
2563. Talerman A (1979). Gonadal tumours composed of germ cells and sex cord stroma derivatives. *Patol Pol* 30: 221-228.
2564. Talerman A (1980). Endodermal sinus (yolk sac) tumor elements in testicular germ-cell tumors in adults: comparison of prospective and retrospective studies. *Cancer* 46: 1213-1217.
2565. Talerman A (1980). Spermatocytic seminoma: clinicopathological study of 22 cases. *Cancer* 45: 2169-2176.
2566. Talerman A (1980). The pathology of gonadal neoplasms composed of germ cell and sex cord stroma derivatives. *Pathol Res Pract* 170: 24-38.
2567. Talerman A (1985). Pure granulosa cell tumour of the testis. Report of a case and review of the literature. *Appl Pathol* 3: 117-122.
2568. Talerman A, Fu YS, Okagaki T (1984). Spermatocytic seminoma. Ultrastructural and microspectrophotometric observations. *Lab Invest* 51: 343-349.
2569. Talerman A, Gratama S, Miranda S, Okagaki T (1978). Primary carcinoid tumor of the testis: case report, ultrastructure and review of the literature. *Cancer* 42: 2696-2706.
2570. Tallarigo C, Baldassarre R, Bianchi G, Comunale L, Olivo G, Pea M, Bonetti F, Martignoni G, Zamboni G, Mobilio G (1992). Diagnostic and therapeutic problems in multicentric renal angiomyolipoma. *J Urol* 148: 1880-1884.
2571. Tamboli P, Amin MB, Mohsin SK, Ben-dor D, Lopez-Beltran A (2000). Plasmacytoid variant of non-papillary urothelial carcinoma. *Mod Pathol* 13: 116A.

2572. Tamboli P, Mohsin SK, Hailemariam S, Amin MB (2002). Colonic adenocarcinoma metastatic to the urinary tract versus primary tumors of the urinary tract with glandular differentiation: a report of 7 cases and investigation using a limited immunohistochemical panel. *Arch Pathol Lab Med* 126: 1057-1063.
2573. Tamboli P, Ro JY, Amin MB, Ligato S, Ayala AG (2000). Benign tumors and tumor-like lesions of the adult kidney. Part II: Benign mesenchymal and mixed neoplasms, and tumor-like lesions. *Adv Anat Pathol* 7: 47-66.
2574. Tamboli P, Tran KP, Ro JY, Ayala AG, Ayala G, Amin MB, Velazquez EF, Cubilla AL (2000). Mixed basaloid-condylomatous (warty) squamous cell carcinoma of the penis: a report of 17 cases. *Lab Invest* 80: 115A.
2575. Tanaka Y, Carney JA, Ijiri R, Kato K, Miyake T, Nakatani Y, Misugi K (2002). Utility of immunostaining for S-100 protein subunits in gonadal sex cord-stromal tumors, with emphasis on the large-cell calcifying Sertoli cell tumor of the testis. *Hum Pathol* 33: 285-289.
2576. Tanaka Y, Sasaki Y, Tachibana K, Suwa S, Terashima K, Nakatani Y (1994). Testicular juvenile granulosa cell tumor in an infant with X/XY mosaicism clinically diagnosed as true hermaphroditism. *Am J Surg Pathol* 18: 316-322.
2577. Tanguay C, Harvey I, Houde M, Srigley JR, Tetu B (2003). Leiomyosarcoma of urinary bladder following cyclophosphamide therapy: report of two cases. *Mod Pathol* 16: 512-514.
2578. Taniguchi S, Inoue A, Hamada T (1994). Angiokeratoma of Fordyce: a cause of scrotal bleeding. *Br J Urol* 73: 589-590.
2579. Tanis PJ, Lont AP, Meinhardt W, Olmos RA, Nieweg OE, Horenblas S (2002). Dynamic sentinel node biopsy for penile cancer: reliability of a staging technique. *J Urol* 168: 76-80.
2580. Tannenbaum M (1975). Transitional cell carcinoma of prostate. *Urology* 5: 674-678.
2581. Tarjan M, Cserni G, Szabo Z (2001). Malignant fibrous histiocytoma of the kidney. *Scand J Urol Nephrol* 35: 518-520.
2582. Tarle M, Ahel MZ, Kovacic K (2002). Acquired neuroendocrine-positivity during maximal androgen blockade in prostate cancer patients. *Anticancer Res* 22: 2525-2529.
2583. Tash JA, Reuter V, Russo P (2002). Metastatic carcinoid tumor of the prostate. *J Urol* 167: 2526-2527.
2584. Tavtigian SV, Simard J, Teng DH, Abtin V, Baumgard M, Beck A, Camp NJ, Carillo AR, Chen Y, Dayananth P, Desrochers M, Dumont M, Farnham JM, Frank D, Frye C, Ghaffari S, Gupte JS, Hu R, Iliev D, Janecki T, Kort EN, Laity KE, Leavitt A, Leblanc G, McArthur-Morrison J, Pederson A, Penn B, Peterson KT, Reid JE, Richards S, Schroeder M, Smith R, Snyder SC, Swedlund B, Swensen J, Thomas A, Tranchant M, Woodland AM, Labrie F, Skolnick MH, Neuhausen S, Rommens J, Cannon-Albright LA (2001). A candidate prostate cancer susceptibility gene at chromosome 17p. *Nat Genet* 27: 172-180.
2585. Tawfik OW, Moral LA, Richardson WP, Lee KR (1993). Multicentric bilateral renal cell carcinomas and a vascular leiomyoma in a child. *Pediatr Pathol* 13: 289-298.
2586. Tay HP, Bidair M, Shabaik A, Gilbaugh JH3rd, Schmidt JD (1995). Primary yolk sac tumor of the prostate in a patient with Klinefelter's syndrome. *J Urol* 153: 1066-1069.
2587. Taylor DC, Bhagavan BS, Larsen MP, Cox JA, Epstein JI (1996). Papillary urothelial hyperplasia. A precursor to papillary neoplasms. *Am J Surg Pathol* 20: 1481-1488.
2588. Taylor MD, Gokgoz N, Andrulis IL, Mainprize TG, Drake JM, Rutka JT (2000). Familial posterior fossa brain tumors of infancy secondary to germline mutation of the hSNF5 gene. *Am J Hum Genet* 66: 1403-1406.
2589. Tefilli MV, Gheiler EL, Tiguert R, Banerjee M, Sakr W, Grignon DJ, Pontes JE, Wood DPJr (1998). Prognostic indicators in patients with seminal vesicle involvement following radical prostatectomy for clinically localized prostate cancer. *J Urol* 160: 802-806.
2590. Tefilli MV, Gheiler EL, Tiguert R, Sakr W, Grignon DJ, Banerjee M, Pontes JE, Wood DPJr (1999). Should Gleason score 7 prostate cancer be considered a unique grade category? *Urology* 53: 372-377.
2591. Teilum G (1943). Arrhenoblastoma-androblastoma. Homologous ovarian and testicular tumours. II. Including the so-called luteomas and adrenal tumors of the ovary and the interstitial cell tumors of the testis. *Acta Pathol Microbiol Scand* 23: 252-264.
2592. Teilum G (1944). Homologous tumors in the ovary and testis. *Acta Obstet Gynecol Scand* 24: 480-503.
2593. Teilum G (1959). Endotermal sinus tumors of the ovary and testis. Comparative morphogenesis of the so-called mesonephroma ovarii (Schiller) and extraembryonic (yolk sac-allantoic) structures of the rat placenta. *Cancer* 12: 1092-1105.
2594. Tempany CM, Zhou X, Zerhouni EA, Rifkin MD, Quint LE, Piccoli CW, Ellis JH, McNeil BJ (1994). Staging of prostate cancer: results of Radiology Diagnostic Oncology Group project comparison of three MR imaging techniques. *Radiology* 192: 47-54.
2595. Terenziani M, Piva L, Spreafico F, Salvioni R, Massimino M, Luksch R, Cefalo G, Casanova M, Ferrari A, Polastri D, Mazza E, Bellani FF, Nicolai N (2002). Clinical stage I nonseminomatous germ cell tumors of the testis in childhood and adolescence: an analysis of 31 cases. *J Pediatr Hematol Oncol* 24: 454-458.
2596. Terracciano L, Richter J, Tornillo L, Beffa L, Diener PA, Maurer R, Gasser TC, Moch H, Mihatsch MJ, Sauter G (1999). Chromosomal imbalances in small cell carcinomas of the urinary bladder. *J Pathol* 189: 230-235.
2597. Terrier-Lacombe MJ, Martinez-Madrigal F, Porta W, Rahal J, Droz JP (1990). Embryonal rhabdomyosarcoma arising in a mature teratoma of the testis: a case report. *J Urol* 143: 1232-1234.
2598. Terris MK, Pham TQ, Issa MM, Kabalin JN (1997). Routine transition zone and seminal vesicle biopsies in all patients undergoing transrectal ultrasound guided prostate biopsies are not indicated. *J Urol* 157: 204-206.
2599. Tetu B, Allard P, Fradet Y, Roberge N, Bernard P (1996). Prognostic significance of nuclear DNA content and S-phase fraction by flow cytometry in primary papillary superficial bladder cancer. *Hum Pathol* 27: 922-926.
2600. Tetu B, Ro JY, Ayala AG, Johnson DE, Logothetis CJ, Ordonez NG (1987). Small cell carcinoma of the prostate. Part I. A clinicopathologic study of 20 cases. *Cancer* 59: 1803-1809.
2601. Tetu B, Ro JY, Ayala AG, Ordonez NG, Johnson DE (1987). Small cell carcinoma of the kidney. A clinicopathologic, immunohistochemical, and ultrastructural study. *Cancer* 60: 1809-1814.
2602. Tetu B, Vaillancourt L, Camilleri JP, Bruneval P, Bernier L, Tourigny R (1993). Juxtaglomerular cell tumor of the kidney: report of two cases with a papillary pattern. *Hum Pathol* 24: 1168-1174.
2603. Thackray AC, Crane WA (1976). Seminoma. In: *Pathology of the Testis*, RC Pugh, ed. Blackwell Scientific: Oxford, pp. 164-198.
2604. The European Chromosome 16 Tuberous Sclerosis Consortium (1993). Identification and characterization of the tuberous sclerosis gene on chromosome 16. *Cell* 75: 1305-1315.
2605. Theodorescu D (2001). Preoperative magnetic resonance imaging for prostate cancer may be cost effective for men with a risk of extracapsular disease. *Evidence-based Oncology* 2: 51-52.
2606. Thiede T, Christensen BC (1969). Bladder tumours induced by chlornaphazine. A five-year follow-up study of chlornaphazine-treated patients with polycythaemia. *Acta Med Scand* 185: 133-137.
2607. Thiel RP, Oesterling JE, Wojno KJ, Partin AW, Chan DW, Carter HB, Stamey TA, Prestigiacomo AR, Brawer MK, Petteway JC, Carlson G, Luderer AA (1996). Multicenter comparison of the diagnostic performance of free prostate-specific antigen. *Urology* 48: 45-50.
2608. Thoenes W, Storkel S, Rumpelt HJ (1985). Human chromophobe cell renal carcinoma. *Virchows Arch B Cell Pathol Incl Mol Pathol* 48: 207-217.
2609. Thoenes W, Storkel S, Rumpelt HJ (1986). Histopathology and classification of renal cell tumors (adenomas, oncocytomas and carcinomas). The basic cytological and histopathological elements and their use for diagnostics. *Pathol Res Pract* 181: 125-143.
2610. Thoenes W, Storkel S, Rumpelt HJ, Moll R, Baum HP, Werner S (1988). Chromophobe cell renal carcinoma and its variants—a report on 32 cases. *J Pathol* 155: 277-287.
2611. Thogersen VB, Jorgensen PE, Sorensen BS, Bross P, Orntoft T, Wolf H, Nexo E (1999). Expression of transforming growth factor alpha and epidermal growth factor receptor in human bladder cancer. *Scand J Clin Lab Invest* 59: 267-277.
2612. Thomas DG, Ward AM, Williams JL (1971). A study of 52 cases of adenocarcinoma of the bladder. *Br J Urol* 43: 4-15.
2613. Thompson GJ (1942). Transurethral resection of malignant lesions of the prostatic gland. *JAMA* 120: 1105-1109.
2614. Thrash-Bingham CA, Greenberg RE, Howard S, Bruzel A, Bremer M, Goll A, Salazar H, Freed JJ, Tartof KD (1995). Comprehensive allelotyping of human renal cell carcinomas using microsatellite DNA probes. *Proc Natl Acad Sci USA* 92: 2854-2858.
2615. Tian Q, Frierson HFJr, Krystal GW, Moskaluk CA (1999). Activating c-kit gene mutations in human germ cell tumors. *Am J Pathol* 154: 1643-1647.
2616. Tickoo SK, Hutchinson B, Bacik J, Mazumdar M, Motzer RJ, Bajorin DF, Bosl GJ, Reuter VE (2002). Testicular seminoma: a clinicopathologic and immunohistochemical study of 105 cases with special reference to seminomas with atypical features. *Int J Surg Pathol* 10: 23-32.
2617. Tickoo SK, Lee MW, Eble JN, Amin M, Christopherson T, Zarbo RJ, Amin MB (2000). Ultrastructural observations on mitochondria and microvesicles in renal oncocytoma, chromophobe renal cell carcinoma, and eosinophilic variant of conventional (clear cell) renal cell carcinoma. *Am J Surg Pathol* 24: 1247-1256.
2618. Tickoo SK, Reuter VE, Amin MB, Srigley JR, Epstein JI, Min KW, Rubin MA, Ro JY (1999). Renal oncocytosis: a morphologic study of fourteen cases. *Am J Surg Pathol* 23: 1094-1101.
2619. Tiguert R, Bianco FJJr, Oskanian P, Li Y, Grignon DJ, Wood DPJr, Pontes JE, Sarkar FH (2001). Structural alteration of p53 protein in patients with muscle invasive bladder transitional cell carcinoma. *J Urol* 166: 2155-2160.
2620. Tiguert R, Lessard A, So A, Fradet Y (2002). Prognostic markers in muscle invasive bladder cancer. *World J Urol* 20: 190-195.
2621. Tognon C, Garnett M, Kenward E, Kay R, Morrison K, Sorensen PH (2001). The chimeric protein tyrosine kinase ETV6-NTRK3 requires both Ras-Erk1/2 and PI3-kinase-Akt signaling for fibroblast transformation. *Cancer Res* 61: 8909-8916.
2622. Toh KL, Tan PH, Cheng WS (1999). Primary extraskeletal Ewing's sarcoma of the external genitalia. *J Urol* 162: 159-160.
2623. Tolley E, Craig I (1975). Presence of two forms of fumarase (fumarate hydratase E.C. 4.2.1.2) in mammalian cells: immunological characterization and genetic analysis in somatic cell hybrids. Confirmation of the assignment of a gene necessary for the enzyme expression to human chromosome 1. *Biochem Genet* 13: 867-883.
2624. Tomaszewski JE, Korat OC, LiVolsi VA, Connor AM, Wein A (1986). Paget's disease of the urethral meatus following transitional cell carcinoma of the bladder. *J Urol* 135: 368-370.
2625. Tomic S, Warner TF, Messing E, Wilding G (1995). Penile Merkel cell carcinoma. *Urology* 45: 1062-1065.
2626. Tomlinson GE, Nisen PD, Timmons CF, Schneider NR (1991). Cytogenetics of a renal cell carcinoma in a 17-month-old child. Evidence for Xp11.2 as a recurring breakpoint. *Cancer Genet Cytogenet* 57: 11-17.
2627. Tomlinson IP, Alam NA, Rowan AJ, Barclay E, Jaeger EE, Kelsell D, Leigh I, Gorman P, Lamlum H, Rahman S, Roylance RR, Olpin S, Bevan S, Barker K, Hearle N, Houlston RS, Kiuru M, Lehtonen R, Karhu A, Vilkki S, Laiho P, Eklund C, Vierimaa O, Aittomaki K, Hietala M, Sistonen P, Paetau A, Salovaara R, Herva R, Launonen V, Aaltonen LA (2002). Germline mutations in FH predispose to dominantly inherited uterine fibroids, skin leiomyomata and papillary renal cell cancer. *Nat Genet* 30: 406-410.
2628. Tong YC, Chieng PU, Tsai TC, Lin SN (1990). Renal angiomyolipoma: report of 24 cases. *Br J Urol* 66: 585-589.
2629. Torenbeek R, Lagendijk JH, van Diest PJ, Bril H, van de Molengraft FJ, Meijer CJ (1998). Value of a panel of antibodies to identify the primary origin of adenocarcinomas presenting as bladder carcinoma. *Histopathology* 32: 20-27.

2630. Torikata C (1994). Papillary cystadenoma of the epididymis. An ultrastructural and immunohistochemical study. *J Submicrosc Cytol Pathol* 26: 387-393.

2631. Toro JR, Glenn G, Duray P, Darling T, Weirich G, Zbar B, Linehan M, Turner ML (1999). Birt-Hogg-Dube syndrome: a novel marker of kidney neoplasia. *Arch Dermatol* 135: 1195-1202.

2632. Toro JR, Nickerson ML, Wei MH, Warren MB, Glenn GM, Turner ML, Stewart L, Duray P, Tourre O, Sharma N, Choyke P, Stratton P, Merino M, Walther MM, Linehan WM, Schmidt LS, Zbar B (2003). Mutations in the fumarate hydratase gene cause hereditary leiomyomatosis and renal cell cancer in families in North America. *Am J Hum Genet* 73: 95-106.

2633. Tosoni I, Wagner U, Sauter G, Egloff M, Knonagel H, Alund G, Bannwart F, Mihatsch MJ, Gasser TC, Maurer R (2000). Clinical significance of interobserver differences in the staging and grading of superficial bladder cancer. *BJU Int* 85: 48-53.

2634. Townsend MF3rd, Gal AA, Thoms WW, Newman JL, Eble JN, Graham SDJr (1999). Ureteral rhabdomyosarcoma. *Urology* 54: 561.

2635. Tozzini A, Bulleri A, Orsitto E, Morelli G, Pieri L (1999). Hodgkin's lymphoma: an isolated case of involvement of the ureter. *Eur Radiol* 9: 344-346.

2636. Tran KP, Epstein JI (1996). Mucinous adenocarcinoma of urinary bladder type arising from the prostatic urethra. Distinction from mucinous adenocarcinoma of the prostate. *Am J Surg Pathol* 20: 1346-1350.

2637. Tran TT, Sengupta E, Yang XJ (2001). Prostatic foamy gland carcinoma with aggressive behavior: clinicopathologic, immunohistochemical, and ultrastructural analysis. *Am J Surg Pathol* 25: 618-623.

2638. Trapman J, Cleutjens KB (1997). Androgen-regulated gene expression in prostate cancer. *Semin Cancer Biol* 8: 29-36.

2639. Trent JM, Stanisic T, Olson S (1984). Cytogenetic analysis of urologic malignancies: study of tumor colony forming cells and premature chromosome condensation. *J Urol* 131: 146-151.

2640. Trias I, Algaba F, Condom E, Espanol I, Segui J, Orsola I, Villavicencio H, Garcia Del Muro X (2001). Small cell carcinoma of the urinary bladder. Presentation of 23 cases and review of 134 published cases. *Eur Urol* 39: 85-90.

2641. Tribukait B (1987). Flow cytometry in assessing the clinical aggressiveness of genito-urinary neoplasms. *World J Urol* 5: 108.

2642. Tricker AR, Mostafa MH, Spiegelhalder B, Preussmann R (1989). Urinary excretion of nitrate, nitrite and N-nitroso compounds in Schistosomiasis and bilharzia bladder cancer patients. *Carcinogenesis* 10: 547-552.

2643. Tricker AR, Mostafa MH, Spiegelhalder B, Preussmann R (1991). Urinary nitrate, nitrite and N-nitroso compounds in bladder cancer patients with schistosomiasis (bilharzia). *IARC Sci Publ* 105: 178-181.

2644. Troncoso P, Babaian RJ, Ro JY, Grignon DJ, von Eschenbach AC, Ayala AG (1989). Prostatic intraepithelial neoplasia and invasive prostatic adenocarcinoma in cystoprostatectomy specimens. *Urology* 34: 52-56.

2645. True LD (1994). Surgical pathology examination of the prostate gland. Practice survey by American society of clinical pathologists. *Am J Clin Pathol* 102: 572-579.

2646. True LD, Otis CN, Delprado W, Scully RE, Rosai J (1988). Spermatocytic seminoma of testis with sarcomatous transformation. A report of five cases. *Am J Surg Pathol* 12: 75-82.

2647. Truong LD, Caraway N, Ngo T, Laucirica R, Katz R, Ramzy I (2001). Renal lymphoma. The diagnostic and therapeutic roles of fine-needle aspiration. *Am J Clin Pathol* 115: 18-31.

2648. Tsai YC, Nichols PW, Hiti AL, Williams Z, Skinner DG, Jones PA (1990). Allelic losses of chromosomes 9, 11, and 17 in human bladder cancer. *Cancer Res* 50: 44-47.

2649. Tsang WY, Chan JK, Lee KC, Fisher C, Fletcher CD (1992). Aggressive angiomyxoma. A report of four cases occurring in men. *Am J Surg Pathol* 16: 1059-1065.

2650. Tsuchiya K, Reijo R, Page DC, Disteche CM (1995). Gonadoblastoma: molecular definition of the susceptibility region on the Y chromosome. *Am J Hum Genet* 57: 1400-1407.

2651. Tsuda K, Narumi Y, Nakamura H, Nonomura I, Okuyama A (2000). [Staging urinary bladder cancer with dynamic MR imaging]. *Hinyokika Kiyo* 46: 835-839.

2652. Tsuji M, Murakami Y, Kanayama H, Sano T, Kagawa S (1999). A case of renal metanephric adenoma: histologic, immunohistochemical and cytogenetic analyses. *Int J Urol* 6: 203-207.

2653. Tsurusaki M, Mimura F, Yasui N, Minayoshi K, Sugimura K (2001). Neurilemoma of the renal capsule: MR imaging and pathologic correlation. *Eur Radiol* 11: 1834-1837.

2654. Tu SM, Reyes A, Maa A, Bhowmick D, Pisters LL, Pettaway CA, Lin SH, Troncoso P, Logothetis CJ (2002). Prostate carcinoma with testicular or penile metastases. Clinical, pathologic, and immunohistochemical features. *Cancer* 94: 2610-2617.

2655. Tungekar MF, Heryet A, Gatter KC (1991). The L1 antigen and squamous metaplasia in the bladder. *Histopathology* 19: 245-250.

2656. Tyrkus M, Powell I, Fakr W (1992). Cytogenetic studies of carcinoma in situ of the bladder: prognostic implications. *J Urol* 148: 44-46.

2657. Uchibayashi T, Hisazumi H, Hasegawa M, Shiba N, Muraishi Y, Tanaka T, Nonomura A (1997). Squamous cell carcinoma of the prostate. *Scand J Urol Nephrol* 31: 223-224.

2658. Uchida T, Shimoda T, Miyata H, Shikata T, Iino S, Suzuki H, Oda T, Hirano K, Sugiura M (1981). Immunoperoxidase study of alkaline phosphatase in testicular tumor. *Cancer* 48: 1455-1462.

2659. Uchida T, Wada C, Shitara T, Egawa S, Mashimo S, Koshiba K (1993). Infrequent involvement of p53 mutations and loss of heterozygosity of 17p in the tumorigenesis of renal cell carcinoma. *J Urol* 150: 1298-1301.

2660. Uchijima Y, Ito H, Takahashi M, Yamashina M (1990). Prostate mucinous adenocarcinoma with signet ring cell. *Urology* 36: 267-268.

2661. Uehling DT, Smith JE, Logan R, Hafez GR (1987). Newborn granulosa cell tumor of the testis. *J Urol* 138: 385-386.

2662. UICC (2002). *TNM Classification of Malignant Tumours*. 6th Edition. Wiley & Sons: New York.

2663. Ulbright TM (1997). *Neoplasms of the Testis. Urological Pathology.* 2nd Edition. WB Saunders Company: Philadelphia.

2664. Ulbright TM, Amin MB, Young RH (1999). *Tumors of the Testis, Adnexa, Spermatic Cord and Scrotum.* AFIP: Washington.

2665. Ulbright TM, Loehrer PJ, Roth LM, Einhorn LH, Williams SD, Clark SA (1984). The development of non-germ cell malignancies within germ cell tumors. A clinicopathologic study of 11 cases. *Cancer* 54: 1824-1833.

2666. Ulbright TM, Michael H, Loehrer PJ, Donohue JP (1990). Spindle cell tumors resected from male patients with germ cell tumors. A clinicopathologic study of 14 cases. *Cancer* 65: 148-156.

2667. Ulbright TM, Orazi A, de Riese W, de Riese C, Messemer JE, Foster RS, Donohue JP, Eble JN (1994). The correlation of P53 protein expression with proliferative activity and occult metastases in clinical stage I non-seminomatous germ cell tumors of the testis. *Mod Pathol* 7: 64-68.

2668. Ulbright TM, Roth LM (1999). Testicular and paratesticular tumours. In: *Diagnostic Surgical Pathology*, SS Sternberg, ed. 3rd Edition. Lippincott Williams and Wilkins: Philadelphia, p. 2000.

2669. Ulbright TM, Roth LM, Brodhecker CA (1986). Yolk sac differentiation in germ cell tumors. A morphologic study of 50 cases with emphasis on hepatic, enteric, and parietal yolk sac features. *Am J Surg Pathol* 10: 151-164.

2670. Ulbright TM, Srigley JR (2001). Dermoid cyst of the testis: a study of five postpubertal cases, including a pilomatrixoma-like variant, with evidence supporting its separate classification from mature testicular teratoma. *Am J Surg Pathol* 25: 788-793.

2671. Ulbright TM, Srigley JR, Reuter VE, Wojno K, Roth LM, Young RH (2000). Sex cord-stromal tumors of the testis with entrapped germ cells: a lesion mimicking unclassified mixed germ cell sex cord-stromal tumors. *Am J Surg Pathol* 24: 535-542.

2672. Ulbright TM, Young RH, Scully RE (1997). Trophoblastic tumors of the testis other than classic choriocarcinoma: "monophasic" choriocarcinoma and placental site trophoblastic tumor: a report of two cases. *Am J Surg Pathol* 21: 282-288.

2673. Ullmann AS, Ross OA (1967). Hyperplasia, atypism, and carcinoma in situ in prostatic periurethral glands. *Am J Clin Pathol* 47: 497-504.

2674. Umbas R, Schalken JA, Aalders TW, Carter BS, Karthaus HF, Schaafsma HE, Debruyne FM, Isaacs WB (1992). Expression of the cellular adhesion molecule E-cadherin is reduced or absent in high-grade prostate cancer. *Cancer Res* 52: 5104-5109.

2675. Underwood M, Bartlett J, Reeves J, Gardiner DS, Scott R, Cooke T (1995). C-erbB-2 gene amplification: a molecular marker in recurrent bladder tumors? *Cancer Res* 55: 2422-2430.

2676. Uno H, Shima T, Maeda K, Katakami H, Tsubouchi H (1998). Hypercalcemia associated with parathyroid hormone-related protein produced by B-cell type primary malignant lymphoma of the kidney. *Ann Hematol* 76: 221-224.

2677. Urban BA, Fishman EK (2000). Renal lymphoma: CT patterns with emphasis on helical CT. *Radiographics* 20: 197-212.

2678. Urist MJ, di Como CJ, Lu ML, Charytonowicz E, Verbel D, Crum CP, Ince TA, McKeon FD, Cordon-Cardo C (2002). Loss of p63 expression is associated with tumor progression in bladder cancer. *Am J Pathol* 161: 1199-1206.

2679. Utz DC, Farrow GM, Rife CC, Segura JW, Zincke H (1980). Carcinoma in situ of the bladder. *Cancer* 45: 1842-1848.

2680. Vahlensieck WJr, Riede U, Wimmer B, Ihling C (1991). Beta-human chorionic gonadotropin-positive extragonadal germ cell neoplasia of the renal pelvis. *Cancer* 67: 3146-3149.

2681. Vailancourt L, Ttu B, Fradet Y, Dupont A, Gomez J, Cusan L, Suburu ER, Diamond P, Candas B, Labrie F (1996). Effect of neoadjuvant endocrine therapy (combined androgen blockade) on normal prostate and prostatic carcinoma. A randomized study. *Am J Surg Pathol* 20: 86-93.

2682. Vakar-Lopez F, Abrams J (2000). Basaloid squamous cell carcinoma occurring in the urinary bladder. *Arch Pathol Lab Med* 124: 455-459.

2683. Val-Bernal JF, Azcarretazabal T, Torio B, Mayorga M (1999). Primary pure intratesticular fibrosarcoma. *Pathol Int* 49: 185-189.

2684. Val-Bernal JF, Garijo MF (2000). Pagetoid dyskeratosis of the prepuce. An incidental histologic finding resembling extramammary Paget's disease. *J Cutan Pathol* 27: 387-391.

2685. Val-Bernal JF, Hernandez-Nieto E (2000). Benign mucinous metaplasia of the penis. A lesion resembling extramammary Paget's disease. *J Cutan Pathol* 27: 76-79.

2686. van den Berg E, Buys CH (1997). Involvement of multiple loci on chromosome 3 in renal cell cancer development. *Genes Chromosomes Cancer* 19: 59-76.

2687. van den Berg E, Dijkhuizen T, Storkel S, de la Riviere GB, Dam A, Mensink HJ, Oosterhuis JW, de Jong B (1995). Chromosomal changes in renal oncocytomas. Evidence that t(5;11)(q35;q13) may characterize a second subgroup of oncocytomas. *Cancer Genet Cytogenet* 79: 164-168.

2688. van den Berg E, Gouw AS, Oosterhuis JW, Storkel S, Dijkhuizen T, Mensink HJ, de Jong B (1995). Carcinoid in a horseshoe kidney. Morphology, immunohistochemistry, and cytogenetics. *Cancer Genet Cytogenet* 84: 95-98.

2689. van den Berg E, Hulsbeek MF, de Jong D, Kok K, Veldhuis PM, Roche J, Buys CH (1996). Major role for a 3p21 region and lack of involvement of the t(3;8) breakpoint region in the development of renal cell carcinoma suggested by loss of heterozygosity analysis. *Genes Chromosomes Cancer* 15: 64-72.

2690. van den Berg E, van der Hout AH, Oosterhuis JW, Storkel S, Dijkhuizen T, Dam A, Zweers HM, Mensink HJ, Buys CH, de Jong B (1993). Cytogenetic analysis of epithelial renal-cell tumors: relationship with a new histopathological classification. *Int J Cancer* 55: 223-227.

2691. van der Hout AH, van der Vlies P, Wijmenga C, Li FP, Oosterhuis JW, Buys CH (1991). The region of common allelic losses in sporadic renal cell carcinoma is bordered by the loci D3S2 and THRB. *Genomics* 11: 537-542.

2692. van Echten J, Oosterhuis JW, Looijenga LH, van de Pol M, Wiersema J, te Meerman GJ, Schaffordt Koops H, Sleijfer DT, de Jong B (1995). No recurrent structural abnormalities apart from i(12p) in primary germ cell tumors of the adult testis. *Genes Chromosomes Cancer* 14: 133-144.

2693. van Echten J, Timmer A, van der Veen AY, Molenaar WM, de Jong B (2002). Infantile and adult testicular germ cell tumors. a different pathogenesis? *Cancer Genet Cytogenet* 135: 57-62.

2694. van Echten J, van Gurp RJ, Stoepker M, Looijenga LH, de Jong J, Oosterhuis W (1995). Cytogenetic evidence that carcinoma in situ is the precursor lesion for invasive testicular germ cell tumors. *Cancer Genet Cytogenet* 85: 133-137.

2695. Van Erp F, Van Ravenswaaij C, Bodmer D, Eleveld M, Hoogerbrugge N, Mulders P, Geurts vK (2003). Chromosome 3 translocations and the risk to develop renal cell cancer: a Dutch intergroup study. *Genet Couns* 14: 149-154.

2696. van Gelder T, Michiels JJ, Mulder AH, Klooswijk AI, Schalekamp MA (1992). Renal insufficiency due to bilateral primary renal lymphoma. *Nephron* 60: 108-110.

2697. van Gurp RJ, Oosterhuis JW, Kalscheuer V, Mariman EC, Looijenga LH (1994). Biallelic expression of the H19 and IGF2 genes in human testicular germ cell tumors. *J Natl Cancer Inst* 86: 1070-1075.

2698. van Iersel MP, Witjes WP, de la Rosette JJ, Oosterhof GO (1995). Prostate-specific antigen density: correlation with histological diagnosis of prostate cancer, benign prostatic hyperplasia and prostatitis. *Br J Urol* 76: 47-53.

2699. van Poppel H, De Ridder D, Elgamal AA, van de Voorde W, Werbrouck P, Ackaert K, Oyen R, Pittomvils G, Baert L (1995). Neoadjuvant hormonal therapy before radical prostatectomy decreases the number of positive surgical margins in stage T2 prostate cancer: interim results of a prospective randomized trial. The Belgian Uro-Oncological Study Group. *J Urol* 154: 429-434.

2700. van Rhijn BW, Lurkin I, Radvanyi F, Kirkels WJ, van der Kwast TH, Zwarthoff EC (2001). The fibroblast growth factor receptor 3 (FGFR3) mutation is a strong indicator of superficial bladder cancer with low recurrence rate. *Cancer Res* 61: 1265-1268.

2701. van Rhijn BW, Montironi R, Zwarthoff EC, Jobsis AC, van der Kwast TH (2002). Frequent FGFR3 mutations in urothelial papilloma. *J Pathol* 198: 245-251.

2702. van Savage JG, Carson CC3rd (1994). Primary adenocarcinoma of the penis. *J Urol* 152: 1555-1556.

2703. van Schothorst EM, Mohkamsing S, van Gurp RJ, Oosterhuis JW, van der Saag PT, Looijenga LH (1999). Lack of Bcl10 mutations in testicular germ cell tumours and derived cell lines. *Br J Cancer* 80: 1571-1574.

2704. van Slegtenhorst M, de Hoogt R, Hermans C, Nellist M, Janssen B, Verhoef S, Lindhout D, van den Ouweland A, Halley D, Young J, Burley M, Jeremiah S, Woodward K, Nahmias J, Fox M, Ekong R, Osborne J, Wolfe J, Povey S, Snell RG, Cheadle JP, Jones AC, Tachataki M, Ravine D, Sampson JR, Reeve MP, Richardson P, Wilmer F, Munro CS, Hawkins TL, Sepp T, Ali JBM, Ward S, Green AJ, Yates JR, Kwiatkowska J, Henske EP, Short MP, Haines JH, Jozwiak S, Kwiatkowski DJ (1997). Identification of the tuberous sclerosis gene TSC1 on chromosome 9q34. *Science* 277: 805-808.

2705. Vanatta PR, Silva FG, Taylor WE, Costa JC (1983). Renal cell carcinoma and systemic amyloidosis: demonstration of AA protein and review of the literature. *Hum Pathol* 14: 195-201.

2706. Vang R, Abrams J (2000). A micropapillary variant of transitional cell carcinoma arising in the ureter. *Arch Pathol Lab Med* 124: 1347-1348.

2707. Vang R, Kempson RL (2002). Perivascular epithelioid cell tumor ('PEComa') of the uterus: a subset of HMB-45-positive epithelioid mesenchymal neoplasms with an uncertain relationship to pure smooth muscle tumors. *Am J Surg Pathol* 26: 1-13.

2708. Vang R, Whitaker BP, Farhood AI, Silva EG, Ro JY, Deavers MT (2001). Immunohistochemical analysis of clear cell carcinoma of the gynecologic tract. *Int J Gynecol Pathol* 20: 252-259.

2709. Vanni R, Scarpa RM, Nieddu M, Usai E (1986). Identification of marker chromosomes in bladder tumor. *Urol Int* 41: 403-406.

2710. Vanni R, Scarpa RM, Nieddu M, Usai E (1988). Cytogenetic investigation on 30 bladder carcinomas. *Cancer Genet Cytogenet* 30: 35-42.

2711. Varambally S, Dhanasekaran SM, Zhou M, Barrette TR, Kumar-Sinha C, Sanda MG, Ghosh D, Pienta KJ, Sewalt RG, Otte AP, Chinnaiyan AM (2002). The polycomb group protein EZH2 is involved in progression of prostate cancer. *Nature* 419: 624-629.

2712. Varela-Duran J, Urdiales-Viedma M, Taboada-Blanco F, Cuevas C (1987). Neurofibroma of the ureter. *J Urol* 138: 1425-1426.

2713. Varkarakis MJ, Gaeta J, Moore RH, Murphy GP (1974). Superficial bladder tumor. Aspects of clinical progression. *Urology* 4: 414-420.

2714. Varma M, Morgan M, Jasani B, Tamboli P, Amin MB (2002). Polyclonal anti-PSA is more sensitive but less specific than monoclonal anti-PSA: Implications for diagnostic prostatic pathology. *Am J Clin Pathol* 118: 202-207.

2715. Vazquez JL, Barnewolt CE, Shamberger RC, Chung T, Perez-Atayde AR (1998). Ossifying renal tumor of infancy presenting as a palpable abdominal mass. *Pediatr Radiol* 28: 454-457.

2716. Veeramachaneni DN, Sawyer HR (1998). Carcinoma in situ and seminoma in equine testis. *APMIS* 106: 183-185.

2717. Veeramachaneni DN, Vandewoude S (1999). Interstitial cell tumour and germ cell tumour with carcinoma in situ in rabbit testes. *Int J Androl* 22: 97-101.

2718. Vega F, Medeiros LJ, Abruzzo LV (2001). Primary paratesticular lymphoma: a report of 2 cases and review of literature. *Arch Pathol Lab Med* 125: 428-432.

2719. Velazquez EF (2003). Limitations in the interpretation of biopsies in patients with penile squamous cell carcinomas. *Int J Surg Pathol* (in press).

2720. Velazquez EF (2003). Positive resection margins in partial penectomies: sites of involvement and proposal of local routes of spread in penile squamous cell carcinoma. *Am J Surg Pathol* (in press).

2721. Velickovic M, Delahunt B, Grebe SK (1999). Loss of heterozygosity at 3p14.2 in clear cell renal cell carcinoma is an early event and is highly localized to the FHIT gene locus. *Cancer Res* 59: 1323-1326.

2722. Velickovic M, Delahunt B, McIver B, Grebe SK (2002). Intragenic PTEN/MMAC1 loss of heterozygosity in conventional (clear-cell) renal cell carcinoma is associated with poor patient prognosis. *Mod Pathol* 15: 479-485.

2723. Velickovic M, Delahunt B, Storkel S, Grebe SK (2001). VHL and FHIT locus loss of heterozygosity is common in all renal cancer morphotypes but differs in pattern and prognostic significance. *Cancer Res* 61: 4815-4819.

2724. Veltman I, van Asseldonk M, Schepens M, Stoop H, Looijenga LH, Wouters C, Govaerts L, Suijkerbuijk R, van Kessel A (2002). A novel case of infantile sacral teratoma and a constitutional t(12;15)(q13;q25) pat. *Cancer Genet Cytogenet* 136: 17-22.

2725. Vere White RW, Stapp E (1998). Predicting prognosis in patients with superficial bladder cancer. *Oncology (Huntingt)* 12: 1717-1723.

2726. Verkerk AJ, Ariel I, Dekker MC, Schneider T, van Gurp RJ, de Groot N, Gillis AJ, Oosterhuis JW, Hochberg AA, Looijenga LH (1997). Unique expression patterns of H19 in human testicular cancers of different etiology. *Oncogene* 14: 95-107.

2727. Vermeulen P, Hoekx L, Colpaert C, Wyndaele JJ, van Marck E (2000). Biphasic sarcomatoid carcinoma (carcinosarcoma) of the renal pelvis with heterologous chondrogenic differentiation. *Virchows Arch* 437: 194-197.

2728. Verp MS, Simpson JL (1987). Abnormal sexual differentiation and neoplasia. *Cancer Genet Cytogenet* 25: 191-218.

2729. Versteege I, Sevenet N, Lange J, Rousseau-Merck MF, Ambros P, Handgretinger R, Aurias A, Delattre O (1998). Truncating mutations of hSNF5/INI1 in aggressive paediatric cancer. *Nature* 394: 203-206.

2730. Vessella RL, Blouke KA, Stray JE, Riley DE, Spies AG, Arfman EW, Lange PH (1992). The use of the polymerase chain reaction to detect metastatic prostate cancer in lymph nodes and bone marrow. *Proc Amer Assn Cancer Res* 33: 396.

2731. Viadana E, Bross ID, Pickren JW (1978). An autopsy study of the metastatic patterns of human leukemias. *Oncology* 35: 87-96.

2732. Vieweg J, Gschwend JE, Herr HW, Fair WR (1999). Pelvic lymph node dissection can be curative in patients with node positive bladder cancer. *J Urol* 161: 449-454.

2733. Vieweg J, Gschwend JE, Herr HW, Fair WR (1999). The impact of primary stage on survival in patients with lymph node positive bladder cancer. *J Urol* 161: 72-76.

2734. Villers A, McNeal JE, Freiha FS, Boccon-Gibod L, Stamey TA (1993). Invasion of Denonvilliers' fascia in radical prostatectomy specimens. *J Urol* 149: 793-798.

2735. Villers A, McNeal JE, Redwine EA, Freiha FS, Stamey TA (1989). The role of perineural space invasion in the local spread of prostatic adenocarcinoma. *J Urol* 142: 763-768.

2736. Viola MV, Fromowitz F, Oravez S, Deb S, Schlom J (1985). ras Oncogene p21 expression is increased in premalignant lesions and high grade bladder carcinoma. *J Exp Med* 161: 1213-1218.

2737. Visakorpi T, Kallioniemi AH, Syvanen AC, Hyytinen ER, Karhu R, Tammela T, Isola JJ, Kallioniemi OP (1995). Genetic changes in primary and recurrent prostate cancer by comparative genomic hybridization. *Cancer Res* 55: 342-347.

2738. Visco C, Medeiros LJ, Mesina OM, Rodriguez MA, Hagemeister FB, McLaughlin P, Romaguera JE, Cabanillas F, Sarris AH (2001). Non-Hodgkin's lymphoma affecting the testis: is it curable with doxorubicin-based therapy? *Clin Lymphoma* 2: 40-46.

2739. Vizcaino AP, Parkin DM, Boffetta P, Skinner ME (1994). Bladder cancer: epidemiology and risk factors in Bulawayo, Zimbabwe. *Cancer Causes Control* 5: 517-522.

2740. Vock P, Haertel M, Fuchs WA, Karrer P, Bishop MC, Zingg EJ (1982). Computed tomography in staging of carcinoma of the urinary bladder. *Br J Urol* 54: 158-163.

2741. Voeller HJ, Augustus M, Madike V, Bova GS, Carter KC, Gelmann EP (1997). Coding region of NKX3.1, a prostate-specific homeobox gene on 8p21, is not mutated in human prostate cancers. *Cancer Res* 57: 4455-4459.

2742. Vogelzang NJ, Fremgen AM, Guinan PD, Chmiel JS, Sylvester JL, Sener SF (1993). Primary renal sarcoma in adults. A natural history and management study by the American Cancer Society, Illinois Division. *Cancer* 71: 804-810.

2743. Vogelzang NJ, Yang X, Goldman S, Vijayakumar S, Steinberg G (1998). Radiation induced renal cell cancer: a report of 4 cases and review of the literature. *J Urol* 160: 1987-1990.

2744. Voges GE, McNeal JE, Redwine EA, Freiha FS, Stamey TA (1992). Morphologic analysis of surgical margins with positive findings in prostatectomy for adenocarcinoma of the prostate. *Cancer* 69: 520-526.

2745. Voges GE, McNeal JE, Redwine EA, Freiha FS, Stamey TA (1992). The predictive significance of substaging stage A prostate cancer (A1 versus A2) for volume and grade of total cancer in the prostate. *J Urol* 147: 858-863.

2746. Voges GE, Tauschke E, Stockle M, Alken P, Hohenfellner R (1989). Computerized tomography: an unreliable method for accurate staging of bladder tumors in patients who are candidates for radical cystectomy. *J Urol* 142: 972-974.

2747. Voges GE, Wippermann F, Duber C, Hohenfellner R (1990). Pheochromocytoma in the pediatric age group: the prostate—an unusual location. *J Urol* 144: 1219-1221.

2748. Vollmer RT, Humphrey PA, Swanson PE, Wick MR, Hudson ML (1998). Invasion of the bladder by transitional cell carcinoma: its relation to histologic grade and expression of p53, MIB-1, c-erb B-2, epidermal growth factor receptor, and bcl-2. *Cancer* 82: 715-723.

2749. von der Maase H, Giwercman A, Muller J, Skakkebaek NE (1987). Management of carcinoma-in-situ of the testis. *Int J Androl* 10: 209-220.

2750. von der Maase H, Rorth M, Walbom-Jorgensen S, Sorensen BL, Christophersen IS, Hald T, Jacobsen GK, Berthelsen JG, Skakkebaek NE (1986). Carcinoma in situ of contralateral testis in patients with testicular germ cell cancer: study of 27 cases in 500 patients. *Br Med J (Clin Res Ed)* 293: 1398-1401.

2751. von der Maase H, Specht L, Jacobsen GK, Jakobsen A, Madsen EL, Pedersen M, Rorth M, Schultz H (1993). Surveillance following orchidectomy for stage I seminoma of the testis. *Eur J Cancer* 29A: 1931-1934.

2752. von Hippel E (1904). Uber eine sehr seltene Erkrankung der Netzhaut. *Graefe's Arch* 59: 83-86.

2753. von Hochstetter AR, Hedinger CE (1982). The differential diagnosis of testicular germ cell tumors in theory and practice. A critical analysis of two major systems of classification and review of 389 cases. *Virchows Arch A Pathol Anat Histol* 396: 247-277.
2754. von Krogh G (2001). Management of anogenital warts (condylomata acuminata). *Eur J Dermatol* 11: 598-603.
2755. von Krogh G, Dahlman-Ghozlan K, Syrjanen S (2002). Potential human papillomavirus reactivation following topical corticosteroid therapy of genital lichen sclerosus and erosive lichen planus. *J Eur Acad Dermatol Venereol* 16: 130-133.
2756. von Krogh G, Horenblas S (2000). Diagnosis and clinical presentation of premalignant lesions of the penis. *Scand J Urol Nephrol Suppl* 205: 201-214.
2757. Vousden KH, Lu X (2002). Live or let die: the cell's response to p53. *Nat Rev Cancer* 2: 594-604.
2758. Vujanic GM, Delemarre JF, Moeslichan S, Lam J, Harms D, Sandstedt B, Voute PA (1993). Mesoblastic nephroma metastatic to the lungs and heart—another face of this peculiar lesion: case report and review of the literature. *Pediatr Pathol* 13: 143-153.
2759. Vujanic GM, Harms D, Sandstedt B, Weirich A, de Kraker J, Delemarre JF (1999). New definitions of focal and diffuse anaplasia in Wilms tumor: the International Society of Paediatric Oncology (SIOP) experience. *Med Pediatr Oncol* 32: 317-323.
2760. Wagner JR, Honig SC, Siroky MB (1993). Non-Hodgkin's lymphoma can mimic renal adenocarcinoma with inferior vena caval involvement. *Urology* 42: 720-723.
2761. Wagner U, Sauter G, Moch H, Novotna H, Epper R, Mihatsch MJ, Waldman FM (1995). Patterns of p53, erbB-2, and EGF-r expression in premalignant lesions of the urinary bladder. *Hum Pathol* 26: 970-978.
2762. Wagner U, Suess K, Luginbuhl T, Schmid U, Ackermann D, Zellweger T, Maurer R, Alund G, Knonagel H, Rist M, Jordan P, Moch H, Mihatsch MJ, Gasser TC, Sauter G (1999). Cyclin D1 overexpression lacks prognostic significance in superficial urinary bladder cancer. *J Pathol* 188: 44-50.
2763. Wahren B, Holmgren PA, Stigbrand T (1979). Placental alkaline phosphatase, alphafetoprotein and carcinoembryonic antigen in testicular tumors. Tissue typing by means of cytologic smears. *Int J Cancer* 24: 749-753.
2764. Wai DH, Knezevich SR, Lucas T, Jansen B, Kay RJ, Sorensen PH (2000). The ETV6-NTRK3 gene fusion encodes a chimeric protein tyrosine kinase that transforms NIH3T3 cells. *Oncogene* 19: 906-915.
2765. Waisman J, Adolfsson J, Lowhagen T, Skoog L (1991). Comparison of transrectal prostate digital aspiration and ultrasound-guided core biopsies in 99 men. *Urology* 37: 301-307.
2766. Waldman FM, Carroll PR, Kerschmann R, Cohen MB, Field FG, Mayall BH (1991). Centromeric copy number of chromosome 7 is strongly correlated with tumor grade and labeling index in human bladder cancer. *Cancer Res* 51: 3807-3813.
2767. Walker AN, Mills SE, Jones PF, Stanley CM (1988). Borderline serous cystadenoma of the tunica vaginalis testis. *Surg Pathol* 1: 431-436.
2768. Walker BF, Someren A, Kennedy JC, Nicholas EM (1992). Primary carcinoid tumor of the urinary bladder. *Arch Pathol Lab Med* 116: 1217-1220.
2769. Walley VM, Veinot JP, Tazelaar H, Courtice RW (1999). Lesions described as nodular mesothelial hyperplasia. *Am J Surg Pathol* 23: 994-995.
2770. Walsh IK, Keane PF, Herron B (1993). Benign urethral polyps. *Br J Urol* 72: 937-938.
2771. Walt H, Oosterhuis JW, Stevens LC (1993). Experimental testicular germ cell tumorigenesis in mouse strains with and without spontaneous tumours differs from development of germ cell tumours of the adult human testis. *Int J Androl* 16: 267-271.
2772. Walther M, O'Brien DP3rd, Birch HW (1986). Condylomata acuminata and verrucous carcinoma of the bladder: case report and literature review. *J Urol* 135: 362-365.
2773. Walther MM, Lubensky IA, Venzon D, Zbar B, Linehan WM (1995). Prevalence of microscopic lesions in grossly normal renal parenchyma from patients with von Hippel-Lindau disease, sporadic renal cell carcinoma and no renal disease: clinical implications. *J Urol* 154: 2010-2014.
2774. Wanderas EH, Fossa SD, Tretli S (1997). Risk of a second germ cell cancer after treatment of a primary germ cell cancer in 2201 Norwegian male patients. *Eur J Cancer* 33: 244-252.
2775. Wanderas EH, Grotmol T, Fossa SD, Tretli S (1998). Maternal health and pre- and perinatal characteristics in the etiology of testicular cancer: a prospective population- and register-based study on Norwegian males born between 1967 and 1995. *Cancer Causes Control* 9: 475-486.
2776. Wang DS, Rieger-Christ K, Latini JM, Moinzadeh A, Stoffel J, Pezza JA, Saini K, Libertino JA, Summerhayes IC (2000). Molecular analysis of PTEN and MXI1 in primary bladder carcinoma. *Int J Cancer* 88: 620-625.
2777. Wang HL, Lu DW, Yerian LM, Alsikafi N, Steinberg G, Hart J, Yang XJ (2001). Immunohistochemical distinction between primary adenocarcinoma of the bladder and secondary colorectal adenocarcinoma. *Am J Surg Pathol* 25: 1380-1387.
2778. Wang J, Arber DA, Frankel K, Weiss LM (2001). Large solitary fibrous tumor of the kidney: report of two cases and review of the literature. *Am J Surg Pathol* 25: 1194-1199.
2779. Wang T, Palazzo JP, Mitchell D, Petersen RO (1993). Renal capsular hemangioma. *J Urol* 149: 1122-1123.
2780. Warde P, Gospodarowicz MK, Banerjee D, Panzarella T, Sugar L, Catton CN, Sturgeon JF, Moore M, Jewett MA (1997). Prognostic factors for relapse in stage I testicular seminoma treated with surveillance. *J Urol* 157: 1705-1709.
2781. Warde P, Specht L, Horwich A, Oliver T, Panzarella T, Gospodarowicz M, von der Maase H (2002). Prognostic factors for relapse in stage I seminoma managed by surveillance: a pooled analysis. *J Clin Oncol* 20: 4448-4452.
2782. Warfel KA, Eble JN (1982). Renal oncocytomatosis. *J Urol* 127: 1179-1180.
2783. Warfel KA, Eble JN (1985). Renomedullary interstitial cell tumors. *Am J Clinic Pathol* 83: 262.
2784. Warren W, Biggs PJ, el Baz M, Ghoneim MA, Stratton MR, Venitt S (1995). Mutations in the p53 gene in schistosomal bladder cancer: a study of 92 tumours from Egyptian patients and a comparison between mutational spectra from schistosomal and non-schistosomal urothelial tumours. *Carcinogenesis* 16: 1181-1189.
2785. Washecka R, Dresner MI, Honda SA (2002). Testicular tumors in Carney's complex. *J Urol* 167: 1299-1302.
2786. Washecka RM, Mariani AJ, Zuna RE, Honda SA, Chong CD (1996). Primary intratesticular sarcoma. Immunohistochemical ultrastructural and DNA flow cytometric study of three cases with a review of the literature. *Cancer* 77: 1524-1528.
2787. Watanabe K, Kurizaki Y, Ogawa A, Ishii K, Kawakami H (1994). Primary malignant lymphoma of the penis: a case report. *Int J Urol* 1: 283-284.
2788. Waterhouse J, Muir C, Shanmugaratnam K, Powell J (1982). *Cancer Incidence in Five Continents. IARC Scientific Publication No 42.* J Waterhouse, C Muir, K Shanmugaratnam, J Powell, eds. IARC Press: Lyon.
2789. Watson P, Lynch HT (1993). Extracolonic cancer in hereditary nonpolyposis colorectal cancer. *Cancer* 71: 677-685.
2790. Watson RB, Civantos F, Soloway MS (1996). Positive surgical margins with radical prostatectomy: detailed pathological analysis and prognosis. *Urology* 48: 80-90.
2791. Wattenberg CA, Beare JB, Tornmey AR (1956). Exstrophy of the urinary bladder complicated by adenocarcinoma. *J Urol* 76: 583-594.
2792. Waxman M, Vuletin JC, Pertschuk LP, Bellamy J, Enu K (1982). Pleomorphic atypical thyroid adenoma arising in struma testis: light microscopic, ultrastructural and immunofluorescent studies. *Mt Sinai J Med* 49: 13-17.
2793. Wazait HD, Chahal R, Sundurum SK, Rajkumar GN, Wright D, Aslam MM (2001). MALT-type primary lymphoma of the urinary bladder: clinicopathological study of 2 cases and review of the literature. *Urol Int* 66: 220-224.
2794. Webber RJ, Alsaffar N, Bissett D, Langlois NE (1998). Angiosarcoma of the penis. *Urology* 51: 130-131.
2795. Weeks DA, Beckwith JB, Mierau GW, Zuppan CW (1991). Renal neoplasms mimicking rhabdoid tumor of kidney. A report from the National Wilms' Tumor Study Pathology Center. *Am J Surg Pathol* 15: 1042-1054.
2796. Weeks DA, Malott RL, Arnesen M, Zuppan C, Aitken D, Mierau G (1991). Hepatic angiomyolipoma with striated granules and positivity with melanoma—specific antibody (HMB-45): a report of two cases. *Ultrastruct Pathol* 15: 563-571.
2797. Weidner IS, Moller H, Jensen TK, Skakkebaek NE (1999). Risk factors for cryptorchidism and hypospadias. *J Urol* 161: 1606-1609.
2798. Weidner N (1991). Myoid gonadal stromal tumor with epithelial differentiation (? testicular myoepithelioma). *Ultrastruct Pathol* 15: 409-416.
2799. Weidner U, Peter S, Strohmeyer T, Hussnatter R, Ackermann R, Sies H (1990). Inverse relationship of epidermal growth factor receptor and HER2/neu gene expression in human renal cell carcinoma. *Cancer Res* 50: 4504-4509.
2800. Weingartner K, Gerharz EW, Neumann K, Pfluger KH, Gruber M, Riedmiller H (1995). Primary osteosarcoma of the kidney. Case report and review of literature. *Eur Urol* 28: 81-84.
2801. Weingartner K, Kozakewich HP, Hendren WH (1997). Nephrogenic adenoma after urethral reconstruction using bladder mucosa: report of 6 cases and review of the literature. *J Urol* 158: 1175-1177.
2802. Weinstein MH, Partin AW, Veltri RW, Epstein JI (1996). Neuroendocrine differentiation in prostate cancer: enhanced prediction of progression after radical prostatectomy. *Hum Pathol* 27: 683-687.
2803. Weinstein RS, Miller AW3rd, Pauli BU (1980). Carcinoma in situ: comments on the pathobiology of a paradox. *Urol Clin North Am* 7: 523-531.
2804. Weirich G, Klein B, Wohl T, Engelhardt D, Brauch H (2002). VHL2C phenotype in a German von Hippel-Lindau family with concurrent VHL germline mutations P81S and L188V. *J Clin Endocrinol Metab* 87: 5241-5246.
2805. Weissbach L, Altwein JE, Stiens R (1984). Germinal testicular tumors in childhood. Report of observations and literature review. *Eur Urol* 10: 73-85.
2806. Weissbach L, Bussar-Maatz R, Lohrs U, Schubert GE, Mann K, Hartmann M, Dieckmann KP, Fassbinder J (1999). Prognostic factors in seminomas with special respect to HCG: results of a prospective multicenter study. Seminoma Study Group. *Eur Urol* 36: 601-608.
2807. Welsh JB, Sapinoso LM, Su AI, Kern SG, Wang-Rodriguez J, Moskaluk CA, Frierson HFJr, Hampton GM (2001). Analysis of gene expression identifies candidate markers and pharmacological targets in prostate cancer. *Cancer Res* 61: 5974-5978.
2808. Westra WH, Grenko RT, Epstein JI (2000). Solitary fibrous tumor of the lower urogenital tract: a report of five cases involving the seminal vesicles, urinary bladder, and prostate. *Hum Pathol* 31: 63-68.
2809. Weterman MJ, van Groningen JJ, Jansen A, van Kessel AG (2000). Nuclear localization and transactivating capacities of the papillary renal cell carcinoma-associated TFE3 and PRCC (fusion) proteins. *Oncogene* 19: 69-74.
2810. Whaley JM, Naglich J, Gelbert L, Hsia YE, Lamiell JM, Green JS, Collins D, Neumann HP, Laidlaw J, Li FP (1994). Germline mutations in the von Hippel-Lindau tumor-suppressor gene are similar to somatic von Hippel-Lindau aberrations in sporadic renal cell carcinoma. *Am J Hum Genet* 55: 1092-1102.
2811. Wheeler JD, Hill WT (1954). Adenocarcinoma involving the urinary bladder. *Cancer* 7: 119-135.
2812. Wheeler TM, Dillioglugil O, Kattan MW, Arakawa A, Soh S, Suyama K, Ohori M, Scardino PT (1998). Clinical and pathological significance of the level and extent of capsular invasion in clinical stage T1-2 prostate cancer. *Hum Pathol* 29: 856-862.
2813. Whitehead ED, Tessler AN (1971). Carcinoma of the urachus. *Br J Urol* 43: 468-476.
2814. Whitehead R, Williams AF (1951). Carcinoma of the epididymis. *Br J Surg* 38: 513-516.
2815. Whittemore AS, Wu AH, Kolonel LN, John EM, Gallagher RP, Howe GR, West DW, Teh CZ, Stamey T (1995). Family history and prostate cancer risk in Black, White, and Asian men in the United States and Canada. *Am J Epidemiol* 141: 732-740.

2816. Wick MR, Berg LC, Hertz MI (1992). Large cell carcinoma of the lung with neuroendocrine differentiation. A comparison with large cell "undifferentiated" pulmonary tumors. *Am J Clin Pathol* 97: 796-805.
2817. Wick MR, Brown BA, Young RH, Mills SE (1988). Spindle-cell proliferations of the urinary tract. An immunohistochemical study. *Am J Surg Pathol* 12: 379-389.
2818. Wick MR, Cherwitz DL, Manivel JC, Sibley R (1990). Immunohistochemical findings in tumors of the kidney. In: *Tumor and Tumor-like Conditions of the Kidneys and Ureters*, JN Eble, ed. Churchill Livingstone: New York, pp. 207-247.
2819. Wick MR, Mills SE, Scheithauer BW, Cooper PH, Davitz MA, Parkinson K (1986). Reassessment of malignant "angioendotheliomatosis". Evidence in favor of its reclassification as "intravascular lymphomatosis". *Am J Surg Pathol* 10: 112-123.
2820. Wiener JS, Coppes MJ, Ritchey ML (1998). Current concepts in the biology and management of Wilms tumor. *J Urol* 159: 1316-1325.
2821. Wiener JS, Liu ET, Walther PJ (1992). Oncogenic human papillomavirus type 16 is associated with squamous cell cancer of the male urethra. *Cancer Res* 52: 5018-5023.
2822. Wiener JS, Walther PJ (1994). A high association of oncogenic human papillomaviruses with carcinomas of the female urethra: polymerase chain reaction-based analysis of multiple histological types. *J Urol* 151: 49-53.
2823. Wilcox G, Soh S, Chakraborty S, Scardino PT, Wheeler TM (1998). Patterns of high-grade prostatic intraepithelial neoplasia associated with clinically aggressive prostate cancer. *Hum Pathol* 29: 1119-1123.
2824. Wiley EL, Davidson P, McIntire DD, Sagalowsky AI (1997). Risk of concurrent prostate cancer in cystoprostatectomy specimens is related to volume of high-grade prostatic intraepithelial neoplasia. *Urology* 49: 692-696.
2825. Wilkins BS, Williamson JM, O'Brien CJ (1989). Morphological and immunohistological study of testicular lymphomas. *Histopathology* 15: 147-156.
2826. Williams JC, Merguerian PA, Schned AR, Amdur RJ (1994). Bilateral testicular carcinoma in situ in persistent mullerian duct syndrome: a case report and literature review. *Urology* 44: 595-598.
2827. Williams SG, Buscarini M, Stein JP (2001). Molecular markers for diagnosis, staging, and prognosis of bladder cancer. *Oncology (Huntingt)* 15: 1461-1476.
2828. Williams TR, Wagner BJ, Corse WR, Vestevich JC (2002). Fibroepithelial polyps of the urinary tract. *Abdom Imaging* 27: 217-221.
2829. Willis TG, Jadayel DM, Du MQ, Peng H, Perry AR, Abdul-Rauf M, Price H, Karran L, Majekodunmi O, Wlodarska I, Pan L, Crook T, Hamoudi R, Isaacson PG, Dyer MJ (1999). Bcl10 is involved in t(1;14)(p22;q32) of MALT B cell lymphoma and mutated in multiple tumor types. *Cell* 96: 35-45.
2830. Wills ML, Hamper UM, Partin AW, Epstein JI (1997). Incidence of high-grade prostatic intraepithelial neoplasia in sextant needle biopsy specimens. *Urology* 49: 367-373.
2831. Wilson BE, Netzloff ML (1983). Primary testicular abnormalities causing precocious puberty Leydig cell tumor, Leydig cell hyperplasia, and adrenal rest tumor. *Ann Clin Lab Sci* 13: 315-320.
2832. Wilson TG, Pritchett TR, Lieskovsky G, Warner NE, Skinner DG (1991). Primary adenocarcinoma of bladder. *Urology* 38: 223-226.
2833. Wirnsberger GH, Ratschek M, Dimai HP, Holzer H, Mandal AK (1999). Post-transplantation lymphoproliferative disorder of the T-cell/B-cell type: an unusual manifestation in a renal allograft. *Oncol Rep* 6: 29-32.
2834. Wishnow KI, Johnson DE, Swanson DA, Tenney DM, Babaian RJ, Dunphy CH, Ayala AG, Ro JY, von Eschenbach AC (1989). Identifying patients with low-risk clinical stage I nonseminomatous testicular tumors who should be treated by surveillance. *Urology* 34: 339-343.
2835. Witjes JA, Kiemeney LA, Schaafsma HE, Debruyn FM (1994). The influence of review pathology on study outcome of a randomized multicentre superficial bladder cancer trial. Members of the Dutch South East Cooperative Urological Group. *Br J Urol* 73: 172-176.
2836. Wolf H, Olsen PR, Fischer A, Hojgaard K (1987). Urothelial atypia concomitant with primary bladder tumour. Incidence in a consecutive series of 500 unselected patients. *Scand J Urol Nephrol* 21: 33-38.
2837. Wood DPJr, Montie JE, Pontes JE, Vanderbrug Medendrop S, Levin HS (1989). Transitional cell carcinoma of the prostate in cystoprostatectomy specimens removed for bladder cancer. *J Urol* 141: 346-349.
2838. Wood EW, Gardner WAJr, Brown FM (1972). Spindle cell squamous carcinoma of the penis. *J Urol* 107: 990-991.
2839. Woodruff JM, Godwin TA, Erlandson RA, Susin M, Martini N (1981). Cellular schwannoma: a variety of schwannoma sometimes mistaken for a malignant tumor. *Am J Surg Pathol* 5: 733-744.
2840. Woolcott CG, King WD, Marrett LD (2002). Coffee and tea consumption and cancers of the bladder, colon and rectum. *Eur J Cancer Prev* 11: 137-145.
2841. World Cancer Research Fund in Association with American Institute for Cancer Research (1997). *Food, Nutrition and the Prevention of Cancer: A Global Perspective.* WCRF: Washington, DC.
2842. World Cancer Research Fund Panel (1997). *Diet, nutrition and the prevention of cancer: a global perspective.* WCRF: Washington, DC.
2843. World Health Organization (2003). World Health Statistics Annual 1997-1999 Edition. http://www.who.int/whosis.
2844. Wright C, Mellon K, Johnston P, Lane DP, Harris AL, Horne CH, Neal DE (1991). Expression of mutant p53, c-erbB-2 and the epidermal growth factor receptor in transitional cell carcinoma of the human urinary bladder. *Br J Cancer* 63: 967-970.
2845. Wright C, Thomas D, Mellon K, Neal DE, Horne CH (1995). Expression of retinoblastoma gene product and p53 protein in bladder carcinoma: correlation with Ki67 index. *Br J Urol* 75: 173-179.
2846. Wright GL, Haley C, Beckett ML, Schellhammer PF (1995). Expression of prostate-specific membrane antigen in normal, benign and malignant tissues. *Urol Oncol* 1: 18-28.
2847. Wright GLJr, Grob BM, Haley C, Grossman K, Newhall K, Petrylak D, Troyer J, Konchuba A, Schellhammer PF, Moriarty R (1996). Upregulation of prostate-specific membrane antigen after androgen-deprivation therapy. *Urology* 48: 326-334.
2848. Wu RL, Osman I, Wu XR, Lu ML, Zhang ZF, Liang FX, Hamza R, Scher H, Cordon-Cardo C, Sun TT (1998). Uroplakin II gene is expressed in transitional cell carcinoma but not in bilharzial bladder squamous cell carcinoma: alternative pathways of bladder epithelial differentiation and tumor formation. *Cancer Res* 58: 1291-1297.
2849. Wu SQ, Hafez GR, Xing W, Newton M, Chen XR, Messing E (1996). The correlation between the loss of chromosome 14q with histologic tumor grade, pathologic stage, and outcome of patients with nonpapillary renal cell carcinoma. *Cancer* 77: 1154-1160.
2850. Wu X, Senechal K, Neshat MS, Whang YE, Sawyers CL (1998). The PTEN/MMAC1 tumor suppressor phosphatase functions as a negative regulator of the phosphoinositide 3-kinase/Akt pathway. *Proc Natl Acad Sci USA* 95: 15587-15591.
2851. Wyatt JK, Craig I (1980). Verrucous carcinoma of urinary bladder. *Urology* 16: 97-99.
2852. Xiao SY, Rizzo P, Carbone M (2000). Benign papillary mesothelioma of the tunica vaginalis testis. *Arch Pathol Lab Med* 124: 143-147.
2853. Xiaoxu L, Jianhong L, Jinfeng W, Klotz LH (2001). Bladder adenocarcinoma: 31 reported cases. *Can J Urol* 8: 1380-1383.
2854. Xipell JM (1971). The incidence of benign renal nodules (a clinicopathologic study). *J Urol* 106: 503-506.
2855. Xu J, Meyers D, Freije D, Isaacs S, Wiley K, Nusskern D, Ewing C, Wilkens E, Bujnovszky P, Bova GS, Walsh P, Isaacs W, Schleutker J, Matikainen M, Tammela T, Visakorpi T, Kallioniemi OP, Berry R, Schaid D, French A, McDonnell S, Schroeder J, Blute M, Thibodeau S, Gronberg H, Emanuelsson M, Damber JE, Bergh A, Jonsson BA, Smith J, Bailey-Wilson J, Carpten J, Stephan D, Gillanders E, Amundson I, Kainu T, Freas-Lutz D, Baffoe-Bonnie A, Van Aucken A, Sood R, Collins F, Brownstein M, Trent J (1998). Evidence for a prostate cancer susceptibility locus on the X chromosome. *Nat Genet* 20: 175-179.
2856. Xu J, Stolk JA, Zhang X, Silva SJ, Houghton RL, Matsumura M, Vedvick TS, Leslie KB, Badaro R, Reed SG (2000). Identification of differentially expressed genes in human prostate cancer using subtraction and microarray. *Cancer Res* 60: 1677-1682.
2857. Xu J, Zheng SL, Komiya A, Mychaleckyj JC, Isaacs SD, Hu JJ, Sterling D, Lange EM, Hawkins GA, Turner A, Ewing CM, Faith DA, Johnson JR, Suzuki H, Bujnovszky P, Wiley KE, de Marzo AM, Bova GS, Chang B, Hall MC, McCullough DL, Partin AW, Kassabian VS, Carpten JD, Bailey-Wilson JE, Trent JM, Ohar J, Bleecker ER, Walsh PC, Isaacs WB, Meyers DA (2002). Germline mutations and sequence variants of the macrophage scavenger receptor 1 gene are associated with prostate cancer risk. *Nat Genet* 32: 321-325.
2858. Xu J, Zheng SL, Turner A, Isaacs SD, Wiley KE, Hawkins GA, Chang BL, Bleecker ER, Walsh PC, Meyers DA, Isaacs WB (2002). Associations between hOGG1 sequence variants and prostate cancer susceptibility. *Cancer Res* 62: 2253-2257.
2859. Xu X, Stower MJ, Reid IN, Garner RC, Burns PA (1996). Molecular screening of multifocal transitional cell carcinoma of the bladder using p53 mutations as biomarkers. *Clin Cancer Res* 2: 1795-1800.
2860. Yachia D, Auslaender L (1989). Primary leiomyosarcoma of the testis. *J Urol* 141: 955-956.
2861. Yagi H, Igawa M, Shiina H, Shigeno K, Yoneda T, Wada Y, Urakami S (1999). Inverted papilloma of the urinary bladder in a girl. *Urol Int* 63: 258-260.
2862. Yalla SV, Ivker M, Burros HM, Dorey F (1975). Cystitis glandularis with perivesical lipomatosis. Frequent association of two unusual proliferative conditions. *Urology* 5: 383-386.
2863. Yamamoto T, Ito K, Suzuki K, Yamanaka H, Ebihara K, Sasaki A (2002). Rapidly progressive malignant epithelioid angiomyolipoma of the kidney. *J Urol* 168: 190-191.
2864. Yaman O, Baltaci S, Arikan N, Yilmaz E, Gogus O (1996). Staging with computed tomography, transrectal ultrasonography and transurethral resection of bladder tumour: comparison with final pathological stage in invasive bladder carcinoma. *Br J Urol* 78: 197-200.
2865. Yang CH, Krzyzaniak K, Brown WJ, Kurtz SM (1985). Primary carcinoid tumor of urinary bladder. *Urology* 26: 594-597.
2866. Yang CW, Park JH, Park JH, Cho SG, Kim YS, Bang BK (2001). Acute graft dysfunction due to Kaposi sarcoma involving the bladder in a renal transplant recipient. *Nephrol Dial Transplant* 16: 625-627.
2867. Yang RM, Naitoh J, Murphy M, Wang HJ, Phillipson J, Dekernion JB, Loda M, Reiter RE (1998). Low p27 expression predicts poor disease-free survival in patients with prostate cancer. *J Urol* 159: 941-945.
2868. Yang XJ, McEntee M, Epstein JI (1998). Distinction of basaloid carcinoma of the prostate from benign basal cell lesions by using immunohistochemistry for bcl-2 and Ki-67. *Hum Pathol* 29: 1447-1450.
2869. Yang XJ, Wu CL, Woda BA, Dresser K, Tretiakova M, Fanger GR, Jiang Z (2002). Expression of alpha-Methylacyl-CoA racemase (P504S) in atypical adenomatous hyperplasia of the prostate. *Am J Surg Pathol* 26: 921-925.
2870. Yashi M, Hashimoto S, Muraishi O, Tozuka K, Tokue A (2000). Leiomyoma of the ureter. *Urol Int* 64: 40-42.
2871. Yashi M, Muraishi O, Kobayashi Y, Tokue A, Nanjo H (2002). Elevated serum progastrin-releasing peptide (31-98) in metastatic and androgen-independent prostate cancer patients. *Prostate* 51: 84-97.
2872. Yasukawa S, Aoshi H, Takamatsu M (1987). Ectopic prostatic adenoma in retrovesical space. *J Urol* 137: 998-999.
2873. Yasunaga Y, Shin M, Fujita MQ, Nonomura N, Miki T, Okuyama A, Aozasa K (1998). Different patterns of p53 mutations in prostatic intraepithelial neoplasia and concurrent carcinoma: analysis of microdissected specimens. *Lab Invest* 78: 1275-1279.
2874. Yatani R, Chigusa I, Akazaki K, Stemmermann GN, Welsh RA, Correa P (1982). Geographic pathology of latent prostatic carcinoma. *Int J Cancer* 29: 611-616.
2875. Yazaki T, Takahashi S, Ogawa Y, Kanoh S, Kitagawa R (1985). Large renal hemangioma necessitating nephrectomy. *Urology* 25: 302-304.
2876. Ylagan LR, Humphrey PA (2001). Micropapillary variant of transitional cell carcinoma of the urinary bladder: a report of three cases with cytologic diagnosis in urine specimens. *Acta Cytol* 45: 599-604.
2877. Yong EL, Lim J, Qi W, Ong V, Mifsud A (2000). Molecular basis of androgen receptor diseases. *Ann Med* 32: 15-22.

2878. Yoo J, Park S, Jung Lee H, Jin Kang S, Kee Kim B (2002). Primary carcinoid tumor arising in a mature teratoma of the kidney: a case report and review of the literature. *Arch Pathol Lab Med* 126: 979-981.

2879. Yoon DS, Li L, Zhang RD, Kram A, Ro JY, Johnston D, Grossman HB, Scherer S, Czerniak B (2001). Genetic mapping and DNA sequence-based analysis of deleted regions on chromosome 16 involved in progression of bladder cancer from occult preneoplastic conditions to invasive disease. *Oncogene* 20: 5005-5014.

2880. Yoshida SO, Imam A, Olson CA, Taylor CR (1986). Proximal renal tubular surface membrane antigens identified in primary and metastatic renal cell carcinomas. *Arch Pathol Lab Med* 110: 825-832.

2881. Yoshida T, Hirai S, Horii Y, Yamauchi T (2001). Granular cell tumor of the urinary bladder. *Int J Urol* 8: 29-31.

2882. Yoshida T, Ogawa T, Fujinaga T, Kusuyama Y (1990). [A case of carcinosarcoma originating from the renal pelvis]. *Nippon Hinyokika Gakkai Zasshi* 81: 1739-1742.

2883. Yoshimura I, Kudoh J, Saito S, Tazaki H, Shimizu N (1995). p53 gene mutation in recurrent superficial bladder cancer. *J Urol* 153: 1711-1715.

2884. Yoshimura K, Arai Y, Fujimoto H, Nishiyama H, Ogura K, Okino T, Ogawa O (2002). Prognostic impact of extensive parenchymal invasion pattern in pT3 renal pelvic transitional cell carcinoma. *Cancer* 94: 3150-3156.

2885. Yoshimura S, Ito Y (1951). Malignant transformation of endometriosis of the urinary bladder: a case report. *Gann* 42: 2.

2886. Younes M, Sussman J, True LD (1990). The usefulness of the level of the muscularis mucosae in the staging of invasive transitional cell carcinoma of the urinary bladder. *Cancer* 66: 543-548.

2887. Young AN, Amin MB, Moreno CS, Lim SD, Cohen C, Petros JA, Marshall FF, Neish AS (2001). Expression profiling of renal epithelial neoplasms: a method for tumor classification and discovery of diagnostic molecular markers. *Am J Pathol* 158: 1639-1651.

2888. Young BW, Lagios MD (1973). Endometrial (papillary) carcinoma of the prostatic utricle—response to orchiectomy. A case report. *Cancer* 32: 1293-1300.

2889. Young RH (1990). Spindle cell lesions of the urinary bladder. *Histol Histopathol* 5: 505-512.

2890. Young RH (1992). Nephrogenic adenomas of the urethra involving the prostate gland: a report of two cases of a lesion that may be confused with prostatic adenocarcinoma. *Mod Pathol* 5: 617-620.

2891. Young RH, Eble JN (1991). Unusual forms of carcinoma of the urinary bladder. *Hum Pathol* 22: 948-965.

2892. Young RH, Finlayson N, Scully RE (1989). Tubular seminoma. Report of a case. *Arch Pathol Lab Med* 113: 414-416.

2893. Young RH, Frierson HFJr, Mills SE, Kaiser JS, Talbot WH, Bhan AK (1988). Adenoid cystic-like tumor of the prostate gland. A report of two cases and review of the literature on "adenoid cystic carcinoma" of the prostate. *Am J Clin Pathol* 89: 49-56.

2894. Young RH, Koelliker DD, Scully RE (1998). Sertoli cell tumors of the testis, not otherwise specified: a clinicopathologic analysis of 60 cases. *Am J Surg Pathol* 22: 709-721.

2895. Young RH, Lawrence WD, Scully RE (1985). Juvenile granulosa cell tumor—another neoplasm associated with abnormal chromosomes and ambiguous genitalia. A report of three cases. *Am J Surg Pathol* 9: 737-743.

2896. Young RH, Oliva E (1996). Transitional cell carcinomas of the urinary bladder that may be underdiagnosed. A report of four invasive cases exemplifying the homology between neoplastic and non-neoplastic transitional cell lesions. *Am J Surg Pathol* 20: 1448-1454.

2897. Young RH, Oliva E, Garcia JA, Bhan AK, Clement PB (1996). Urethral caruncle with atypical stromal cells simulating lymphoma or sarcoma—a distinctive pseudoneoplastic lesion of females. A report of six cases. *Am J Surg Pathol* 20: 1190-1195.

2898. Young RH, Parkhurst EC (1984). Mucinous adenocarcinoma of bladder. Case associated with extensive intestinal metaplasia of urothelium in patient with nonfunctioning bladder for twelve years. *Urology* 24: 192-195.

2899. Young RH, Proppe KH, Dickersin GR, Scully RE (1987). Myxoid leiomyosarcoma of the urinary bladder. *Arch Pathol Lab Med* 111: 359-362.

2900. Young RH, Rosenberg AE (1987). Osteosarcoma of the urinary bladder. Report of a case and review of the literature. *Cancer* 59: 174-178.

2901. Young RH, Scully RE (1985). Clear cell adenocarcinoma of the bladder and urethra. A report of three cases and review of the literature. *Am J Surg Pathol* 9: 816-826.

2902. Young RH, Scully RE (1986). Testicular and paratesticular tumors and tumor-like lesions of ovarian common epithelial and mullerian types. A report of four cases and review of the literature. *Am J Clin Pathol* 86: 146-152.

2903. Young RH, Scully RE (1987). Pseudosarcomatous lesions of the urinary bladder, prostate gland, and urethra. A report of three cases and review of the literature. *Arch Pathol Lab Med* 111: 354-358.

2904. Young RH, Scully RE (1990). *Testicular Tumors.* ASCP Press: Chicago.

2905. Young RH, Srigley JR, Amin MB, Ulbright TM, Cubilla AL (2000). *Tumors of the Prostate Gland, Seminal Vesicles, Male Urethra and Penis (fascicle 28).* 3rd Edition. AFIP: Washington, DC.

2906. Young RH, Talerman A (1987). Testicular tumors other than germ cell tumors. *Semin Diagn Pathol* 4: 342-360.

2907. Young S, Gooneratne S, Straus FH, Zeller WP, Bulun SE, Rosenthal IM (1995). Feminizing Sertoli cell tumors in boys with Peutz-Jeghers syndrome. *Am J Surg Pathol* 19: 50-58.

2908. Yu GS, Nseyo UO, Carson JW (1989). Primary penile lymphoma in a patient with Peyronie's disease. *J Urol* 142: 1076-1077.

2909. Yu J, Astrinidis A, Henske EP (2001). Chromosome 16 loss of heterozygosity in tuberous sclerosis and sporadic lymphangiomyomatosis. *Am J Respir Crit Care Med* 164: 1537-1540.

2910. Yu KK, Hricak H, Alagappan R, Chernoff DM, Bacchetti P, Zaloudek CJ (1997). Detection of extracapsular extension of prostate carcinoma with endorectal and phased-array coil MR imaging: multivariate feature analysis. *Radiology* 202: 697-702.

2911. Yu KK, Scheidler J, Hricak H, Vigneron DB, Zaloudek CJ, Males RG, Nelson SJ, Carroll PR, Kurhanewicz J (1999). Prostate cancer: prediction of extracapsular extension with endorectal MR imaging and three-dimensional proton MR spectroscopic imaging. *Radiology* 213: 481-488.

2912. Yuan JM, Castelao JE, Gago-Dominguez M, Ross RK, Yu MC (1998). Hypertension, obesity and their medications in relation to renal cell carcinoma. *Br J Cancer* 77: 1508-1513.

2913. Yum M, Ganguly A, Donohue JP (1984). Juxtaglomerular cells in renal angiomyolipoma. Ultrastructural observation. *Urology* 24: 283-286.

2914. Zafarana G, Gillis AJ, van Gurp RJ, Olsson PG, Elstrodt F, Stoop H, Millan JL, Oosterhuis JW, Looijenga LH (2002). Coamplification of DAD-R, SOX5, and EKI1 in human testicular seminomas, with specific overexpression of DAD-R, correlates with reduced levels of apoptosis and earlier clinical manifestation. *Cancer Res* 62: 1822-1831.

2915. Zafarana G, Grygalewicz B, Gillis AJ, Vissers LE, van de Vliet W, van Gurp RJ, Stoop H, Debiec-Rychter M, Oosterhuis JW, van Kessel AG, Schoenmakers EF, Looijenga LH, Veltman JA (2003). 12p-amplicon structure analysis in testicular germ cell tumors of adolescents and adults by array CGH. *Oncogene* 22: 7695-7701.

2916. Zaidi SZ, Mor Y, Scheimberg I, Quimby GF, Mouriquand PD (1998). Renal haemangioma presenting as an abdominal mass in a neonate. *Br J Urol* 82: 763-764.

2917. Zajaczek S, Gronwald J, Kata G, Borowka A, Lubinski J (1999). Familial renal cell cancer (CRCC) associated with a constitutional reciprocal translocation t(2;3)(q33;q21). *Cytogenet Cell Genet* 85: 172.

2918. Zaky Ahel M, Kovacic K, Kraljic I, Tarle M (2001). Oral estramustine therapy in serum chromogranin A-positive stage D3 prostate cancer patients. *Anticancer Res* 21: 1475-1479.

2919. Zaloudek C, Williams JW, Kempson RL (1976). "Endometrial" adenocarcinoma of the prostate: a distinctive tumor of probable prostatic duct origin. *Cancer* 37: 2255-2262.

2920. Zamboni G, Pea M, Martignoni G, Zancanaro C, Faccioli G, Gilioli E, Pederzoli P, Bonetti F (1996). Clear cell "sugar" tumor of the pancreas. A novel member of the family of lesions characterized by the presence of perivascular epithelioid cells. *Am J Surg Pathol* 20: 722-730.

2921. Zapzalka DM, Krishnamurti L, Manivel JC, di Sandro MJ (2002). Lymphangioma of the renal capsule. *J Urol* 168: 220.

2922. Zavala-Pompa A, Folpe AL, Jimenez RE, Lim SD, Cohen C, Eble JN, Amin MB (2001). Immunohistochemical study of microphthalmia transcription factor and tyrosinase in angiomyolipoma of the kidney, renal cell carcinoma, and renal and retroperitoneal sarcomas: comparative evaluation with traditional diagnostic markers. *Am J Surg Pathol* 25: 65-70.

2923. Zavala-Pompa A, Ro JY, el-Naggar A, Ordonez NG, Amin MB, Pierce PD, Ayala AG (1993). Primary carcinoid tumor of testis. Immunohistochemical, ultrastructural, and DNA flow cytometric study of three cases with a review of the literature. *Cancer* 72: 1726-1732.

2924. Zbar B, Alvord WG, Glenn G, Turner M, Pavlovich CP, Schmidt L, Walther M, Choyke P, Weirich G, Hewitt SM, Duray P, Gabril F, Greenberg C, Merino MJ, Toro J, Linehan WM (2002). Risk of renal and colonic neoplasms and spontaneous pneumothorax in the Birt-Hogg-Dube syndrome. *Cancer Epidemiol Biomarkers Prev* 11: 393-400.

2925. Zbar B, Brauch H, Talmadge C, Linehan M (1987). Loss of alleles of loci on the short arm of chromosome 3 in renal cell carcinoma. *Nature* 327: 721-724.

2926. Zbar B, Glenn G, Lubensky I, Choyke P, Walther MM, Magnusson G, Bergerheim US, Pettersson S, Amin M, Hurley K (1995). Hereditary papillary renal cell carcinoma: clinical studies in 10 families. *J Urol* 153: 907-912.

2927. Zbar B, Kishida T, Chen F, Schmidt L, Maher ER, Richards FM, Crossey PA, Webster AR, Affara NA, Ferguson-Smith MA, Brauch H, Glavac D, Neumann HP, Tisherman S, Mulvihill JJ, Gross DJ, Shuin T, Whaley J, Seizinger B, Kley N, Olschwang S, Boisson C, Richard S, Lips CH, Linehan WM, Lerman M (1996). Germline mutations in the Von Hippel-Lindau disease (VHL) gene in families from North America, Europe, and Japan. *Hum Mutat* 8: 348-357.

2928. Zbar B, Tory K, Merino M, Schmidt L, Glenn G, Choyke P, Walther MM, Lerman M, Linehan WM (1994). Hereditary papillary renal cell carcinoma. *J Urol* 151: 561-566.

2929. Zeeman AM, Stoop H, Boter M, Gillis AJ, Castrillon DH, Oosterhuis JW, Looijenga LH (2002). VASA is a specific marker for both normal and malignant human germ cells. *Lab Invest* 82: 159-166.

2930. Zein TA, Huben R, Lane W, Pontes JE, Englander LS (1985). Secondary tumors of the prostate. *J Urol* 133: 615-616.

2931. Zhang FF, Arber DA, Wilson TG, Kawachi MH, Slovak ML (1997). Toward the validation of aneusomy detection by fluorescence in situ hybridization in bladder cancer: comparative analysis with cytology, cytogenetics, and clinical features predicts recurrence and defines clinical testing limitations. *Clin Cancer Res* 3: 2317-2328.

2932. Zhang HM (1991). [Immunohistochemical demonstration of neurohormonal polypeptides in primary carcinoid tumor of testis]. *Zhonghua Bing Li Xue Za Zhi* 20: 41-43.

2933. Zhang XM, Elhosseiny A, Melamed MR (2002). Plasmacytoid urothelial carcinoma of the bladder. A case report and the first description of urinary cytology. *Acta Cytol* 46: 412-416.

2934. Zhao J, Richter J, Wagner U, Roth B, Schraml P, Zellweger T, Ackermann D, Schmid U, Moch H, Mihatsch MJ, Gasser TC, Sauter G (1999). Chromosomal imbalances in noninvasive papillary bladder neoplasms (pTa). *Cancer Res* 59: 4658-4661.

2935. Zhou M, Chinnaiyan AM, Kleer CG, Lucas PC, Rubin MA (2002). Alpha-Methylacyl-CoA racemase: a novel tumor marker over-expressed in several human cancers and their precursor lesions. *Am J Surg Pathol* 26: 926-931.

2936. Zhou M, Jiang Z, Epstein JI (2003). Expression and diagnostic utility of alpha-methylacyl-CoA-racemase (P504S) in foamy gland and pseudohyperplastic prostate cancer. *Am J Surg Pathol* 27: 772-778.

2937. Zhuang Z, Park WS, Pack S, Schmidt L, Vortmeyer AO, Pak E, Pham T, Weil RJ, Candidus S, Lubensky IA, Linehan WM, Zbar B, Weirich G (1998). Trisomy 7-harbouring non-random duplication of the mutant MET allele in hereditary papillary renal carcinomas. *Nat Genet* 20: 66-69.

2938. Zietman AL, Coen JJ, Ferry JA, Scully RE, Kaufman DS, McGovern FG (1996). The management and outcome of stage IAE nonHodgkin's lymphoma of the testis. *J Urol* 155: 943-946.

2939. Zippel L (1942). Zur Kenntnis der Oncocytome. *Virchows Arch [A] Pathol Anat* 308: 360-382.

2940. Zisman A, Pantuck AJ, Dorey F, Said JW, Shvarts O, Quintana D, Gitlitz BJ, Dekernion JB, Figlin RA, Belldegrun AS (2001). Improved prognostication of renal cell carcinoma using an integrated staging system. *J Clin Oncol* 19: 1649-1657.

2941. Zlotta AR, Djavan B, Marberger M, Schulman CC (1997). Prostate specific antigen density of the transition zone: a new effective parameter for prostate cancer prediction. *J Urol* 157: 1315-1321.

2942. Zlotta AR, Noel JC, Fayt I, Drowart A, van Vooren JP, Huygen K, Simon J, Schulman CC (1999). Correlation and prognostic significance of p53, p21WAF1/CIP1 and Ki-67 expression in patients with superficial bladder tumors treated with bacillus Calmette-Guerin intravesical therapy. *J Urol* 161: 792-798.

2943. Zorn B, Virant-Klun I, Sinkovec J, Vraspir-Porenta O, Meden-Vrtovec H (1999). [Carcinoma in situ of the testis in infertile men. Experience in a medically assisted reproduction program]. *Contracept Fertil Sex* 27: 41-46.

2944. Zouhair A, Weber D, Belkacemi Y, Ketterer N, Dietrich PY, Villa S, Scandolaro L, Bieri S, Studer G, Delacretaz F, Girardet C, Mirimanoff RO, Ozsahin M (2002). Outcome and patterns of failure in testicular lymphoma: a multicenter Rare Cancer Network study. *Int J Radiat Oncol Biol Phys* 52: 652-656.

2945. Zucca E, Conconi A, Mughal TI, Sarris AH, Vitolo U, Gospodarowicz MK (2000). Patterns of survival in primary diffuse large B-cell lymphoma (DLCL) of the testis: an international survey of 373 patients. 42nd Annual Meeting of the American Society of Hematology, 2000, San Francisco. *Blood* 96: 1443.

2946. Zuckman MH, Williams G, Levin HS (1988). Mitosis counting in seminoma: an exercise of questionable significance. *Hum Pathol* 19: 329-335.

2947. Zuk RJ, Rogers HS, Martin JE, Baithun SI (1988). Clinicopathological importance of primary dysplasia of bladder. *J Clin Pathol* 41: 1277-1280.

2948. Zukerberg LR, Armin AR, Pisharodi L, Young RH (1990). Transitional cell carcinoma of the urinary bladder with osteoclast-type giant cells: a report of two cases and review of the literature. *Histopathology* 17: 407-411.

2949. Zukerberg LR, Harris NL, Young RH (1991). Carcinomas of the urinary bladder simulating malignant lymphoma. A report of five cases. *Am J Surg Pathol* 15: 569-576.

2950. Zukerberg LR, Young RH (1990). Primary testicular sarcoma: a report of two cases. *Hum Pathol* 21: 932-935.

2951. Zukerberg LR, Young RH, Scully RE (1991). Sclerosing Sertoli cell tumor of the testis. A report of 10 cases. *Am J Surg Pathol* 15: 829-834.

2952. Zuppan CW, Beckwith JB, Luckey DW (1988). Anaplasia in unilateral Wilms' tumor: a report from the National Wilms' Tumor Study Pathology Center. *Hum Pathol* 19: 1199-1209.

Subject index

Multiple leiomyomas of the skin, 18
Multiple renal tumours, 20
MYBL2, 108, 226
MYCL1, 226
MYCN, 226
Myf4, 277
MyoD1, 139, 276, 277
Myointimoma, 293-297
Myxofibrosarcoma, 293, 297
Myxoid chondrosarcoma, 37
Myxoma, 57

N

N-acetyltransferase 2, 13
Nelson syndrome, 252
Neonatal jaundice, 223
Nephroblastic tumours, 10
Nephroblastoma, 12, 48-56, 87, 213, 218, 247, 263, 279
Nephroblastomatosis, 53, 54
Nephrogenic adenoma, 78, 99, 133, 156, 172
Nephrogenic metaplasia, 99
Nephrogenic rests, 10, 53
Nested variant of urothelial carcinoma, 99, 138
Neuroblastoma, 10, 39, 52, 84, 160, 213, 214, 247, 279
Neuroendocrine carcinoma, 10, 82, 135, 136, 248
Neuroendocrine tumours, 10, 16, 90, 153, 160, 172, 207
Neurofibroma, 145, 153, 258, 274, 293-297
Neurofibromatosis, 51
Neurofibromatosis type 1, 145
Neuron specific enolase, 51, 66, 84, 138, 207, 273
NF2, 296
Nodular mesothelial hyperplasia, 270
Non-invasive papillary urothelial carcinoma, high grade, 90, 117
Non-invasive papillary urothelial carcinoma, low grade, 90, 104, 116
Non-invasive papillary urothelial neoplasm of low malignant potential, 90
Non-invasive urothelial neoplasia, 123
Non-invasive urothelial tumours, 110
Non-keratinizing squamous metaplasia, 114
NonO (p54NRB), 37
Normal urothelium, 112

Normocytic anaemia, 13
NRC-1, 25
NSE, 84, 274
NTRK3, 60
Nuclear grooves, 41, 258

O

Obesity, 9, 13, 95, 164
Omphalocele, 52
Oncocyte, 42
Oncocytic tumour, 18, 21
Oncocytic variant, prostate carcinoma, 177
Oncocytoma, 10, 15, 39, 42, 43, 65, 66
Oncocytomatosis, 43
Oncocytosis, 43
Orchioblastoma, 238
ORTI, 62
Osseous metaplasia, 26, 44, 142
Ossifying renal tumour of infancy, 62
Ossifying renal tumour of infants, 10
Osteosarcoma, 63, 90, 102, 103, 142, 144, 153, 178, 209, 211, 247, 293, 297
Overweight, 12

P

p14ARF, 121, 123
p15, 103, 107, 108, 121, 228
p16, 21, 107, 121, 130
p27, 17, 109, 122, 186, 187, 197
p63, 117, 118, 123, 174
Paget disease, 172, 281, 282, 285, 290, 291
PAP, See Prostatic acid phosphatase
Papillary adenoma, 10, 41
Papillary carcinoma, 28, 281, 284, 287
Papillary necrosis, 151
Papillary renal adenomas, 41
Papillary renal cell carcinoma, 10, 15, 18, 27-29
Papillary serous carcinoma of the ovary, 100
Papillary urothelial neoplasm of low malignant potential, 104, 115, 116
Paraganglioma, 85, 90, 99, 136-138, 160, 213, 218, 263
Paraneoplastic endocrine syndromes, 13

Paratesticular liposarcoma, 275, 276
Paratesticular rhabdomyosarcoma, 275, 277
Parity, 13
Penile melanosis, 292
Perilobar nephrogenic rest, 53
Peripheral neuroectodermal tumour, 52
Peripheral neuroepithelioma, 247
Peritumoural fibrous pseudocapsule, 49, 53, 54
Perlman syndrome, 51
Pesticides, 12
Peutz-Jeghers syndrome, 253-255
Peyrone disease, 298
Phaeochromocytoma, 10, 15, 17, 85, 136, 153, 214
Phenacetin, 13, 94, 151
Phosphatidyl inositol-3-kinase (PI3K), 61
PI3/Akt, 186
PIN, See Prostatic intraepithelial neoplasia
Placental alkaline phosphatase, 100, 229-238, 243, 245, 247, 249, 255, 256, 260, 261
Placental site trophoblastic tumour, 218, 243
PLAP, See Placental alkaline phosphatase
Plasmacytoid carcinoma, 135
Plasmacytoid variant, urothelial carcinoma, 101
Plasmacytoma, 10, 86, 90, 101, 102, 147, 153, 157, 264, 265
Platelet-derived growth factor beta, 17
Pleuropulmonary blastoma, 76
PNET, 58, 59, 83, 84, 245-248, 279
Pneumothorax, 15, 20
Polycyclic aromatic hydrocarbons, 13
Polycythemia, 44, 48
Polyembryoma, 221, 247, 248, 250
Polyvesicular vitelline, 240, 242
Post-atrophic hyperplasia, prostate, 173, 175
Postoperative spindle cell nodule/tumour, 140, 145
Posttransplant lymphoproliferative disease, 147
PRCC, 15, 27, 28, 37
PRCC-TFE3 renal carcinomas, 37
Priapism, 298, 299
Primitive neuroectodermal tumour, 10, 83, 245, 246
Prolactin, 14
Promontory sign, 296

Promoter methylation, 21

Prostate specific antigen, 154, 159, 161, 163-169, 172, 174, 177-179, 188-190, 192, 194, 198, 199, 201-208, 212-214, 278

Prostate specific membrane antigen, 167, 172

Prostatic acid phosphatase, 81, 167, 172, 177, 178, 201, 204, 205, 208, 214

Prostatic intraepithelial neoplasia, 160, 174, 180, 186-188, 193-198

Protein degredation, 17

PSA, See Prostate specific antigen

Psammoma bodies, 37, 41, 44, 45, 100, 252

Pseudoglandular spaces, 98

Pseudohermaphroditism, 51

Pseudohyperparathyroidism, 13

Pseudohyperplastic prostate cancer, 175

Pseudosarcomatous stromal reaction, 97

PTEN, 25, 32, 107, 185, 187

Pulmonary cysts, 20, 21

PUNLMP, 110, 113, 115-117, 122

Purkinje cells, 16

Pushing margin, 23

pVHL, 15, 16, 17

Pyogenic granuloma, 141

R

Ras, 61, 122

RASSF1A, 25

RB1, 107

Rbx1, 17

RCC17, 37

Reactive atypia, 112

Reinke crystals, 251, 252

Renal adenomatosis, 41

Renal angiosarcoma, 64

Renal carcinoid tumour, 81

Renal carcinoma, 30, 52

Renal cell cancer, 12-31, 38, 39, 65, 299

Renal cell carcinoma, 14-34, 39, 41, 43, 65, 68, 75, 212, 279, 299

Renal Cell Carcinoma Marker antigen, 37

Renal cell carcinoma, unclassified, 10, 43

Renal failure, 67, 85, 147

Renal medullary carcinoma, 10, 35

Renal oncocytoma, 20, 42

Renal osteosarcoma, 63

Renin, 13, 48, 67, 72, 73

Renomedullary interstitial cell tumour, 10, 74

Retained placenta, 223

Rete adenomas, 256

Rete testis carcinoma, 266

Retina, 15, 16

Retinal anlage tumour, 272

Retinoblastoma, 107, 109, 122

Retrograde metastasis, 23

Rhabdoid cells, 79

Rhabdoid tumour, 10, 52, 58, 59, 160, 213

Rhabdoid tumour of the kidney (RTK), 58

Rhabdomyosarcoma, 102, 139, 145, 153, 160, 178, 209-211, 236, 248, 270, 274-277, 293, 296, 297

RNASEL, 184, 186

RTK, 58, 59

S

S. haematobium, 124, 125, 130

S100 protein, 27, 47, 57, 66, 84, 137, 145, 146, 206, 247, 252, 254, 256-259, 271, 273, 295

Sarcomatoid carcinoma, 64, 102, 108, 140, 142, 144, 153, 155, 157, 160, 178, 179, 236, 287, 288

Sarcomatoid change, 23, 43

Sarcomatoid variant, urothelial carcinoma, 102

Schiller-Duval bodies, 240

Schistosoma haematobium, 94, 124, 125, 130

Schistosoma japonicum, 124

Schistosoma mansoni, 124

Schistosomiasis, 124-127, 130, 142, 147, 205

Schwannoma, 56, 75, 153, 274, 293, 294, 295, 297

Sclerosing adenosis, 173

Sclerosing Sertoli cell tumour, 218, 253, 255

Sebaceous carcinoma, 281, 288

Seminoma, 160, 221-240, 244-249, 255, 256, 260

Seminoma with syncytiotrophoblastic cells, 218, 233

Serotonin, 138, 207

Serous carcinoma, 218

Serous tumour of borderline malignancy, 218

Sertoli cell tumour, 218, 232, 238, 253-256, 258, 266

Sertoli cell tumour, lipid rich variant, 218

Serum alkaline phosphatase, 13

Sickle cell trait, 35

Signet-ring variant, 195

Simpson-Golabi-Behmel syndrome, 51

SIOP, 48, 49, 52

Skene glands, 90, 155

SMAD4, 225

Small cell carcinoma, 90, 135, 136, 153, 160, 207, 208, 281, 288

Small cell neuroendocrine carcinoma, 207

Small cell neuroendocrine variant, PIN, 196

Smooth muscle actin, 66, 69, 102, 144, 206, 257, 258, 259, 295, 296

Soft tissue alveolar soft part sarcoma, 37

Solitary fibrous tumour, 10, 75, 144, 160, 209, 211, 215, 258

Sotos syndrome, 51

Soya bean agglutinins, 40

Spermatocytic seminoma, 218, 221, 223-225, 229, 234-237

Spermatocytic seminoma with sarcoma, 218, 236, 237

Spermatogenesis, 230

Spermatogenic arrest, 231

Spermatogonia, 223, 230, 231

Spindle cell rhabdomyosarcoma, 275, 277

Squamous cell carcinoma, 90, 124-127, 153-156, 160, 205, 281-290

Squamous cell papilloma, 90, 127

SRD5A2, 164

SSX family gene, 80

Steroid 5-alpha reductase type II, 164

Stromal proliferations of uncertain malignant potential of the prostate, 209

Stromal sarcoma, 160, 209

Stromal tumour of uncertain malignant potential, 160, 209

STUMP, 209, 210

Sturge-Weber syndrome, 71, 146

Sustentacular cells, 85, 136, 137

Synaptophysin, 81, 82, 84, 85, 137, 138, 196, 207, 247, 273

Syncytiotrophoblastic cells, 103, 238, 243, 244, 249